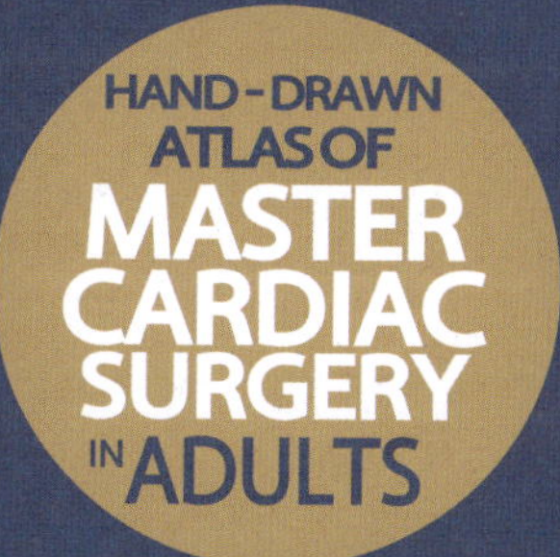
HAND-DRAWN
ATLAS OF
MASTER
CARDIAC
SURGERY
IN ADULTS

U0922787

谨以此书
纪念我们的良师挚友
翁渝国 医生

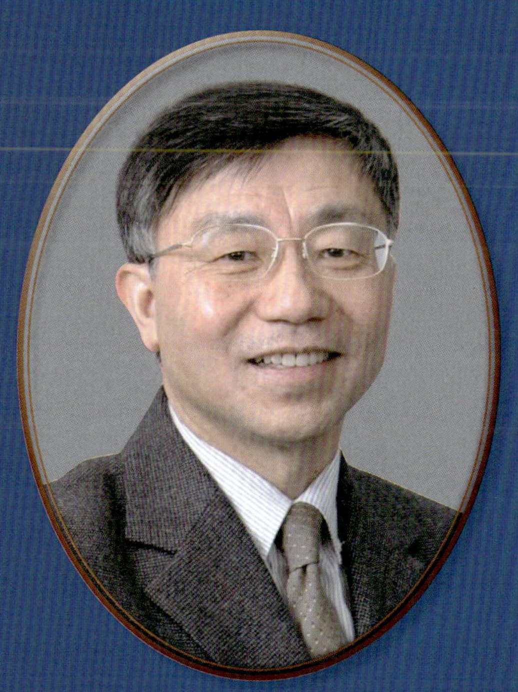

1946.09.06 — 2017.06.26

This book commemorates
Dr. Weng Yuguo,
our good teacher and friend.

汉英对照

成人心脏外科
名家手术
手绘图解

HAND-DRAWN ATLAS OF MASTER CARDIAC SURGERY IN ADULTS

主　编 | 刘中民　翁渝国　李颖则

副主编 | 李铁岩　华一飞

译　者 | 陈水平　吕　桂

绘　图 | 朱丽萍

人民卫生出版社

·北　京·

图书在版编目（CIP）数据

成人心脏外科名家手术手绘图解：汉英对照 / 刘中民，翁渝国，李颖则主编．—北京：人民卫生出版社，2024.8

ISBN 978-7-117-36264-1

Ⅰ. ①成… Ⅱ. ①刘…②翁…③李… Ⅲ. ①心脏外科手术－图解 Ⅳ. ①R654.2-64

中国国家版本馆 CIP 数据核字（2024）第 089376 号

人卫智网	www.ipmph.com	医学教育、学术、考试、健康， 购书智慧智能综合服务平台
人卫官网	www.pmph.com	人卫官方资讯发布平台

成人心脏外科名家手术手绘图解（汉英对照）

Chengren Xinzang Waike Mingjia Shoushu Shouhui Tujie

（Han-Ying Duizhao）

主　　编：刘中民　翁渝国　李颖则
出版发行：人民卫生出版社（中继线 010-59780011）
地　　址：北京市朝阳区潘家园南里 19 号
邮　　编：100021
E - mail：pmph @ pmph.com
购书热线：010-59787592　010-59787584　010-65264830
印　　刷：北京盛通印刷股份有限公司印刷
经　　销：新华书店
开　　本：889 × 1194　1/16　　印张：37
字　　数：1008 千字
版　　次：2024 年 8 月第 1 版
印　　次：2024 年 9 月第 1 次印刷
标准书号：ISBN 978-7-117-36264-1
定　　价：498.00 元

打击盗版举报电话：010-59787491　E-mail：WQ @ pmph.com
质量问题联系电话：010-59787234　E-mail：zhiliang @ pmph.com
数字融合服务电话：4001118166　E-mail：zengzhi @ pmph.com

痛失敬爱的翁医生

The loss of our beloved Dr. Weng

1986年春，奥格斯堡的Struck教授给我电话，说他有一位非常优秀的外科同事因为巴伐利亚州政府不能再延长他的居留权，必须要回中国，问我是否有办法帮忙。我当时正在组建德国心脏中心（柏林），需要有经验的外科医生。由于我的同事多是年轻人，不太有经验，我必须亲自动手术。因此，Struck教授的电话来得恰逢其时。柏林那时仍被封锁，但西柏林是没问题的。在给卫生和建设部的Ara博士打过电话后，我马上开始办理翁医生和他夫人及女儿到柏林的手续。1986年秋，他到达了我院。

In the spring of 1986, Professor Struck called from Augsburg to ask if I could accommodate one of his colleagues, an excellent surgeon, who otherwise had to go back to China because his right of abode could not be extended by the Bayern government. At that time, I was setting up the German Heart Center (Berlin) and needed experienced surgeons. Since most of my colleagues were young and inexperienced, I had to perform all the operations myself. Therefore, Professor Struck's phone call came at the right time. Berlin was still cordoned off, but West Berlin was fine. After a call to Dr. Ara at the Ministry of Health and Construction, I immediately started to go through the formalities for Dr. Weng, his wife, and his daughter to go to Berlin. In the autumn of 1986, Dr. Weng arrived at our hospital.

我很快发现，他是一位非常有经验的外科医生，于是很快升他为我的副手。他不仅会全部的心脏外科手术，还对新生儿先天性心脏病、胸腔外科、大血管以及其他器官疾病皆有所能。据我所知，他之所能全学自于中国，很多的经验来自当"赤脚医生"的经历。没有他的勤奋和才华，我的工作会很困难。德国心脏中心（柏林）（Deutschen Herzzentrum Berlin，DHZB）也不可能发展成为欧洲最大、手术量最多的中心，手术包括一些复杂手术，如

Dr. Weng was soon found to be a very experienced surgeon and was promoted to be my assistant. He specialized not only in all cardiac surgeries, but also in infantile and congenital atrial septal defect, thoracic surgeries, as well as macrovascular and other organ diseases. As far as I know, he had developed his expertise in China, which mainly came from his experiences as a "barefoot doctor". Without his diligence and talent, my work would not have progressed so smoothly, and the German Heart Center (Berlin)(Deutschen Herzzentrum Berlin, DHZB) could not have developed into the largest center with the largest number of

冠心病手术、小儿先天性心脏病手术、主动脉手术、各种器官移植和人工心脏辅助装置的安装。除此以外，如遇新的或罕见病例，我会请教翁医生，经常需要他的帮忙。一直以来，我对他的团结合作与忠诚非常信任。在他的协助下，我才有勇气不拒绝那些疑难病例，而是尽我们最大的努力医治病患。这样，患者在被其他心脏中心拒绝后，仍然会对 DHZB 抱有一线希望。也因此，无数的尝试和首次进行的手术获得成功。直到今天我仍能见到数年前由翁医生主刀的那位患者，而当时若没有他那双“能手”，那位患者早已经离我们远去了。正因为如此，德国心脏中心成为了世界顶尖的医院。

operations in Europe, covering complex operations such as surgery for coronary heart disease, surgery for pediatric congenital heart disease, aortic surgery, various organ transplants and the installation of artificial heart assist devices. I used to consult Dr. Weng for some novel or rare cases, and I always trusted his teamwork, cooperation and loyalty. With his assistance, I had the courage not to turn down those difficult cases but rather try our best to treat them. In this way, patients would still have a gleam of hope in DHZB after being rejected by other heart centers. It was also with his assistance that countless attempts and trials had been proved to be successful. To this day, I can still see the patient, who would have already passed away but for the superb operation performed by Dr. Weng a few years ago. Because of this, the German Heart Center has become one of the top hospitals in the world.

他的伟大还在于帮助他的祖国中国和德国建立了合作交流的纽带。德国心脏中心与刘中民院长所在的上海市东方医院的合作始于 2000 年（那也正是翁医生走完人生最后旅程的地方）。2001 年 5 月，时任上海市副市长周禹鹏先生亲自到柏林为双方合作揭牌，从此开启了我们与中国医院合作的新里程。超过 1 000 名中国医生和其他部门的工作人员曾数月甚至多年在我院工作进修，给院里增添了很多色彩。经过翁医生以及我的助手 Norbert Franz 和 Meizhu 的共同努力，中国成为我们最大的友好国家。有时我到一个手术室，发现那里工作的都是中国人，而且手术医生、助手、护士都用中文交流。

His greatness also lies in helping to establish ties between his motherland China and Germany. The cooperation between the German Heart Center and Shanghai East Hospital, where Director Liu Zhongmin works, began in 2000. Shanghai East Hospital is also the place where Dr. Weng completed his last journey. In May 2001, Mr. Zhou Yupeng, then vice mayor of Shanghai, personally came to Berlin to launch a bilateral cooperation, and since then, we have embarked on a new journey of cooperation with Chinese hospitals. More than 1000 Chinese doctors and staff from other departments have worked and studied in our hospital for months or even years, which really added a lot of color to the German Heart Center. Through the joint efforts of Dr. Weng, as well as my assistants Norbert Franz and Meizhu, China has become our greatest friendly country. Sometimes, I went to an operating theatre only to find that the people there were all Chinese, and surgeons, assistants and nurses all communicated in Chinese.

翁医生编著了许多的心脏外科教学书籍，我们也一起制作过图解，这本《心脏外科名家手术手绘图解》凝聚了翁医生毕生的经验和心血，历经三十年磨砺，终于在翁医生家人和刘中民院长以及他的同事们的努力下全部完成。翁医生不会被忘记，他的学识和教导将永世流传。

Dr. Weng had written a lot of course books on cardiac surgery, and we had also drawn atlas together. *Hand-drawn Atlas of Master Cardiac Surgery*, having been honed by Dr. Weng for 30 years, is finally completed with the help of Dr. Weng's family, his friend Director Liu Zhongmin and his colleagues. The book, embodying Dr. Weng's lifelong experiences and painstaking effort. Dr. Weng will not be forgotten, and his knowledge and instructions will be handed down from generation to generation.

让我们难过的是，一场重病侵袭了翁医生，也让他数年来受尽煎熬。好一阵子，他不以介怀，因为他的家人和国内的友人们是他的安慰。他用他的一生在帮助和启迪身边每一个人。

To our sadness, a serious illness hit Dr. Weng, which made him suffer for years. For a long time, he didn't take his illness to heart, for his family and friends in China were his comfort. Dr. Weng had dedicated his entire life to helping and enlightening everyone around him.

谨向我们伟大的外科医生、朋友和同伴，架起中德两国友谊桥梁的翁渝国医生致敬！

Tribute to our great surgeon, friend and companion, Dr. Weng Yuguo, who built the bridge of friendship between China and Germany.

Ronald Hetzer

德国心脏中心（柏林）原院长

2017 年 12 月

Ronald Hetzer

Former Director of
the German Heart Center (Berlin)

December, 2017

主编简介

Introduction to editor-in-chief

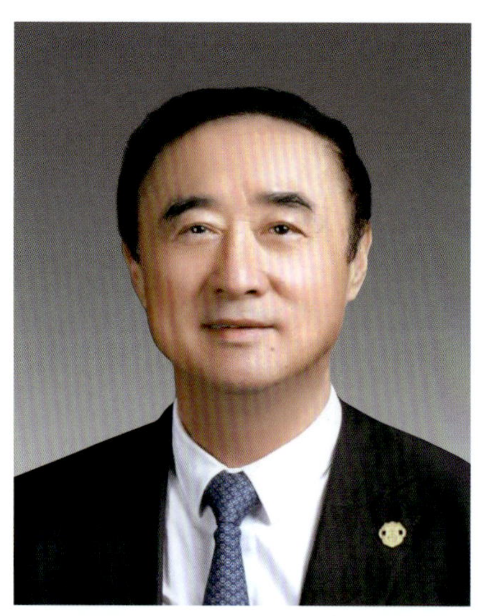

刘中民

主任医师、教授、博士研究生导师，教育部长江学者，俄罗斯工程院外籍院士，法国荣誉军团军官勋章获得者。

刘中民教授从事急危重症和心脏外科工作 40 余年。2000 年初在国内率先开展“柏林人工心脏”和心肺移植治疗终末期心力衰竭的临床研究；同时坚持自主设计研发新型人工心脏，着力推动人工心脏的国产化。

近年来，针对心脏移植供体匮乏、移植后患者生活质量不够理想的现状，他率先进行干细胞治疗心力衰竭的临床研究，以推动心力衰竭治疗从“有创”到“微创”，乃至“无创”的细胞治疗，并获得国家多种类、多途径、多项目的临床备案批准，也获得国家食品药品监督管理局细胞新药的转化和审批。

刘中民教授牵头建设心力衰竭专科和心脏外科 2 个上海市医学重点专科，获批上海市心力衰竭中心和上海人工心脏与心衰医学工程技术研究中心；承担国家高技术研究发展计划(863 计划)和国家干细胞重大研发专项、国家自然科学基金等国家项目 20 余项。作为第一发明人，2 项人工心脏发明专利技术获得授权并分别实施转让。作为第一完成人获国家科技进步奖二等奖 1 项、省部级奖 5 项、上海医学科技奖二等奖 3 项和中华医学科技奖二等奖 1 项，授权发明专利 10 多项(转移转化 5 项)。主编《实用心脏外科学》等专著 13 部，主编国家级规划教材 2 部，发表 SCI 论文 83 篇(影响因子 408)，他引 1 283 次。被评为上海领军人才和上海市医学领军人才。

现任职务：

同济大学灾难医学工程研究院院长

同济大学附属东方医院终身教授、名誉院长

同济大学学术委员会和校务委员会委员

学术兼职：

中国医师协会心血管外科医师分会第五届会长

中华医学会灾难医学分会主任委员、创始主任委员

中华预防医学会灾难预防医学分会创始主任委员

世界灾难与急救医学会理事

亚太灾难医学协会副主席

中国整形美容协会副会长

中国干细胞产业联盟理事长

国家干细胞转化资源库临床级干细胞资源库负责人

中国整形美容协会干细胞研究与应用分会会长

中国中西医结合学会干细胞与再生医学专业委员会主任委员

中国医药生物技术协会再生医学专业委员会副主任委员

上海市医学会干细胞与再生医学分会创始主任委员

上海干细胞临床转化研究院院长

上海市干细胞临床诊疗工程研究中心主任

上海干细胞转化医学工程技术研究中心专家委员会主任委员

湖南湘江实验室副主任、智慧医疗与计算生物研究院院长

海南省干细胞工程中心主任

海南博鳌乐城先行区干细胞专家顾问委员会主任委员

国家级成果奖励：

国家科技进步奖二等奖

何梁何利基金科学与技术进步奖

光华工程科技奖

主编简介

Introduction to editor-in-chief

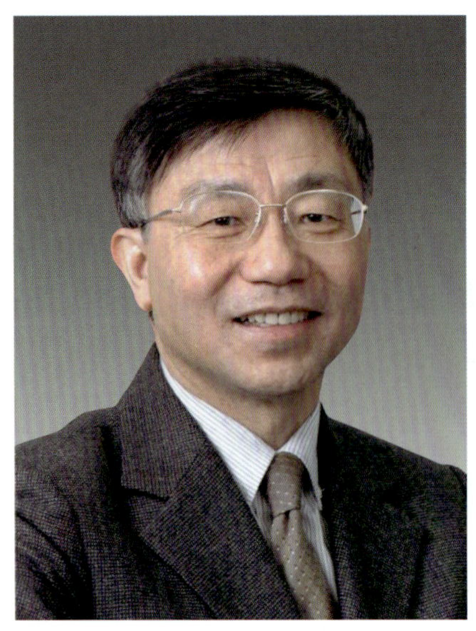

翁渝国

主任医师、教授、博士研究生导师。

翁渝国医生是世界上开展心脏辅助装置植入手术最多的心脏外科医生之一，也是世界上首先使用小儿心脏辅助装置的医生，给四百余位心力衰竭临终患者安装不同的心脏辅助装置，成功率达 80% 以上；在上海开展了亚洲第一例人工心脏手术；为一万余例患者做心内直视手术包括肺移植、心脏移植、心肺联合移植。曾应邀去剑桥大学附属医院，斯坦福大学附属医院，中国香港、澳门、台湾等地区医院进行疑难心脏病手术。

作为炎黄子孙翁渝国医生身居德国，心系祖国故土，关注中国心脏外科的学术进展；他经常回国参加学术会议，做学术报告，手术演示；和中国北京、上海、厦门、昆明、福州、青岛、镇江、台北等地的医院建立各种形式的合作关系，定期为国内数十家医院讲学示范手术义诊；为国内近千名心脏外科医生提供到柏林心脏中心进修学习的机会，现在这些医生都已成为当地医院的心胸外科主干力量。

学术兼职：

德国心胸血管外科协会会员，欧洲心胸血管外科协会会员；

Journal of Thoracic and Cardiovascular Surgery 审稿人，《中国心血管病研究》名誉主编；

先后聘为上海第二医科大学（现上海交通大学医学院）、同济大学附属东方医院、北京医科大学北京医院、广东省心血管研究所、福建医科大学、江苏理工大学、镇江医学院、宁波大学医学院、中山医科大学、第三军医大学、第四军医大学、兰州医学院、青岛医学院、暨南大学名誉教授；沈阳军区总院北方医院心脏外科顾问；中德心脏中心（北京）教授。

工作经历：

1964—1970　北京协和医学院医疗系求学；

1970—1978　陕西省人民医院普通外科、外科轮转住院医生及心胸血管外科主治医师；

1979—1981　考入中国医学科学院心血管研究所、中国协和医科大学研究生院，北京阜外医院心胸外科主治医师；

1982—1985　德国心脏中心（慕尼黑）心胸血管外科主治医生并攻读博士学位；

1985—1987　德国奥格斯堡中心医院心胸科副主任医生；

1987—2008　德国心脏中心（柏林）副院长，德国洪堡大学教授；

2008　洪堡大学终身教授，退休。

学术业绩：

1984 年起开展新生儿大动脉转位的根治手术（Switch），完成 400 余例；

1986 年起临床开展同种主动脉移植物手术，完成 600 余例；

1987 年起开展心脏移植，完成 1 300 余例；

1988 年成功开展主动脉弓部及胸腹主动脉瘤手术；

1989 年起开展肺移植及心肺联合移植，完成 300 余例；

1989 年起临床使用心脏辅助装置或人工心脏，柏林人工心脏，体外型；

1990 年开展背阔肌动力性心肌成形手术；

1991 年改良 Norwood 手术治疗新生儿左心发育不全综合征；

1992 年开展体内植入型心脏辅助装置（Novacor）技术，4 位患者已经带泵存活 4 年；

1993 年开展激光在冠心病外科上的使用；开展体内植入型心脏辅助装置（TCI）技术；为 1 位患者一次替换四个心脏瓣膜成功；

1994 年世界首次采用心脏辅助装置降低左心负荷治疗终末期扩张型心肌病成功；

1995 年为体重仅 1 600 克的早产儿成功进行完全肺静脉畸形引流心下型根治手术；

1997 年为患者做体外携带人工心脏手术，创造存活长达 4 年的世界纪录；

1998 年完成世界首例体内植入型轴流心脏辅助装置（De Bakey-VAD）；

1999 年开展机器人在心外科手术中的应用；

1999 年完成体内全植入型人工心脏，患者存活 3.5 年；

2001 年领导开发新型微型轴流泵 Incor Ⅰ 的动物实验和临床试验成功，并获得欧洲共同体 CE 证书；

2002 年开始在临床上使用 Incor Ⅰ，患者最长健康生活已经超过 2 年；

2003 年开始第三代心脏辅助装置 Dura Heart 的临床试验；

2004 年临床应用全人工心脏（CardioWest）；开始干细胞临床使用治疗终末期心力衰竭。

主编简介

Introduction to editor-in-chief

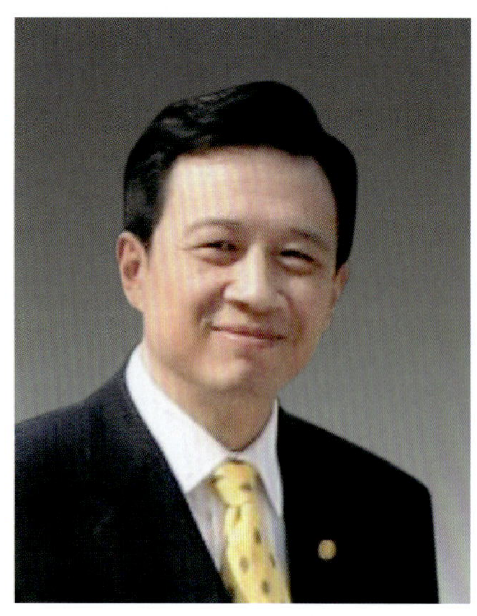

李颖则

主任医师，教授，国务院政府特殊津贴获得者。

在心血管外科领域具有深厚的理论知识和临床造诣，对冠心病、心脏瓣膜病、先天性心脏病、大血管病、心律失常、心包疾病、心脏肿瘤等各种心脏病的诊断和手术治疗均有丰富的经验，并取得了优良的治疗效果。

职　　务： 曾任上海市胸科医院心血管外科主任，并兼任心外科教研室主任。曾任上海市胸科医院业务副院长，并兼任院学术委员会主任、首任院伦理委员会主任、首任药物临床试验机构主任、首任专科医师培训基地主任。

学术兼职： 亚洲胸心血管外科医师协会（ATCSA）理事、中国医师协会心血管外科医师分会第一届及第二届副会长、上海市医学会外科专业委员会委员、上海市医学会胸心外科专业委员会委员、上海市卫生系列高级专业技术职务任职资格评审委员会委员、美国胸外科医师学会（STS）会员。

序

Preface

德国心脏中心（柏林）原副院长翁渝国教授是一位享誉世界的优秀心外科医生，他在心血管外科的专业领域有极高的造诣，而且是一个心外科医生中少有的“多面手”，涉足了包括冠心病、心脏瓣膜疾病、大动脉疾病、心律失常、终末期心脏病、先天性心脏病等各种心脏病的外科治疗，并形成了自己独特的手术技术风格和患者管理方式，其治疗结果显示出国际顶尖水平，特别是在心脏移植、肺移植、心肺联合移植和各种心脏辅助装置植入方面成为经验最多的心外科医生之一。

Professor Weng Yuguo, former Vice Chairman of the German Heart Center (Berlin), was a world-renowned cardiac surgeon with high attainments in the field of cardiovascular surgery. Besides, he was a rare “generalist” among cardiac surgeons with a wide professional field involving the surgical treatment of various heart diseases such as coronary heart disease, valvular heart disease, large artery disease, arrhythmia, end-stage heart disease, and congenital heart disease. He had developed his own unique surgical technique and patient management style, which have produced world-leading clinical results. Furthermore, he was one of the most experienced cardiac surgeons in heart transplantation, lung transplantation, combined heart-lung transplantation, and implantation of various cardiac assist devices.

心血管外科的进步离不开创新和传承。上海市东方医院院长刘中民教授长期与翁渝国教授合作，在上海市东方医院建立了中德心脏中心，借鉴德国模式发展心血管外科。此次在翁教授实际工作的基础上，两位教授精心策划身体力行，将各种真实实施过的成人心脏手术彩绘成图，加以文字说明，分门别类汇集成册，历经数载付梓问世，可喜可贺，为心血管外科医生提供了一本专业参考书，让更多的人从翁教授的经验中得到借鉴和获益。

The progress of cardiovascular surgery is based on innovation and information that is passed down from previous experience. Professor Liu Zhongmin, Dean of Shanghai East Hospital, has cooperated with Professor Weng Yuguo for many years. They established the Sino-German Heart Center at Shanghai East Hospital with the aim of drawing on the German model to develop cardiovascular surgery in China. Again, it is their joint efforts that make this book possible. The book, based on Professor Weng’s clinical experiences, includes illustrations of various adult cardiac surgeries with text to explain the procedures. The illustrations are all compiled and organized by category. After many years of effort, this professional reference book for cardiovascular surgeons will finally be published, allowing more people to learn and benefit from Professor Weng's experiences.

该书图文并茂，按手术步骤详细图解，使读者可以很直观地了解手术过程，极具指导意义，本人推荐此书，并乐为之序。相信该书的出版会对我国的心血管外科事业起到促进作用。同时，也借此机会表达对翁渝国教授的怀念。

With excellent writing and vivid illustrations, this book will be an invaluable guide. It includes detailed, step-by-step instructions, making it easy for learners to grasp the surgical procedure. I highly recommend this book and am honored to write a preface for it. I believe that the publication of this book will promote the development of cardiovascular surgery in China. At the same time, I would also like to take this opportunity to pay tribute to Professor Weng Yuguo.

主任医师 教授
中国工程院院士
国家心血管病中心主任
中国医学科学院阜外医院院长
心血管疾病国家重点实验室主任
国家心血管疾病临床医学研究中心主任
法国医学科学院外籍院士

Hu Shengshou

Chief Surgeon, Professor
Academician of Chinese Academy of Engineering
Director of National Center for Cardiovascular Diseases
President of Fuwai Hospital, Chinese Academy of Medical Sciences
Director of State Key Laboratory of Cardiovascular Disease
Director of National Clinical Research Center for Cardiovascular Diseases
Foreign Academician of National Academy of Medicine of France

2024 年 3 月

March, 2024

前言

Foreword

翁渝国医生是享誉世界的华人心脏外科医生。20 世纪 80 年代，时任汉诺威心脏中心院长的 Ronald Hetzer 教授盛邀他一同创立德国心脏中心（柏林），从此开辟了德国乃至欧洲心脏大血管外科的一个崭新时代。他是世界上少有的个人手术过万例的医生，被德国媒体誉为“拥有一双金手的医生”；也是被德国政府规定不能同时离开德国的三个医生之一；他有很多个“世界第一”，看过他手术的人无不为他的精湛技艺所折服，所谓“化繁为简”“出神入化”“化腐朽为神奇”，在他的手里体现得淋漓尽致！除了高超的医术，他为人极其谦和、热情，为中国培养了一千余名心脏外科医生和心肺转流术灌注师、护理人员等。很多医生如今已经成为中国心脏外科领域的大家，他为中国心血管事业的发展作出了不可磨灭的贡献。

Dr. Weng Yuguo, a world-renowned Chinese cardiologist, co-founded the German Heart Institute in Berlin at the invitation of Professor Roland Hatzer, the then Director at Hanover Heart Center, in the 1980s, ushering in a new era for cardiac vascular surgery in Germany, and even the whole of Europe. He was acclaimed by the German media as "Der Arzt mit den goldenen Händens" (the doctor with golden hands), for he was one of the few doctors worldwide to have personally performed more than 10 000 surgeries. He was also one of three doctors who were prohibited by the German government from leaving Germany simultaneously. He developed many of the world's firsts, and those who observed his operations were deeply impressed by his superb surgical skills. These skills are worthy of the praise they have received, which is the so-called "simplifying the complex" "reaching the acme of perfection" and "turning the bad into good". Despite his achievements, he was very modest and enthusiastic to help others. He trained more than 1 000 cardiac surgeons, cardiopulmonary bypass perfusionists, and nurses for his country. Most of these trainees have become masters in the field in China. He has truly made indelible contributions to the development of Chinese cardiovascular research and practice !

我与翁医生的相识是在 20 世纪 90 年代初期，当时我还在仁济医院任心胸外科副主任，翁医生指导我完成了心脏外科生涯的第一例搭桥手术。从那之后，我们可谓亦师亦友。1998 年春节刚过，我第一次前往柏林进修学习，翁医生夫妇亲自开车到泰格尔机场接机。那年冬天也是少有的寒冷，到处冰天雪地，虽然我从上海出发时做了充足的准备，仍然无法抵挡柏林的严寒。翁医生看在眼里，第二天就让他的夫人陈家大姐送来了又厚又暖的皮夹克，这种他乡雪中送炭的温暖至今还铭刻在我的心里。

It was in the early 1990s that I became acquainted with Dr. Weng. At that time, I was the deputy director of cardiothoracic surgery at Renji Hospital. Under Dr. Weng's instruction, I completed my first bypass surgery as a cardiac surgeon. Since then, he has become my teacher and friend. Just after the Lunar New Year in 1998, I went to Berlin for the first time for further study, and Dr. Weng and his wife drove to Tegel Airport to pick me up. It was, indeed, an extremely cold winter, with everything covered in heavy snow, and I could not still almost cope with the bitter cold here in Berlin, albeit full preparations before my departure from Shanghai. His wife brought a warm leather jacket on the second day. That is still in my mind today.

在柏林学习期间，翁医生在生活上无微不至地关心我和每一个到柏林学习的中国医护人员。考虑到很多人初到柏林，人生地不熟，他常常利用手术的间隙亲自驾车去机场接机。在手术技巧上，他不厌其烦、细心讲解、耐心带教，总是能把复杂的手术变得很简单，把危重的患者处理得很安全，德国的医生和护士都喜欢跟他上台。也正是由于翁医生的言传身教，使我（还包括很多先后去柏林的中国医生）在很短时间里，就学习和掌握了当时在国内看不到的病例和没有的技术，例如极低体重（不到 500g）早产儿先天性心脏病的手术、多种品牌人工心脏的植入和心肺联合移植等，当然还有现代化医院的建设和管理。为了把德国心脏中心（柏林）的信息系统复制回来，我专门买了一台笔记本

During my study in Berlin, Dr. Weng took meticulous care of me, as well as every Chinese medical staff member at the Center. Considering that many of us were new to Berlin and had no friends, he would often take advantage of any spare moment, even a break between surgeries, to pick us up at the airport. When conveying instructions, he would go to great lengths to explain every surgical technique and patiently demonstrate them. He could always simplify complicated operations and handle critically ill patients safely. Therefore, doctors and nurses in Germany all enjoyed working with him in the surgical theater. Dr. Weng's clear explanations and operation demonstrations enabled me (as well as many Chinese doctors who went to the Center) to quickly understand the cases unseen and master the techniques unavailable in China at that time, such as surgery for premature congenital heart disease infants weighing less

电脑，翁医生帮我和分管院长打招呼，破例让我全部下载，使上海市东方医院的信息系统在国内较早地与国际接轨。由于有翁医生的穿针引线和积极推动，上海市东方医院成为国内第一个中德合作医院，时任德国心脏中心（柏林）院长 Hetzer 教授 2000 年 5 月第一次到上海，看到浦东的发展深有感触地说："我们来得太晚了！"自此之后的 20 年间，由于翁医生的辛勤耕耘和精心呵护，上海市东方医院和德国心脏中心（柏林）的合作都被双方政府称为中德合作的典范。我也送了很多年轻医生、护士和学生前往柏林学习，他们在翁医生的指导下如今也都成为了业务骨干。

than 500 g, the implantation of various brands of artificial hearts, combined heart-lung transplantations, and the construction and management of modern hospitals. I specially bought a laptop to copy the information system used by the German Heart Center. Dr. Weng communicated with the director in charge, who finally made an exception for me to download the system so that the information system at Shanghai East Hospital, where I worked, could be in line with international standards early on. Thanks to Dr. Weng's communication and promotion, Shanghai East Hospital became the first Sino-German cooperative hospital in China. Later, when Professor Hetzer, the then director of the German Heart Center (Berlin), visited Shanghai for the first time in May 2000, he was deeply impressed by the development of Pudong and sighed that they came too late. In the two decades since then, through Dr. Weng's efforts, the cooperation between Shanghai East Hospital and the German Heart Center (Berlin) has been regarded as a model of Sino-German cooperation by both governments. I also sent many young doctors, nurses, and students to study in Berlin. Thanks to Dr. Weng's guidance, they are now the backbones of this field.

早在柏林学习期间，我和翁医生就在探讨如何把翁医生自己的手术经验通过图解的形式出版，让更多热爱心脏外科专业的医生学习。开始先是采用线条图的方式，但是很难体现翁医生的手术精髓。后来又采用先进的计算机绘图技术，翁医生仍然不满意，因为计算机操作人员难以理解翁医生手术的原

As early as when I was studying in Berlin, Dr. Weng and I had discussed sharing his personal surgical experiences in the form of a medical atlas to allow more cardiac surgeons to learn from him. Unfortunately, the line drawings used previously could not reflect the essence of Dr. Weng's surgery. Although advanced computer graphics technology was later adopted, Dr. Weng was still unsatisfied because the computer operators could not understand the

创性，不能把翁医生的手术理念和操作要点原汁原味地传授给年轻医生。最后，我在国内专门请了一位人体解剖绘图专家朱女士并送到德国，全程陪同翁医生，按照翁医生画的每一个手术步骤的草图，一边理解一边画图，这一待就是六年。2008 年翁医生患病，我前往柏林看望，那个时候他已经决定放下手术刀，全身心投入书稿的撰写和绘图当中，书中的每一幅图稿从翁医生手绘起稿、画师修稿，到最后定稿、上色都要经过一遍遍打磨，直到能完全反映翁医生的手术技巧和思路。我们俩也经常就图稿细节讨论到深夜。可以说每一幅图解都是翁医生一生学术的总结和经验的凝练，都反映了他对心血管外科的热爱和对患者的负责。

originality of the surgeries, and the graphics could not accurately impart his surgical concepts and operations. Finally, Ms. Zhu, a Chinese specialist in human anatomy illustration, was invited to come over here with these drawings and cooperated with Dr. Weng in Germany. She studied and made sense of all the sketches of the surgical operation procedures by Dr. Weng throughout the following six years. In 2008, when Dr. Weng became ill, I went to Berlin to visit him. At that time, he decided to stop performing any more surgery and devote himself to the writing and drawing of the atlas. Each illustration in the book was hand-painted by Dr. Weng, revised by Ms. Zhu, and finally finalized and colored. Each illustration has been polished over and over until it fully reflects the essence of Dr. Weng's surgery. Dr. Weng and I often discussed the details of the atlas late into the night. It can be said that each illustration is a summary of Dr. Weng's lifelong academic experience, reflecting his passion for cardiovascular surgery and his responsibility to patients.

2015 年翁医生的身体状况变差了，我把他从德国接回来，住在上海市东方医院里，一是方便照顾他的健康，二是方便我们讨论书稿，住院期间他仍然绘图到深夜，不过我们的讨论倒是方便了很多，不用再通过邮件或者越洋电话了。那时，我有一个想法，就是把这套图谱命名为《翁渝国心脏外科手术图谱》，但他婉言拒绝，理由是这里面除了他本人的经验和创新，还有德国同事的配合，以及前人的经验教训，所以还是通俗一点，就定位在“心脏外科手术图解”。全书初稿共有

In 2015, Dr. Weng's health deteriorated. I invited him to return from Germany and hospitalized him at Shanghai East Hospital, which made it convenient for me to care for him and discuss the atlas simultaneously. During his hospitalization, he continued to draw illustrations late into the night, but we were finally able to communicate face-to-face rather than through emails or overseas phone calls. I had suggested the book be titled *Weng Yuguo Cardiac Surgery Atlas*, but he politely refused my proposal. He explained that in addition to his own experiences and innovations, there were also contributions from German colleagues and pre-

手绘彩图 2 000 余幅，均为原创，汇聚了翁医生毕生的心血。2017 年 5 月，翁医生弥留之际，拉着我的手做了最后的嘱托，希望这本图解能够早日出版，供更多的心脏外科医生、医学生、公众学习、参考、科普。2017 年 6 月 26 日 13 时 48 分，我的良师挚友翁渝国医生仙逝，我和翁医生的家人一起陪伴他走完了最后一程。追悼会上，翁医生的同学、同事、学生 500 多人前来送行，斯人虽逝，往事如烟，历历在目，潸然泪下。为了完成翁医生的遗愿，在他走后的几年里，我又邀请刘锦纷教授、李颖则教授共同完善本图解的撰写，并按翁医生的要求将图解分为小儿和成人两册，分别恭请丁文祥教授和胡盛寿院士作序。出于对翁医生的了解和尊敬，两位心脏外科大家欣然命笔，为本书出版增添了浓墨重彩，在此表示衷心感谢！经人民卫生出版社慎重批准，将本书分为《成人心脏外科名家手术手绘图解》和《小儿心脏外科名家手术手绘图解》两册，按中英文对照形式出版，以此告慰翁医生在天之灵。也希望更多的年轻医生从中感悟到心脏外科的深奥和技巧，收获更多前人的经验和爱心。

decessors, so *Atlas of Cardiac Surgery* was a more appropriate title. The book boasts more than 2 000 original hand-drawn color illustrations, all of which embody Dr. Weng's lifelong efforts. In May 2017, shortly before Dr. Weng passed away, he took my hand and made a final request. He hoped that this atlas could be published quickly for cardiac surgeons, medical students, and public learning and reference. At 13: 48 on 26th, June, 2017, Dr. Weng Yuguo, my close teacher and friend, passed away. Dr. Weng's family and I accompanied him on his last journey. At the memorial service, more than 500 of Dr. Weng's classmates, colleagues, and students came to see him off. Although Dr. Weng passed away, my memories of him are still vivid and make me shed tears unconsciously. To realize Dr. Weng's unfinished wish, I worked hard over the following years with Professor Liu Jinfen and Professor Li Yingze on improving the collection of drawings, which, at the request of Dr. Weng, is classified into two volumes: Children and Adults. I have invited Professor Ding Wenxiang and the Chinese Academy of Engineering (CAE) Academician Hu Shengshou to write prefaces for these two volumes. Out of understanding and respect for Dr. Weng, these two masters of cardiac surgery agreed without hesitation to write the prefaces, adding luster to the publication of this book. I would like to express my heartfelt thanks to them here. After careful consideration, the People's Medical Publishing House has approved the publication of this book in both Chinese and English, and it is divided into two volumes: *Hand-drawn Atlas of Master Cardiac Surgery in Adults* and *Hand-drawn Atlas of Master Cardiac Surgery in Children*. It is hoped that the publication of the book will comfort Dr. Weng in heaven and that more young doctors will realize the profoundness of cardiac surgery skills and gain more experience and compassion from their predecessors.

刘中民
中国医师协会心血管外科
医师分会会长
俄罗斯工程院外籍院士
上海市东方医院 / 同济大学
附属东方医院名誉院长
2024 年 2 月

Dr. Liu Zhongmin
President of Cardiovascular Surgeon Branch,
Chinese Medical Doctor Association
Foreign Academician of Russian Academy of Engineering
Honorary President of Shanghai East Hospital/
East Hospital Affiliated to Tongji University
February, 2024

目 录

第一章 基本方法

Chapter 1 General Procedure

Contents

第一章
基本方法

Chapter 1
General Procedure

第一节　胸部切口
Section 1　Chest Incision

图 1-1-1　胸骨正中切口
Figure 1-1-1　Median sternotomy

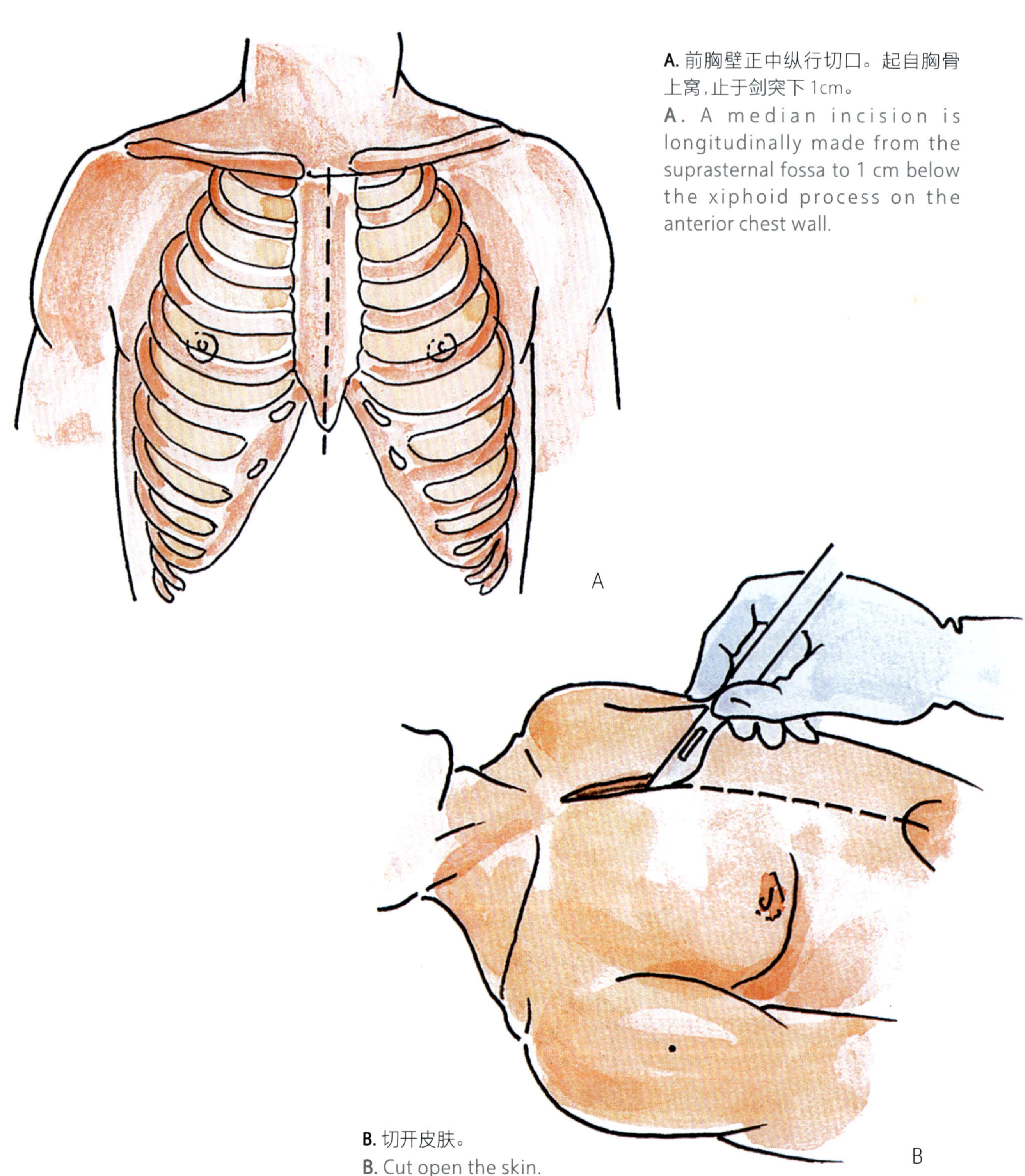

A. 前胸壁正中纵行切口。起自胸骨上窝，止于剑突下 1cm。

A. A median incision is longitudinally made from the suprasternal fossa to 1 cm below the xiphoid process on the anterior chest wall.

B. 切开皮肤。

B. Cut open the skin.

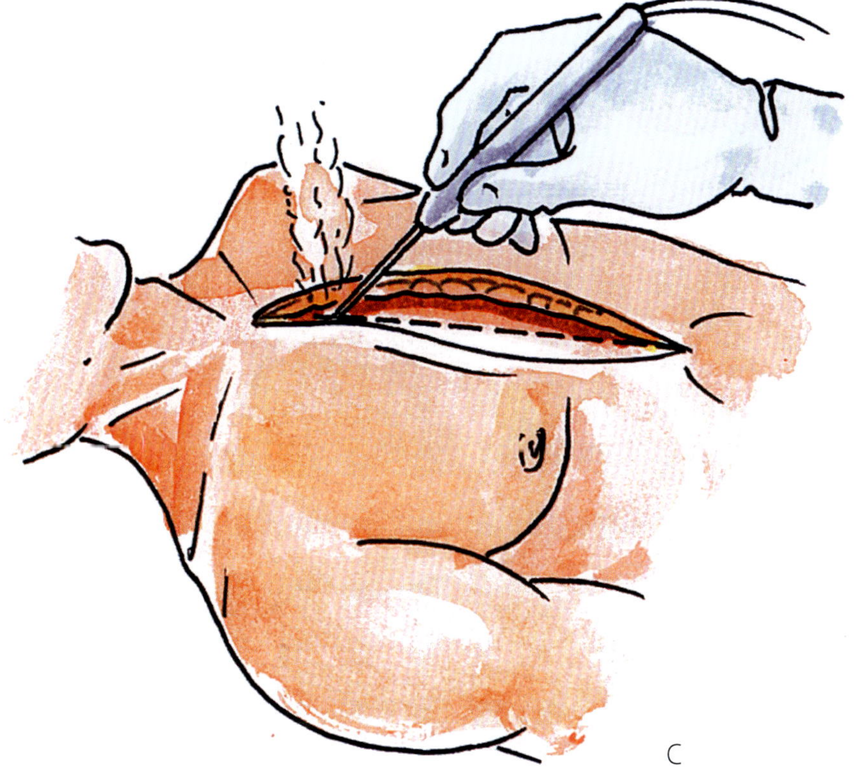

C

C. 电刀切开皮下组织、肌肉和胸骨骨膜。

C. Cut open the subcutaneous tissue, muscle, and sternal periosteum with an electrotome.

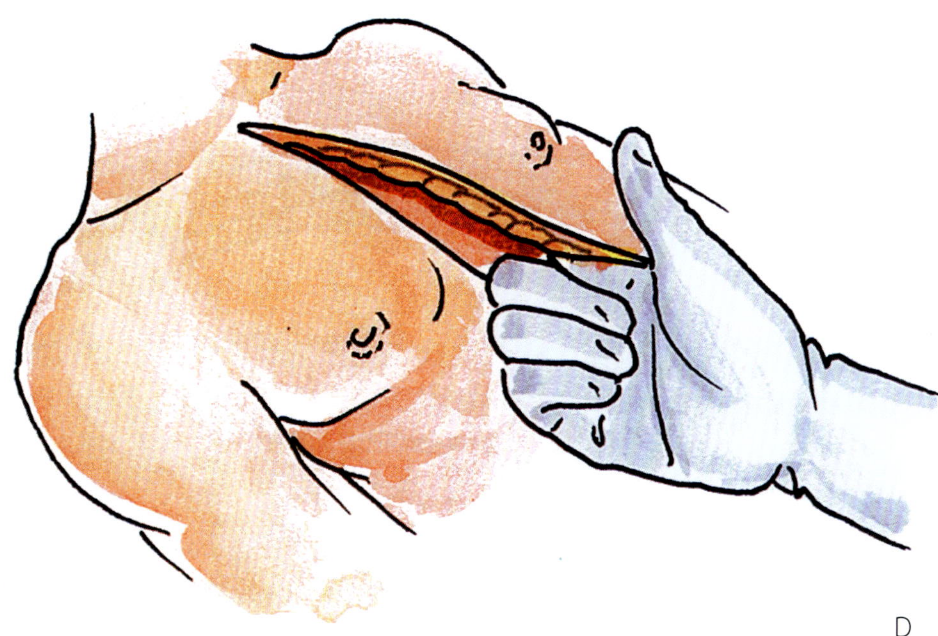

D

D. 手指由剑突下进入胸骨后，钝性分离前纵隔疏松组织。

D. Gain access to the posterior surface of the sternum from below the xiphoid process and bluntly separate the loose tissue from the anterior mediastinum with fingers.

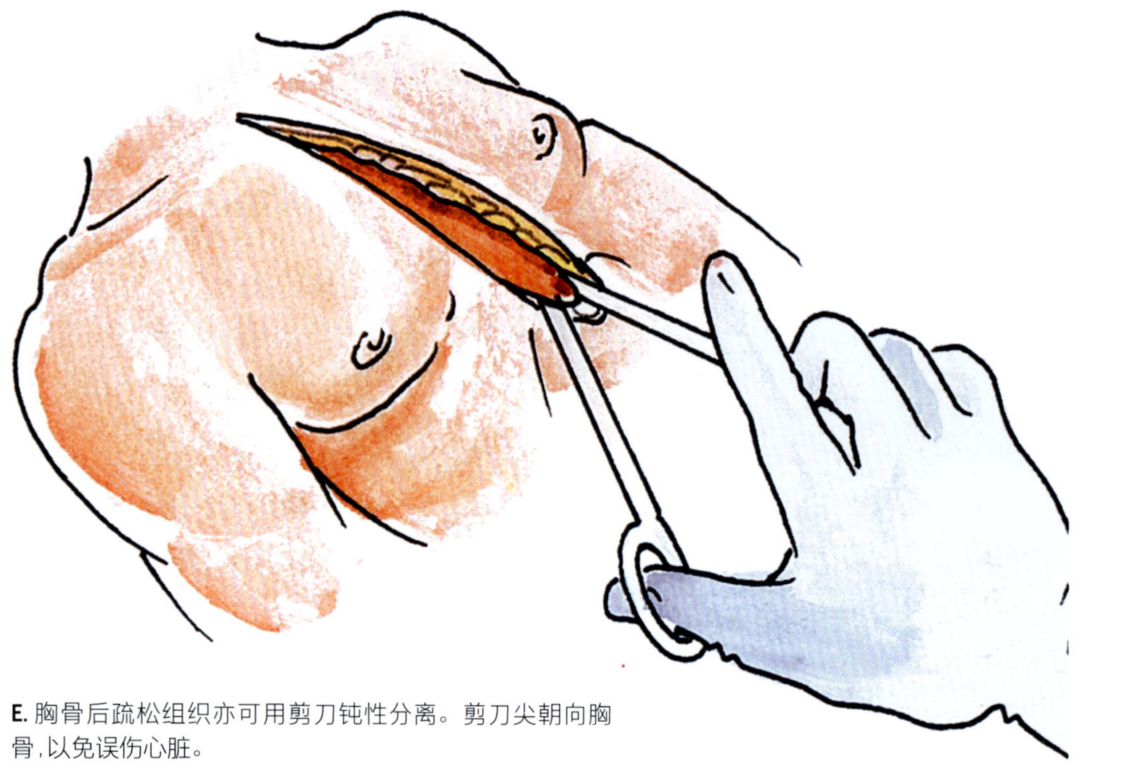

E

E. 胸骨后疏松组织亦可用剪刀钝性分离。剪刀尖朝向胸骨，以免误伤心脏。

E. The retrosternal loose tissues can also be separated bluntly by scissors with the point toward the sternum to avoid any injuries to the heart.

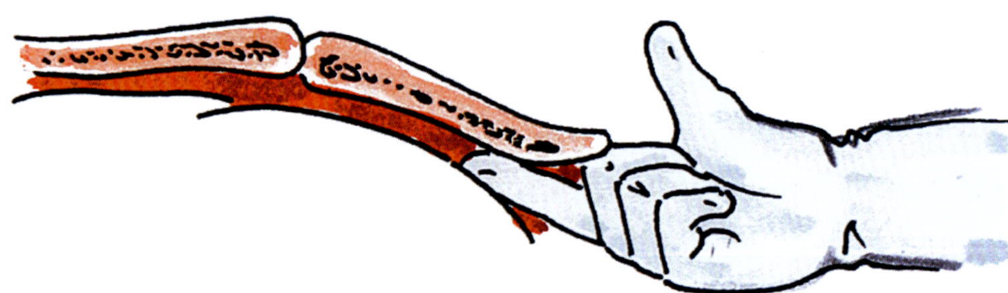

F

F. 钝性分离的解剖层面在胸骨和心包之间，分离紧贴胸骨进行。

F. Anatomically, blunt dissection between the sternum and pericardium should be performed adjacent to the sternum.

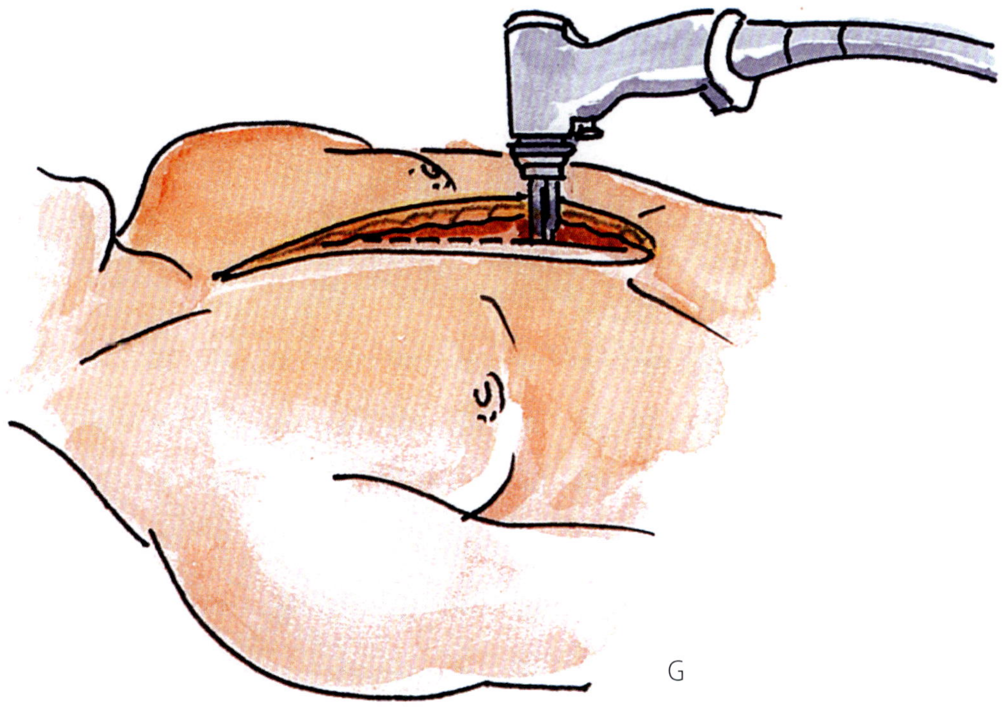

G. 胸骨锯纵行锯开胸骨。胸骨切开面骨髓腔渗血用骨蜡止血。

G. Cut through the sternum longitudinally with a sternal saw, and control bleeding from the incision of the medullary canal with bone wax.

图 1-1-2 心包切开

Figure 1-1-2 Pericardiotomy

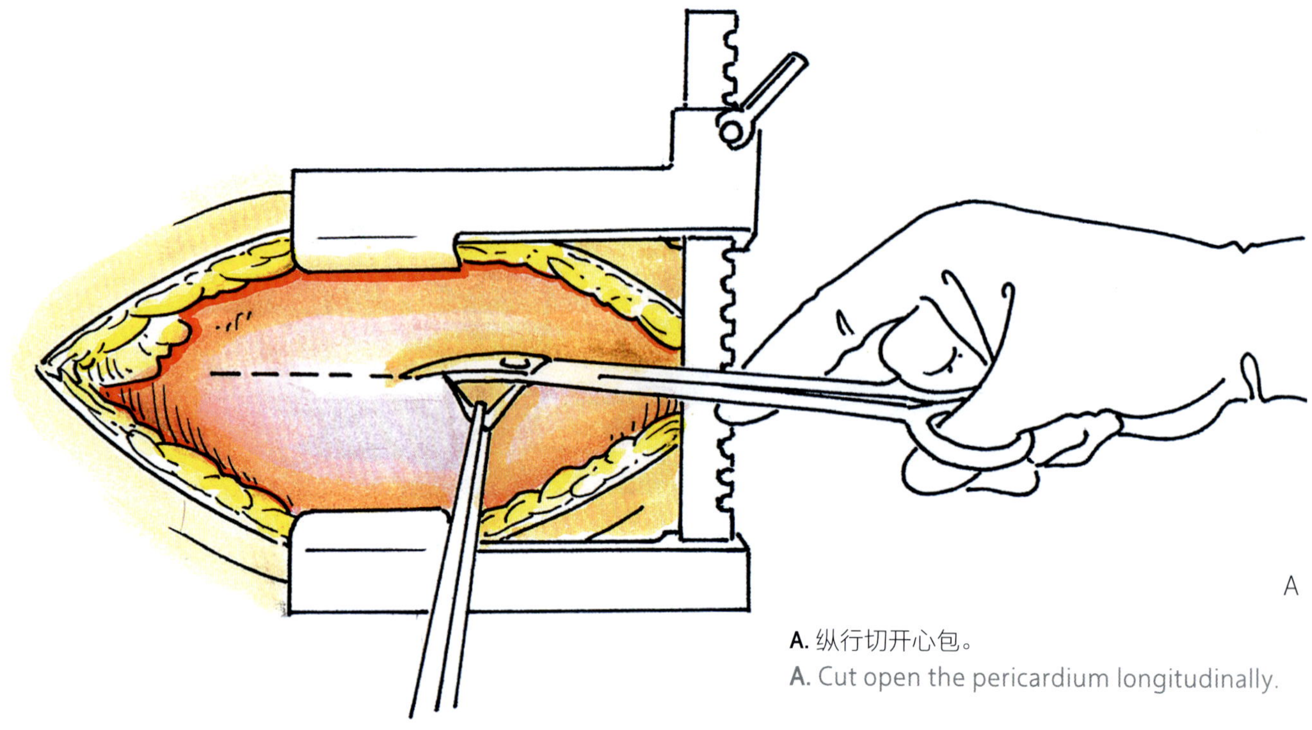

A. 纵行切开心包。

A. Cut open the pericardium longitudinally.

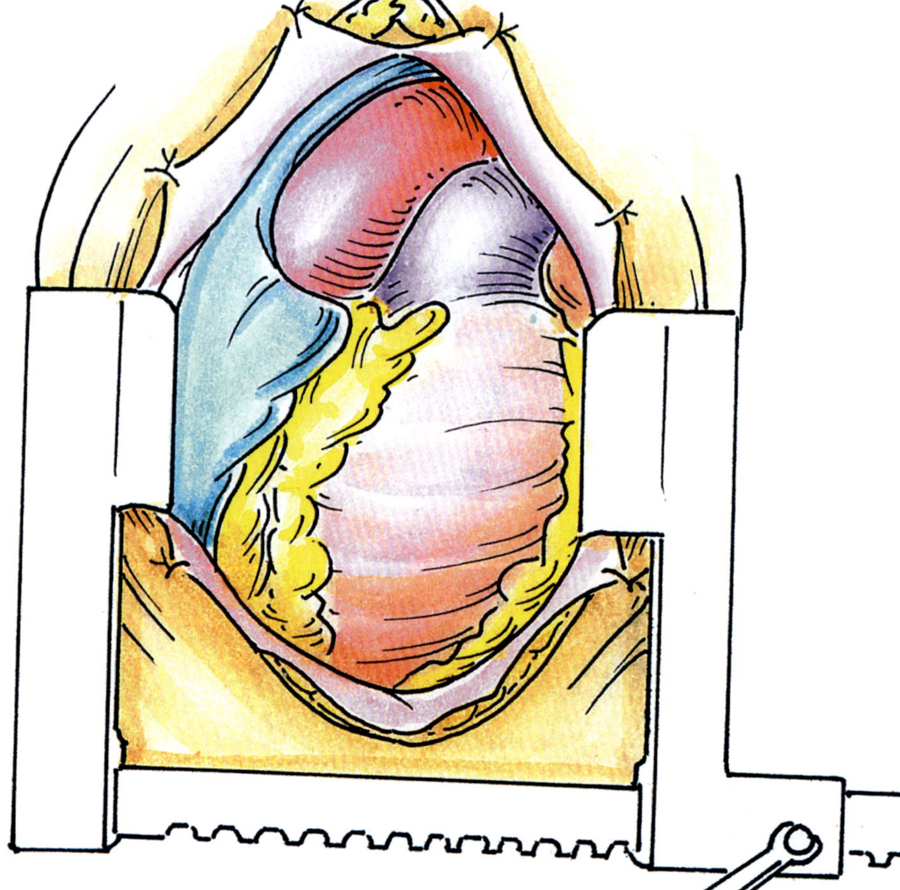

B. 将切开的心包缝吊于胸壁，两侧各缝 3 针。

B. The incised pericardium is suspended to the chest wall with 3 stitches on both sides of the pericardium.

图 1-1-3 再次胸骨切开
Figure 1-1-3 Redo-sternotomy

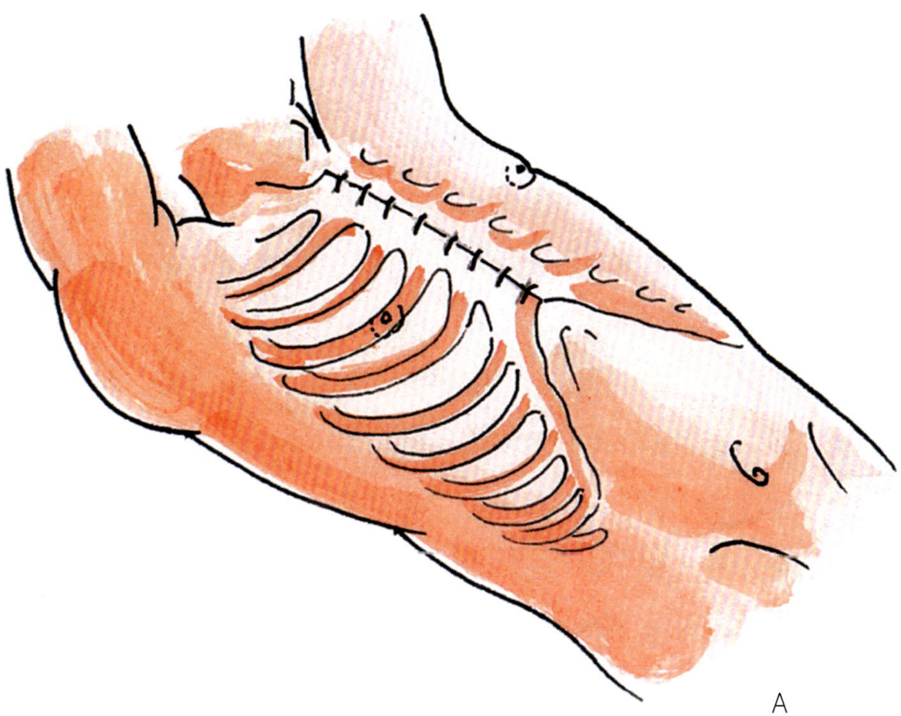

A

A. 仍由原胸部正中切口进入。

A. The heart is accessed through the original sternotomy.

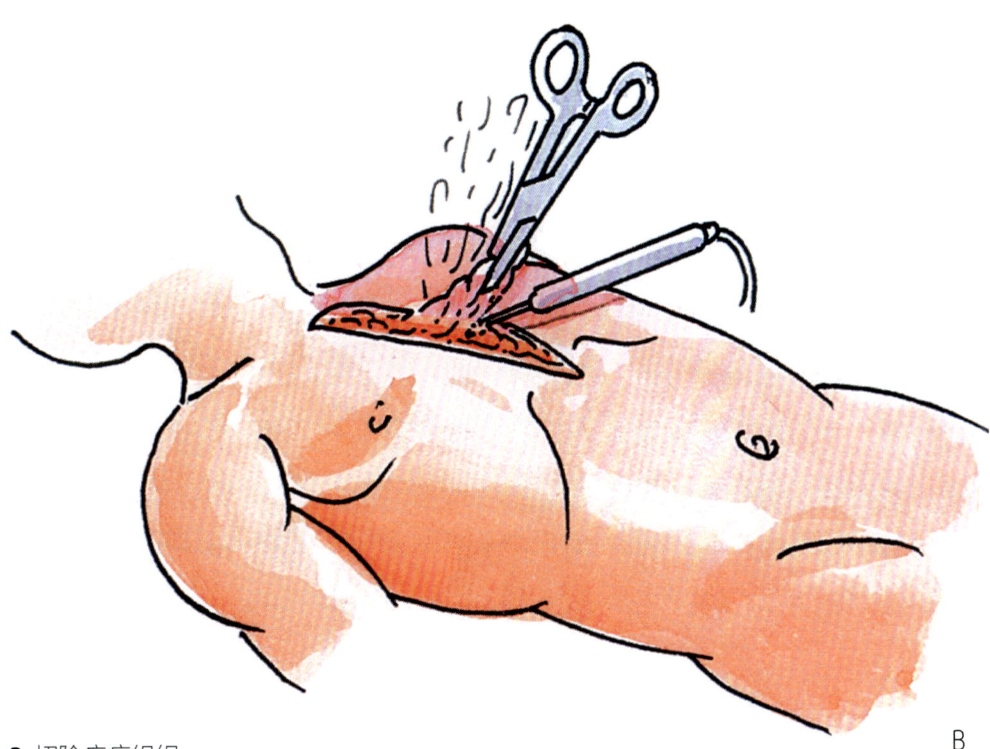

B

B. 切除瘢痕组织。

B. Excise the scar tissues.

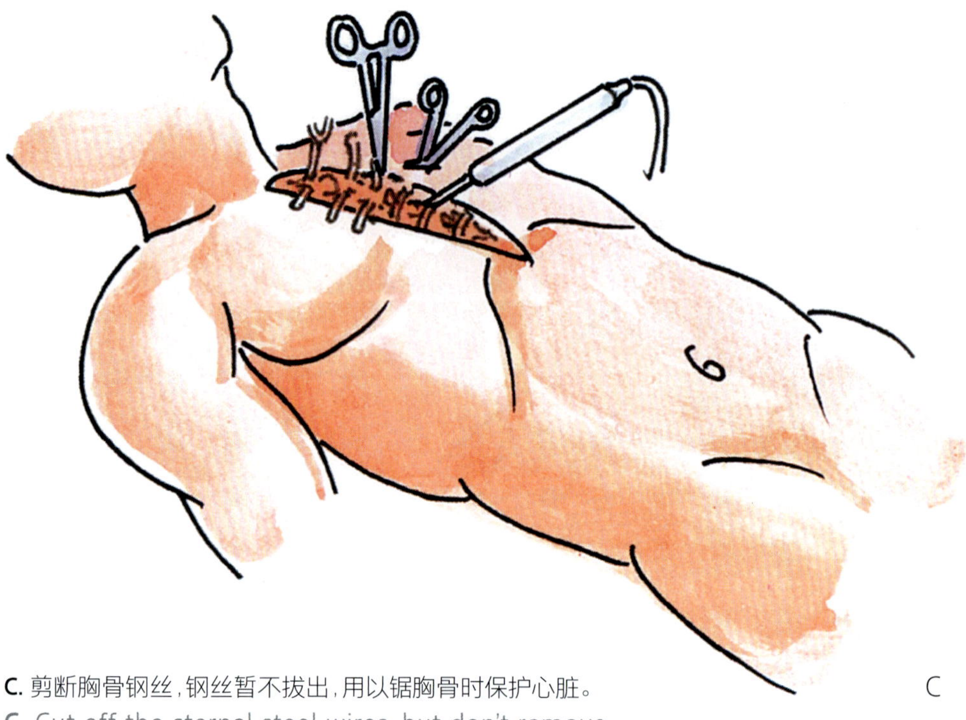

C. 剪断胸骨钢丝，钢丝暂不拔出，用以锯胸骨时保护心脏。

C. Cut off the sternal steel wires, but don't remove them until the sternum is incised, in order to protect the heart.

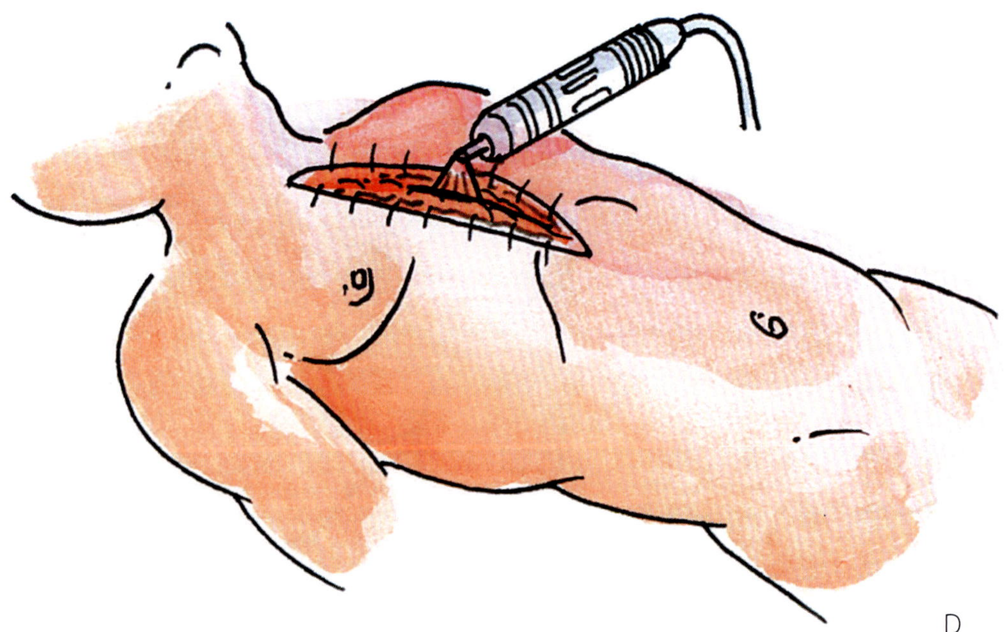

D. 摇摆锯锯开胸骨。

D. Cut through the sternum with an oscillating saw.

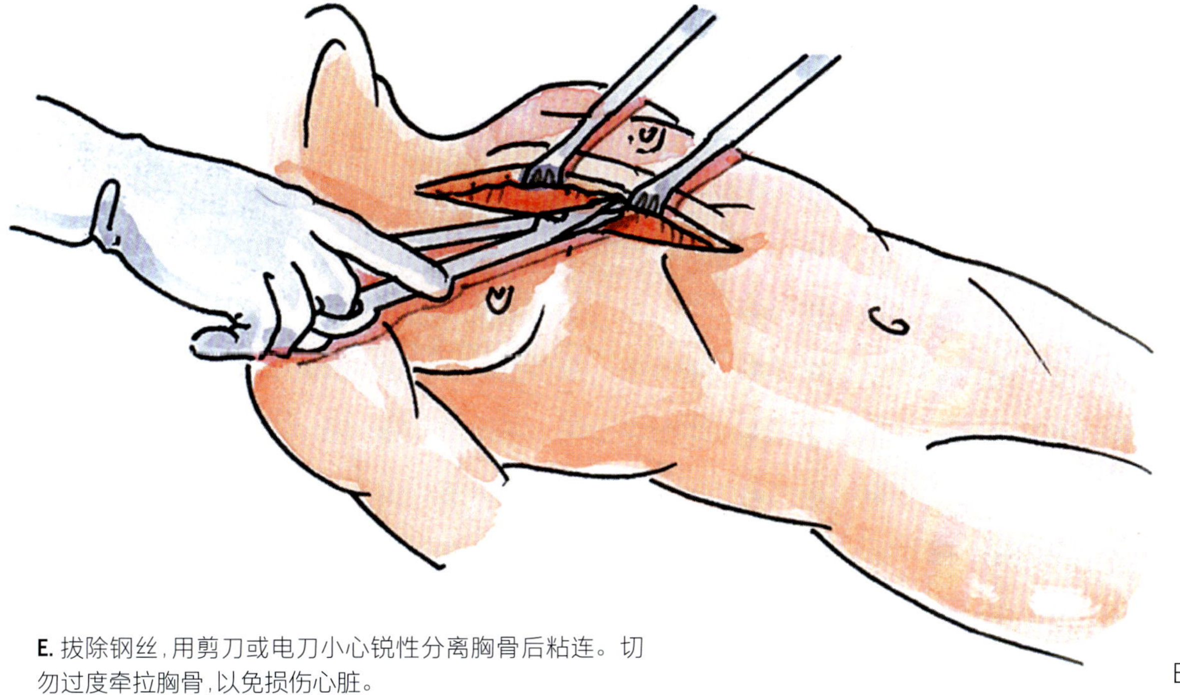

E. 拔除钢丝，用剪刀或电刀小心锐性分离胸骨后粘连。切勿过度牵拉胸骨，以免损伤心脏。

E. The wires are removed now, and the substernal adhesions are dissected sharply with scissors or electrotomes carefully. The sternum should not be overstretched to avoid any injuries to the heart.

图 1-1-4 标准胸部外侧切口

Figure 1-1-4 Standard lateral thoracotomy

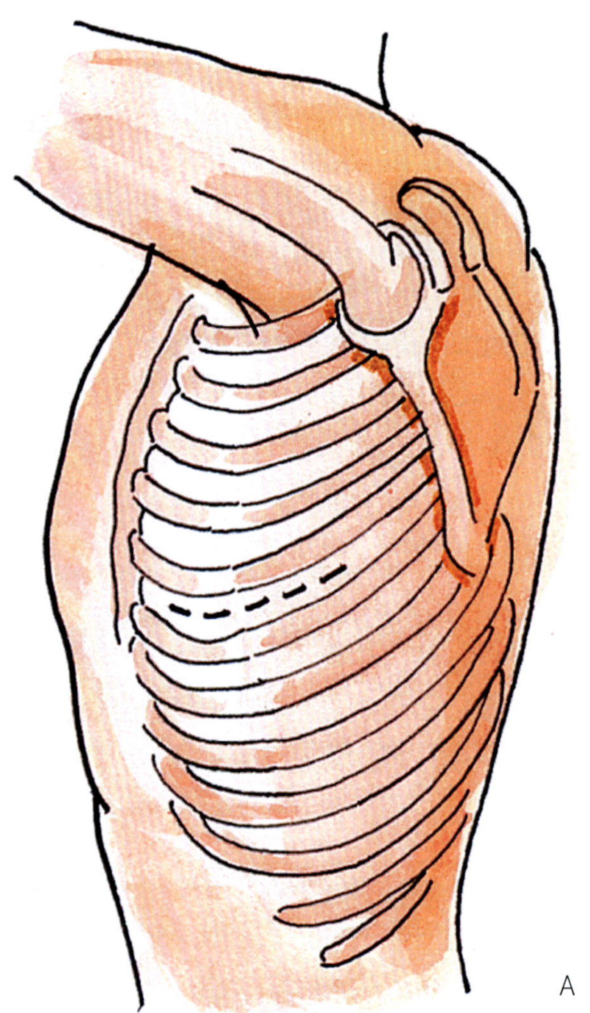

A. 以腋中线为中心沿第 5 肋间做切口。

A. An incision is made in the fifth intercostal space along the midaxillary line.

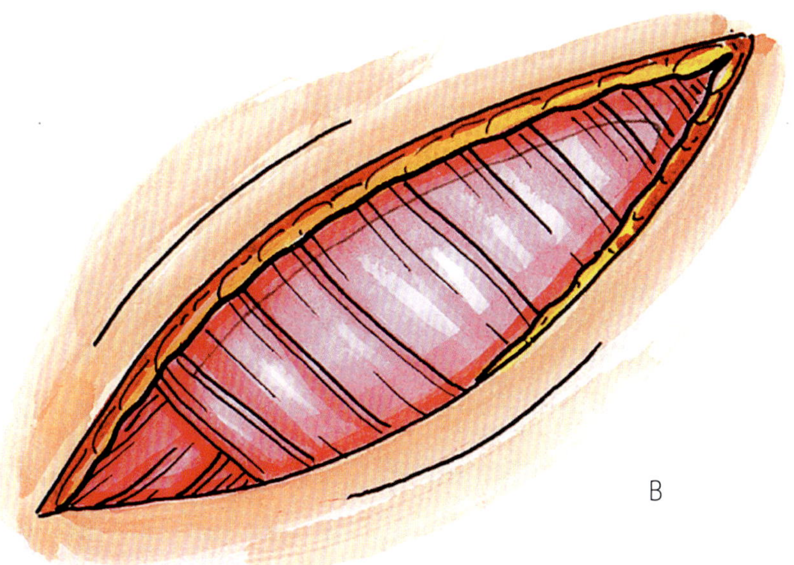

B. 切开皮肤、皮下组织。

B. Cut open the skin and subcutaneous tissues.

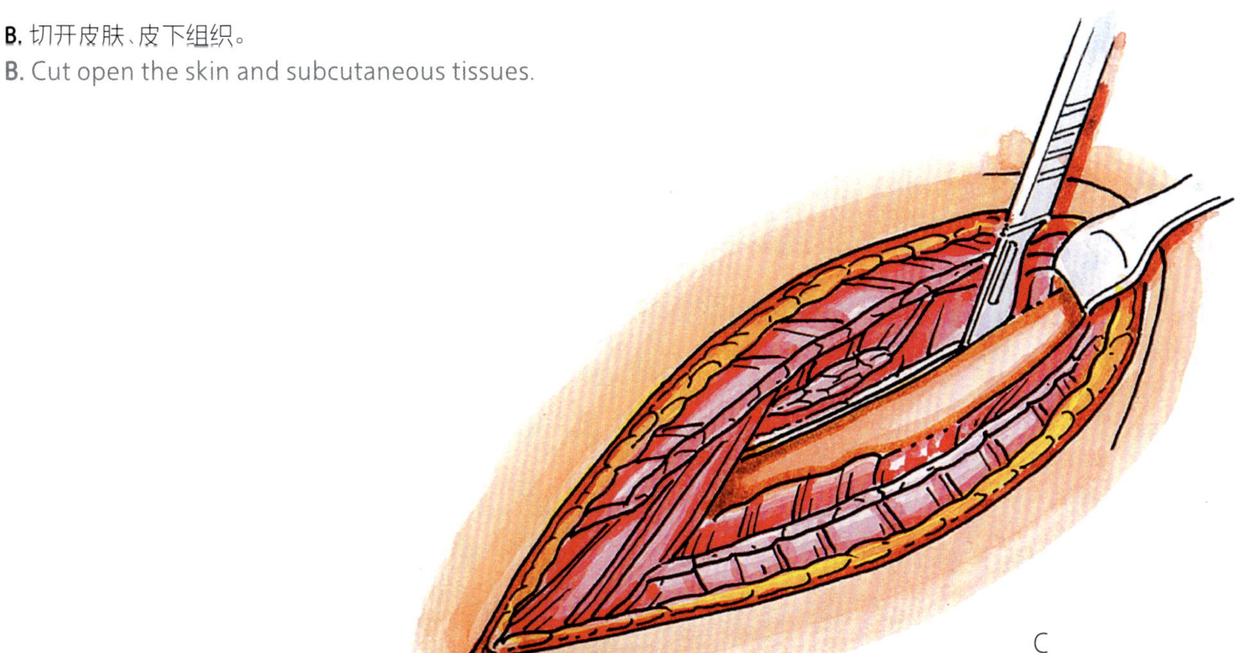

C. 切开背阔肌和前锯肌，沿第 6 肋骨上缘切开肋间内肌和肋间外肌，打开胸膜进胸。

C. The incision is carried in the latissimus dorsi and serratus anterior muscles, and extended to the internal and external intercostal muscles along the upper edge of the sixth rib. Open the pleura, and the chest is accessed.

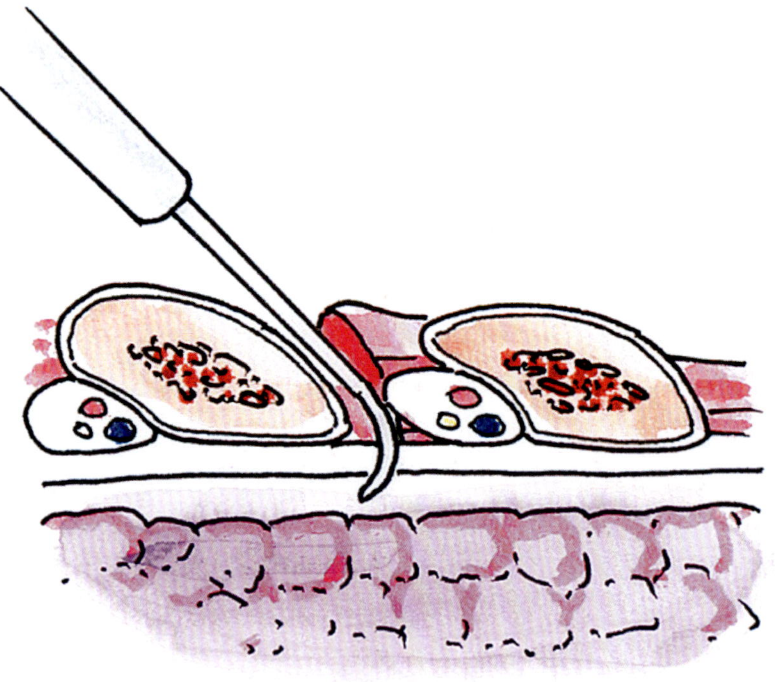

D. 肋间血管走行于肋骨下缘，沿肋骨上缘切开可避免损伤肋间血管。

D. As the intercostal vessels travel along the lower edge of the ribs, incisions along the upper edge of the ribs can avoid injury to the intercostal vessels.

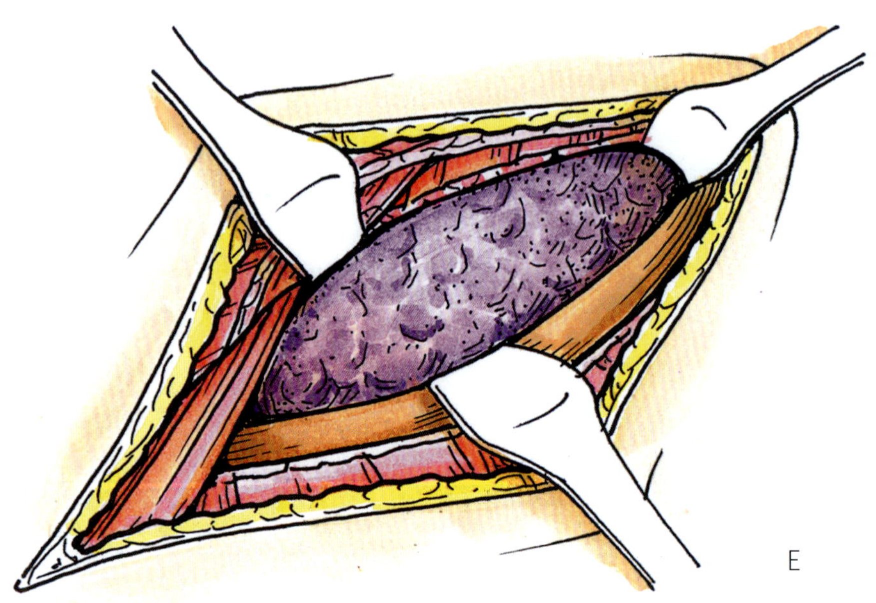

E. 牵开肋骨，显露胸腔内的肺脏。

E. The ribs are retracted to expose the lungs in the chest cavity.

图 1-1-5　胸部后外侧切口

Figure 1-1-5　Posterolateral thoracotomy

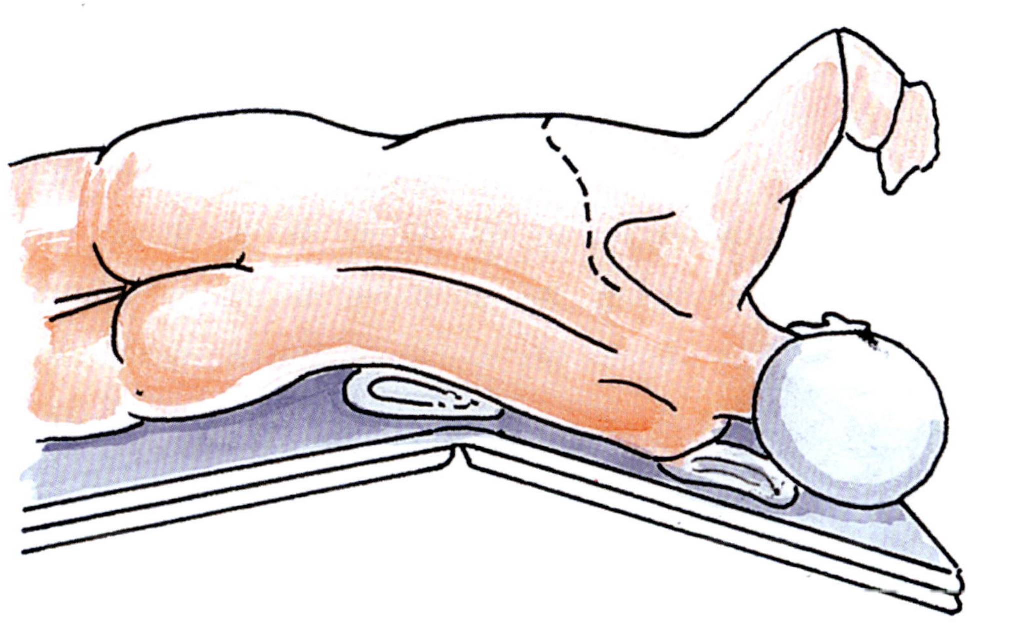

A

A. 患者取侧卧位，患侧朝上。切口自肩胛骨内缘和棘突的中线向下，于肩胛骨下角下方绕向前至腋前线。

A. With patients in the lateral recumbent position, an arcuate incision is made downward from the medial margin between the scapulae and the spinal process and is detoured to the anterior axillary line below the inferior angle of the scapula.

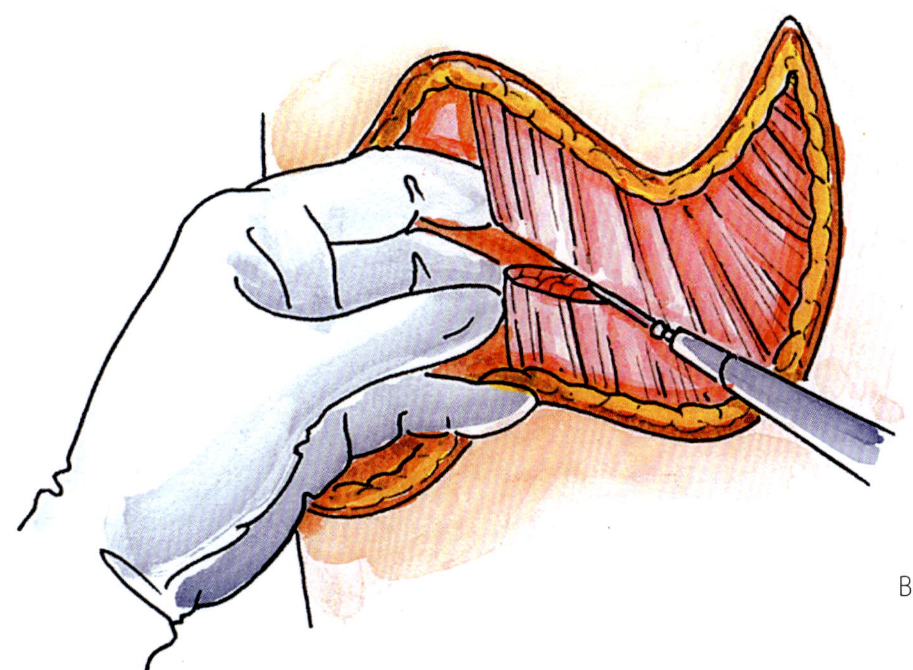

B

B. 在肩胛骨下角筋膜三角处切开至肋骨表面，分别向前和后上全层切开胸壁肌层，包括背阔肌、前锯肌、斜方肌和菱形肌。

B. The incision is made from the subscapular fascial triangle to the rib surface, and extended upwards and backwards to cut the muscle layer on the chest in full thickness, including the latissimus dorsi, serratus anterior, trapezius, and rhomboid.

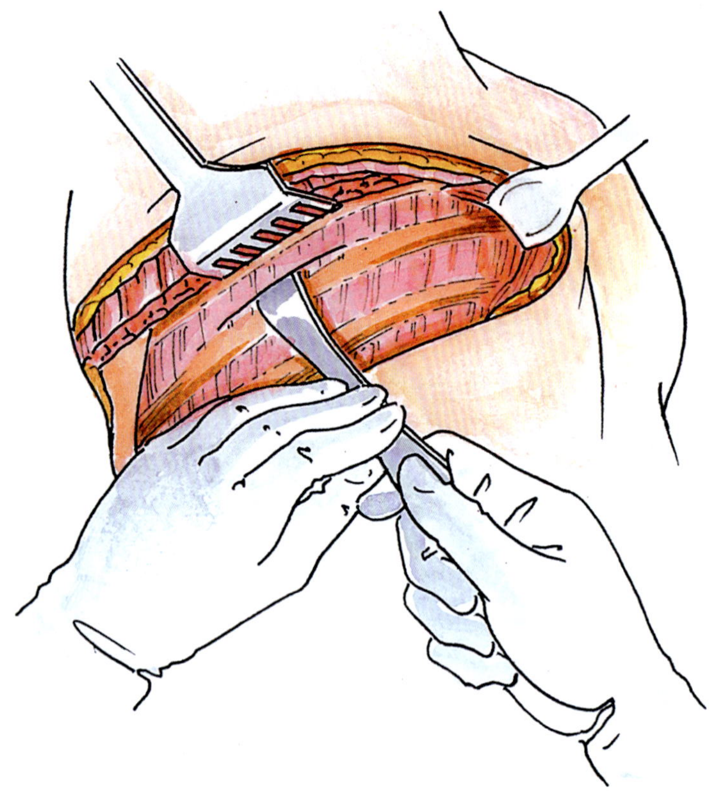
C

C. 在预定肋间的下一肋上缘切开肋间外肌、肋间内肌和胸膜。

C. The external intercostal muscles, internal intercostal muscles, and pleura are dissected along the upper edge of the rib below the predetermined intercostal space.

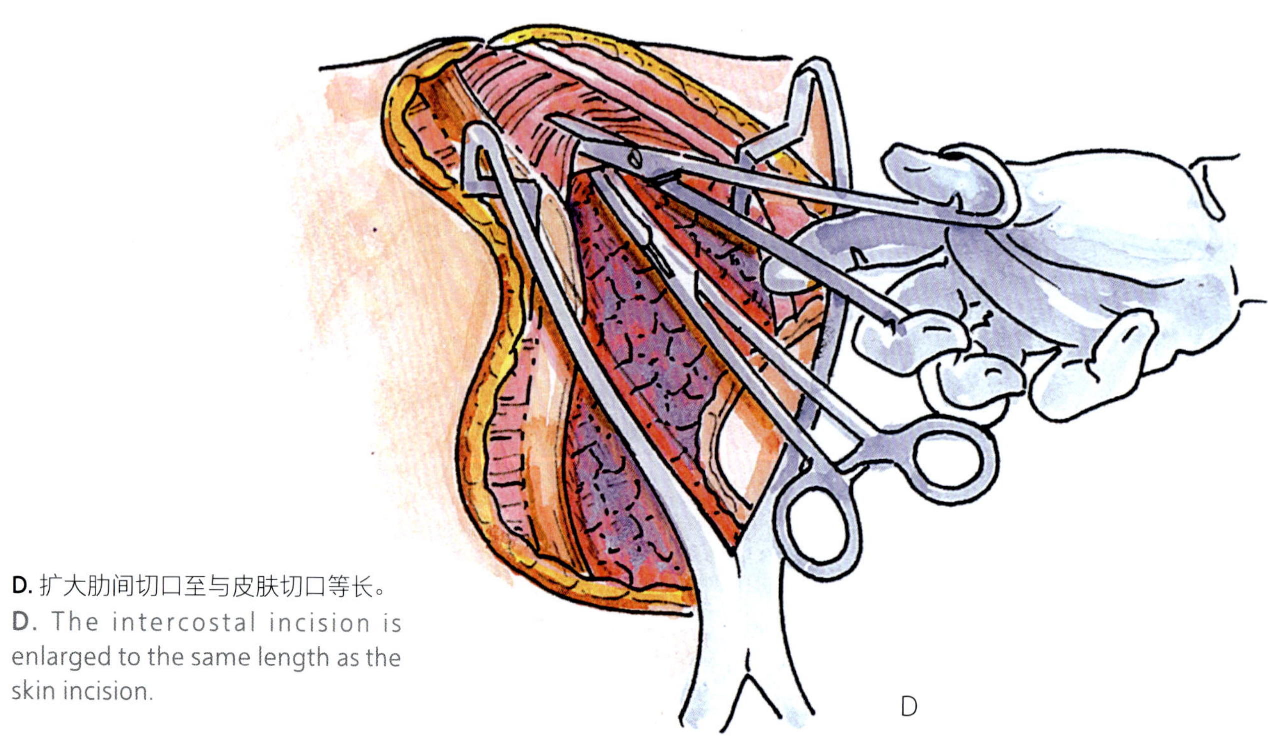
D

D. 扩大肋间切口至与皮肤切口等长。

D. The intercostal incision is enlarged to the same length as the skin incision.

图 1-1-6 胸部前外侧切口
Figure 1-1-6 Anterolateral thoracotomy

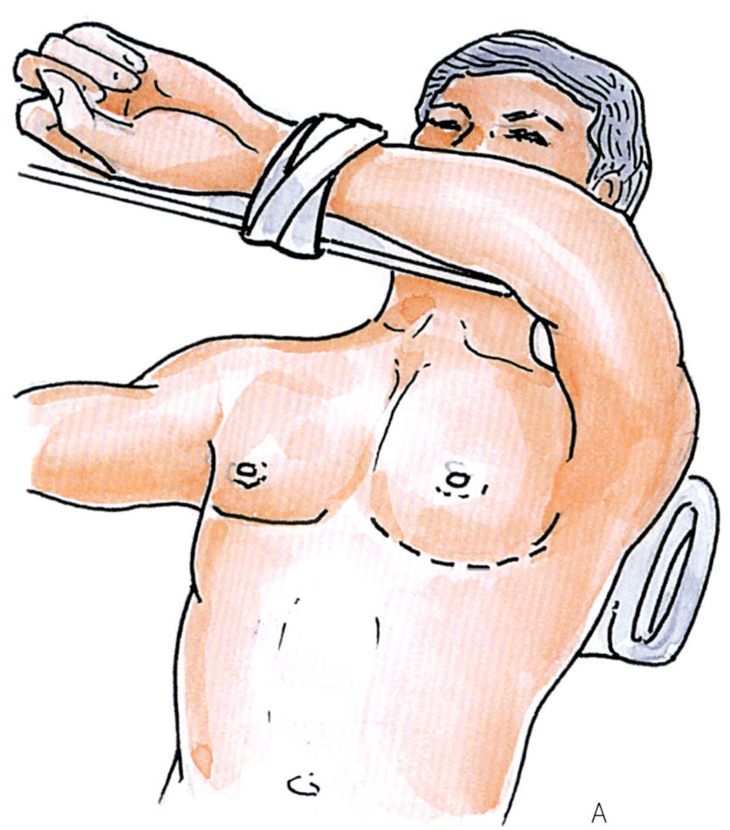

A. 仰卧位，患侧垫高 30°~45°。

A. The patient is in a supine position, with the affected side elevated 30 to 45 degrees.

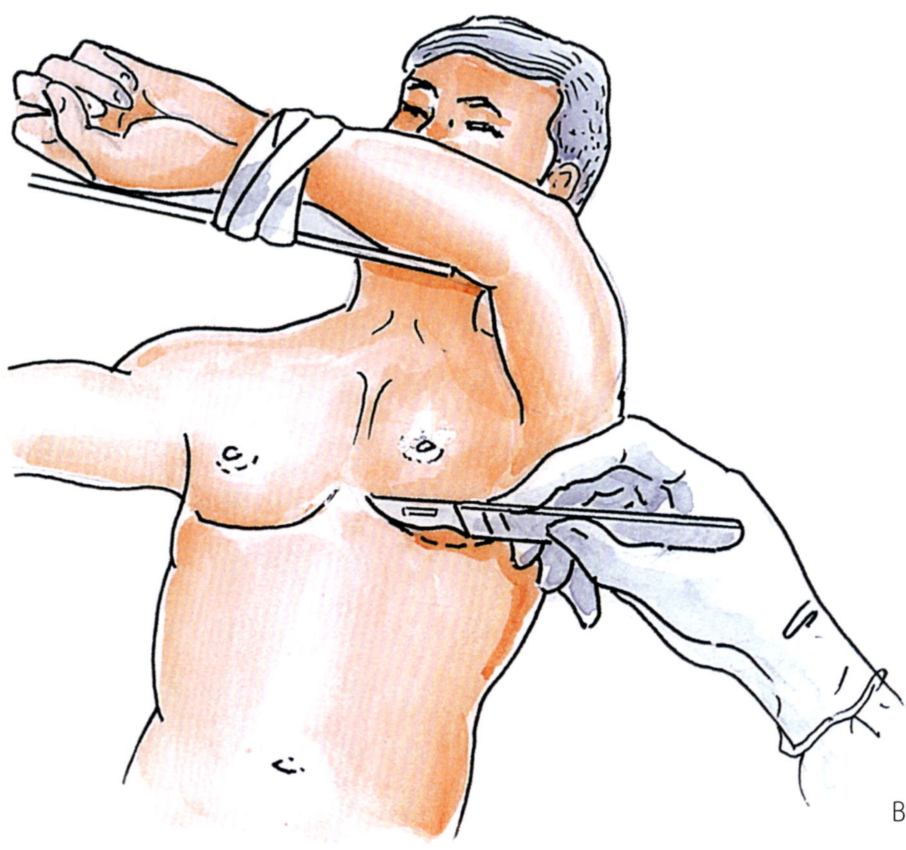

B. 于第 4 或第 5 肋间做切口。男性在相应肋间表面切开皮肤和皮下组织。切口起自胸骨外缘，循肋间走向切至腋前线或腋中线。女性的皮肤切口应在乳房下方。

B. Make an incision in the fourth or fifth intercostal space. In male, skin incisions can be made on the corresponding intercostal surface, starting from the outer edge of the sternum and extending to the anterior axillary line or midaxillary line along the intercostal direction. In female, incisions should be made below the breasts.

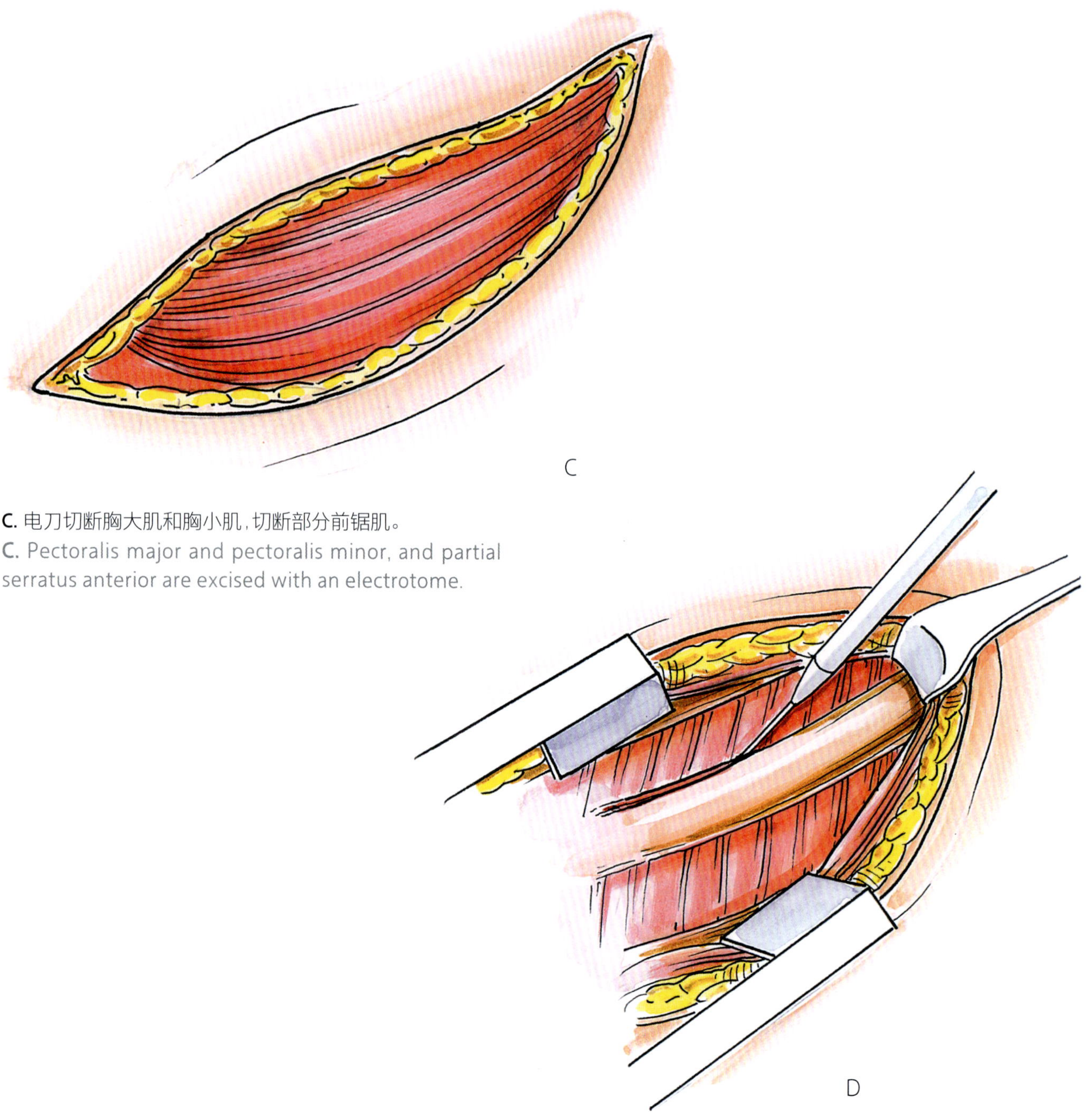

C. 电刀切断胸大肌和胸小肌，切断部分前锯肌。

C. Pectoralis major and pectoralis minor, and partial serratus anterior are excised with an electrotome.

D. 在第 4 或第 5 肋间切开肋间外肌和肋间内肌，切开胸膜进胸。切口内侧有胸廓内动静脉经过，注意保护，若损伤予以结扎。

D. The external and internal intercostal muscles are incised at the fourth or fifth intercostal space. Thoracic cavity can be accessed after an incision of the pleura. Take care to avoid any injuries since there are the internal thoracic artery and vein near the incision. Ligation is needed in the case of injury.

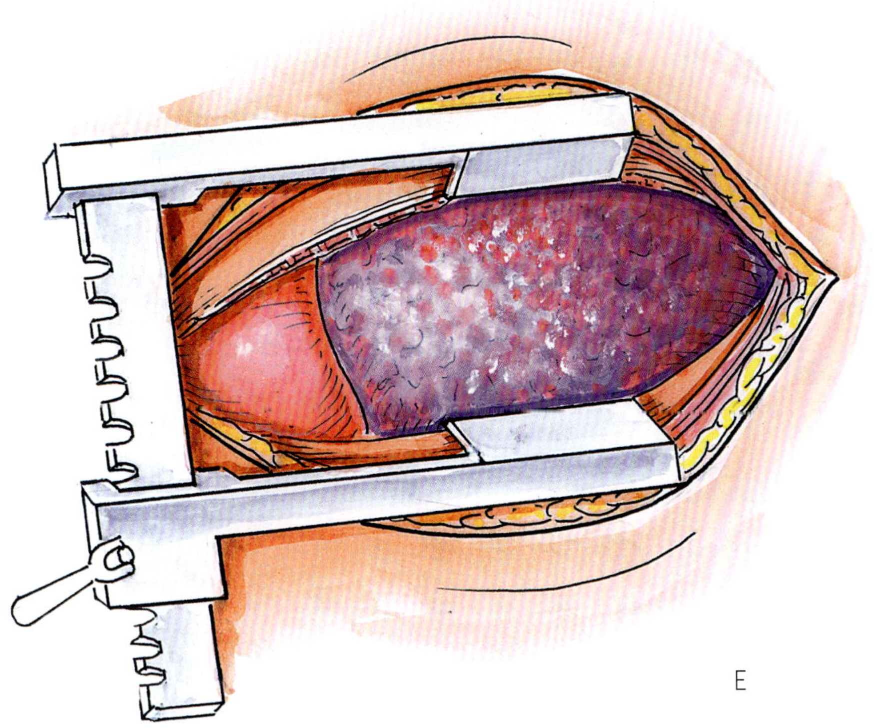

E. 撑开器撑开肋骨，显露左肺及内侧的心包。

E. Ribs are retracted by a spreader for the exposure of the left lung and medial pericardium.

图 1-1-7　双侧胸部横断切口
Figure 1-1-7　Bilateral transverse thoracosternotomy

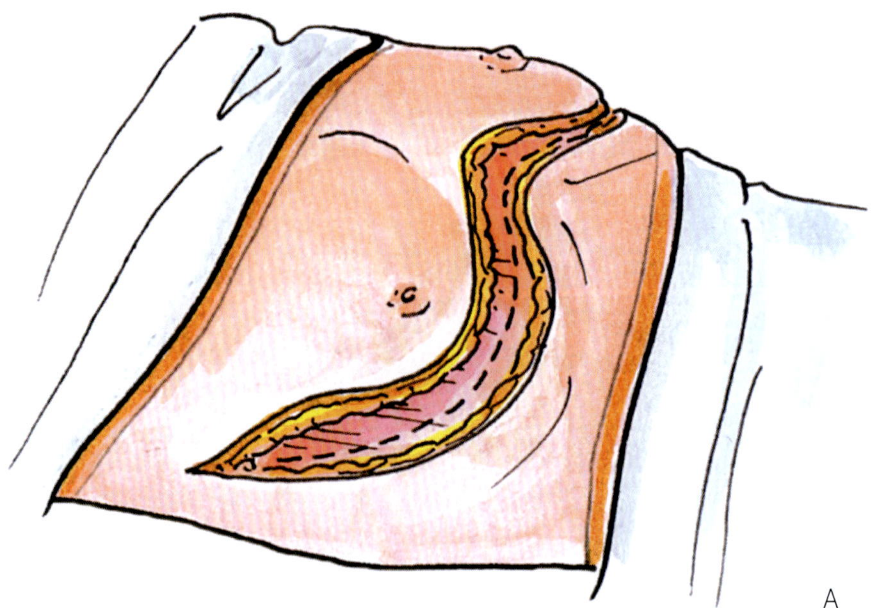

A

A. 仰卧位，沿两侧乳房下缘横过胸骨做波浪式切口。切开皮肤、皮下组织。

A. With the patient lying supine, a wave incision is made across the sternum and along the lower edge of both breasts. Cut open the skin and subcutaneous tissues.

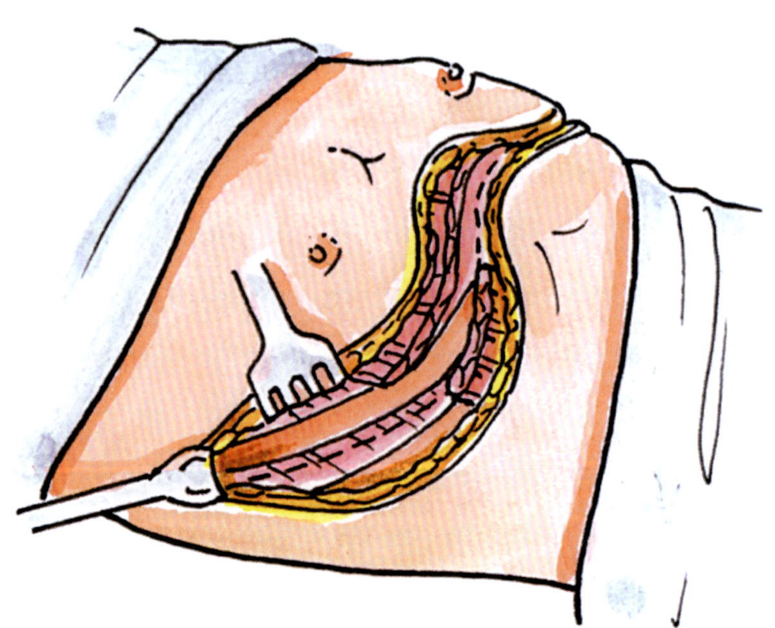

B

B. 右胸经第 3 肋间进胸，左胸由第 4 肋间进胸。

B. The right chest is accessed through the third intercostal space, and the left one through the fourth intercostal space.

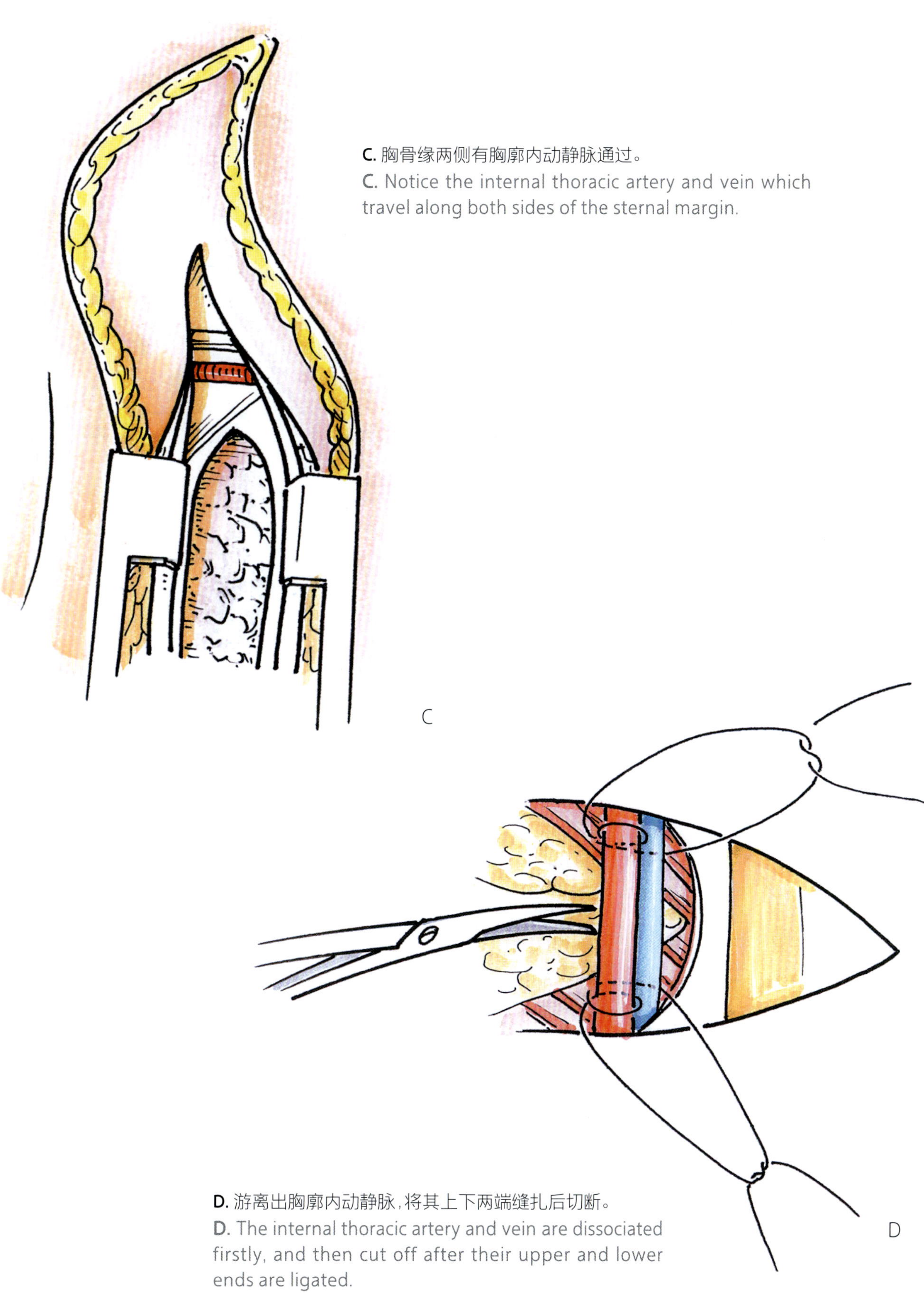

C. 胸骨缘两侧有胸廓内动静脉通过。

C. Notice the internal thoracic artery and vein which travel along both sides of the sternal margin.

D. 游离出胸廓内动静脉，将其上下两端缝扎后切断。

D. The internal thoracic artery and vein are dissociated firstly, and then cut off after their upper and lower ends are ligated.

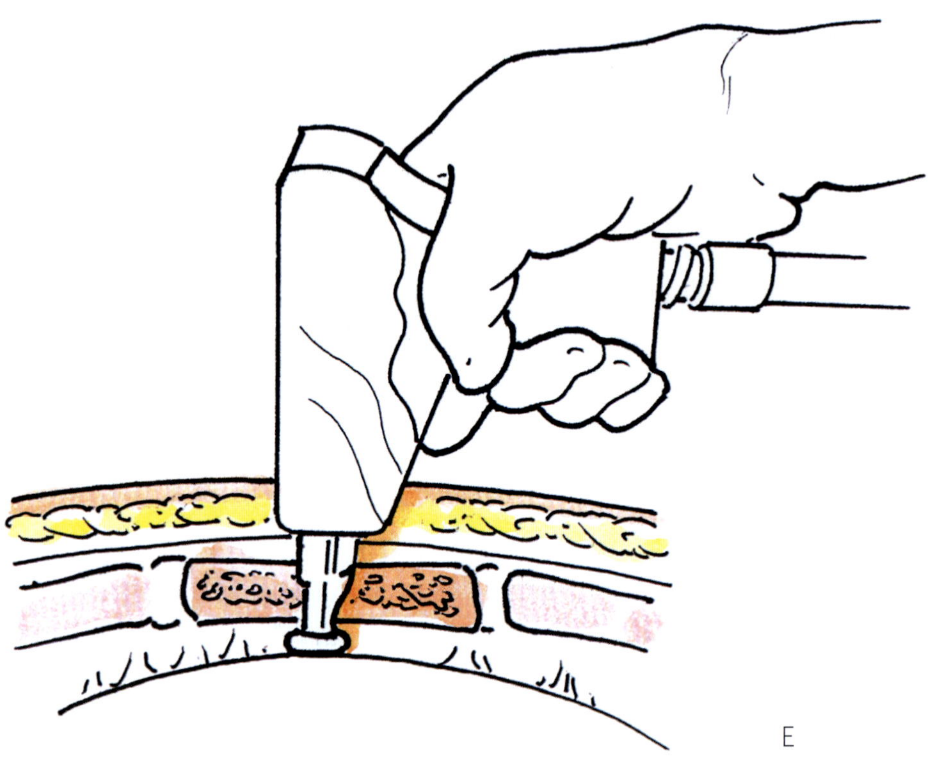

E. 电锯横断胸骨。撑开器分别撑开两侧胸部肋骨，形成一个贯通两侧胸腔的大切口。

E. The sternum is transected by a sternal saw. Bilateral thoracic ribs are retracted with a spreader to obtain a large incision connecting the bilateral thoracic cavities.

图 1-1-8　左胸腹联合切口
Figure 1-1-8　Left thoracoabdominal incision

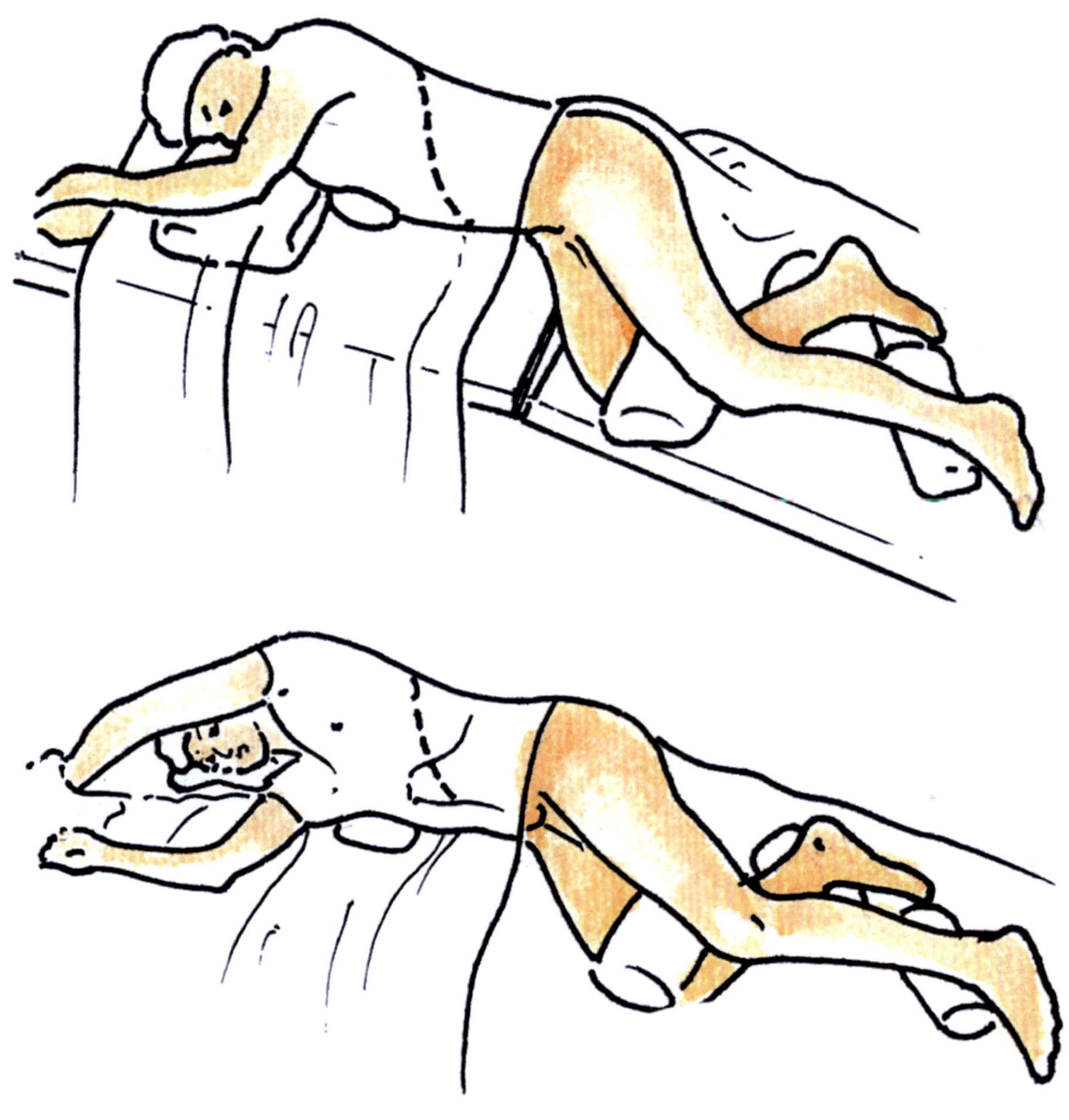

A

A. 右侧卧位，或右侧卧位向后转 30°。沿第 6 或第 7 肋间做切口，切口向前下方至腹直肌旁。必要时切口可按后外侧切口向后上延长，腹部切口可沿腹白线向下延长。

A. The patient is positioned in the full right recumbent position, or the right recumbent position with 30 degrees backward. An incision is made along the sixth or seventh intercostal space and is continued anteriorly and inferiorly to the rectus abdominis. If necessary, the incision can be extended towards the posterosuperior like the posterolateral thoracotomy, and the abdominal incision can be lengthened downwards along the linea alba.

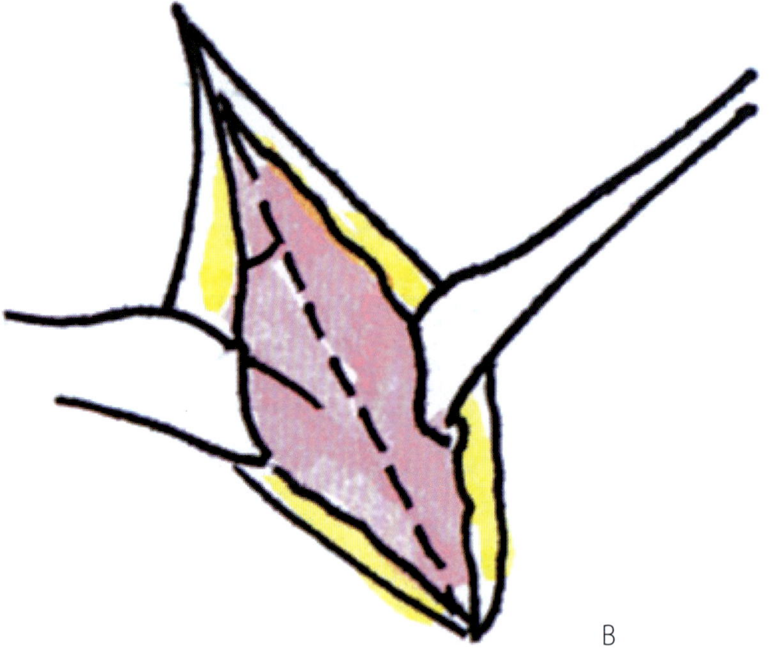

B. 切开皮肤、皮下组织。
B. Cut open the skin and subcutaneous tissues.

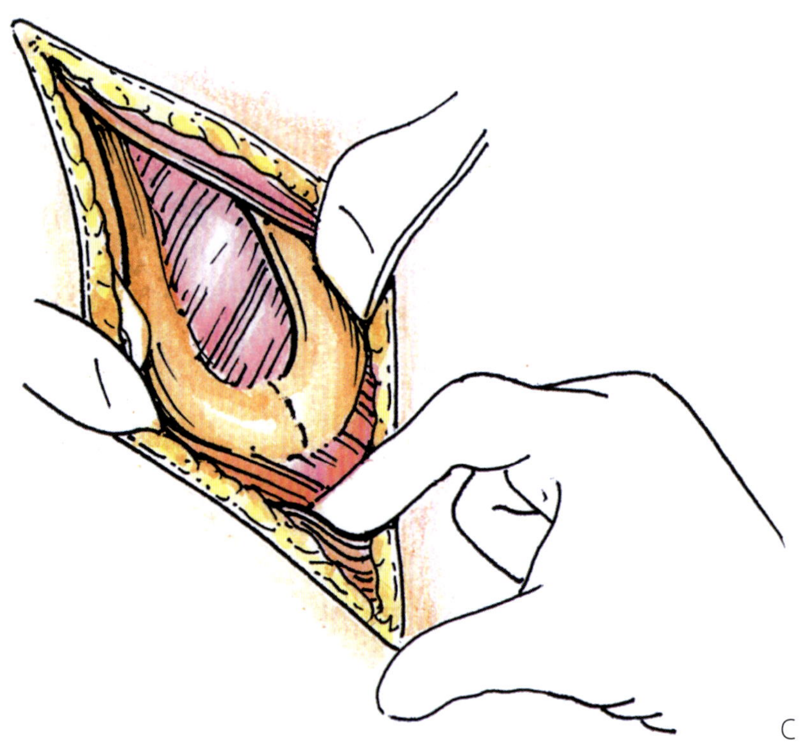

C. 切开胸壁肌层。
C. Open the muscularis of the chest wall.

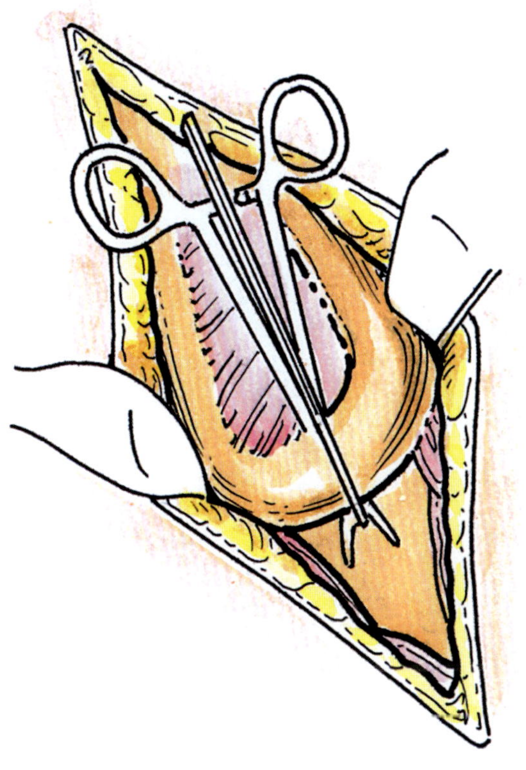

D. 在选定的肋间进胸，循切口打开腹腔，切断肋弓。

D. An incision is made into the chest through the predetermined intercostal, the abdominal cavity is opened along the incision, and the costal arch is severed.

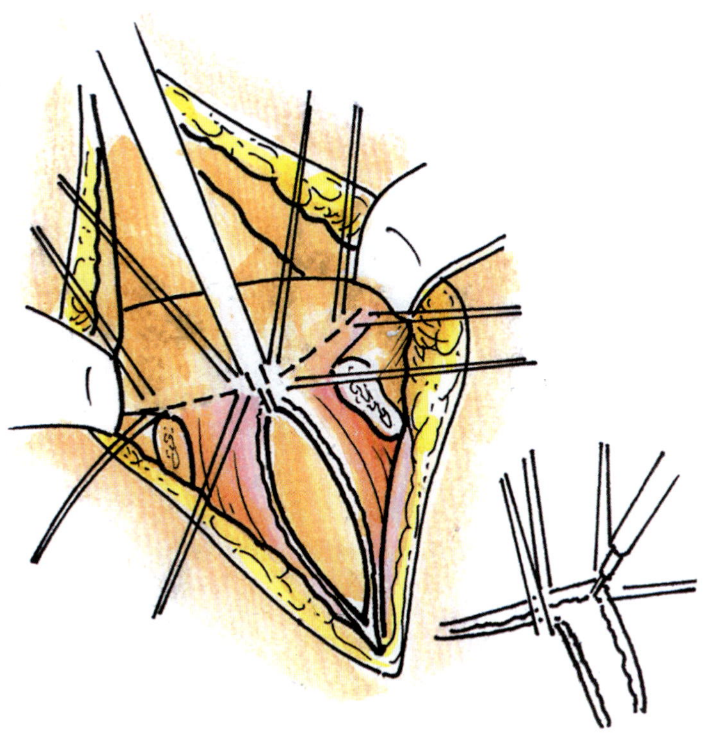

E. 牵引线悬吊后 T 形切开膈肌。

E. Diaphragm is incised in a T-shape manner after its suspension by traction suture.

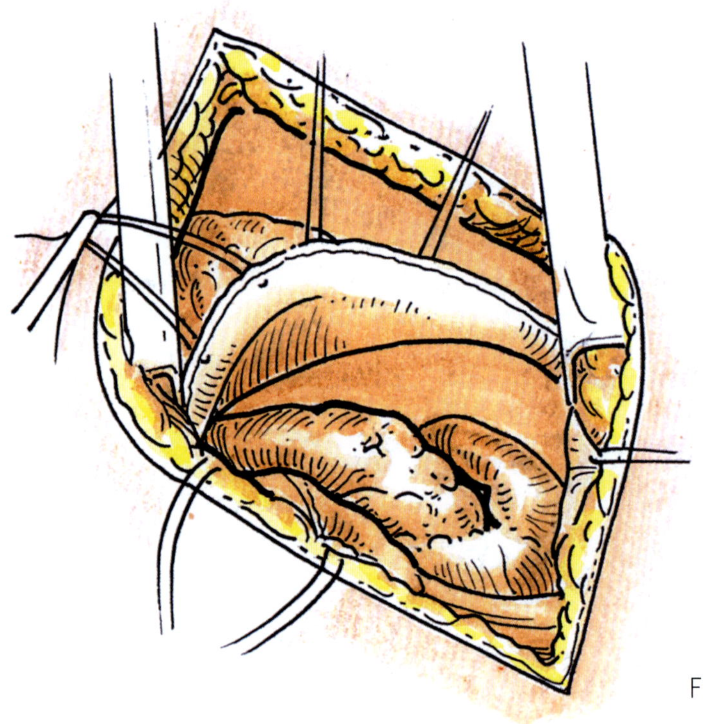

F. 切口完成，可同时显露胸腔和腹腔。

F. After the incision, both the thoracic and abdominal cavities are exposed simultaneously.

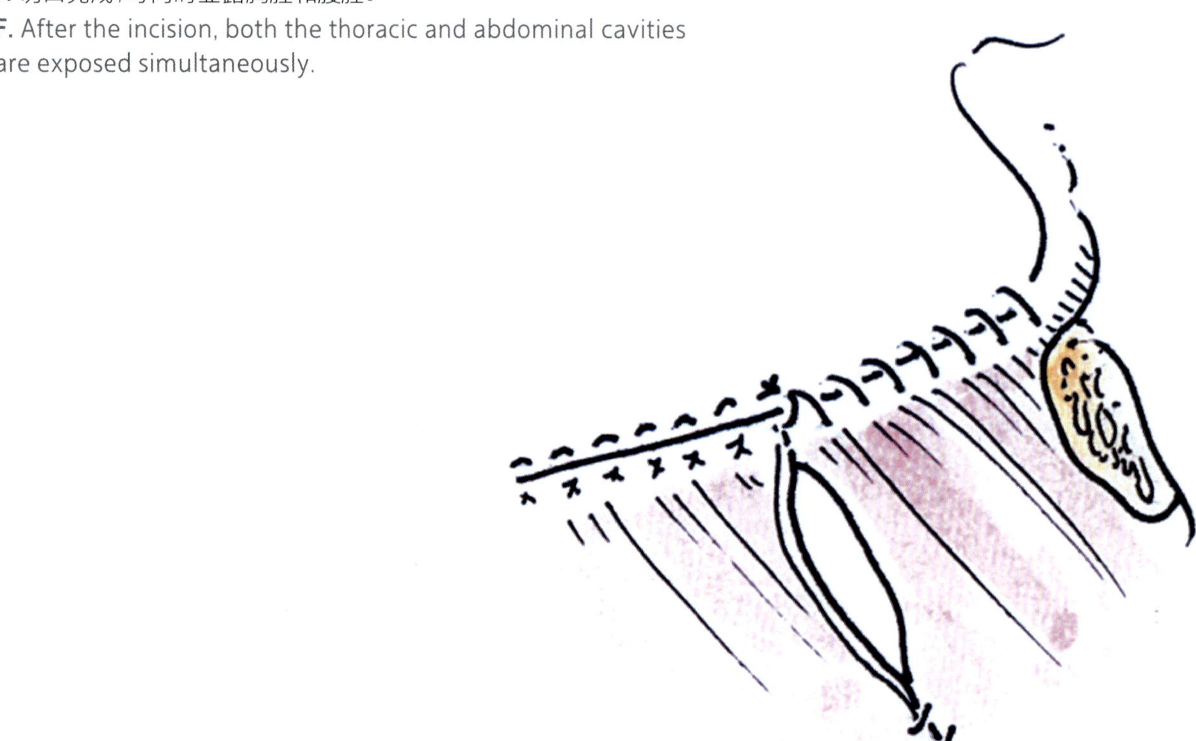

G. 关闭切口前先将膈肌间断水平褥式缝合，再用一层单纯连续缝合加固。

G. Before the closure of the incision, the diaphragm is sutured by horizontal interrupted mattress sutures, and then restrengthened by simple running sutures.

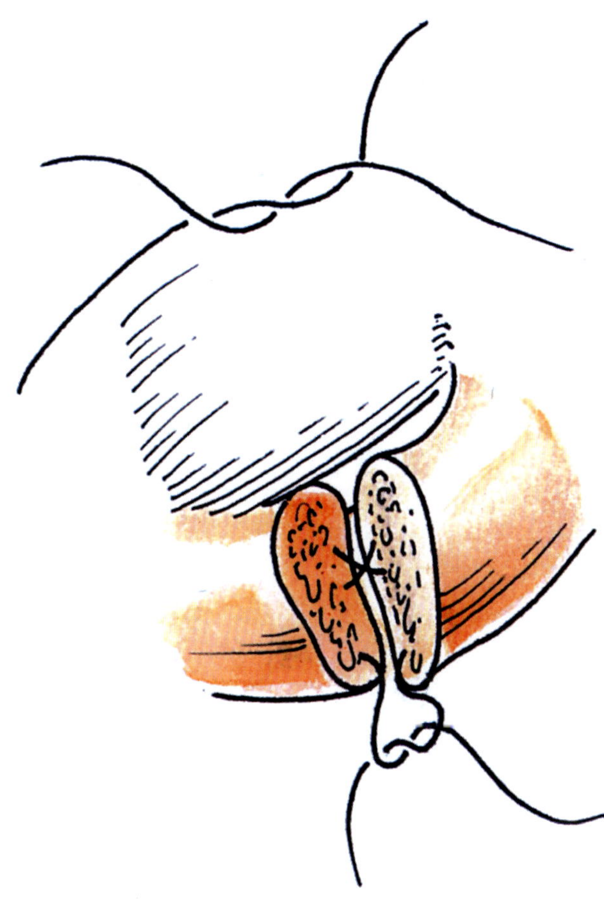

H

H. 肋弓切端剪去一小段，对端缝合。跨肋骨间断缝合肋间。

H. Remove a small segment of the incisal end of the costal arch, and perform the end-to-end anastomosis. The intercostal space closure is performed across the ribs by using interrupted sutures.

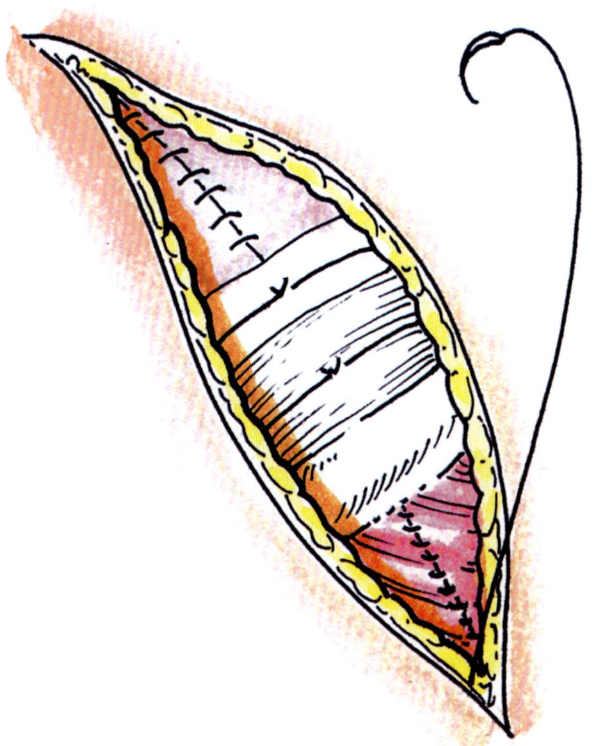

I

I. 缝合胸腹壁肌层，缝合皮下、皮肤。

I. Suture the muscle layer of the thoracic and abdominal wall, and close the subcutaneous tissue and skin.

图 1-1-9 胸骨缝合
Figure 1-1-9 Sternal closure

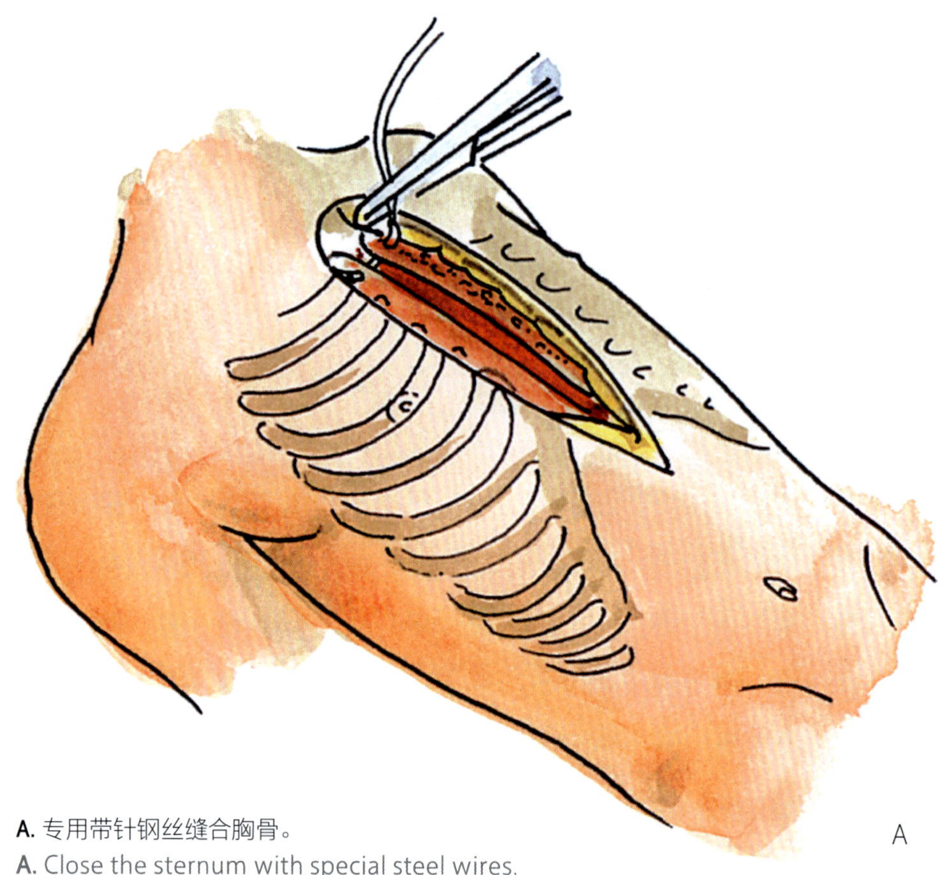

A. 专用带针钢丝缝合胸骨。
A. Close the sternum with special steel wires.

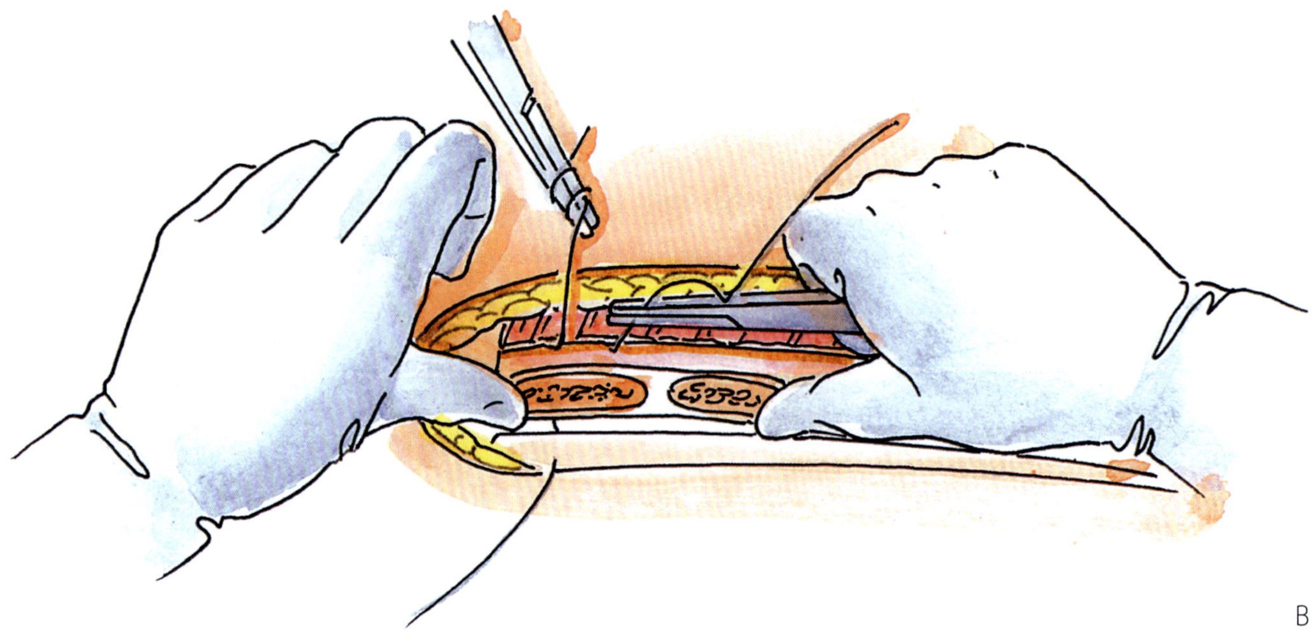

B. 缝针要垂直于胸骨进针。
B. Insert the needle perpendicularly to the sternum.

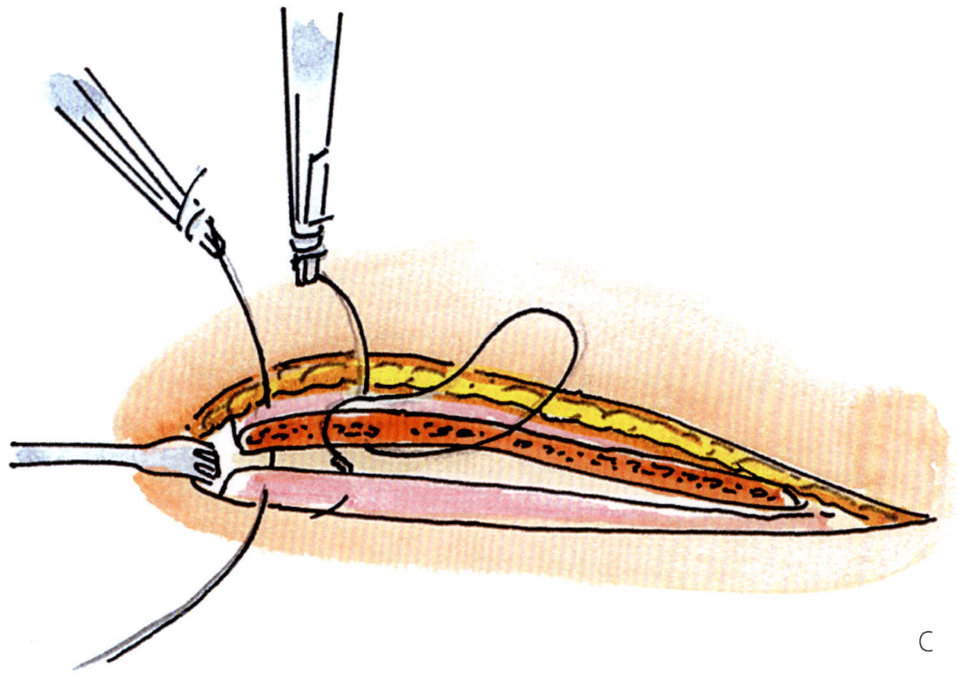

C. 胸骨柄缝 2 针。

C. 2 stitches are placed on the manubrium sterni.

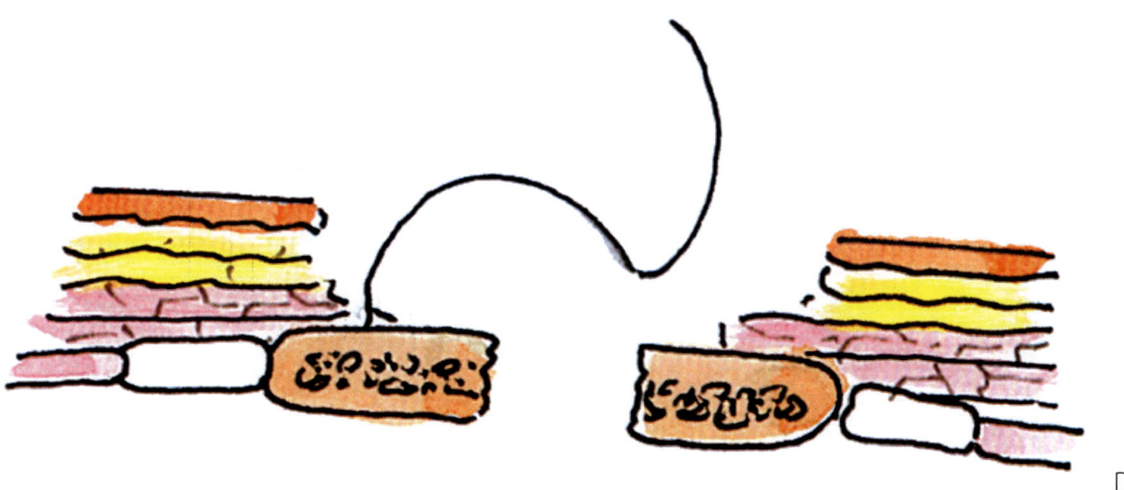

D. 缝合胸骨剖面图。

D. Section view of the sternal closure.

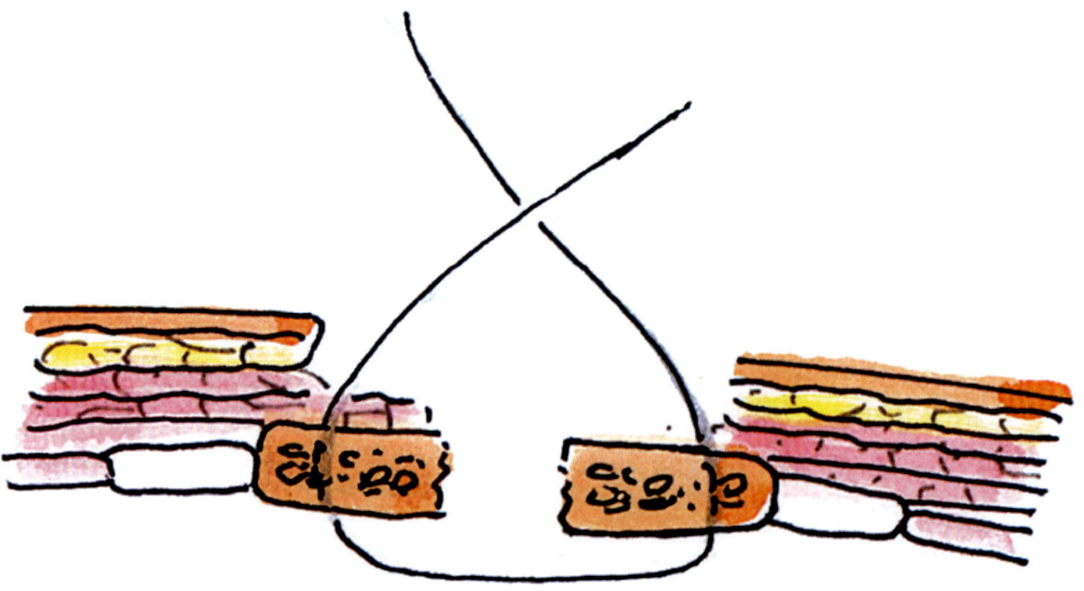

E. 胸骨钢丝缝入后剖面图。

E. Section view when the sternum is sewn with sternal wires.

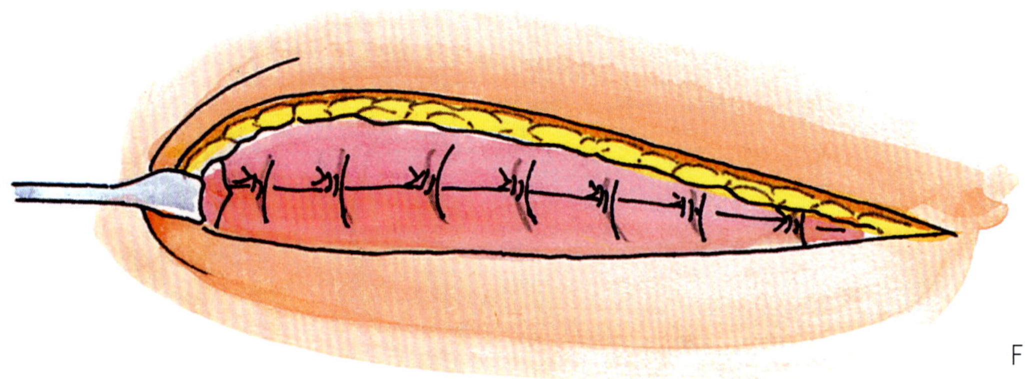

F. 胸骨钢丝缝合针数通常按每 10kg 体重缝 1 针确定。胸骨钢丝安置完毕后再次检查止血，尤其是胸骨后钢丝针眼的止血。拉紧钢丝使胸骨对合，拧紧钢丝。剪去多余钢丝，留约 1cm 长残端。钢丝断端朝向胸骨，避免其刺激皮肤。

F. Usually, the number of steel wire stitches is based on the patient's weight: 1 stitch for 10 kg. After the placement of sternal wires, a double check is performed for possible bleeding, especially in the retrosternal wire needle eyes. The wires are tightened to re-align the sternum. Shear the excess wires, and preserve about 1 cm of the residual ends. Leave the broken ends towards the sternum to avoid irritating the skin.

图 1-1-10 胸壁缝合
Figure 1-1-10 Closure of thorax

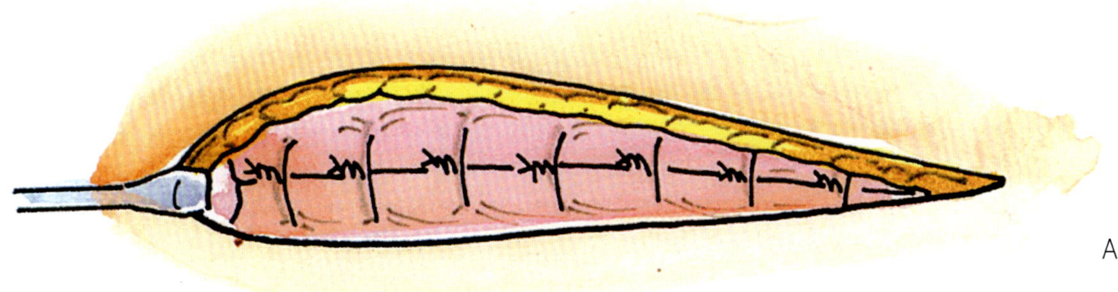

A. 胸骨缝合完毕。
A. Sternum closure is completed.

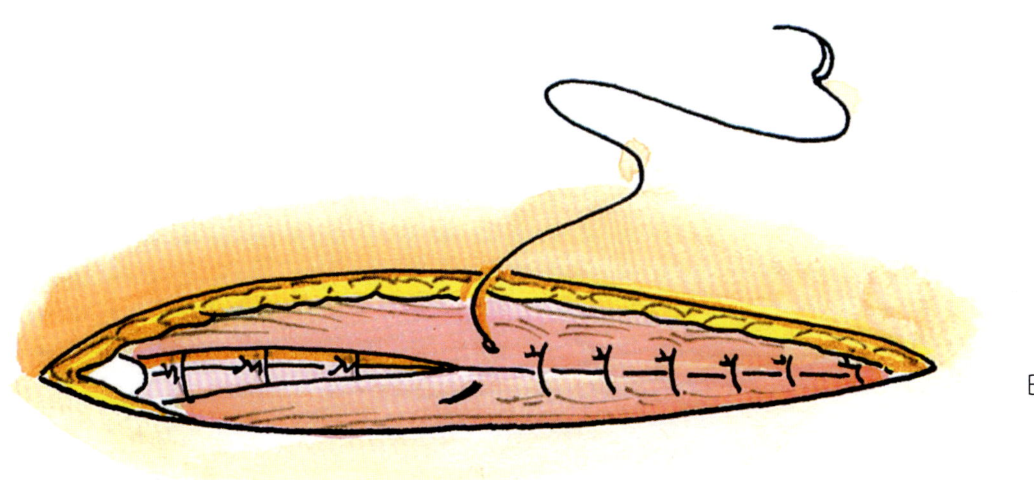

B. 间断缝合肌层。
B. Muscularis is closed with interrupted sutures.

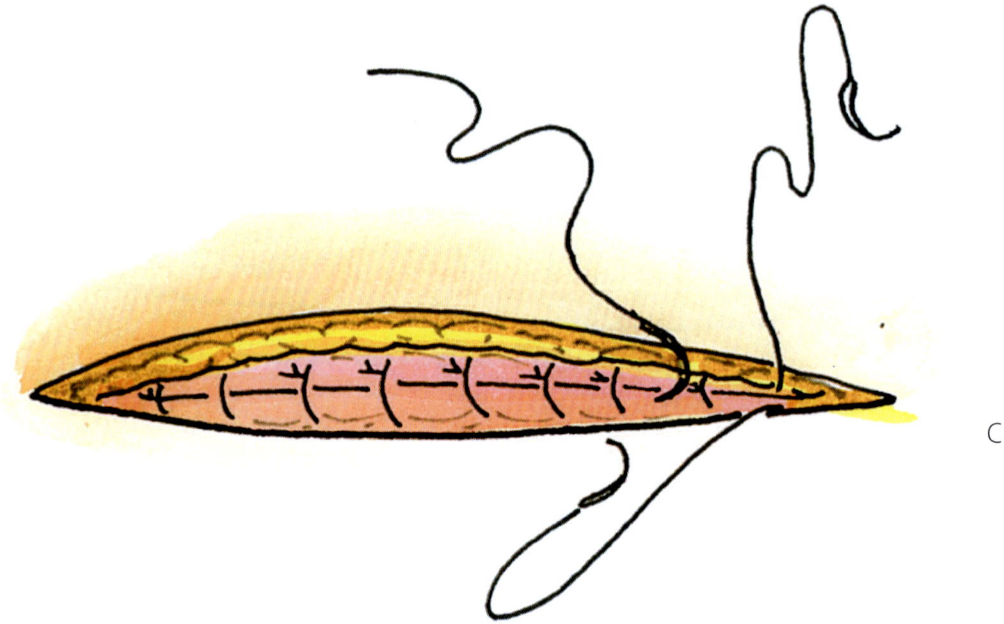

C. 间断缝合皮下组织。

C. Subcutaneous tissues are closed with interrupted sutures.

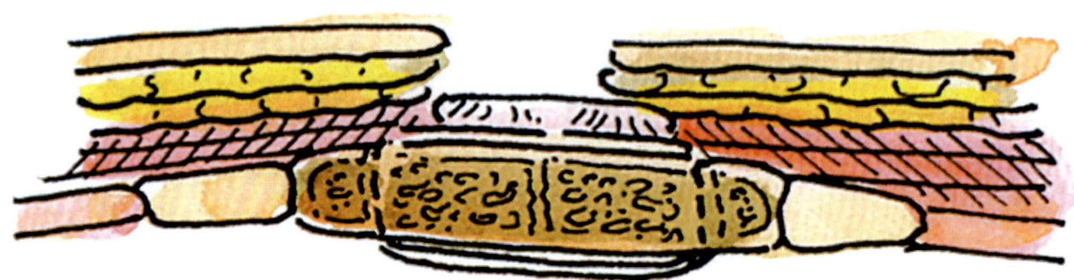

D. 缝合肌层要带到胸骨骨膜，勿使胸骨前留下残腔，避免积液继发感染。

D. The muscularis is to be sutured to the sternal periosteum. Don't leave any residual space in front of the sternum to avoid secondary infection due to fluid accumulation.

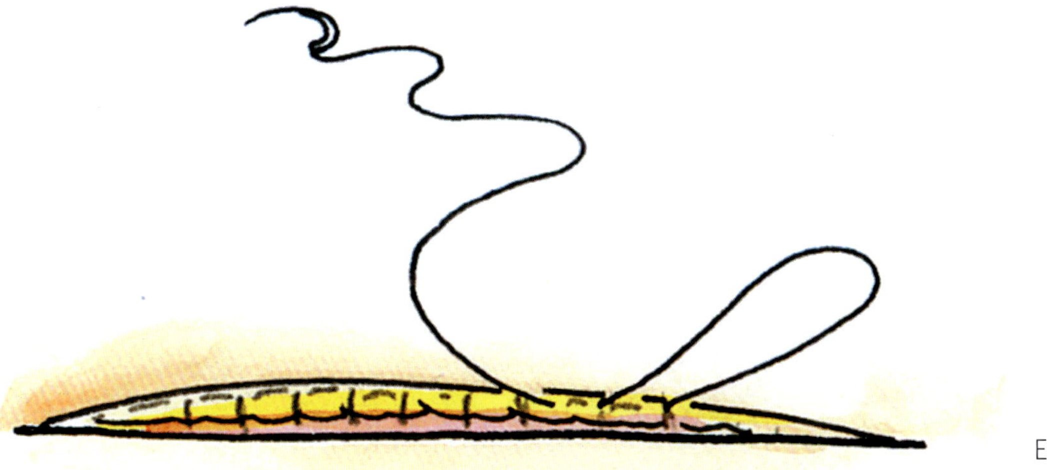

E. 皮内缝合皮肤。

E. Intracutaneous suture is made.

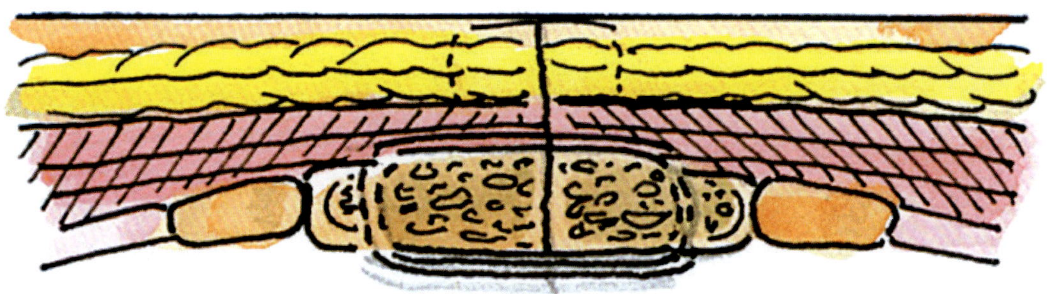

F. 缝合毕剖面图。

F. Section view after the sutures.

图 1-1-11 改良 Robicsek 胸骨缝合法
Figure 1-1-11 Modified Robicsek technique for sternal closure

对于胸骨骨质特别疏松的病例，直接缝合胸骨有钢丝切割胸骨之虞。可采用改良 Robicsek 胸骨缝合法缝合胸骨。

In cases of excessively fragile sternal bones, standard sternal closure is usually associated with the potential risk of bone disruption caused by steel wires, so a modified Robicsek technique can be used instead.

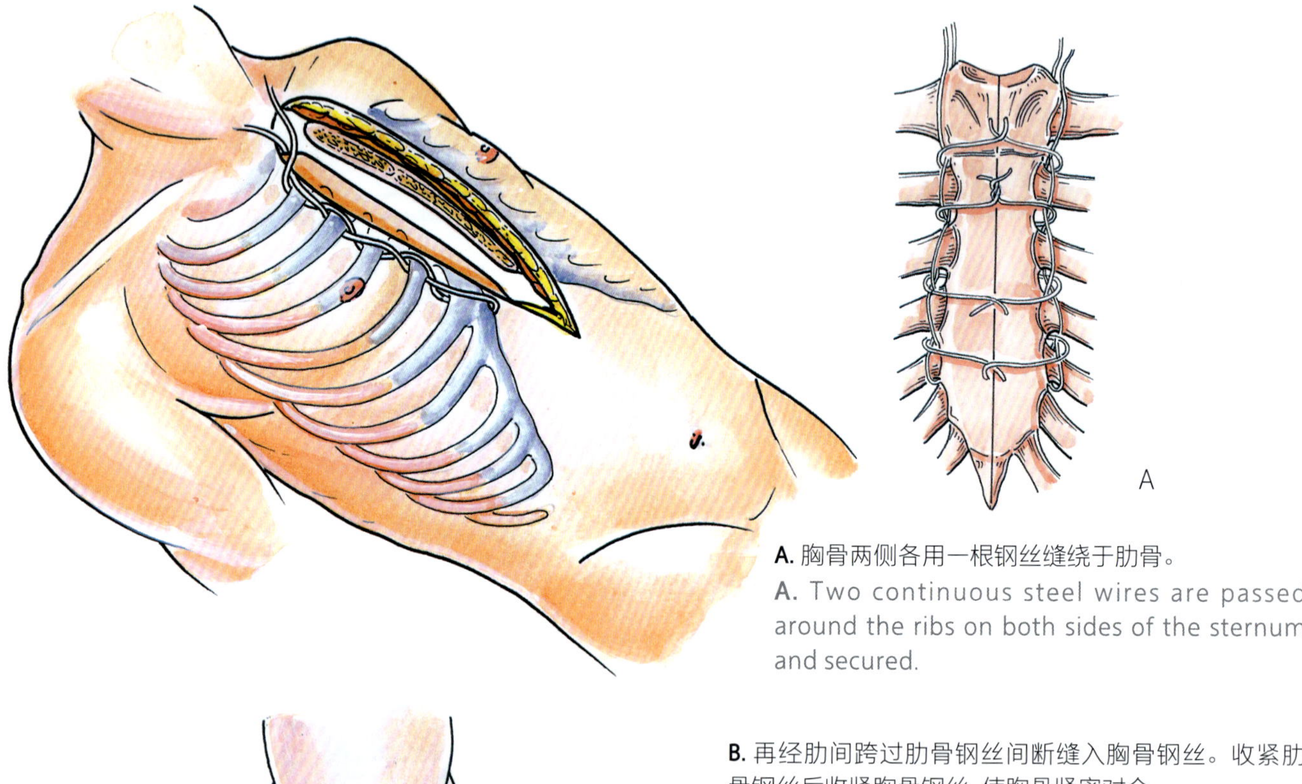

A. 胸骨两侧各用一根钢丝缝绕于肋骨。

A. Two continuous steel wires are passed around the ribs on both sides of the sternum and secured.

B. 再经肋间跨过肋骨钢丝间断缝入胸骨钢丝。收紧肋骨钢丝后收紧胸骨钢丝，使胸骨紧密对合。

B. Other wires are placed around the sternum by intermittently passing through the intercostal space over the rib wires. The rib wires are tightened and then the sternal wires to make sure the sternum is approximated.

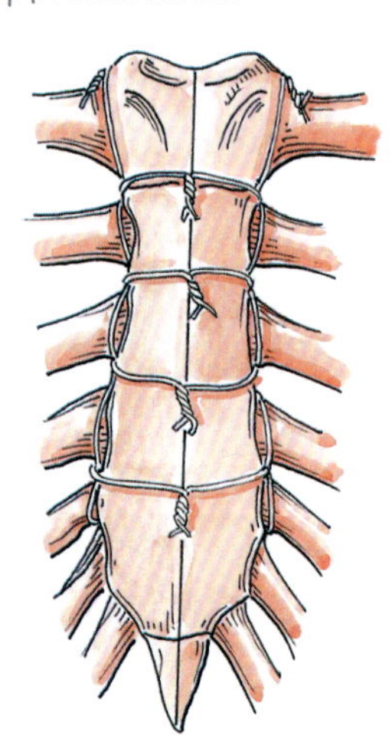

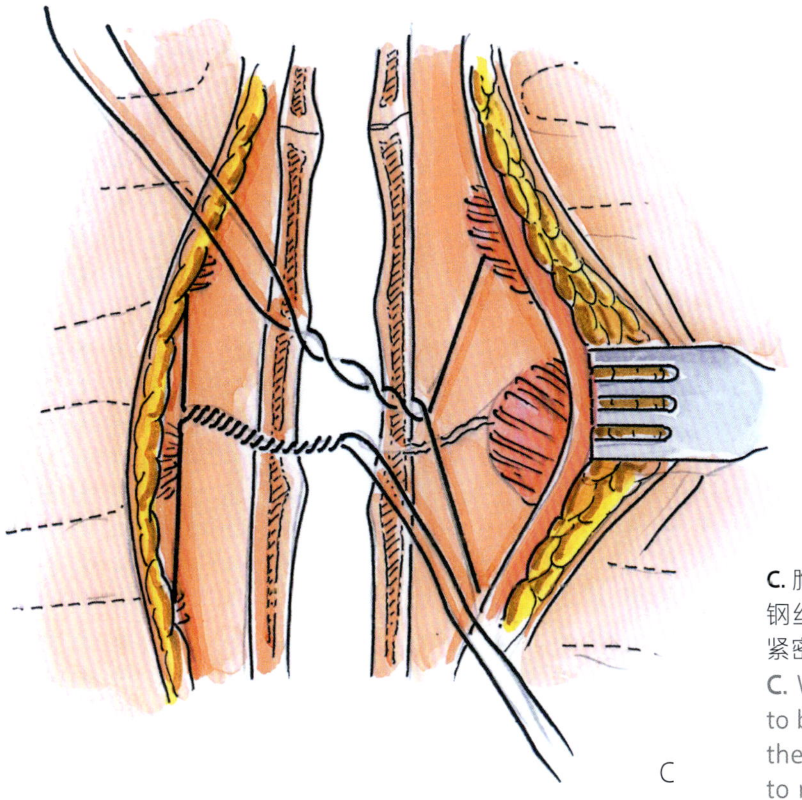

C. 胸骨有断裂处，跨断裂胸骨处上下一根肋骨缝入钢丝，胸骨两侧钢丝缝入后拧紧，使断裂胸骨对合紧密。

C. With ruptures in the sternum, a steel wire is to be passed across the upper and lower ribs of the fractured sternum, and the wire is secured to make the ruptured sternum approximated when the wires at both sides of the sternum are placed.

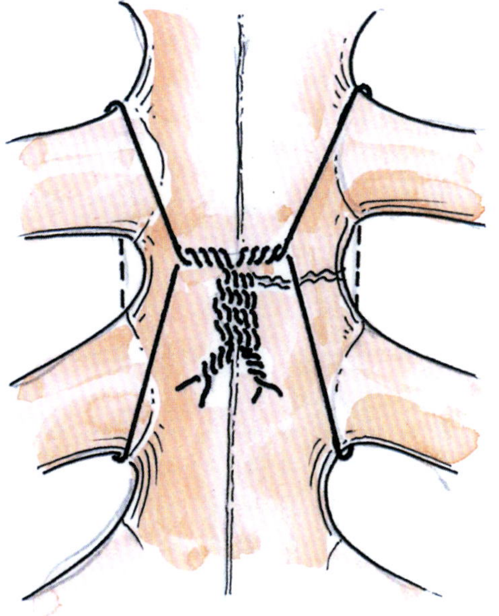

D. 拉紧胸骨两侧钢丝，使胸骨切口对合紧密，拧紧钢丝。

D. The wires on both sides are tightened after making sure the sternum incision is realigned.

第 二 节　体外循环插管

Section 2　Cannulation of Extracorporeal Circulation

图 1-2-1　主动脉插供血管

Figure 1-2-1　Aortic arterial cannulation

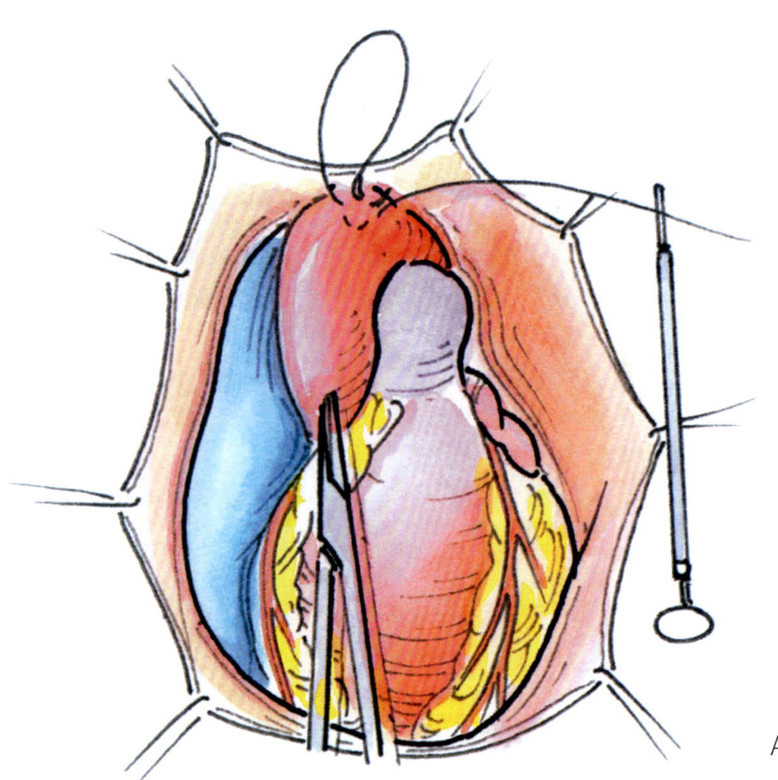

A

A. 钳夹升主动脉外膜向下稍作牵拉，在升主动脉远端动脉插管处做荷包缝合。

A. The adventitia of the ascending aorta is clamped and retracted down slightly, and purse-string sutures are performed at the distal end of the ascending aorta where arterial cannulation is carried out.

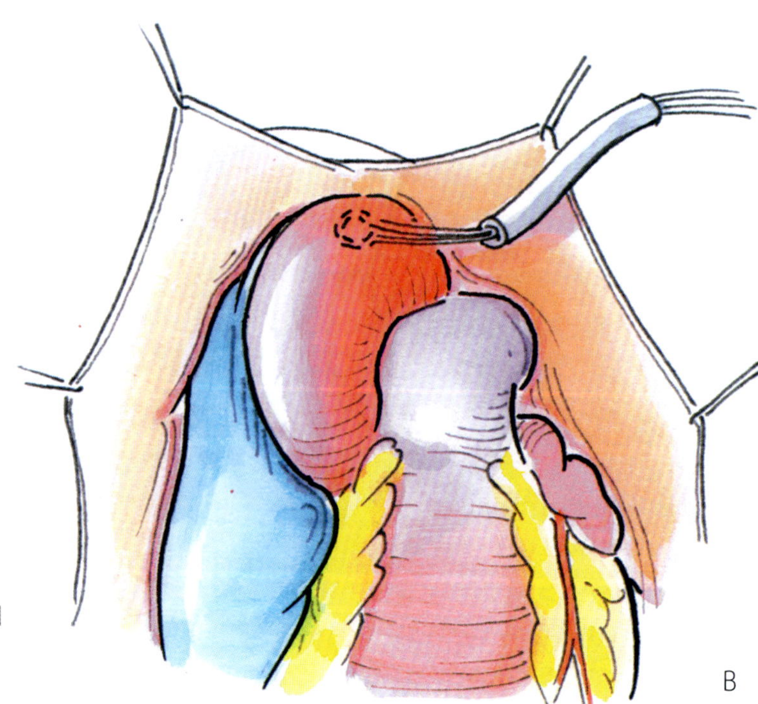

B

B. 双重荷包缝线套入 Rumel 止血器。

B. Double purse-string sutures are passed through the Rumel tourniquets.

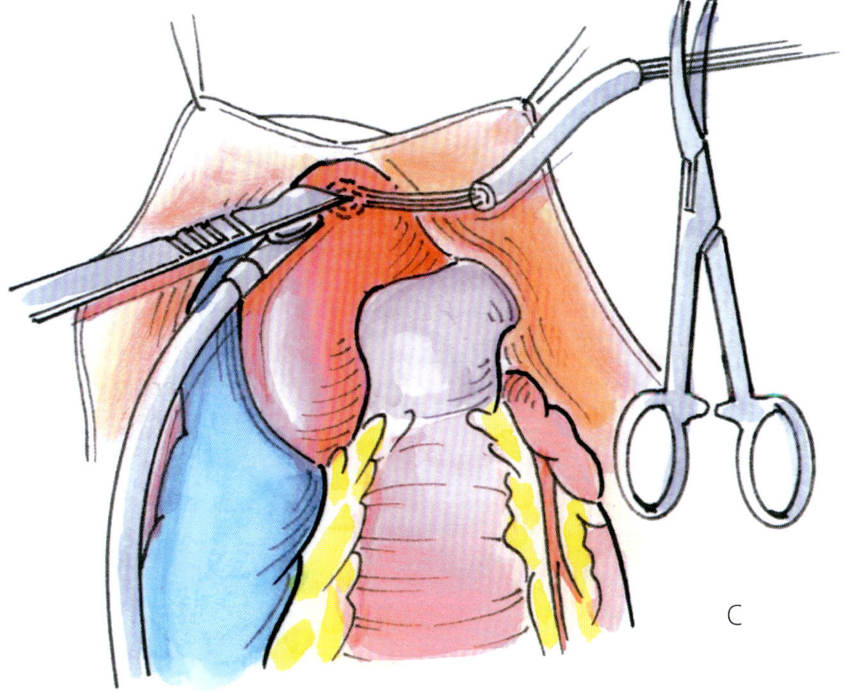

C. 尖头刀刀尖在荷包缝线中间戳口，刀尖勿刺入过深以免损伤主动脉后壁。拔出刀尖时顺势插入主动脉供血管。

C. The scalpel tip pierces in the middle of the purse suture, and it shall not penetrate too deep to avoid damaging the posterior wall of the aorta. The aortic arterial cannulation is inserted when the scalpel is removed.

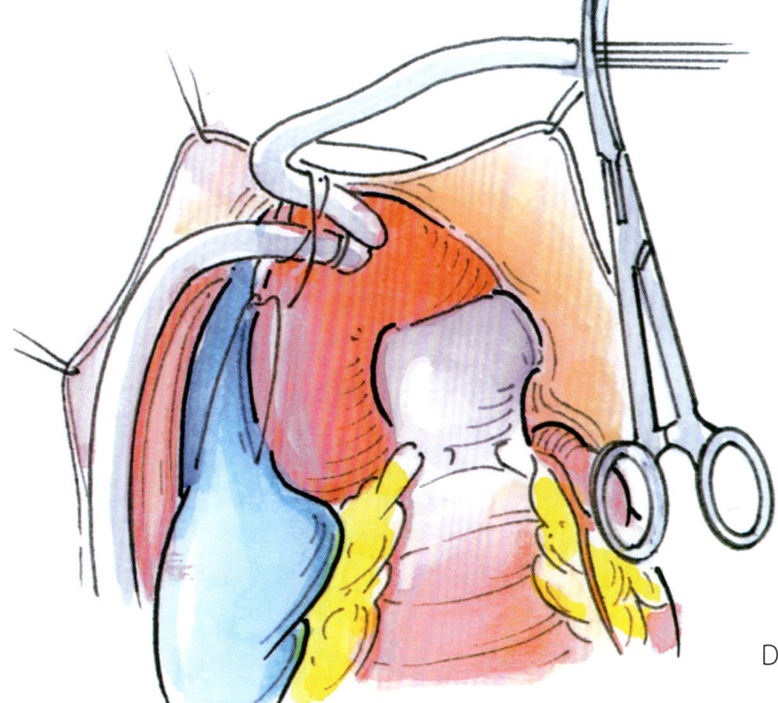

D. 收紧荷包，将动脉插管和 Rumel 止血器并拢结扎，防止主动脉供血管滑脱。

D. The purse-string sutures are tightened and the arterial cannulation and Rumel tourniquets are drawn together and ligated to prevent slippage of the aortic arterial cannulation.

图 1-2-2　腔静脉插管
Figure 1-2-2　Cannulation of venae cava

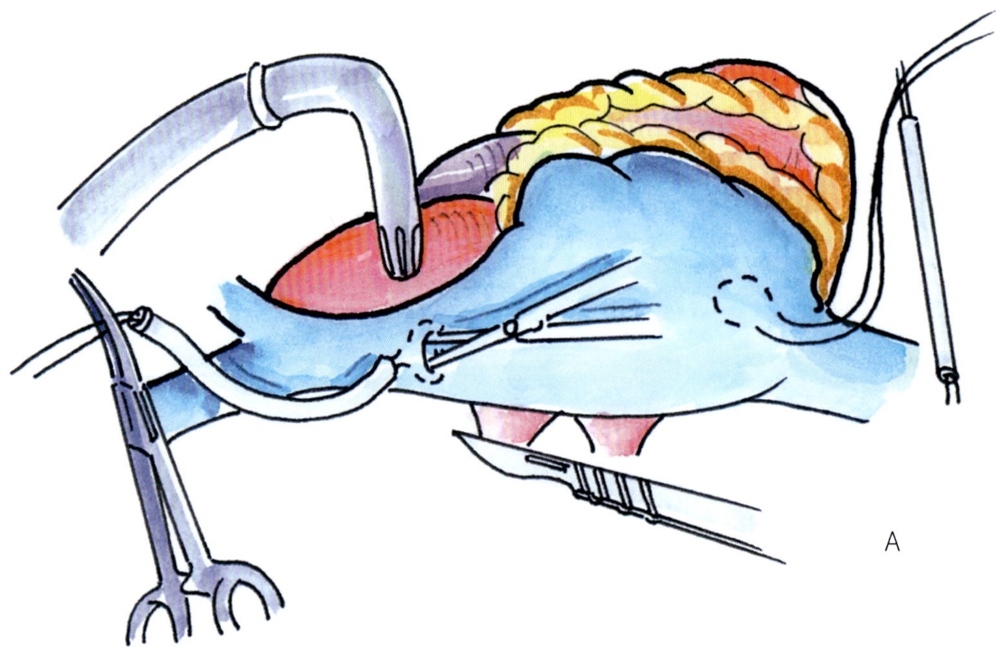

A. 上腔静脉靠近右心房处和右心房靠近下腔静脉处分别做荷包，套入 Rumel 止血器。荷包中间戳口并用剪刀撑大，分别插入上腔静脉引流管和下腔静脉引流管。

A. Purse-string sutures are performed at the superior vena cava proximal to the right atrium and the right atrium proximal to the inferior vena cava through Rumel tourniquets. An opening is made in the middle of the purse and then enlarged with scissors, where cannulas of the superior and inferior vena cava are inserted, respectively.

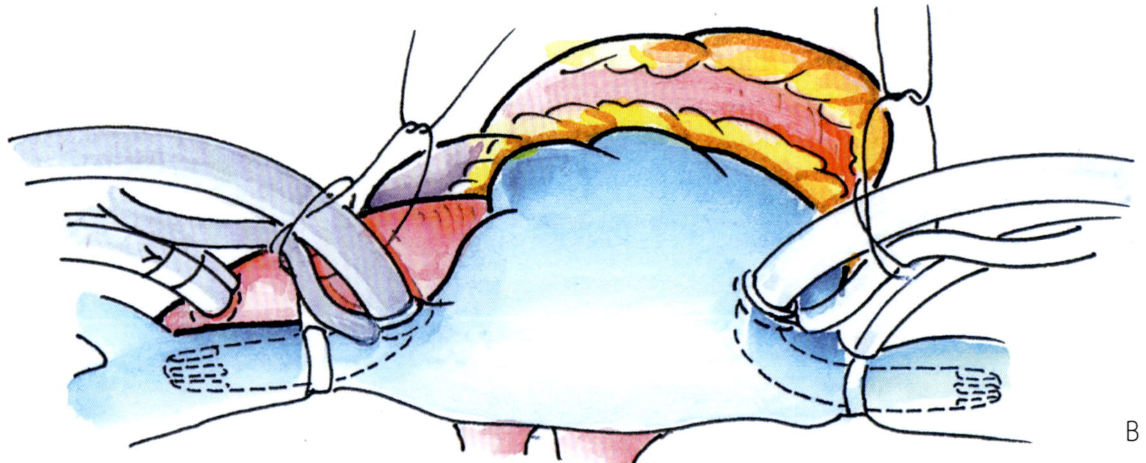

B. 收紧荷包，并分别将上腔静脉引流管和下腔静脉引流管与相应的 Rumel 止血器结扎固定。上、下腔静脉分别游离套纱带，体外循环时束紧阻断回流入心血流。

B. After the purses are tightened, the superior and inferior vena cava cannulas are attached to their corresponding Rumel tourniquets. The superior and inferior vena cava are dissociated and tied with the caval tapes respectively, but only tied tightly to block the reflux of blood from the vena cava to the heart during extracorporeal circulation.

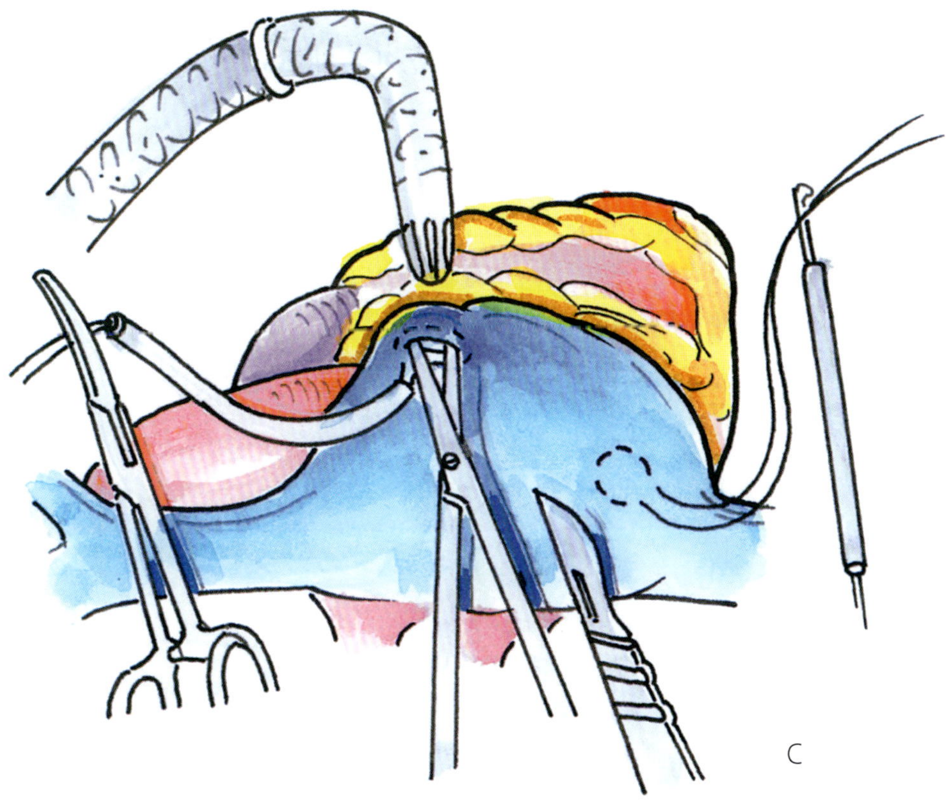

C. 上腔静脉引流管也可从右心耳经右心房插入上腔静脉。

C. The superior vena cava cannula can alternatively be inserted from the right atrial appendage through the right atrium.

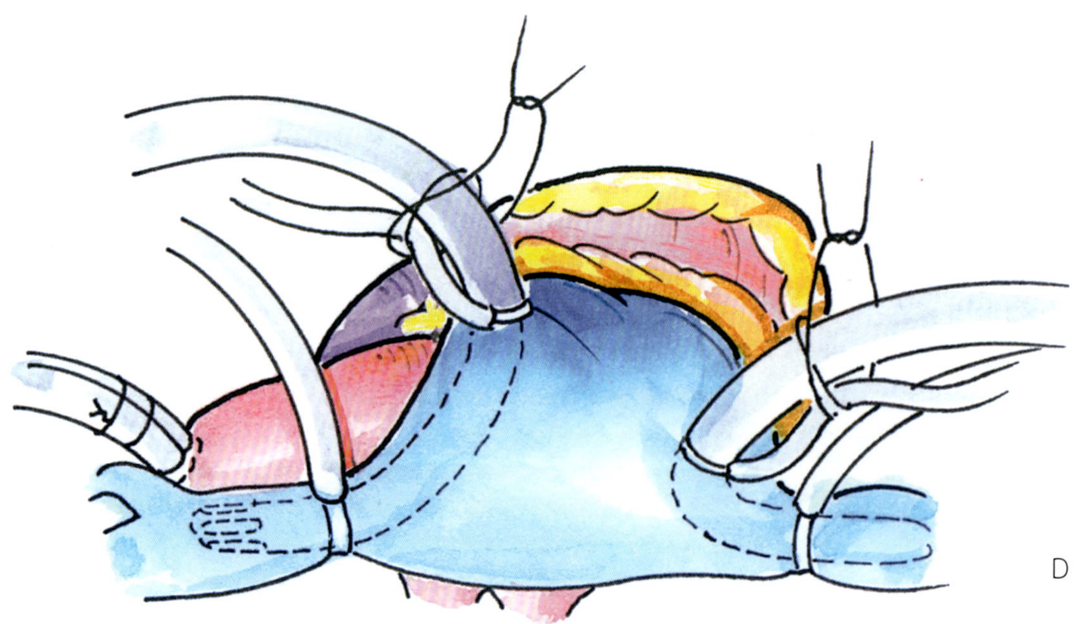

D. 下腔静脉引流管仍由右心房下部插入。

D. The inferior vena cava cannula is still inserted from the lower right atrium.

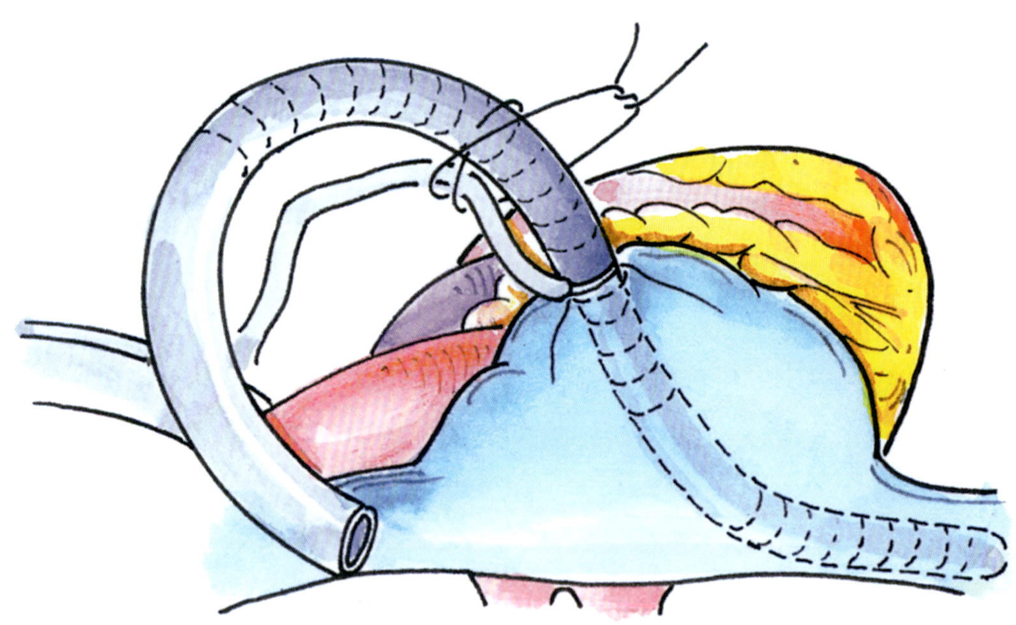

E. 如果术中无须阻断上、下腔静脉，可选择单根插管引流。用二级静脉引流管由右心耳插入，经右心房将尖端送入下腔静脉，其球笼部分留在右心房。

E. If there is no need to block the superior and inferior vena cava intraoperatively, single venous cannulation is another option. A two-stage venous cannula is inserted from the right atrial appendage, and its tip is guided into the inferior vena cava via the right atrium, leaving the cage in the right atrium.

图 1-2-3 股动静脉插管

Figure 1-2-3 Cannulation of femoral artery and vein

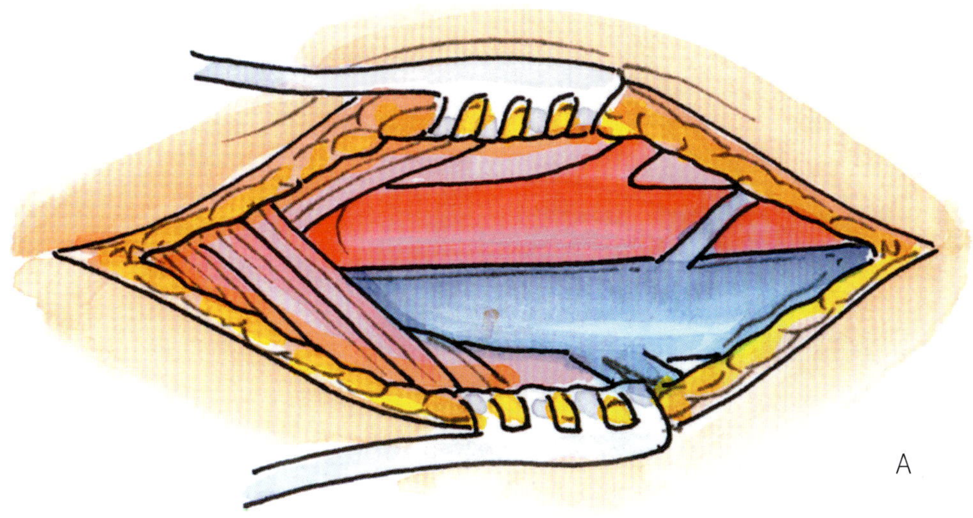

A. 腹股沟沿股动静脉表面切开约 6cm。切口上 1/3 在腹股沟韧带上，下 2/3 在腹股沟韧带下方。显露股动脉及其内侧的股静脉。

A. A 6 cm long incision is made along the surface of the femoral artery and vein to expose the femoral artery and medial femoral vein, with 1/3 incision above the inguinal ligament and 2/3 below the inguinal ligament.

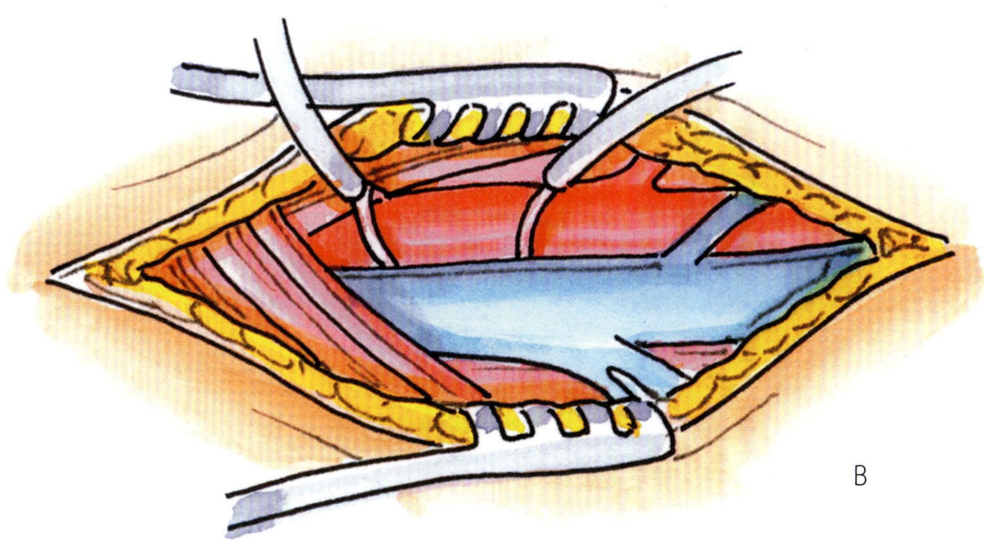

B. 游离股动脉，于股深动脉分支近端套两根细纱带，套入 Rumel 止血器。

B. The femoral artery is freed, and two thin tapes are tied to the proximal end of the profunda femoral artery origin through the Rumel tourniquets.

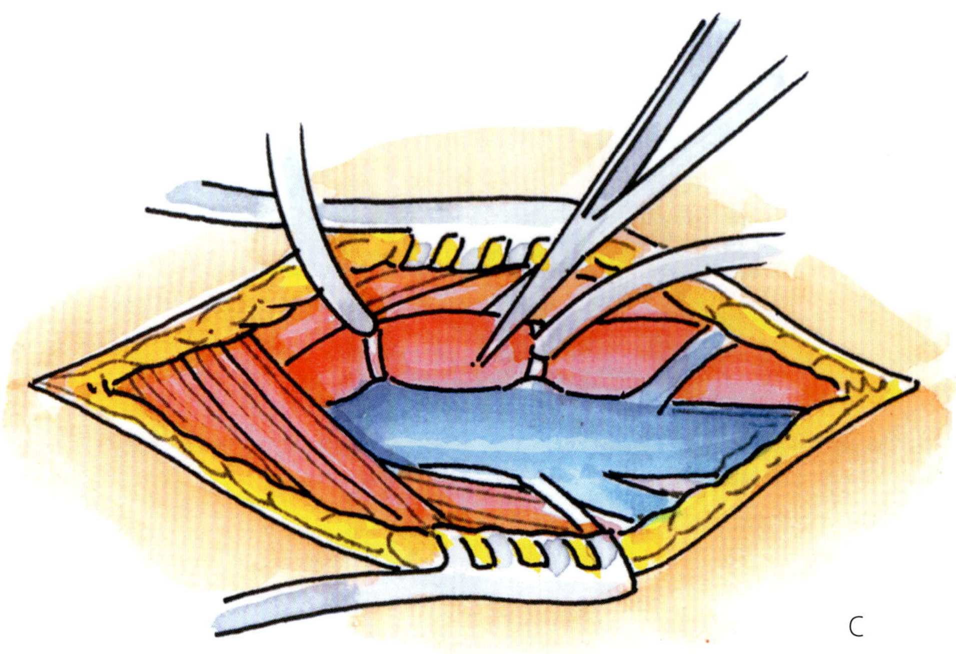

C. 束紧纱带，剪开股动脉前壁。
C. The tapes are tightened, and the anterior wall of the femoral artery is incised.

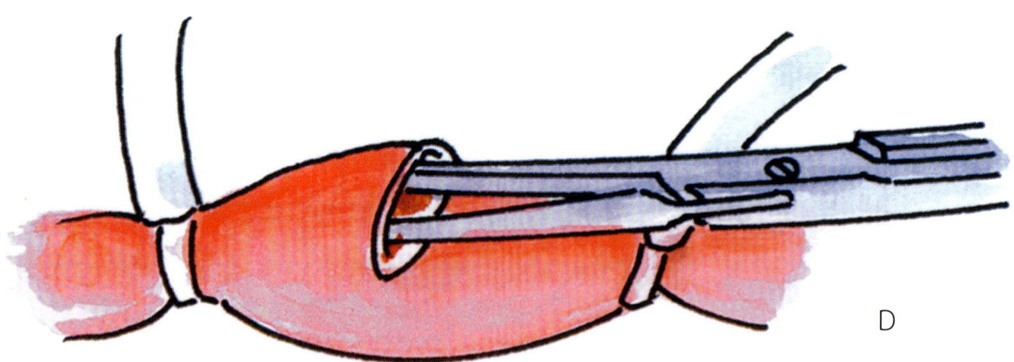

D. 轻柔地将股动脉近端内径略作撑大。
D. The proximal diameter of the femoral artery is slightly enlarged.

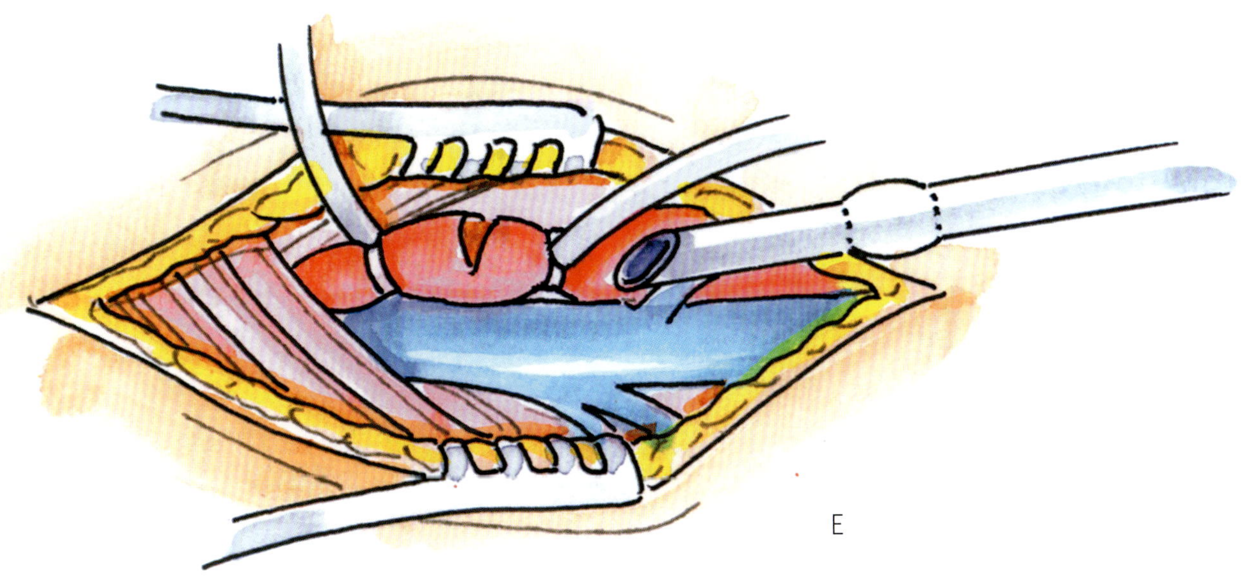

E. 放开近端阻断纱带，插入股动脉供血管。

E. Release the proximal tape, and insert the arterial cannulation in the femoral artery.

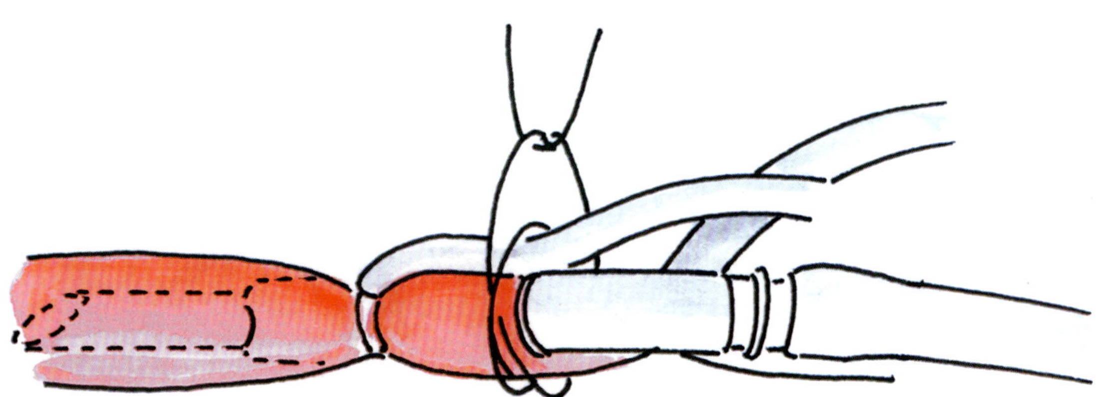

F. 收紧近端纱带，并套线结扎将股动脉供血管与 Rumel 止血器固定。

F. Tighten the proximal blocking tape, and secure the femoral arterial cannulation with the Rumel tourniquets by using a knotted ligation.

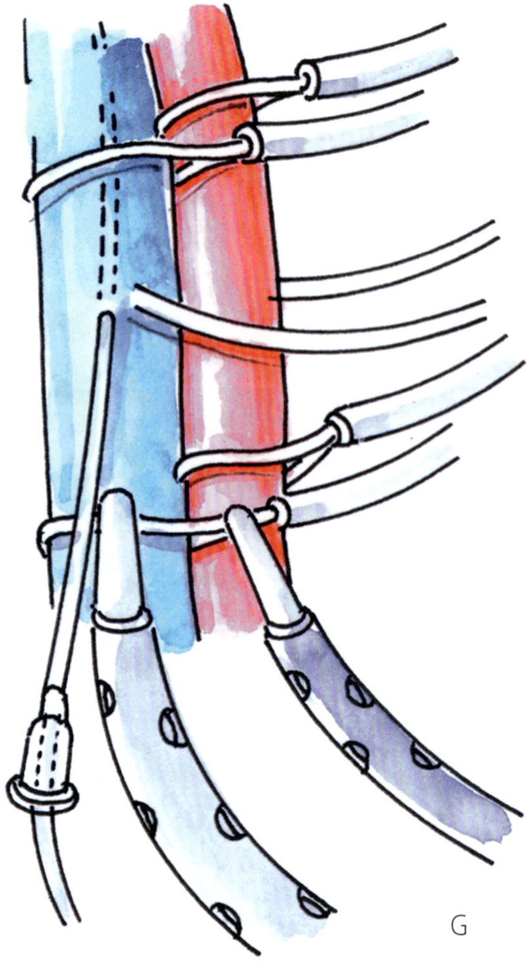

G. 亦可在股动脉前壁做荷包插入供血管。股静脉套纱带，前壁做荷包，穿刺插入引导钢丝，循引导钢丝插入股静脉引流管。

G. The cannula may alternatively be inserted into the anterior wall of the femoral artery after the purse-string suture is made. The femoral vein is tied with tapes, and the anterior wall is subjected to purse-string sutures. The femoral vein cannula is inserted into the wall through a steel guidewire.

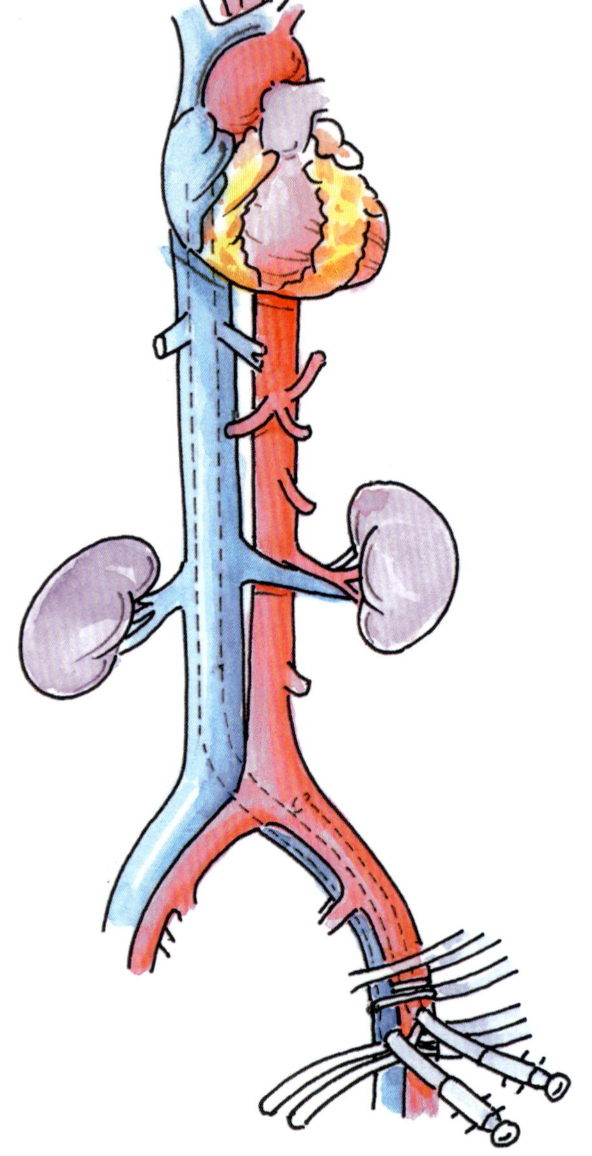

H. 股动静脉插管毕。股静脉引流管尖端要插至右心房。

H. After the arterial and venous cannulation, the tip of the femoral venous cannula is inserted into the right atrium.

图 1-2-4　腋动脉插供血管
Figure 1-2-4　Axillary artery cannulation

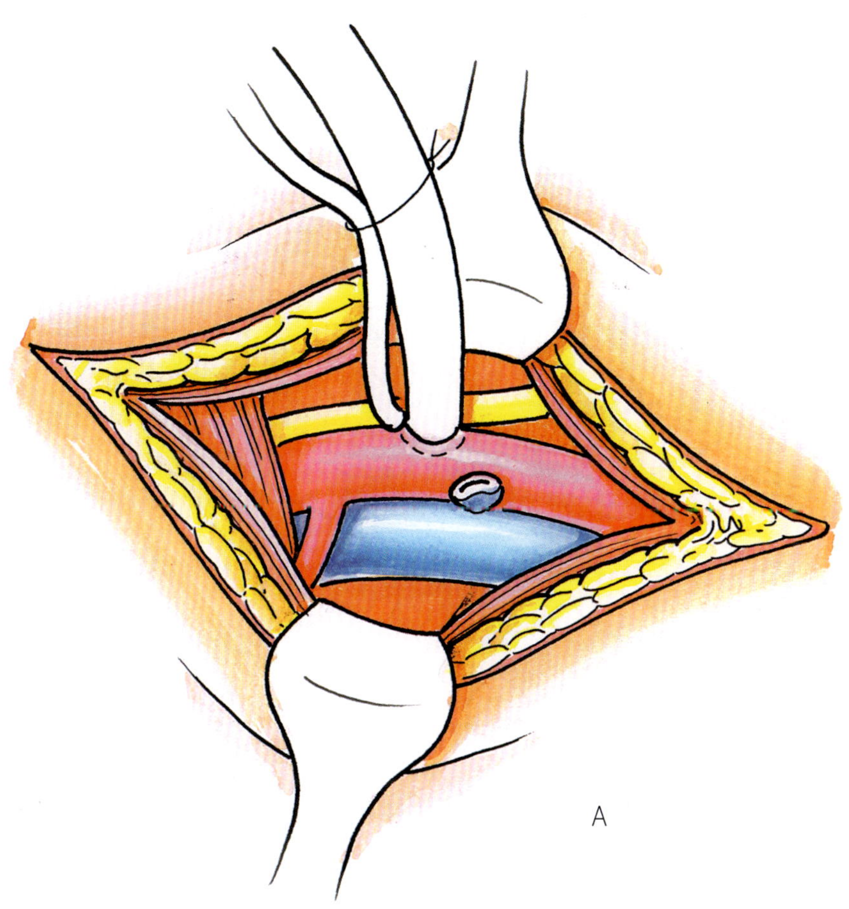

A. 右锁骨下横切口，起自锁骨中点下方 1~2cm 处，向外止于胸大肌和三角肌交界处。切开皮肤、皮下组织、深筋膜，沿胸大肌肌纤维走向钝性分离胸大肌，分次钳夹、切断胸小肌，显露其深层的血管神经鞘。游离腋动脉，注意保护臂丛神经免受损伤。经荷包缝线插入腋动脉供血管并固定。

A. A transverse incision is made below the right clavicle, starting from 1-2 cm below the midpoint of the clavicle and extending outward to the junction of the pectoralis major and deltoid muscle. After the incision of the skin, subcutaneous tissue, and deep fascia, the pectoralis major muscle is bluntly divided along its fibers, and the pectoralis minor muscle is clamped and cut off several times for exposure of the deep-seated vascular sheath. The axillary artery is then dissociated with care to protect the brachial plexus from injury. The axillary arterial cannula is inserted and fixed by using purse-string sutures.

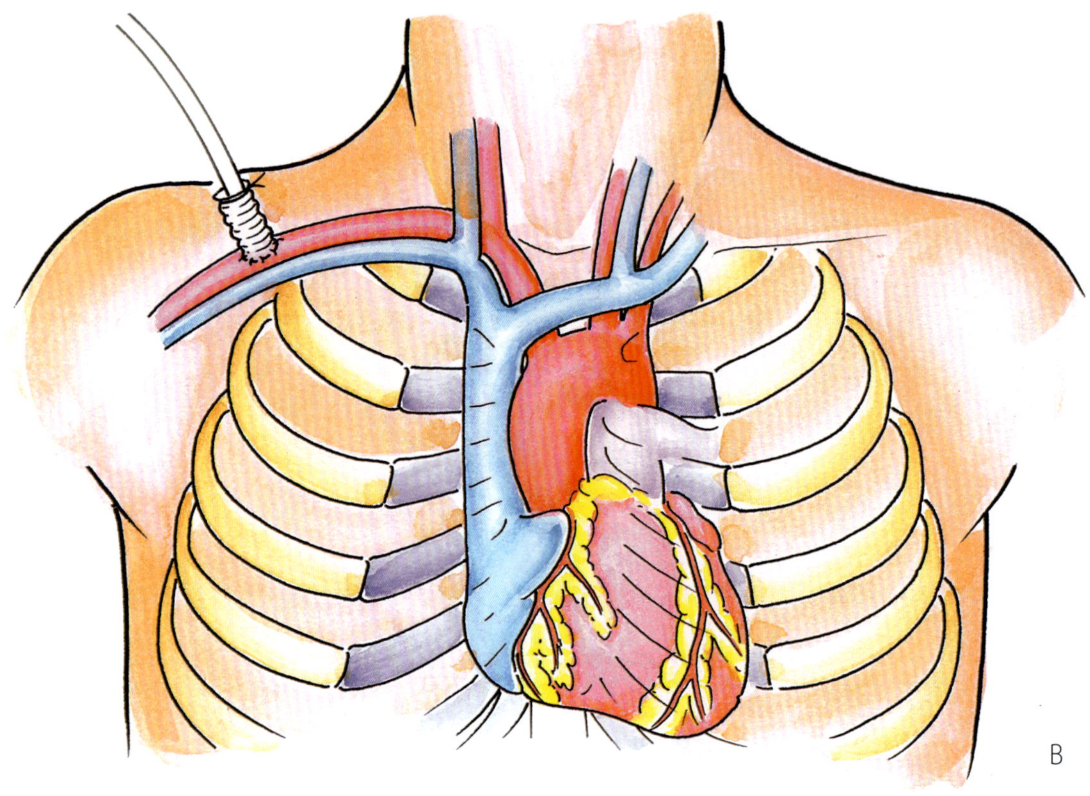

B. 亦可将一段人造血管与腋动脉端侧吻合，经人造血管插入腋动脉供血管。

B. Alternatively, a segment of the artificial blood vessel can be end-to-side anastomosed to the axillary artery, and the axillary arterial cannula is inserted through the artificial vessel.

图 1-2-5　心脏减压管

Figure 1-2-5　Heart venting

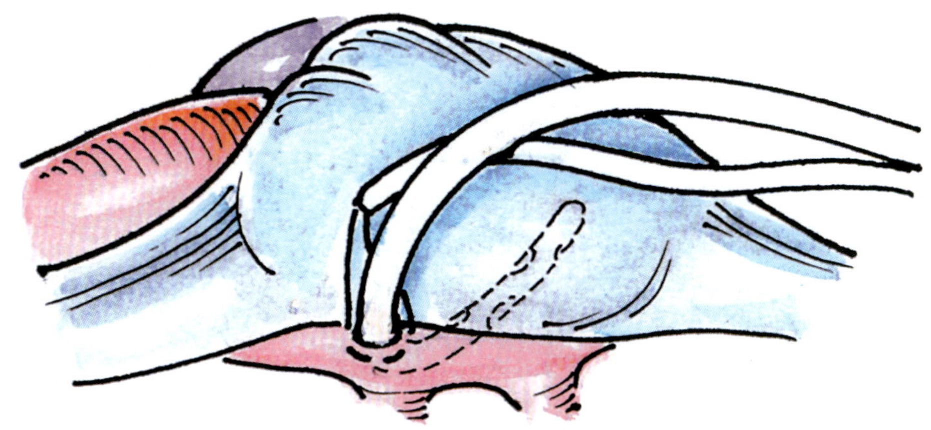

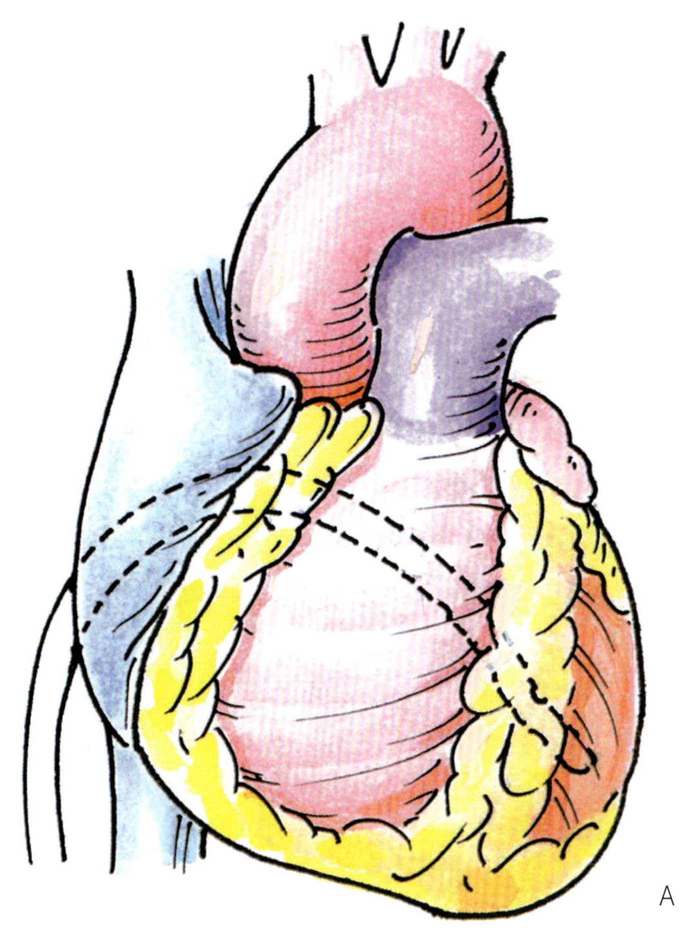

A. 方法一：游离房间沟，左心房靠近右上肺静脉处做荷包，将减压管插入左心房。若左心室减压不满意，可将减压管尖端经二尖瓣口插到左心室。

A. Method 1: The atrial sulcus is freed and purse-string suture is performed at the left atrium close to the right superior pulmonary vein, and the venting catheter is then inserted into the left atrium. If left atrial decompression is not satisfactory, the tip of the venting catheter should be extended to the left ventricle through the mitral orifice.

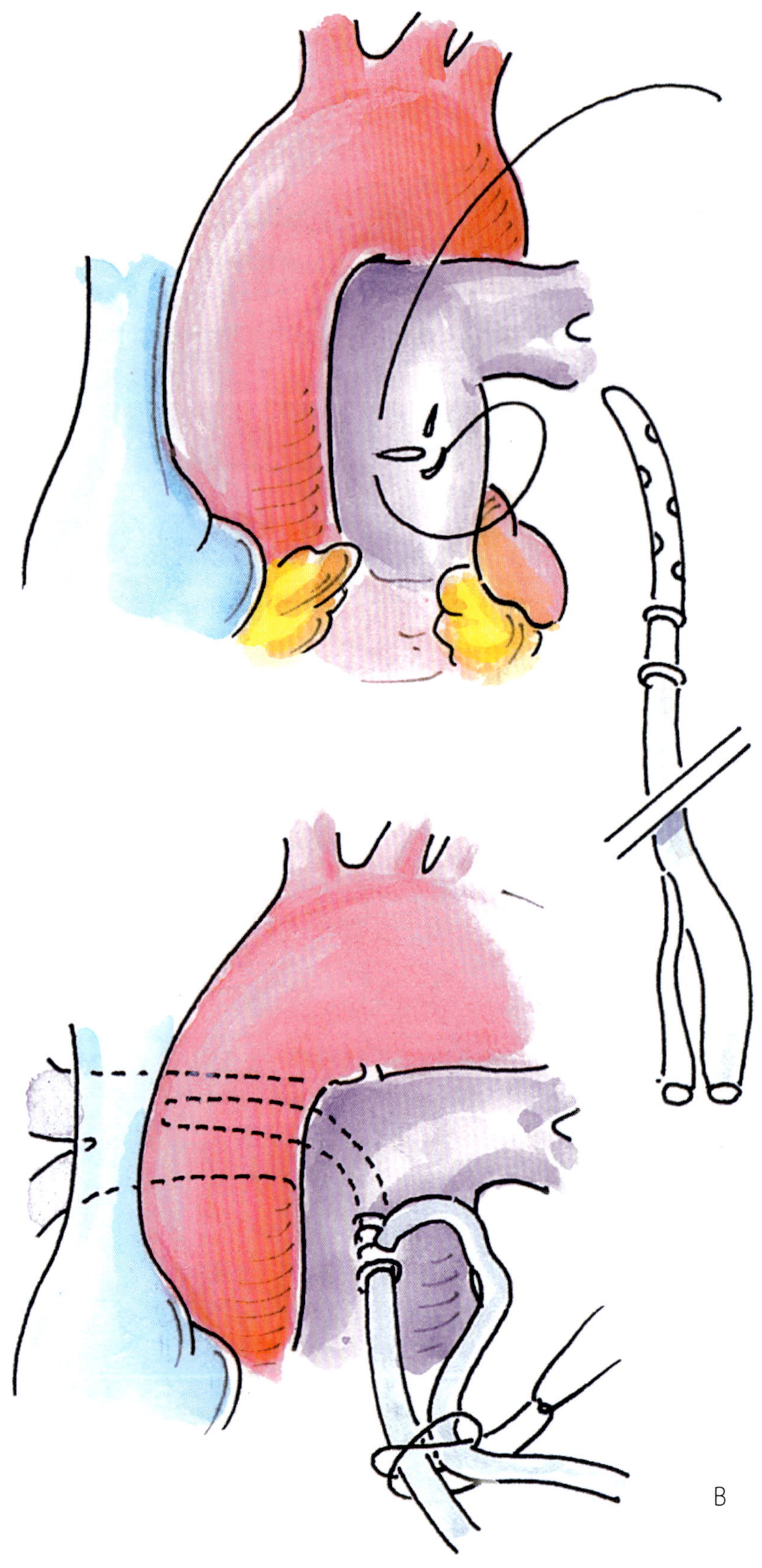

B. 方法二：肺动脉干前壁切开，将减压管插到右肺动脉。肺动脉切口褥式缝线收紧并固定。

B. Method 2: The anterior wall of the common pulmonary trunk is incised, and the venting catheter is inserted into the right pulmonary artery. The pulmonary artery incision is tightened and fixed by mattress sutures.

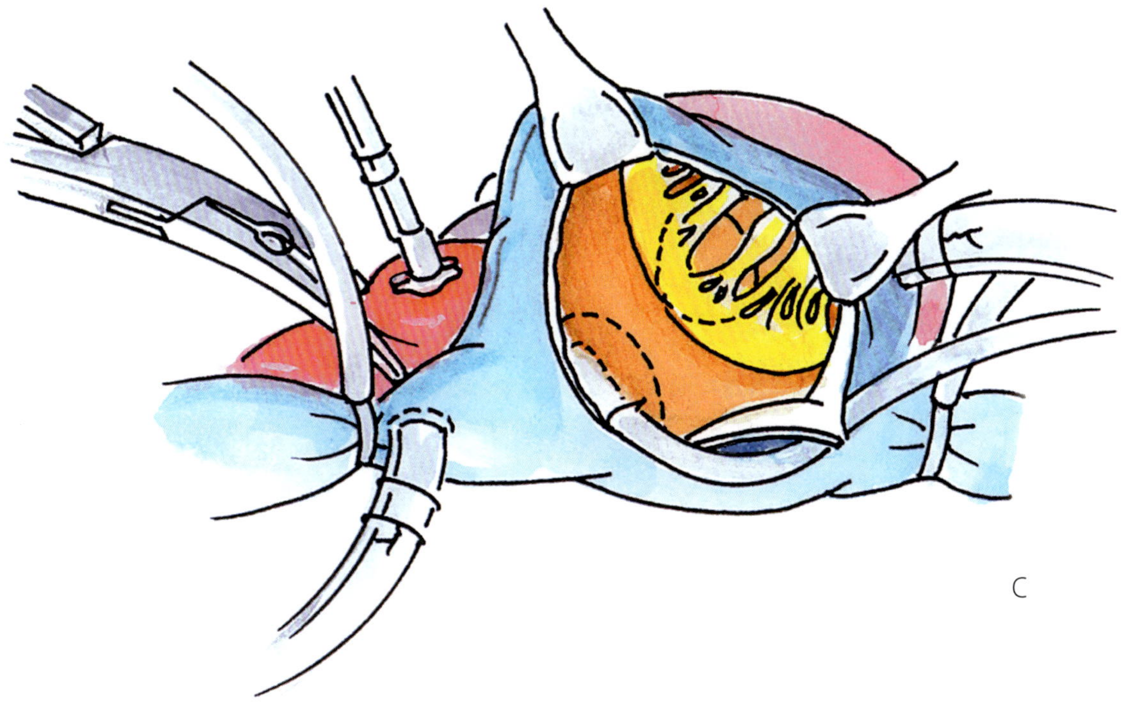

C. 方法三：右心房切开后，经卵圆窝将减压管插入左心房。

C. Method 3: After the incision of the right atrium, the venting catheter is inserted into the left atrium through the oval fossa.

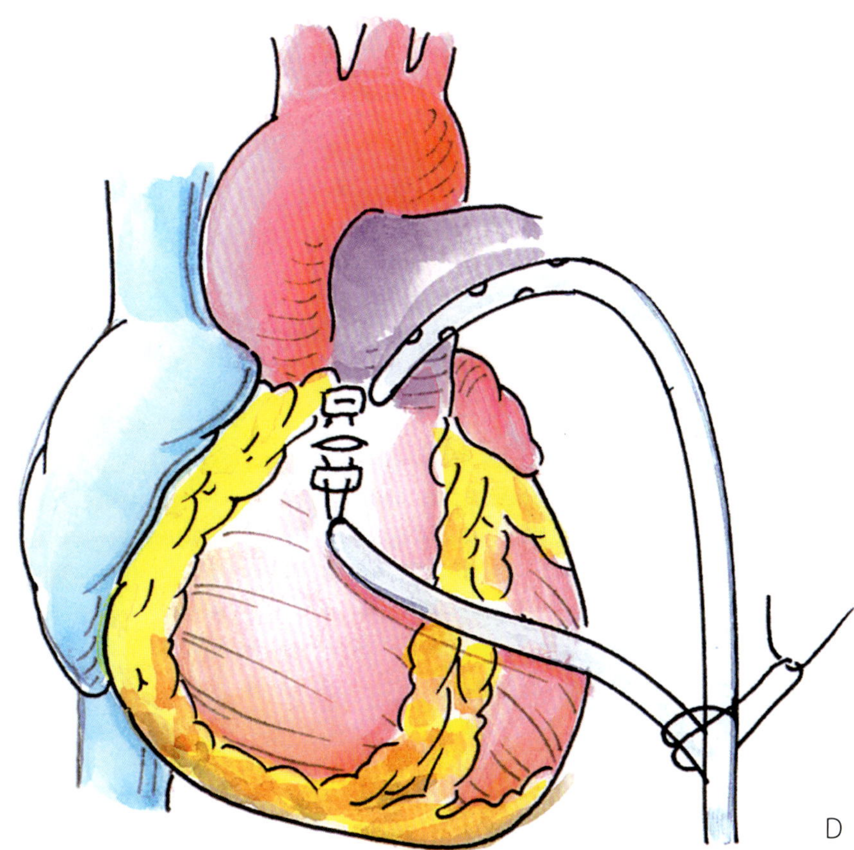

D. 方法四：右心室流出道带垫片褥式缝 1 针，戳口将减压管插入右心室。

D. Method 4: The right ventricular outflow tract is sewn with a pledget-supported mattress suture. The venting catheter is introduced into the right ventricle by a pierced opening.

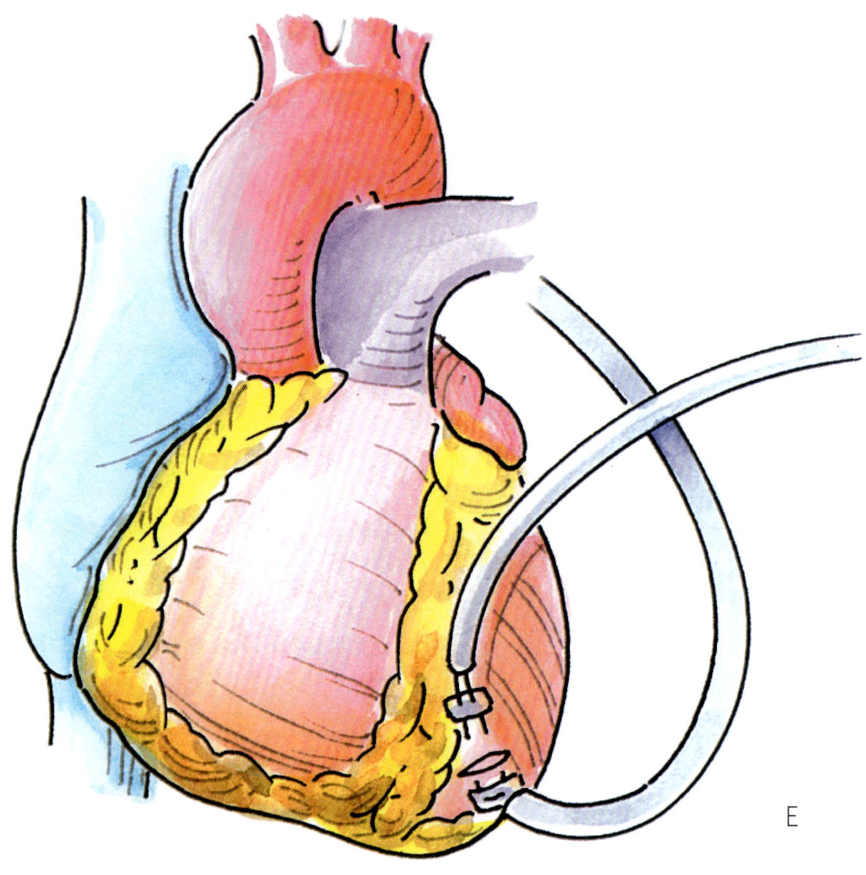

E. 方法五：心尖处带垫片褥式缝 1 针，戳口将减压管插入左心室。

E. Method 5: A pledget-supported mattress suture is passed through a suitable site near the left ventricular apex, and the venting catheter is introduced into the left ventricle through a pierced opening in the apex.

第 三 节 术中心肌保护

Section 3 Intraoperative Myocardial Protection

图 1-3-1 术中心肌保护

Figure 1-3-1 Intraoperative myocardial protection

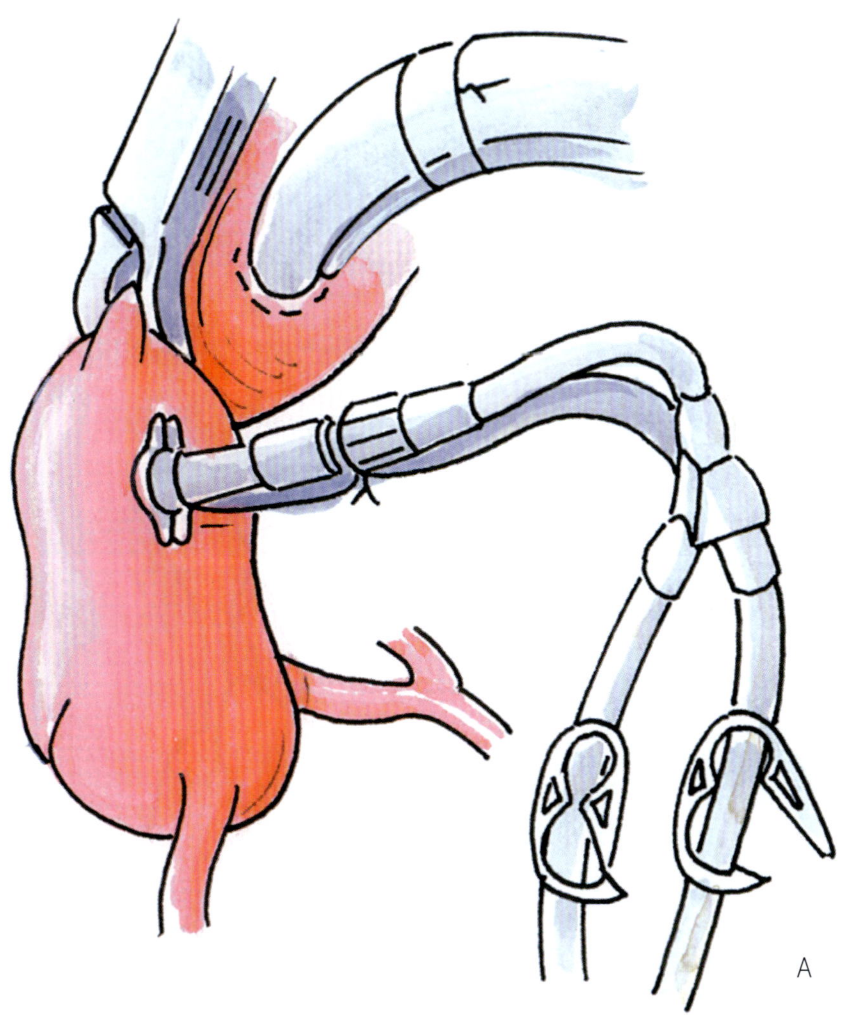

A. 方法一：常用方法是升主动脉根部主动脉阻断钳近端插灌注管，主动脉阻断后灌注心肌保护液。

A. Method 1: Commonly, the cardioplegic cannula is inserted into the ascending aortic root proximal to the aortic clamps, and the cardioplegia is infused after clamping.

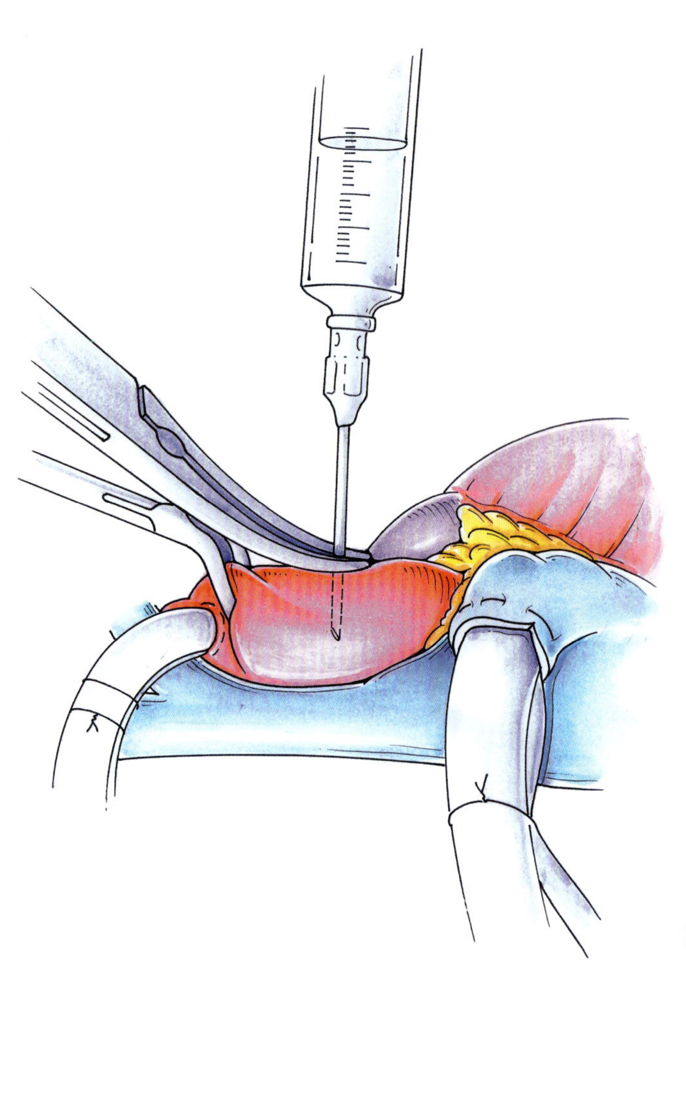

B

B. 方法二：如果只用一次心肌保护液，也可以在升主动脉根部主动脉阻断钳近端穿刺推注心肌保护液。

B. Method 2: If used only once, cardioplegia can also be injected into the ascending aortic root proximal to the aortic clamps after puncturing.

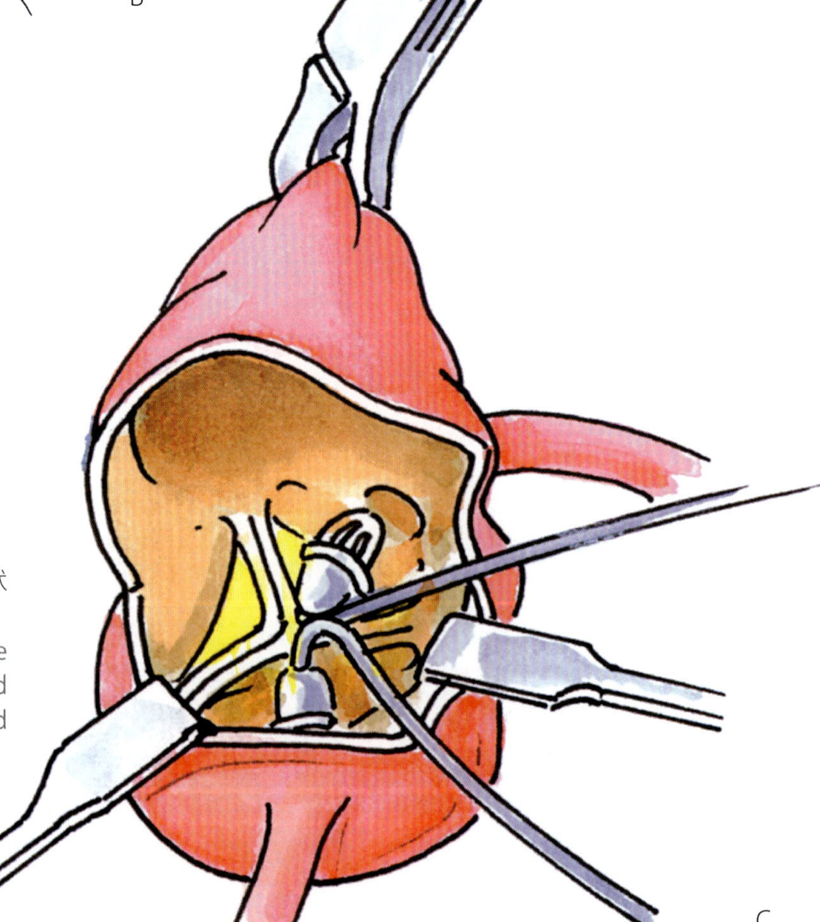

C

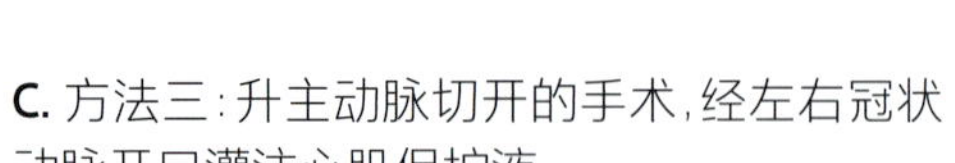

C. 方法三：升主动脉切开的手术，经左右冠状动脉开口灌注心肌保护液。

C. Method 3: During the incision of the ascending aorta, cardioplegia is perfused through the incisions on the left and right coronary arteries.

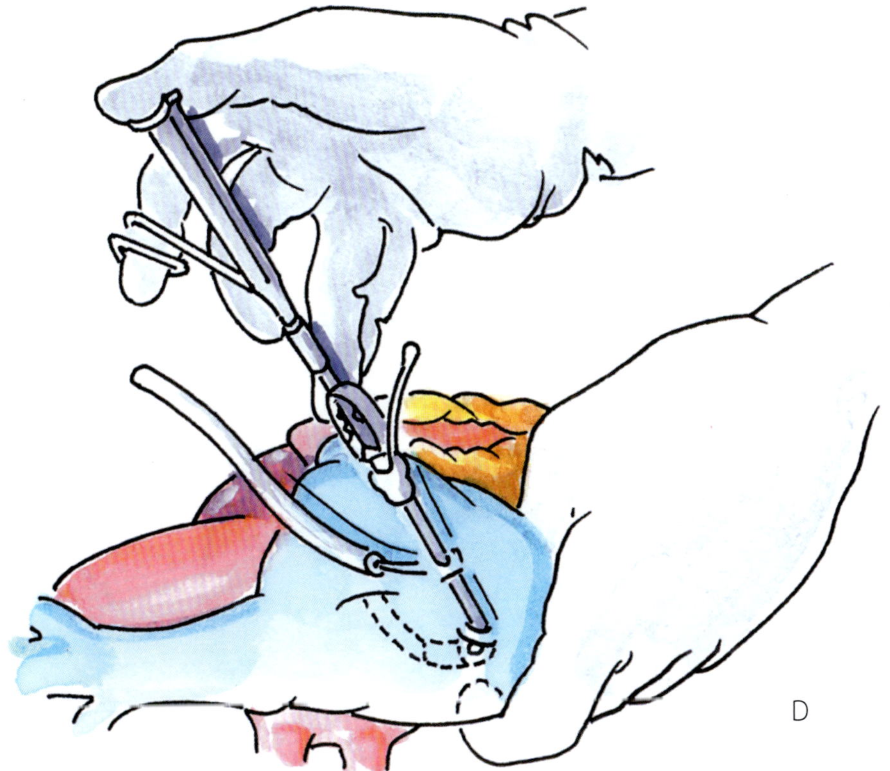

D. 方法四：右心房下部做荷包，插管进入右心房，其尖端插入冠状窦，逆行灌注心肌保护液。冠心病病例常规顺行灌注效果欠佳，可选用此法逆行灌注。

D. Method 4: Purse-string suture is placed on the lower part of the right atrium, through which a cannula is inserted into the right atrium with its tip into the coronary sinus for retrograde cardioplegia. This perfusion can be administrated instead in patients with coronary heart disease when conventional antegrade perfusion is not adequate to meet demands.

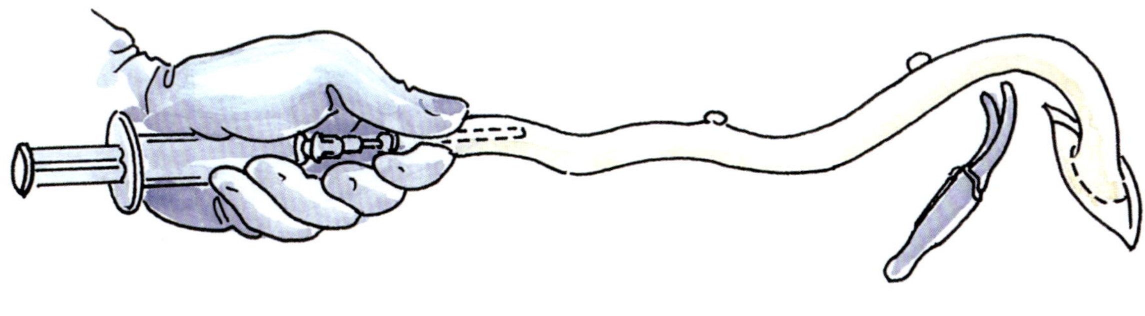

E. 方法五：冠状动脉旁路移植术时，经冠状动脉桥血管注入心肌保护液。

E. Method 5: During coronary artery bypass grafting, cardioplegia is injected through the coronary bridging vein.

第 四 节　胸腔引流

Section 4　Thoracic Drainage

图 1-4-1　纵隔和胸膜腔引流

Figure 1-4-1　Mediastinal and pleural drainage

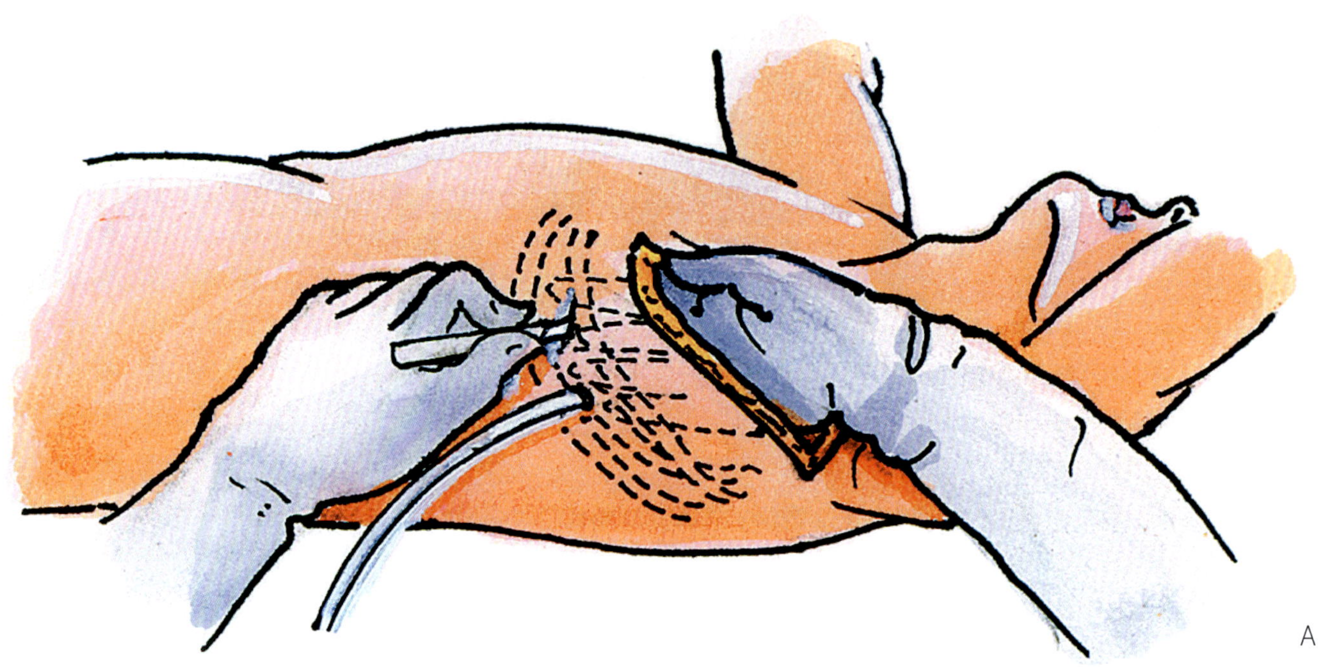

A

A. 开胸手术结束后，经胸部切口或经第 6 肋间腋前线和锁骨中线分别插入胸腔上、下引流管。

A. After thoracic surgeries, the superior and inferior chest drains are inserted through the incision or the anterior axillary line and the midclavicular line in the sixth intercostal space, respectively.

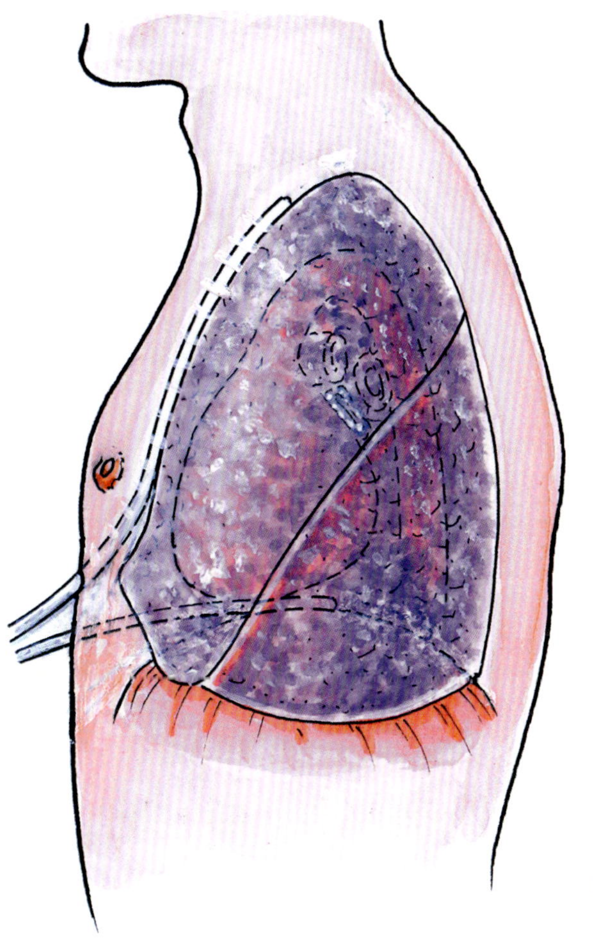

B. 下管经肺底送到后肋膈角，上管由前胸壁和肺之间向上送到胸顶。

B. The inferior drain arrives at the posterior costophrenic angle through the lung base, and the superior drain goes up between the anterior chest wall and the lungs and then arrives at the top of the chest.

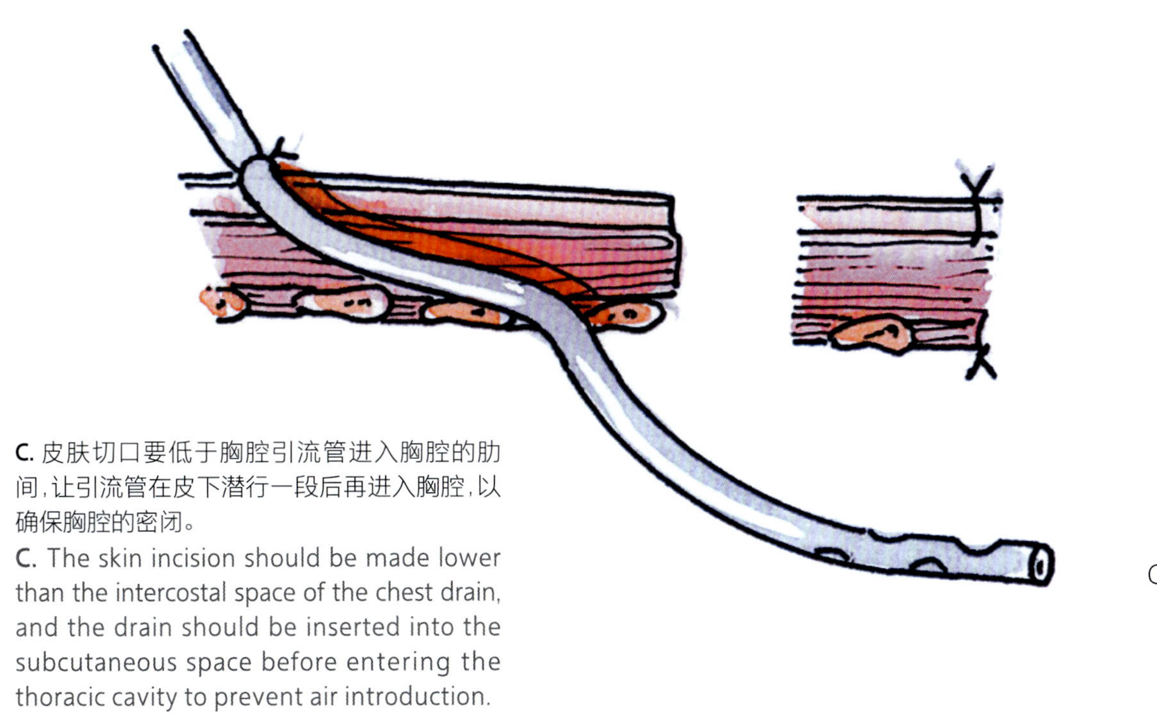

C. 皮肤切口要低于胸腔引流管进入胸腔的肋间，让引流管在皮下潜行一段后再进入胸腔，以确保胸腔的密闭。

C. The skin incision should be made lower than the intercostal space of the chest drain, and the drain should be inserted into the subcutaneous space before entering the thoracic cavity to prevent air introduction.

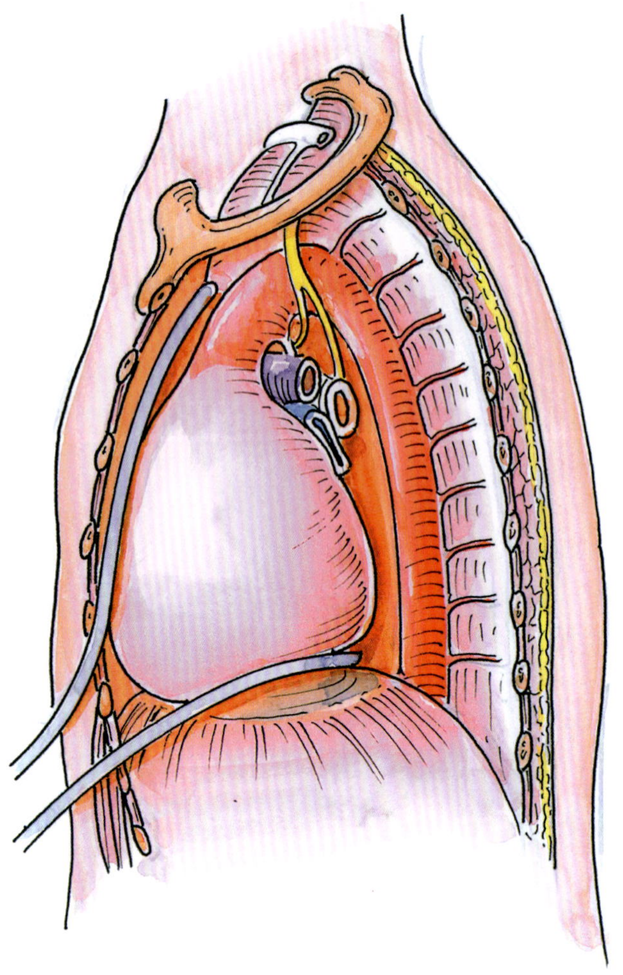

D. 胸骨正中切口心脏手术结束后，须留置纵隔引流管和心包引流管。均由剑突下切小切口引出。

D. Mediastinal and pericardial drains need to be retained after cardiac surgery with sternotomy. The drains are brought out of the body via a stab wound under the xiphoid process.

D

E. 右边是心包引流管，左边是纵隔引流管。

E. Pericardial drain (right) and the mediastinal drain (left).

E

图 1-4-2　纵隔感染的冲洗和引流

Figure 1-4-2　Wash-out and drainage for mediastinitis

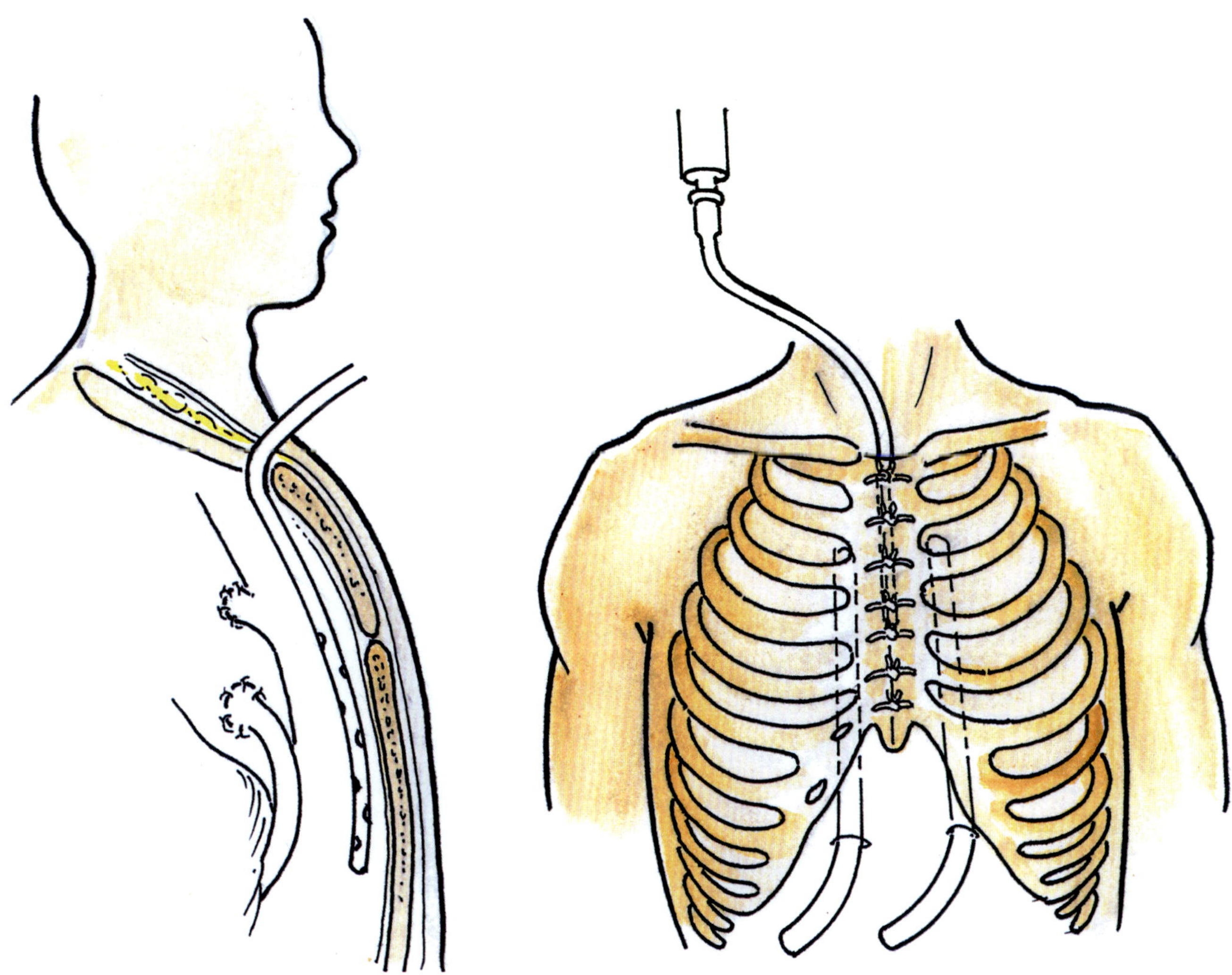

纵隔清创后在前纵隔留置的双引流管由剑突下戳口引出，再由胸骨上置入一多孔管。多孔管持续滴注冲洗液。灌注液由剑突下插入的引流管引出。

After mediastinal debridement, two chest drains placed in the anterior mediastinum are brought out from a stab wound under the xiphoid process, followed by the placement of a porous tube on the sternum. Continuous perfusion of the flushing solution is performed through the porous tube, and the perfusate is then drawn from a drain under the xiphoid process.

第二章
缺血性心脏病

Chapter 2
Ischemic Heart Disease

第 一 节　体外循环冠状动脉旁路移植术

Section 1　Conventional Coronary Artery Bypass Grafting

大隐静脉是最常用的桥血管之一。左胸廓内动脉远端吻合至前降支，大隐静脉在升主动脉和其他病变冠状动脉之间搭桥，是目前最为广泛应用的冠状动脉旁路移植术方式。Chaveg报告大隐静脉桥血管的5年、10年通畅率分别为74%和41%，低于动脉桥血管5年、10年通畅率的97.9%和83%。但大隐静脉容易摘取、有着足够的长度和略粗于冠状动脉的口径且便于行序贯搭桥，是其长处。

The great saphenous vein (GSV) is one of the most common bridging veins for surgery. Here below is the procedure widely used in coronary artery bypass grafting (CABG): the distal end of the left internal thoracic artery is anastomosed to the left anterior descending artery firstly, and then GSV is grafted from the ascending aorta to the diseased coronary arteries. Chaveg reports that the 5 years and 10 years patency rates of GSV grafts are, respectively, 74% and 41%, which is far below artery grafts, 97.9% and 83%. However, GSV has its advantages for it is not only easy to extract but also has enough length. Furthermore, a caliber slightly larger than the coronary artery makes it more suitable for sequential bypass.

摘取大隐静脉的关键技术与摘取其他桥血管一样，是保护血管内膜的完整性，从而保证桥血管良好的长期通畅率。摘取全过程要避免暴力牵拉和过度注液扩张，避免手术器械和电刀直接损伤血管壁。任何血管内膜损伤都会促使桥血管狭窄，直接影响手术远期疗效。

While harvesting GSV, just like other bridging veins, the key point is to make sure the integrity of the tunica intima and keep the long-term patency of the bridging vein. In the whole process, violent pull and excessive injection expansion are strictly forbidden as well as any possible damage to the vascular wall caused by surgical instruments and electric knives, for any intimal injury will cause the stenosis of the bridging vein and then affect the long-term outcome of the surgery.

图 2-1-1 摘取大隐静脉
Figure 2-1-1 Great saphenous vein harvest

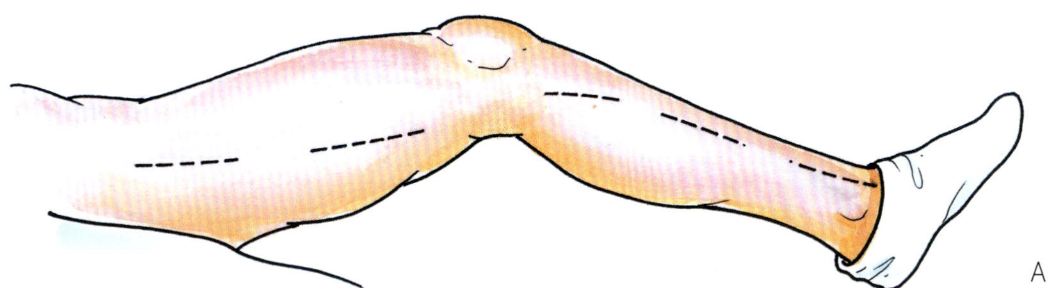

A. 沿大隐静脉分段纵行切开皮肤，大腿、小腿各做 2~3 个小切口，膝关节处皮肤保留完整。也可全程切开腿部皮肤，仅保留膝关节处皮肤不切开。内镜辅助下小切口摘取大隐静脉，由于远期通畅率的劣势，现已不提倡使用。

A. Cut the skin to make 2-3 small segmented incisions along GSV in the thigh and calf respectively, but the skin of the knee joint should be avoided. Alternatively, a continuous incision over the entire length of GSV could be performed with the skin of the knee joint intact. The harvest of GSV is not advocated through a small incision with the help of an endoscope now because of the low patency rate in the long run.

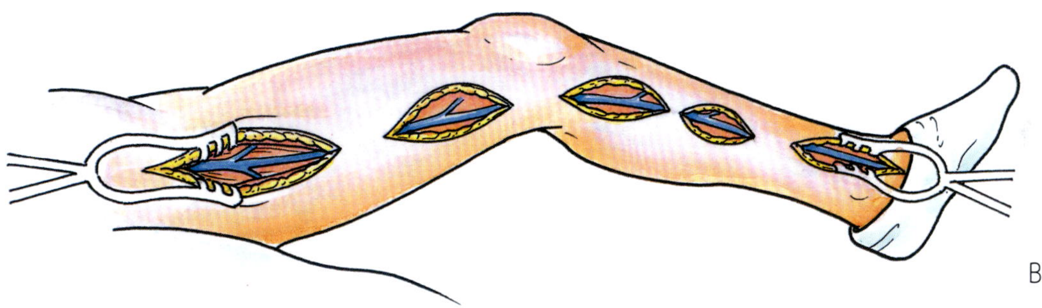

B. 切开皮肤、皮下组织和筋膜，游离大隐静脉。皮肤未切开处通过皮下隧道潜行剥出。

B. Cut open skin, subcutaneous tissues, and fascia. Then, dissociate GSV, and strip out of it by a subcutaneous tunnel where the skin is not incised.

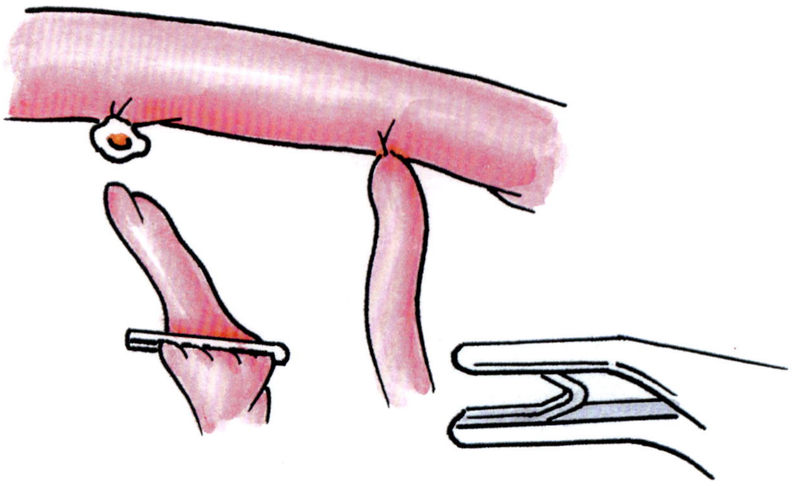

C. 大隐静脉的分支近端 0 号丝线结扎，远端钛夹钳闭。然后剪断分支血管。

C. Ligate the proximal ends of the GSV branches with 0# suture and clamp the distal ends with titanium clips. Then, cut the branch vessels.

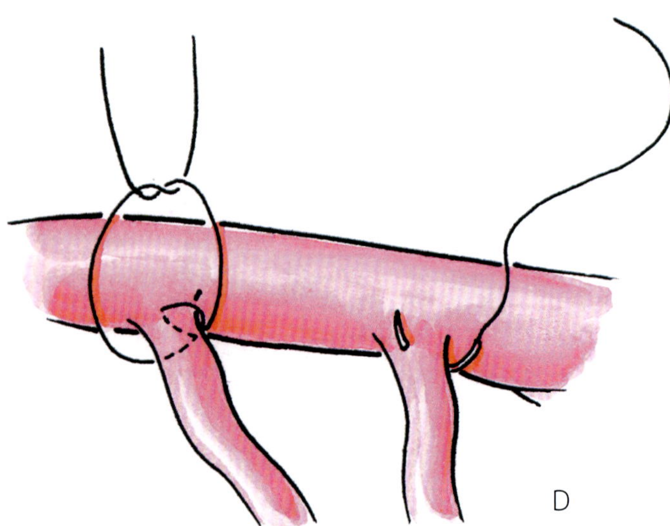

D. 大隐静脉较粗的分支予以缝扎或双重结扎。

D. As to the thicker branches of GSV, sutures or double-loop ligation can be used.

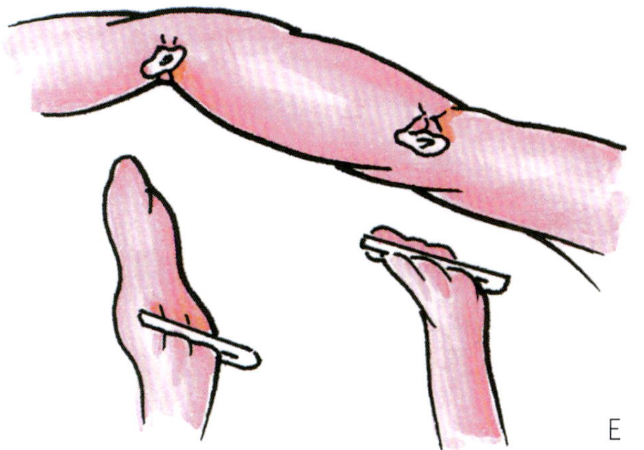

E. 分支的结扎距大隐静脉 1mm 左右，视分支血管的粗细而定。过于贴近大隐静脉会造成大隐静脉狭窄，过远则分支遗留盲端易形成血栓。

E. The ligation location for the branches is usually about 1 mm away from the GSV, and it specifically depends on their thickness. Being too close to the GSV may result in the stenosis of GSV, but if it is too far, diverticula will be formed and it is easy to cause thrombus.

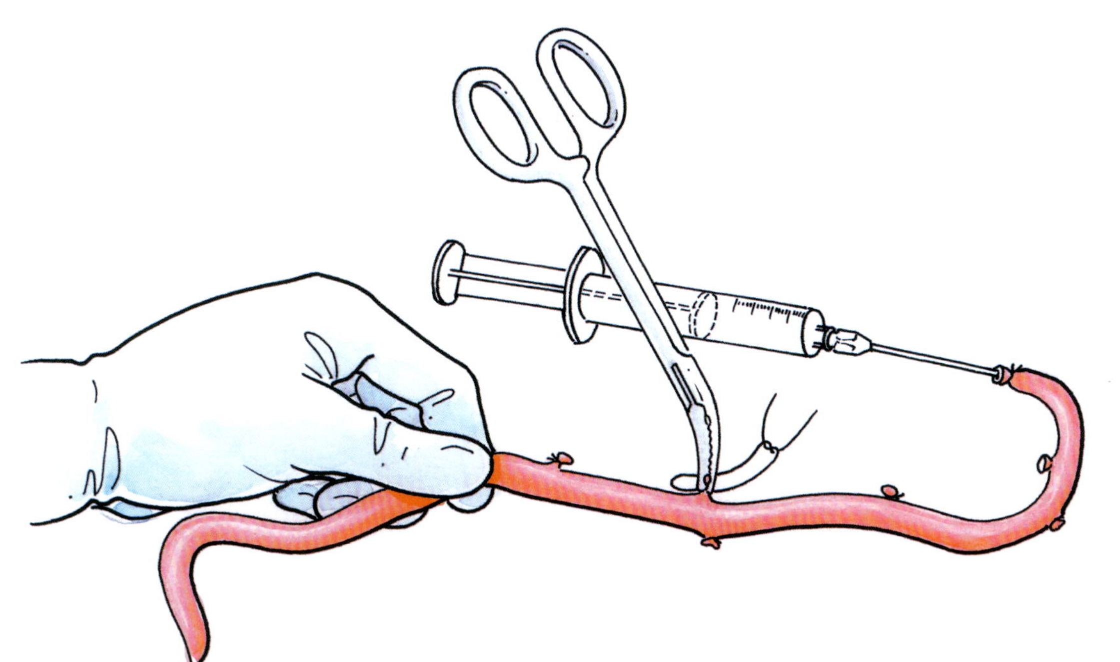

F. 于游离的大隐静脉远心端截断，插入大隐静脉针头结扎固定。缓缓注入含肝素的生理盐水，冲出残留血液并扩张大隐静脉。勿用暴力以免损伤大隐静脉内膜。切断游离的大隐静脉近心端。遗漏的分支予以结扎。生理盐水纱布包覆后备用。

F. Cut off the dissociated GSV at the distal end. Insert the GSV needle, and then ligate and fix it. Slowly, inject some heparinized saline to flush out the residual blood and dilate the GSV. In order to protect the intima of GSV, violence is strictly forbidden. Cut off the proximal end of the dissociated GSV and ligate the remaining branches. The GSV is placed in saline gauze for later use.

胸廓内动脉是远期通畅率最好的桥血管，前降支狭窄通常首选带蒂左胸廓内动脉作为桥血管。

The internal thoracic artery (ITA) is the bridging vein with the highest long-term patency rate, so the pedicled left internal thoracic artery is usually preferred in the case of anterior descending branch stenosis.

摘取胸廓内动脉用胸骨正中切口。锯开胸骨后心包先不打开，用专用撑开器牵起左侧胸骨，抬高手术床并转向左侧。用电刀分离胸膜外和胸骨后之间的疏松组织，显露胸廓内动脉全长。也可纵行切开左纵隔胸膜，于胸膜腔内显露胸廓内动脉。

The ITA is harvested via a median sternotomy. After the sternum is cut through, the pericardium shouldn't be opened. The left side of the sternum is retracted by a special spreader, and the operating table is elevated and rotated to the left. The full length of ITA can be exposed after the loose tissue between the extrapleural area and retrosternal area is separated with an electrotome, or it can be exposed in the pleural cavity after the left mediastinal pleura is longitudinally cut open.

图 2-1-2 摘取左胸廓内动脉
Figure 2-1-2 Left internal thoracic artery harvest

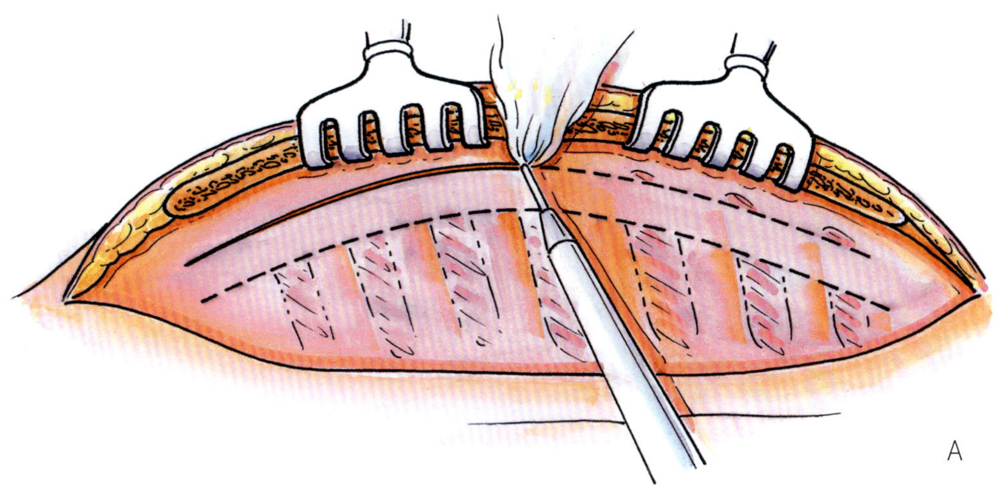

A. 用电凝在胸廓内动脉两侧约 1cm 处切开胸壁筋膜，胸廓内动脉周边注入罂粟碱溶液。

A. Open the pleura of thoracic wall on both sides (about 1 cm) of the ITA by electrocoagulation. Papaverine solution is injected peripherally around the ITA.

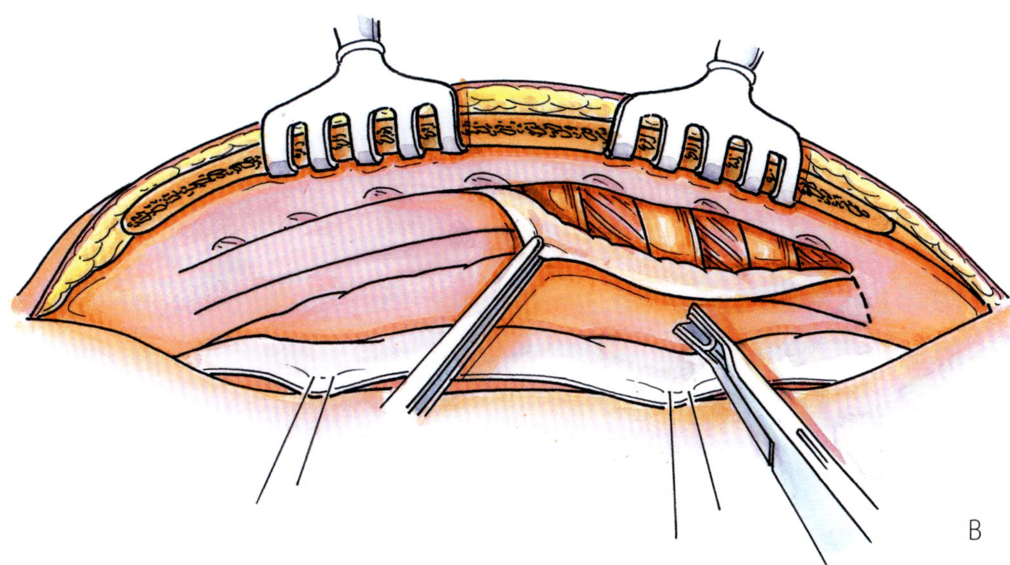

B. 用低功率电凝仔细将胸廓内动脉从胸壁上剥离下来，其分支近端用钛夹夹闭，远端直接电凝止血。胸廓内动脉近端要游离到第 1 肋间，离断第 1 肋间动脉，以保证胸廓内动脉血流量避免肋间动脉窃血。远端游离到第 6 肋间血管分叉处。

B. Carefully dissociate the ITA from the thoracic wall by electrocoagulation at low power. Clip the proximal end of its branch with titanium clips, and control bleeding at the distal end by electrocoagulation. Dissection at the proximal end of ITA is continued to the first rib, and the first intercostal artery should be transected to ensure the blood flow in ITA and avoid the “steal” of blood from the intercostal artery. The distal end of ITA is freed all the way to the bifurcation of the sixth intercostal vessel.

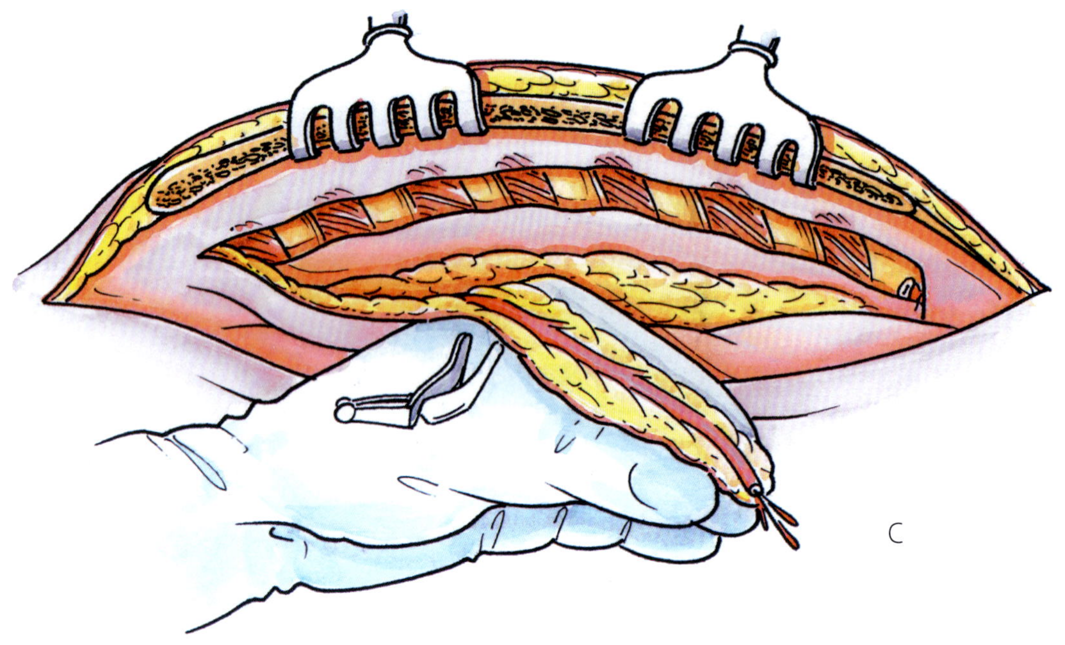

C. 全身肝素化后将胸廓内动脉远端切断，检查血流良好。Bulldog 血管夹控制血流，用含罂粟碱湿纱布包覆后备用。

C. Distal dissection is performed after systemic heparinization. Check the blood flow and control it with a Bulldog clamp if necessary. The harvested ITA is wrapped in the gauze saturated with papaverine solution for later use.

常规冠状动脉旁路移植术在建立体外循环心脏停搏后先做远端吻合。根据术前冠状动脉造影找到靶血管，进行桥血管与冠状动脉的吻合。

Conventional CABG is begun with distal anastomosis under extracorporeal circulation and cardiac arrest. The target vessels are first identified according to preoperative coronary angiography, and then anastomosis between the bridging veins and the coronary arteries is performed.

图 2-1-3 远端吻合——大隐静脉冠状动脉吻合

Figure 2-1-3 Distal anastomosis-anastomosis of GSV to coronary artery

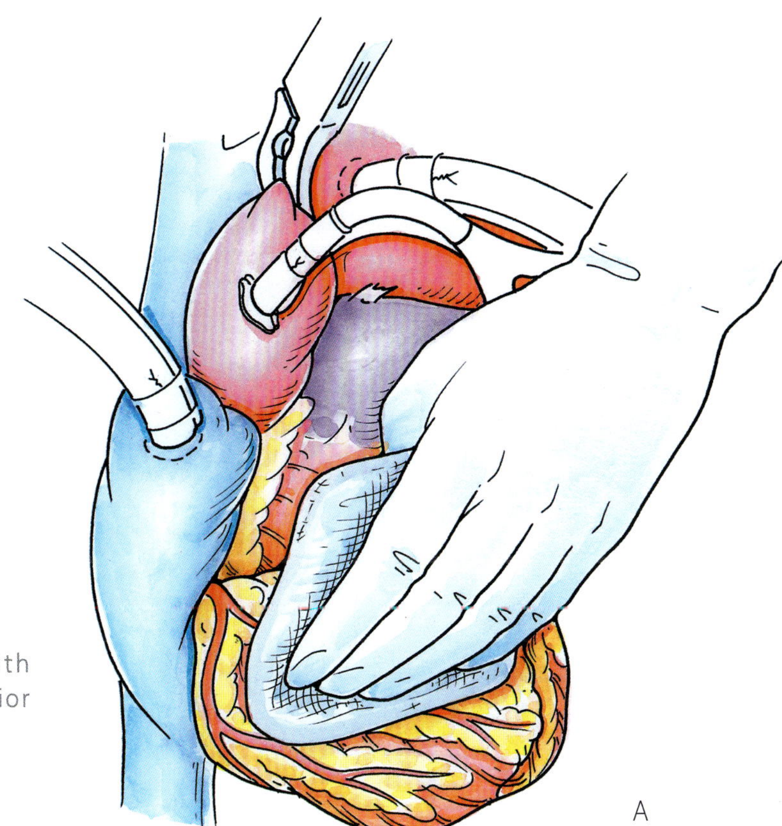

A. 持湿纱布抬起心尖，显露后降支。

A. Lift the apex of the heart with wet gauze to expose the posterior descending branch.

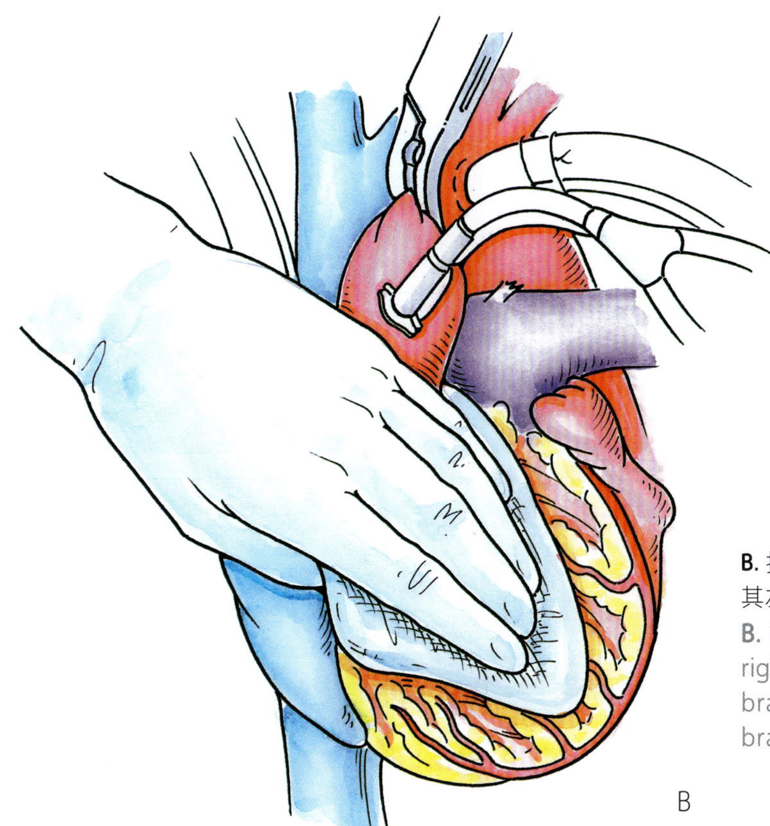

B. 抬高心脏并向右侧翻转，显露前降支及其左后方的回旋支。

B. Elevate the heart and rotate it to the right to expose the anterior descending branch and its left posterior circumflex branch.

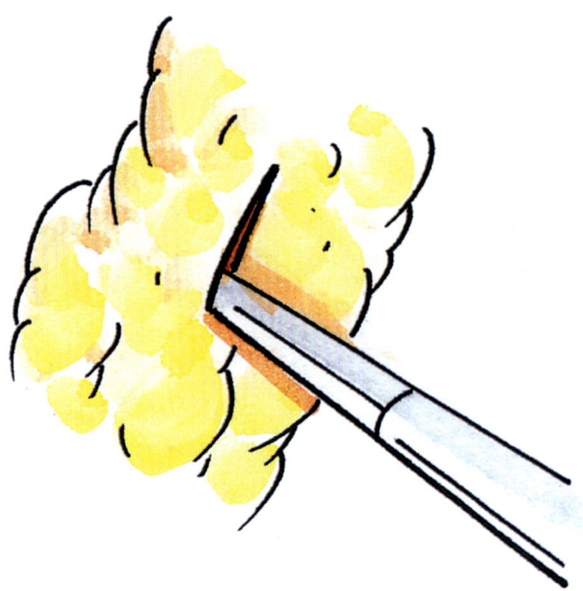

C. 在选定的靶血管，用 15 号刀切开心外膜及脂肪组织约 1cm，暴露冠状动脉。

C. The epicardium and adipose tissue are to be incised by using a 15# blade over the area of the target vessel (about 1 cm long) to expose the coronary artery.

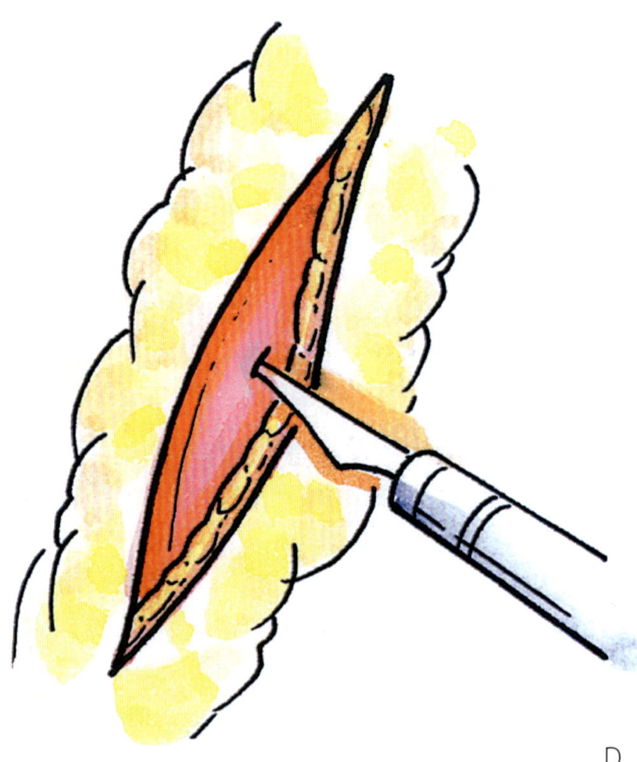

D. 用冠状动脉刀尖在冠状动脉前壁中央纵行挑开，注意勿误伤冠状动脉后壁。

D. The anterior wall of the coronary artery is opened longitudinally in the center with the scalpel blade tip, and any injury to the posterior wall should be avoided.

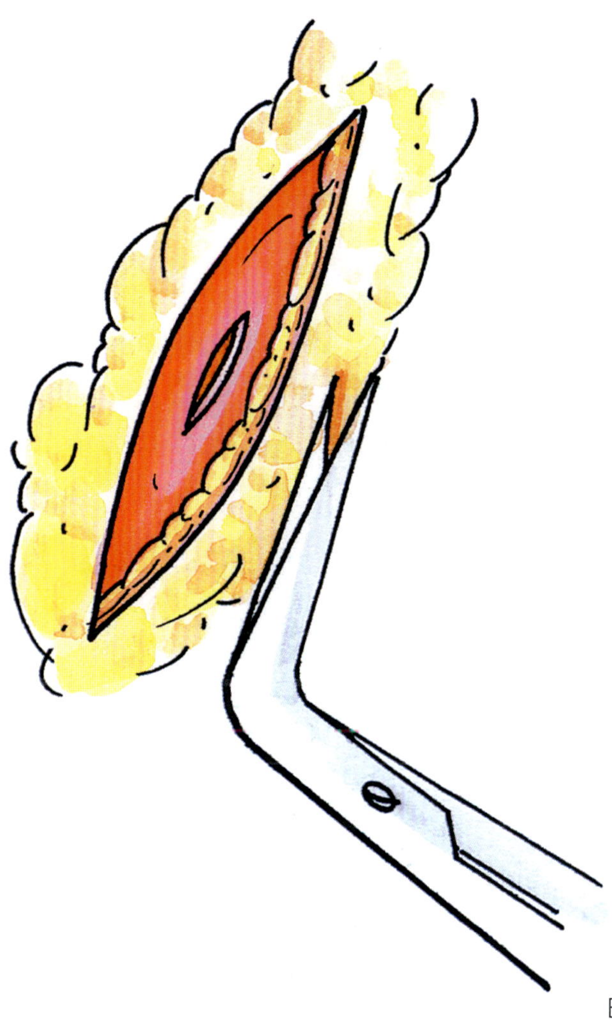

E. 用冠状动脉剪向两端延长冠状动脉切口。切开的长度一般为该冠状动脉直径的 2~3 倍并与桥血管的口径相当。

E. The incision is extended towards two ends with fine angled scissors. The length is usually 2-3 times the diameter of the coronary artery and is about the same as the caliber of the bridging vein.

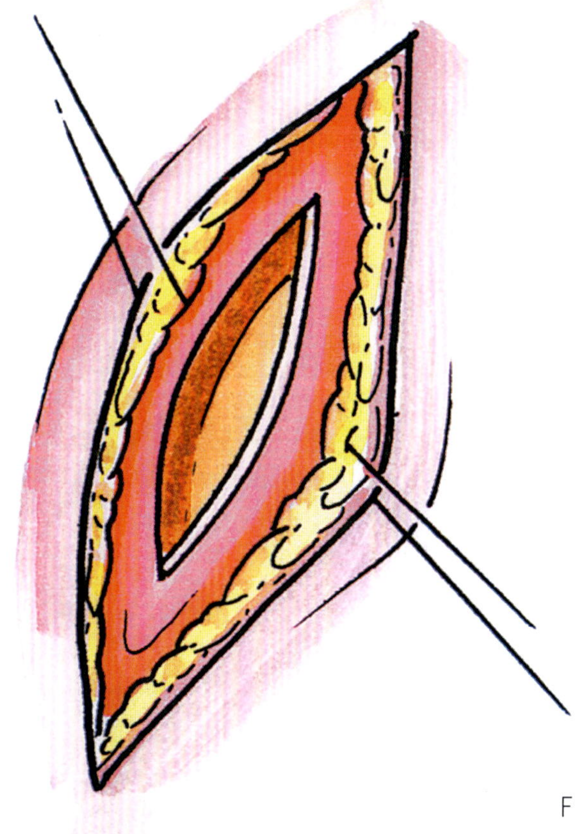

F. 心外膜下脂肪较厚时，以细线悬吊心外膜，借助小蚊式钳向两侧牵拉，帮助显露吻合口。该方法也使冠状动脉切口张开，有利于吻合口的缝合。

F. When the subepicardial fat is thick, the epicardium should be suspended by a fine line and pulled to both sides by small mosquito forceps to help expose the anastomotic stoma. This method also makes the coronary artery incision open, which is conducive to anastomosis.

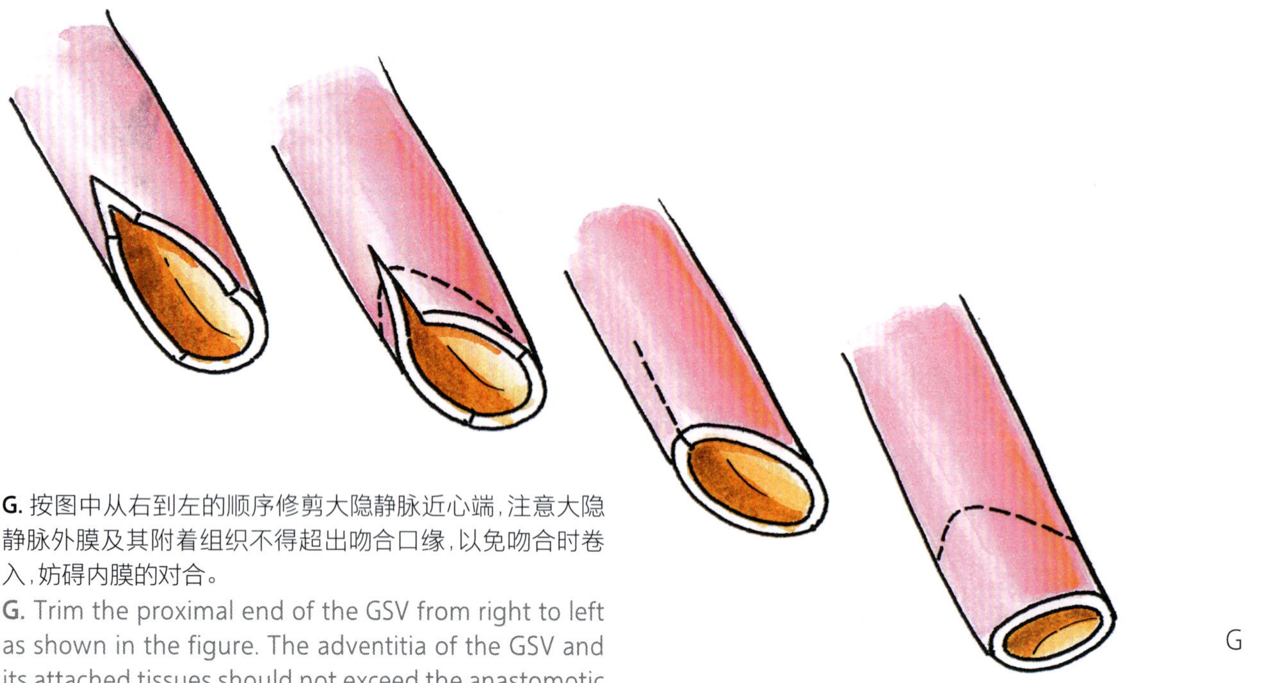

G. 按图中从右到左的顺序修剪大隐静脉近心端，注意大隐静脉外膜及其附着组织不得超出吻合口缘，以免吻合时卷入，妨碍内膜的对合。

G. Trim the proximal end of the GSV from right to left as shown in the figure. The adventitia of the GSV and its attached tissues should not exceed the anastomotic edge to ensure that no extraneous tissue will be incorporated to interfere with the intima alignement.

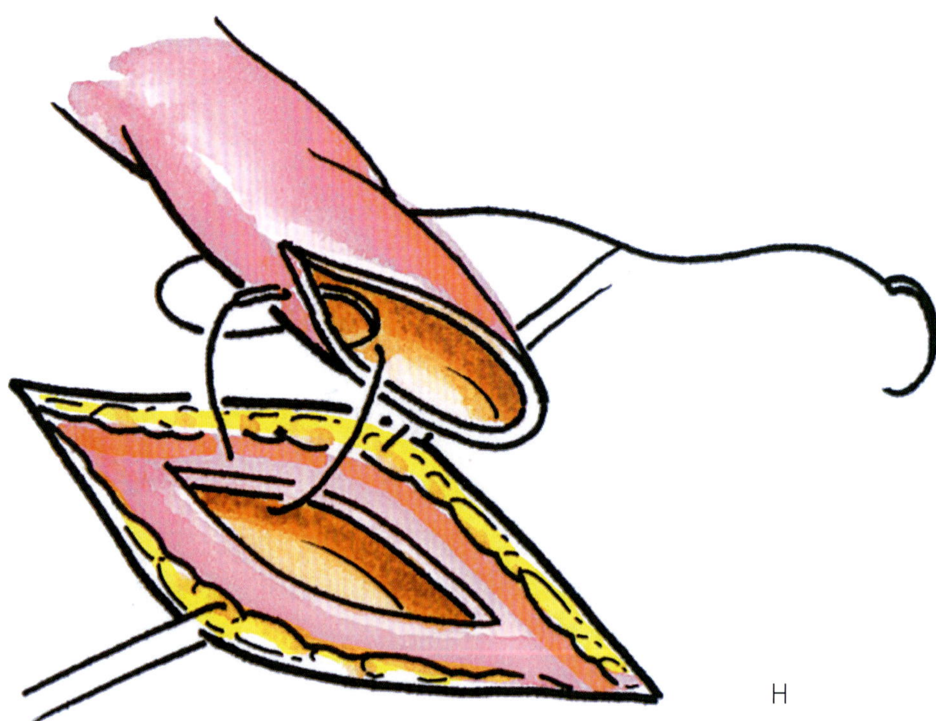

H. 用 7-0 Prolene 双头缝线先缝足跟，由左向右缝，第一针由外向内缝大隐静脉，然后冠状动脉侧由内向外进针，如此较易避免勾住后壁。一般在足跟缝 3 针。

H. Double-armed 7-0 Prolene suture starts from the heel of the anastomosis and travels from left to right. The first suture is passed through the GSV (from outside to inside) and then the coronary artery (from inside to outside), so as to avoid snagging the posterior wall. Three stitches are usually needed at the anastomosis heel.

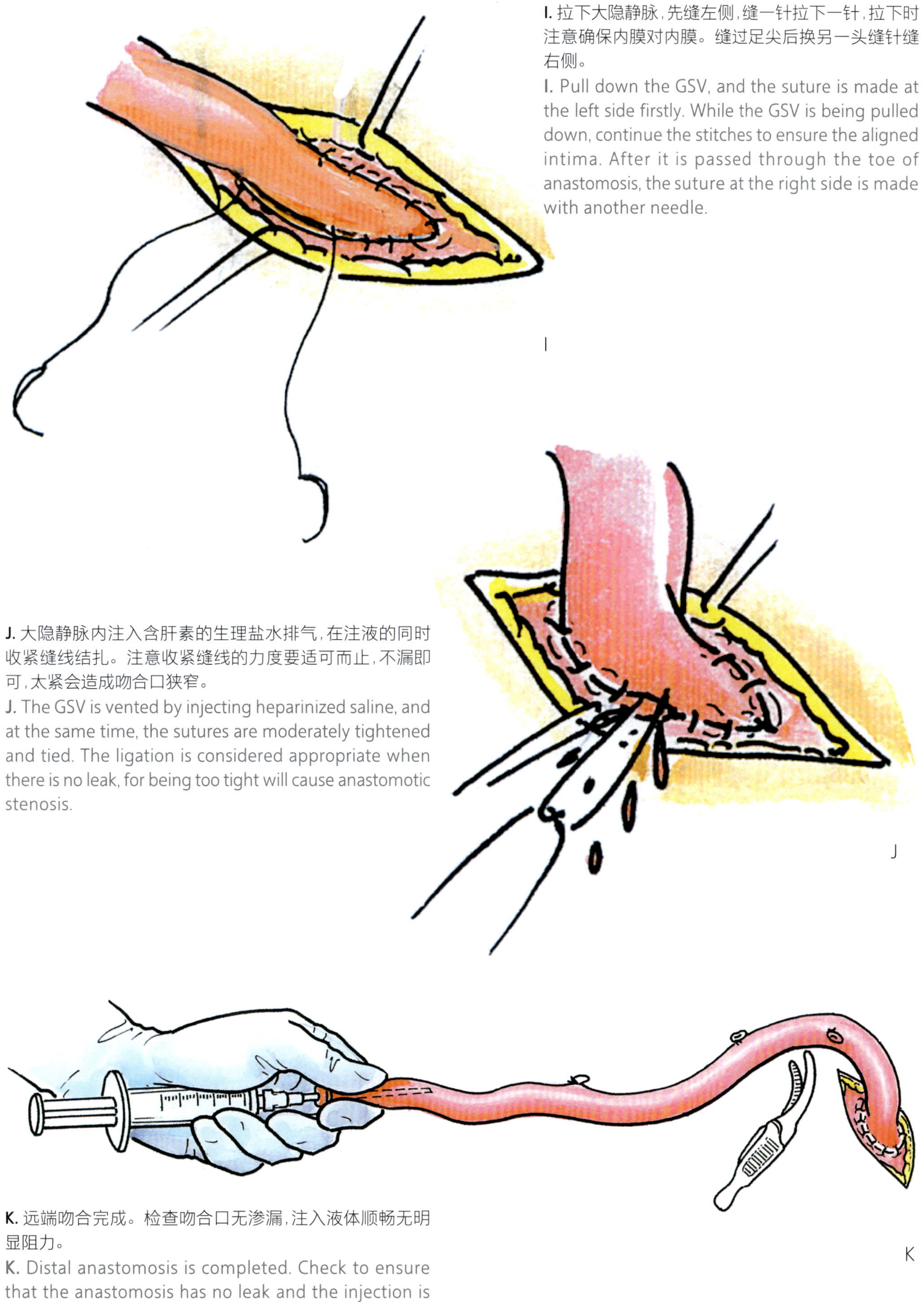

I. 拉下大隐静脉，先缝左侧，缝一针拉下一针，拉下时注意确保内膜对内膜。缝过足尖后换另一头缝针缝右侧。

I. Pull down the GSV, and the suture is made at the left side firstly. While the GSV is being pulled down, continue the stitches to ensure the aligned intima. After it is passed through the toe of anastomosis, the suture at the right side is made with another needle.

I

J. 大隐静脉内注入含肝素的生理盐水排气，在注液的同时收紧缝线结扎。注意收紧缝线的力度要适可而止，不漏即可，太紧会造成吻合口狭窄。

J. The GSV is vented by injecting heparinized saline, and at the same time, the sutures are moderately tightened and tied. The ligation is considered appropriate when there is no leak, for being too tight will cause anastomotic stenosis.

J

K. 远端吻合完成。检查吻合口无渗漏，注入液体顺畅无明显阻力。

K. Distal anastomosis is completed. Check to ensure that the anastomosis has no leak and the injection is smooth without any obvious resistance.

K

图 2-1-4 远端吻合——胸廓内动脉冠状动脉吻合
Figure 2-1-4 Distal anastomosis-anastomosis of ITA to coronary artery

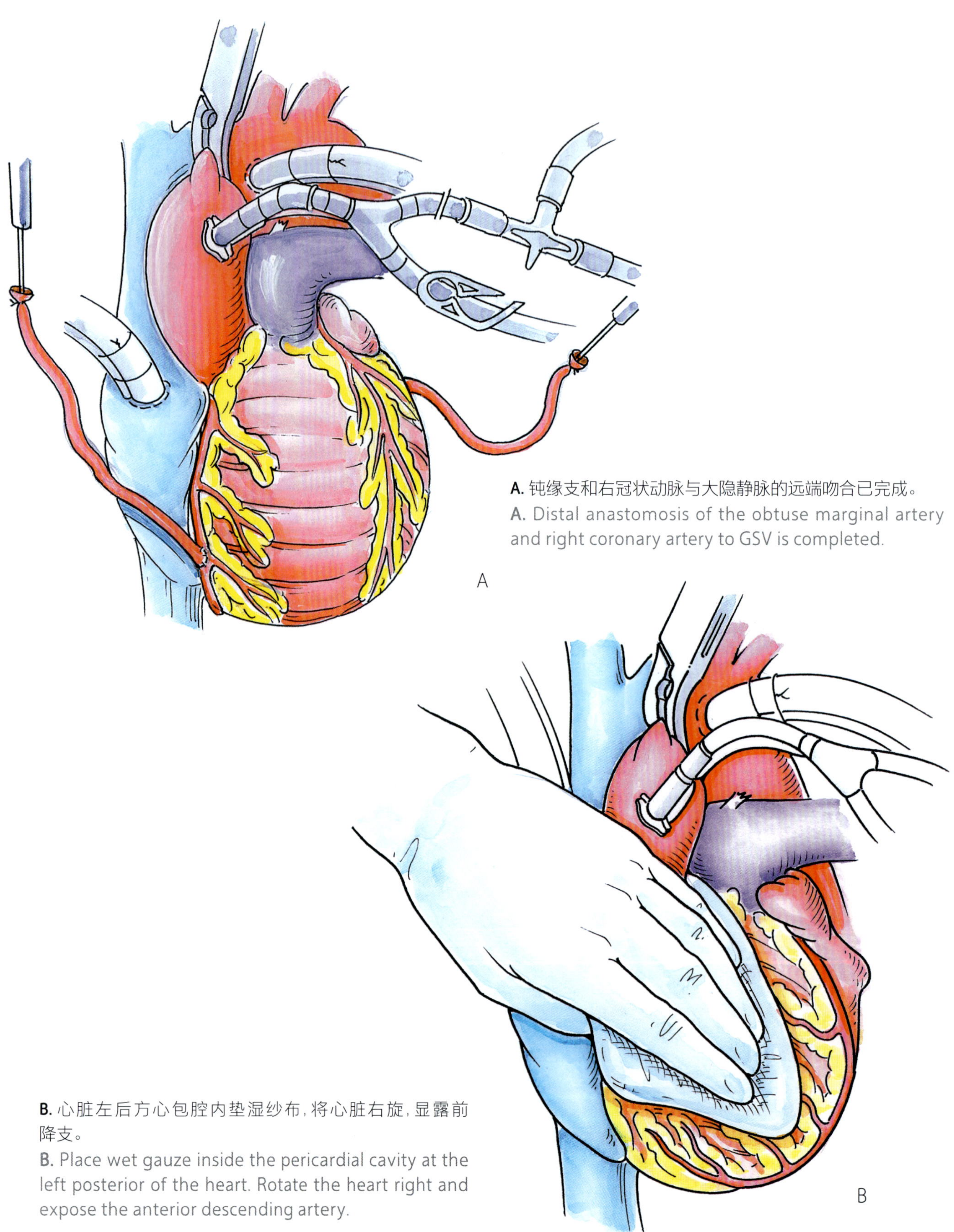

A. 钝缘支和右冠状动脉与大隐静脉的远端吻合已完成。

A. Distal anastomosis of the obtuse marginal artery and right coronary artery to GSV is completed.

B. 心脏左后方心包腔内垫湿纱布，将心脏右旋，显露前降支。

B. Place wet gauze inside the pericardial cavity at the left posterior of the heart. Rotate the heart right and expose the anterior descending artery.

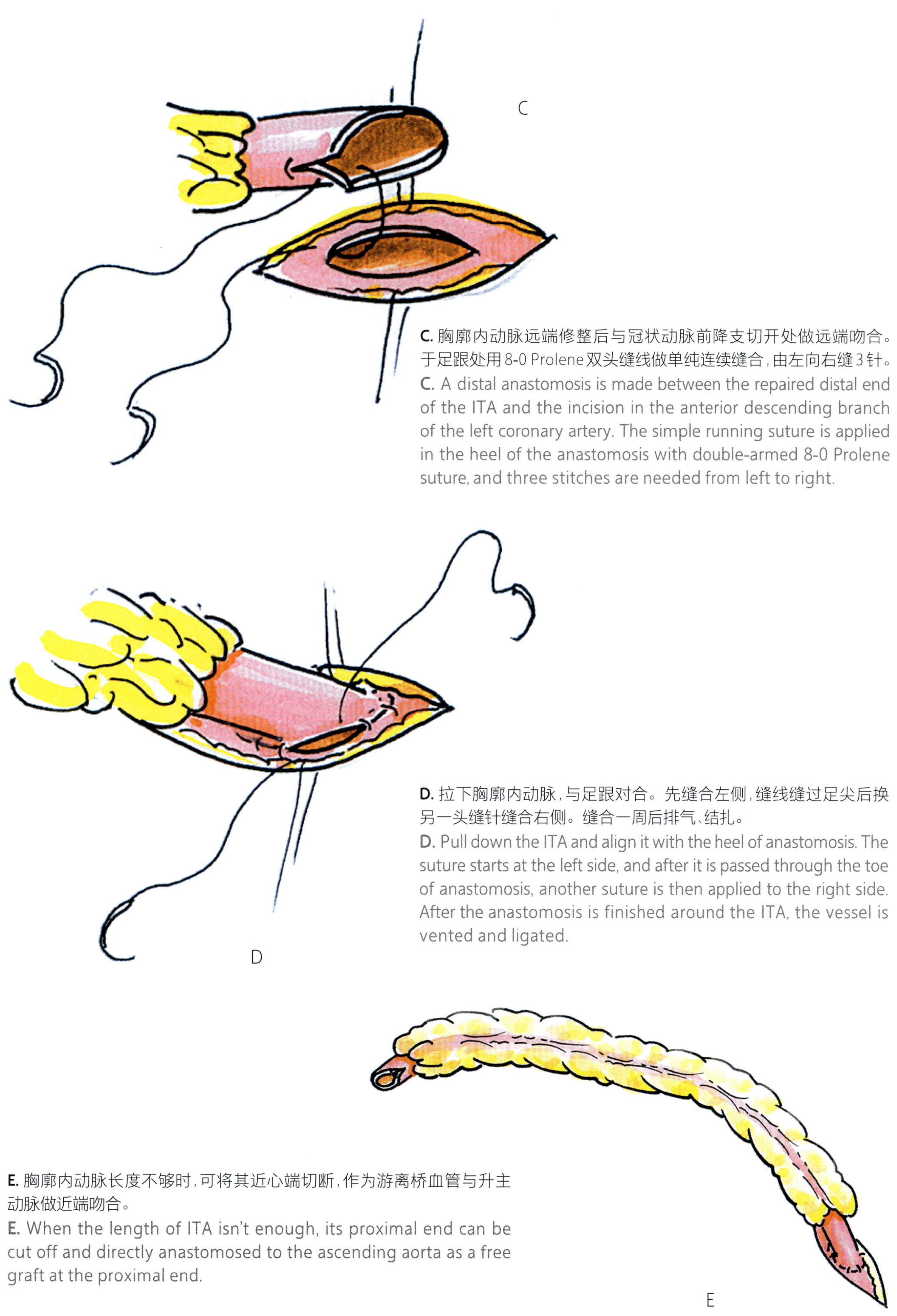

C. 胸廓内动脉远端修整后与冠状动脉前降支切开处做远端吻合。于足跟处用8-0 Prolene双头缝线做单纯连续缝合，由左向右缝3针。

C. A distal anastomosis is made between the repaired distal end of the ITA and the incision in the anterior descending branch of the left coronary artery. The simple running suture is applied in the heel of the anastomosis with double-armed 8-0 Prolene suture, and three stitches are needed from left to right.

D. 拉下胸廓内动脉，与足跟对合。先缝合左侧，缝线缝过足尖后换另一头缝针缝合右侧。缝合一周后排气、结扎。

D. Pull down the ITA and align it with the heel of anastomosis. The suture starts at the left side, and after it is passed through the toe of anastomosis, another suture is then applied to the right side. After the anastomosis is finished around the ITA, the vessel is vented and ligated.

E. 胸廓内动脉长度不够时，可将其近心端切断，作为游离桥血管与升主动脉做近端吻合。

E. When the length of ITA isn't enough, its proximal end can be cut off and directly anastomosed to the ascending aorta as a free graft at the proximal end.

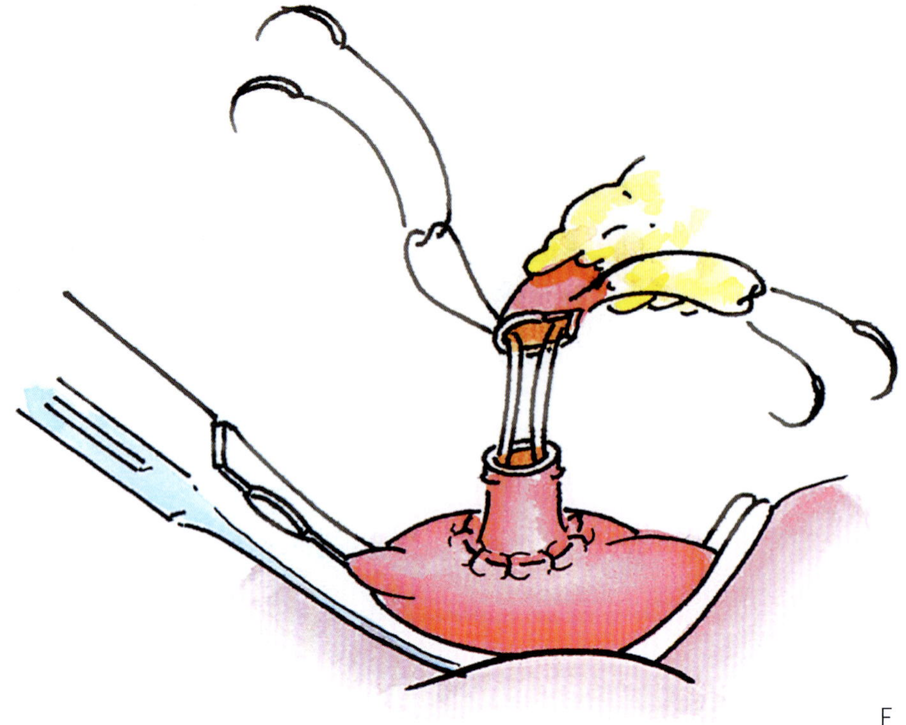

F

F. 游离桥血管须做近端吻合。开放升主动脉阻断钳，心脏复跳。侧壁钳部分阻断升主动脉，打孔器在选定的近端吻合位置打孔。由于升主动脉与胸廓内动脉的管壁厚度相差较大，而且胸廓内动脉管径较细，为便于吻合，可用一段大隐静脉与升主动脉端侧吻合，再将胸廓内动脉近心端与大隐静脉端端吻合。

F. Proximal anastomosis is required for a free graft. Remove the clamp from the ascending aorta, and resume cardiac contractions. Partially block the ascending aorta with an anastomosis clamp, and make a hole with a punch at the selected position for the proximal anastomosis. Since the ascending aorta and ITA have a great difference in the thickness of the wall and the latter's diameter is relatively small, an end-to-side anastomosis between a segment of GSV and the ascending aorta is performed for a better effect. And then, an end-to-end anastomosis is performed between the proximal end of the ITA and the GSV.

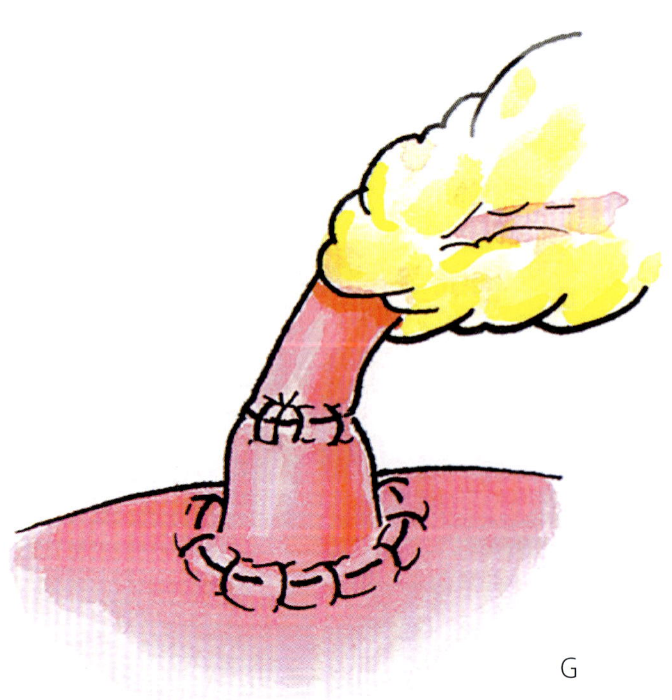

G

G. 吻合完成。

G. Anastomosis is done.

图 2-1-5 近端吻合——大隐静脉升主动脉吻合

Figure 2-1-5 Proximal anastomosis-anastomosis of GSV to ascending aorta

远端吻合全部完成后，开放升主动脉阻断钳，心脏复跳，在并行体外循环下做近端吻合。吻合口的位置通常选择在升主动脉前壁，根据桥血管的根数合理布局。吻合口位置要注意避开主动脉有硬化斑块处。靠近升主动脉起始部的吻合口要开在前壁中部，以远的吻合口则可向左侧或右侧略偏，使吻合完成充盈后的桥血管自然顺畅没有皱褶。左侧心脏有多支桥血管时，近端吻合口应由下而上排列左侧心脏由前至后的桥血管，以避免其交叠受压。

After the completion of distal anastomosis, removal of the aorta clamp, and resumption of cardiac contractions, the proximal anastomosis can be performed under parallel extracorporeal circulation. The anastomosis stoma is usually arranged reasonably on the anterior wall of ascending aorta according to the number of vein grafts, and the atherosclerotic plaques in the aorta should be avoided. In order to make the bridging vessels naturally smooth without twisting after anastomosis, the anastomosis close to the beginning of the ascending aorta should be located in the middle of the anterior wall and the distal anastomosis can slightly deviate to the left or right. When there are multiple bridging vessels in the left heart, the bridging vessels from front to back should be anastomosed from bottom to top at the proximal end to avoid overlapping compression.

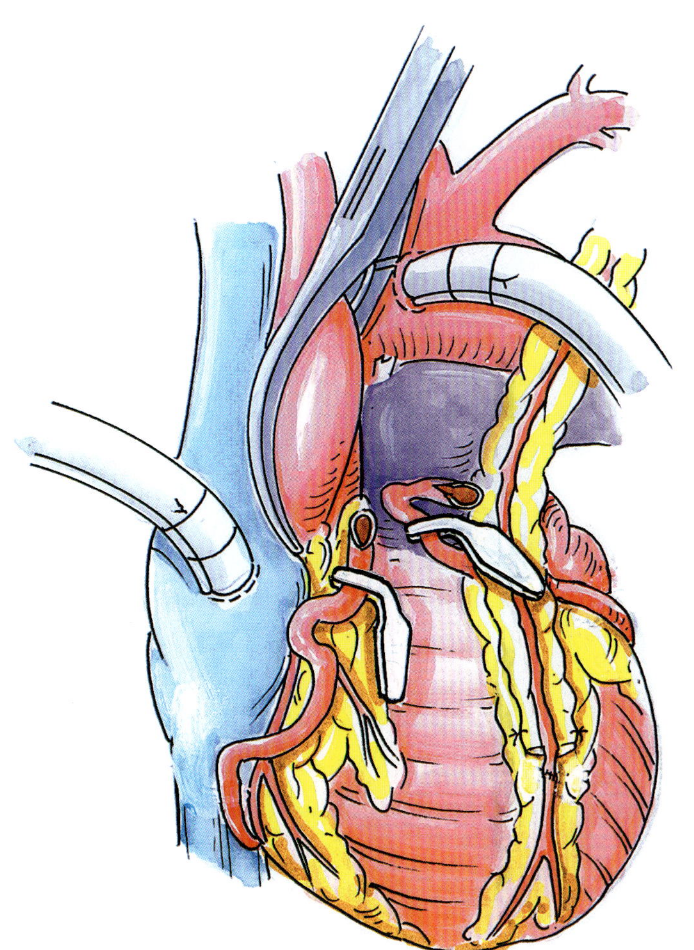

A

A. 剪去选定吻合口表面的升主动脉外膜，侧壁钳钳夹升主动脉。

A. The outer membrane is cut from the selected ascending aorta, and the ascending aorta is clamped by a side-biting clamp.

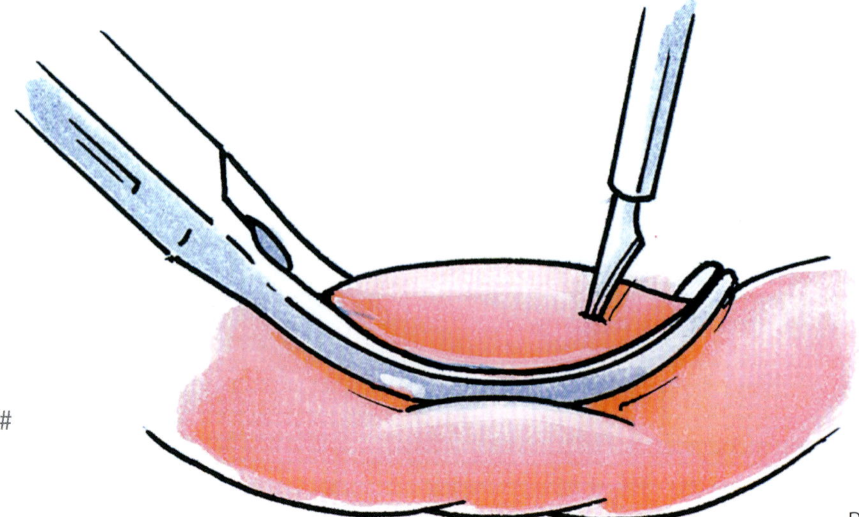

B. 11 号刀刺开主动脉壁全层。

B. Pierce the entire aorta wall with an 11# scalpel blade.

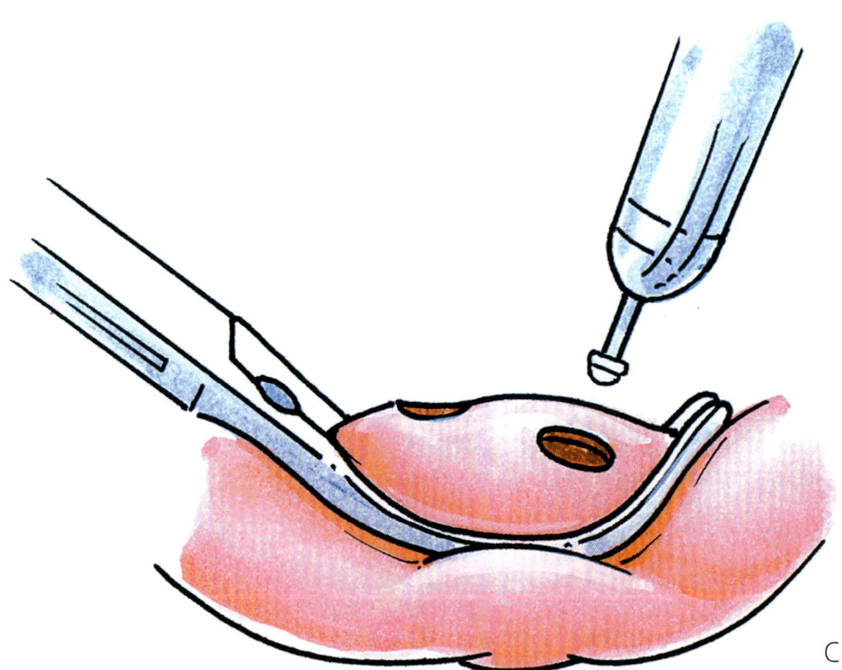

C. 用主动脉打孔器（通常用 5mm 型号）将刺开处主动脉壁打孔，形成圆形的开口。

C. An aortic punch (usually 5 mm) is used to make circular holes in the aortic wall.

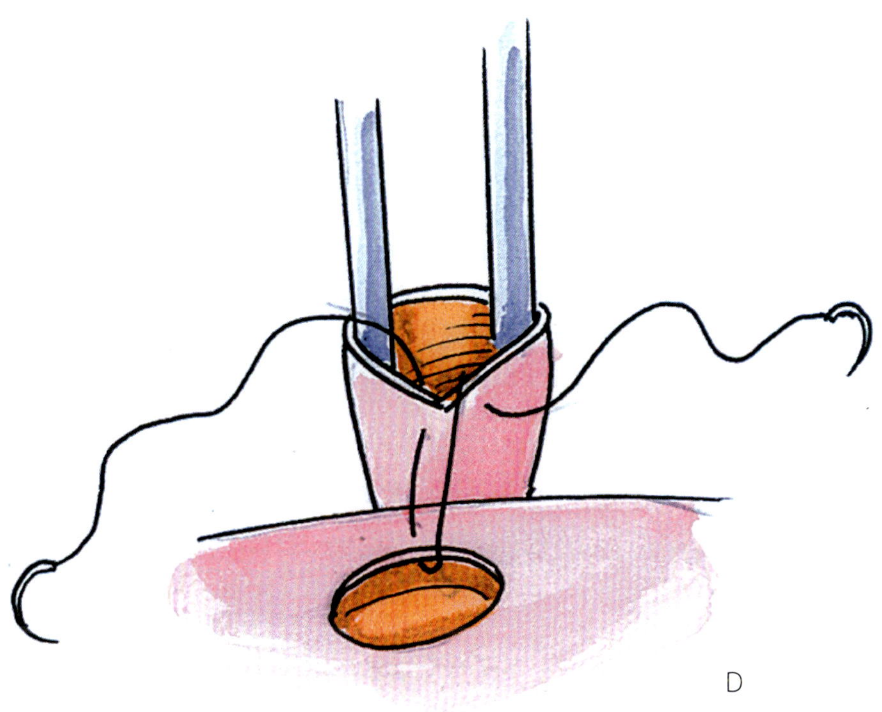

D. 充盈大隐静脉，选择合适的长度剪断。此时心脏未充满，桥血管长度测量应以心包为参照。远心端剪成45°斜面。用5-0 Prolene双头缝线由足跟开始做几个单纯连续缝针。

D. Fill the GSV and harvest it at a suitable length. The length of bridging vessels should be measured with the pericardium as a reference, for the heart is not full. Cut the distal end into a 45° bevel and perform several simple running sutures from the heel with double-armed 5-0 Prolene sutures.

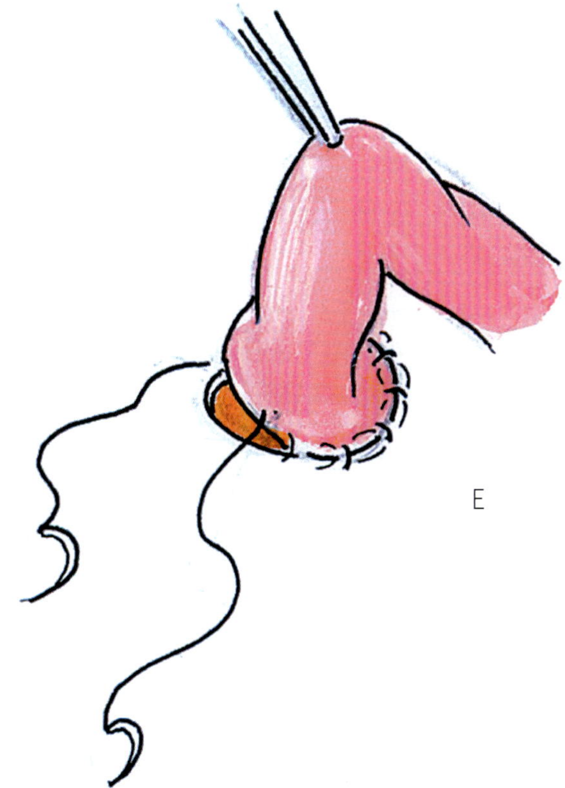

E. 拉下后左侧继续缝合。

E. Pull down the bridging vein and continue sutures at the left side.

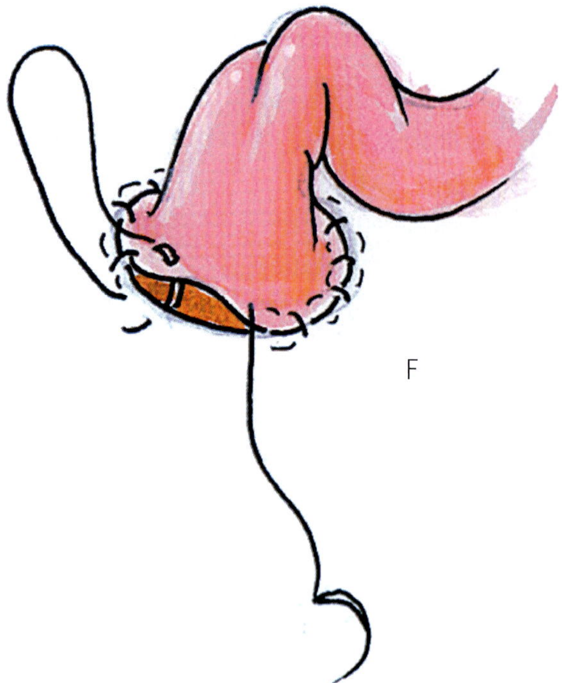

F. 换头缝合右侧。
F. Suture the right side with another needle.

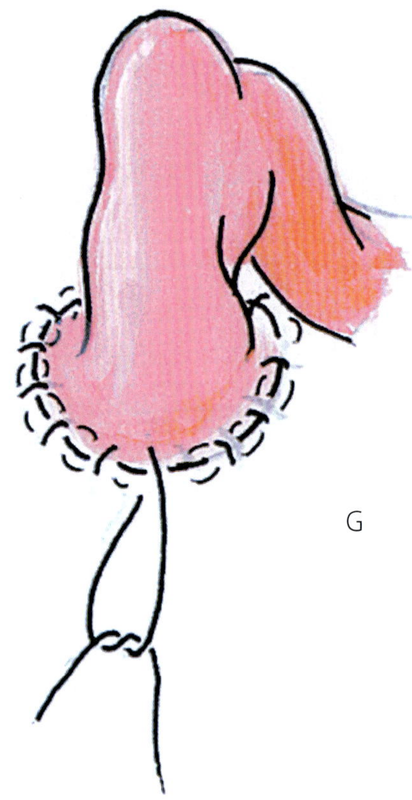

G. 结扎缝线，吻合完成。
G. The ligation is tied and the anastomosis is completed.

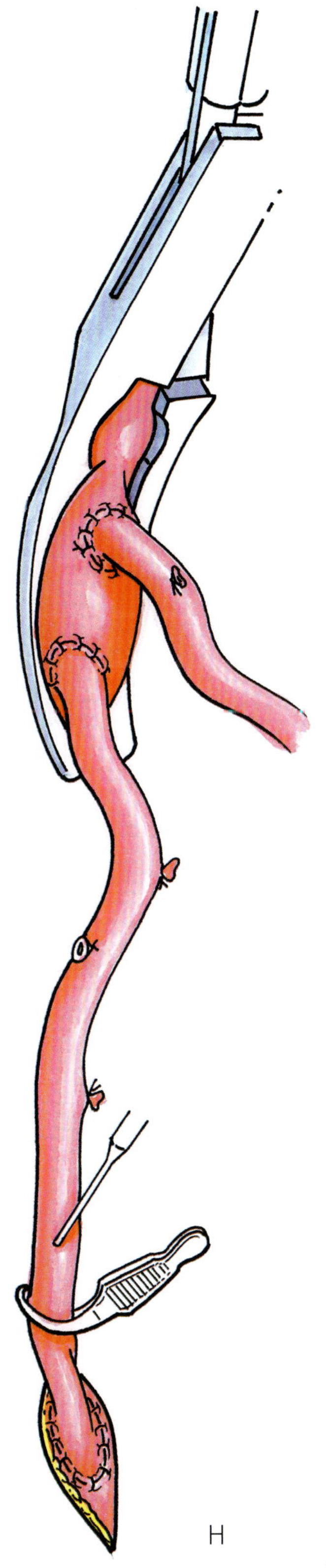

H. 开放侧壁钳，在大隐静脉桥血管靠近 Bulldog 处，用细针刺孔排气。

H. Remove the site-biting clamps and vent the GSV near Bulldog with needle-pierced holes.

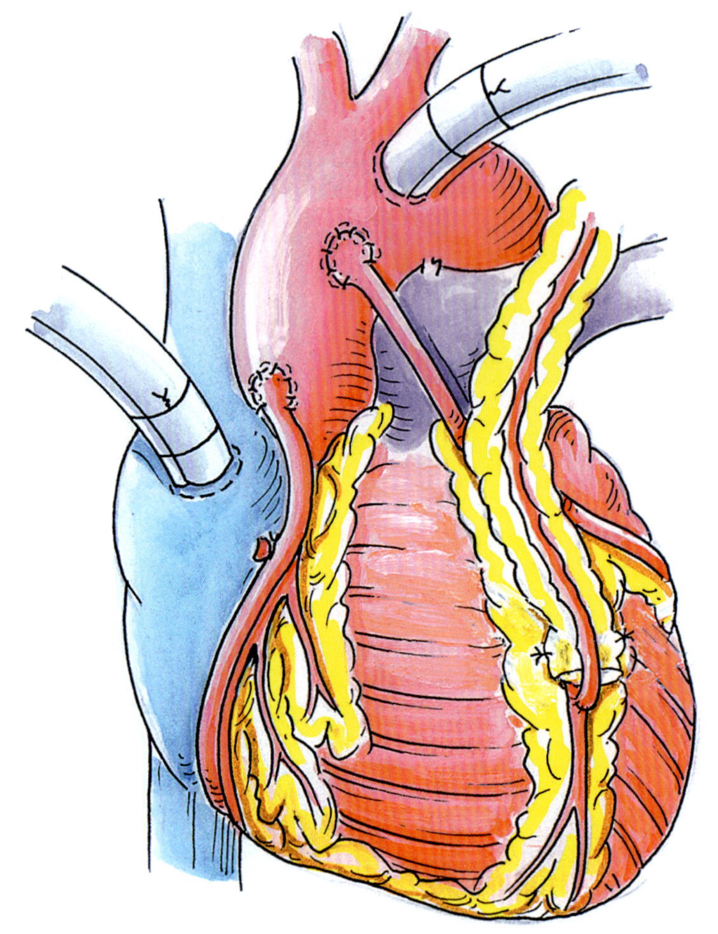

I. 全部吻合完毕。左侧的大隐静脉桥血管由左胸廓内动脉桥血管下穿过。
I. The anastomosis is completed. The GSV graft at the left side is passed under the left ITA graft.

第二节 全动脉冠状动脉旁路移植术

Section 2 Total Arterial Coronary Artery Bypass Grafting

搭桥血管全部用动脉的搭桥手术称全动脉冠状动脉旁路移植术。通常前降支和右冠状动脉分别用左、右胸廓内动脉吻合，其余靶血管选用桡动脉或/和胃网膜右动脉吻合。胃网膜右动脉由肝动脉的分支胃十二指肠动脉在十二指肠后上方发出，在十二指肠后方下行至胃结肠韧带内沿胃大弯左行，至胃大弯约中点处与胃网膜左动脉分支相吻合。通常其远端内径大于1mm，其长度可以到达任一冠状动脉施行吻合。

In total arterial CABG, all the bridging grafts are arteries. Usually, the left and right ITAs are used to be anastomosed with the anterior descending branch and the right coronary artery respectively, and other grafting vessels come from radial arteries or/and right gastroepiploic artery (RGA). The RGA originates from the gastroduodenal artery, a branch of the hepatic artery, at the posterior superior of the duodenum. It descends from the posterior of the duodenum to the gastrocolic ligament, goes leftward along the greater gastric curvature to its middle point, and links with the branch of the left gastroepiploic artery. Usually, the inner diameter of the RGA's distal extremity is larger than 1 mm, and it is also long enough to bypass any coronary artery.

图 2-2-1 胃网膜右动脉与双侧胸廓内动脉全动脉冠状动脉旁路移植术
Figure 2-2-1 Total arterial CABG with RGA and bilateral ITAs

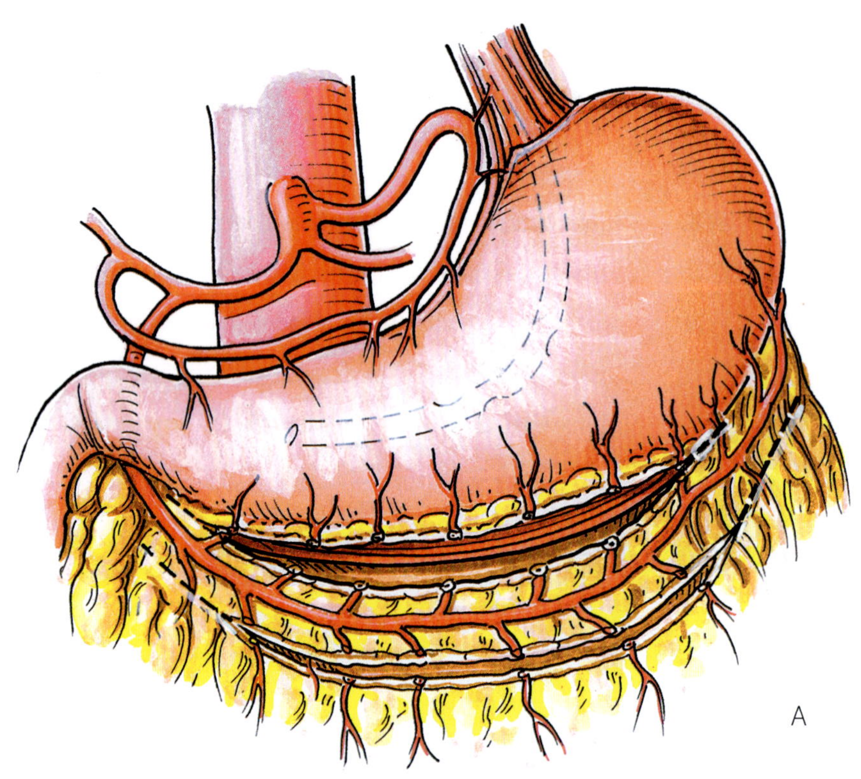

A. 将胸骨正中切口向下延长至剑突下 3~5cm，经腹白线进入腹腔。先从胃大弯中部用电刀分离胃网膜右动脉网膜侧至幽门处，结扎出血点。然后分离胃大弯左侧，逐一结扎其向胃的分支。注意近端分离时勿损伤十二指肠动脉。

A. Make a median sternal incision and extend it downward to 3-5 cm below the xiphoid process until it arrives at the abdominal cavity through linea alba. First, the segment of the RGA in the middle of the greater gastric curvature is freed from the omentum to the pylorus using an electrotome, and ligation is performed at the hemorrhagic spot. Dissection is continued at the left side of the greater gastric curvature, and all the branches of the RGA to the stomach are ligated. Don't damage the duodenal artery during proximal dissection.

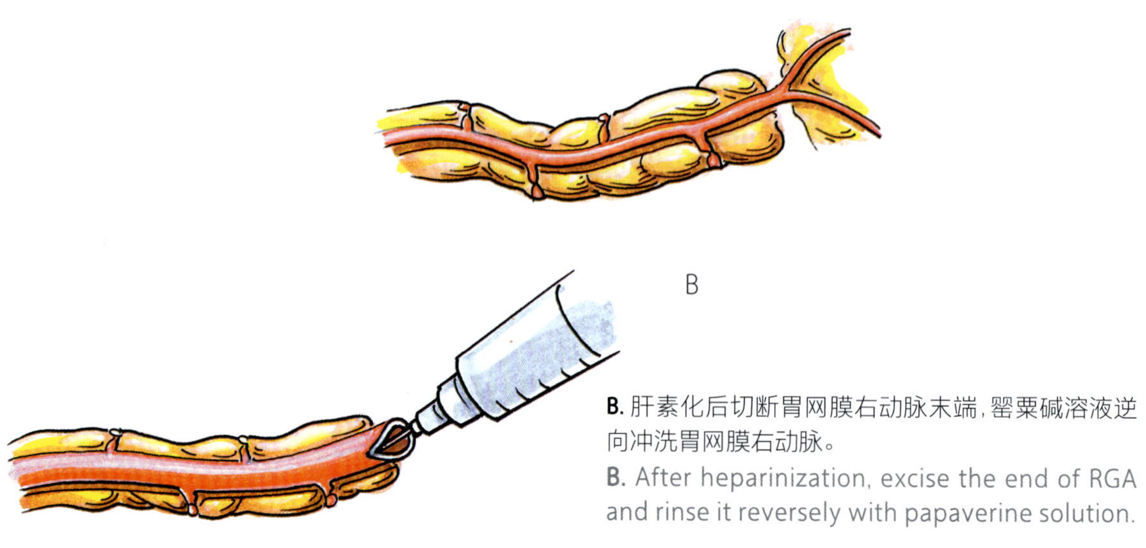

B. 肝素化后切断胃网膜右动脉末端，罂粟碱溶液逆向冲洗胃网膜右动脉。

B. After heparinization, excise the end of RGA and rinse it reversely with papaverine solution.

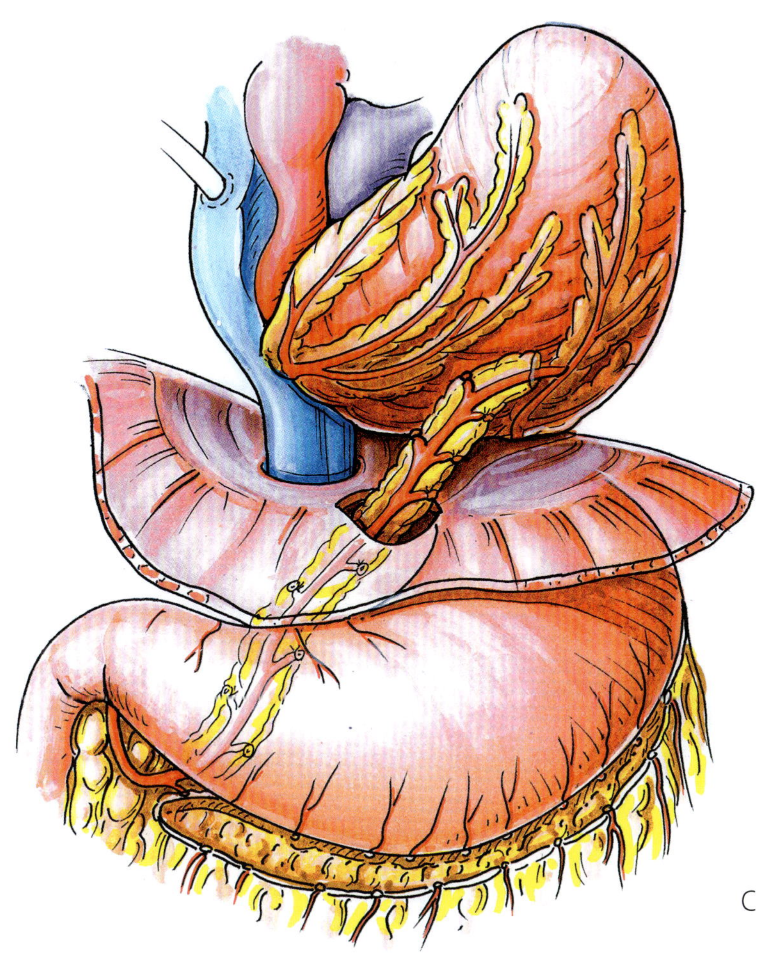

C. 将带蒂胃网膜右动脉由胃后方肝左叶前方经膈肌顶部切口拉入心包腔，与钝缘支端侧吻合。若与前降支端侧吻合，膈肌切口要前移，务使胃网膜右动脉桥血管顺畅无折曲。

C. Pull the pedicled RGA from the anterior left lobe of the liver and the posterior of the stomach into the pericardial cavity through the top incision of the diaphragm. Then, anastomose the artery with the end of the obtuse marginal branch. If the RGA is anastomosed end-to-side to the anterior descending branch, move forward the diaphragm incision, so that the RGA graft is smooth and straight.

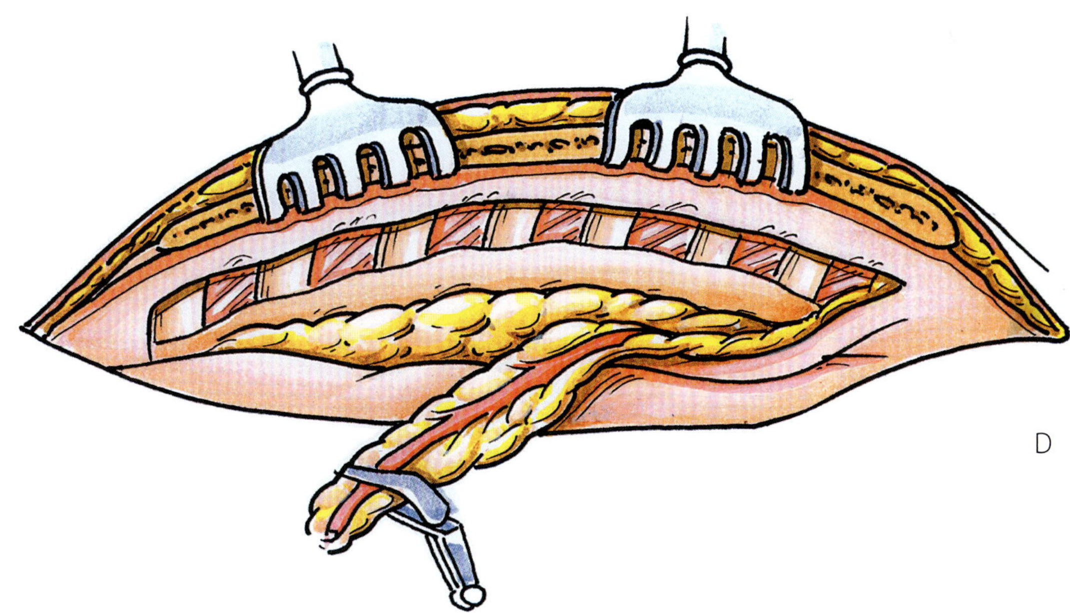

D. 游离带蒂右胸廓内动脉，方法与游离左胸廓内动脉同。

D. Dissociate the right ITA pedicle with the same method as dissociating the left ITA.

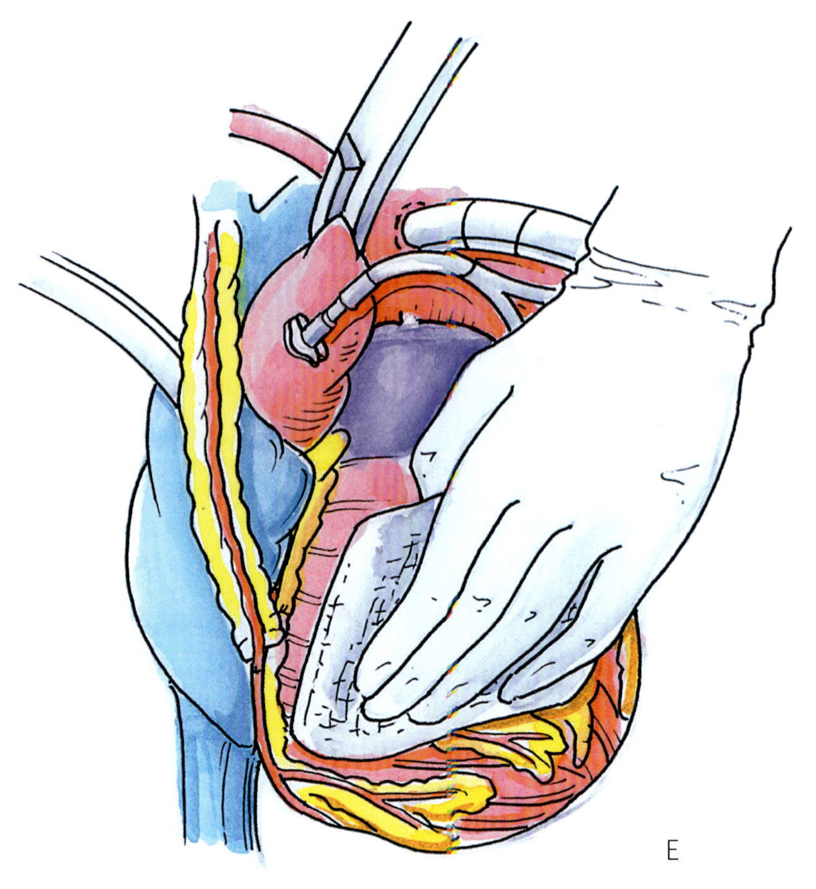

E. 带蒂右胸廓内动脉的长度可以到达右冠状动脉远端，一般不足以到达后降支。将右胸廓内动脉与右冠状动脉远端做端侧吻合。

E. The length of the right ITA pedicle can reach the distal end of the right coronary artery but is generally insufficient to reach the posterior descending artery. The end-to-side anastomose is performed between the right ITA and the distal end of the right coronary artery.

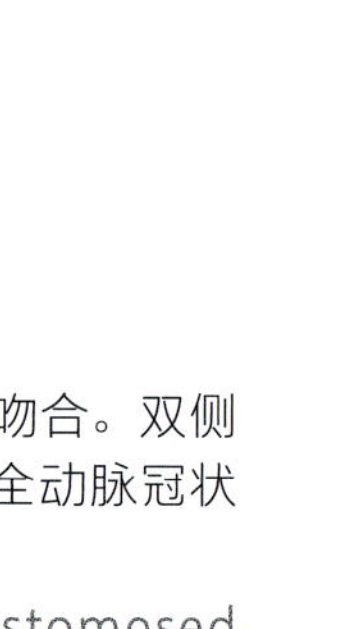

F. 左胸廓内动脉与前降支端侧吻合。双侧胸廓内动脉和胃网膜右动脉的全动脉冠状动脉旁路移植术完成。

F. When the left ITA is anastomosed end-to-side with the end of an anterior descending branch, total arterial CABG with RGA and bilateral ITA is finished.

图 2-2-2 桡动脉与双侧胸廓内动脉全动脉冠状动脉旁路移植术
Figure 2-2-2 Total arterial CABG with radial artery and bilateral ITAs

桡动脉有足够的长度、接近冠状动脉的口径和良好的远期通畅率，是仅次于胸廓内动脉的动脉桥血管选择。桡动脉的平滑肌层厚，容易痉挛，曾一度被放弃使用。钙通道阻滞剂的应用，使其得以再度被用于冠状动脉旁路移植术。

With a sufficient length, a caliber close to the coronary arteries, and a good long-term patency rate, the radial artery is the best choice for artery grafts only next to ITA. However, due to the thick smooth muscle layer, it tends to be spastic easily, and hence had once fallen out of favor. Fortunately, the application of calcium channel blockers allows it to be used again for CABG now.

摘取桡动脉前必须做 Allen 试验测试尺动脉侧支循环是否良好。方法是于腕部压住桡动脉和尺动脉，握拳运动后展开手指，放开尺动脉后观察手掌血色恢复时间，通常 6s 以内恢复者可以安全摘取桡动脉。桡动脉多摘取单侧，右利者取左桡动脉。必要时也可摘取双侧桡动脉。

An Allen test must be performed to test the circulation of the collateral ulnar artery before harvesting. The radial and the ulnar arteries are compressed at the wrist while the patient opens and closes the fist, and the pressure on the ulnar artery is then released to calculate the time when the skin of the palm becomes flushed. Usually, with a time within 6 seconds, the radial artery harvest is safe. The radial artery harvest is often performed on the unilateral side, and for the dextral patients, the left radial artery is chosen, but if necessary, bilateral radial arteries can also be harvested.

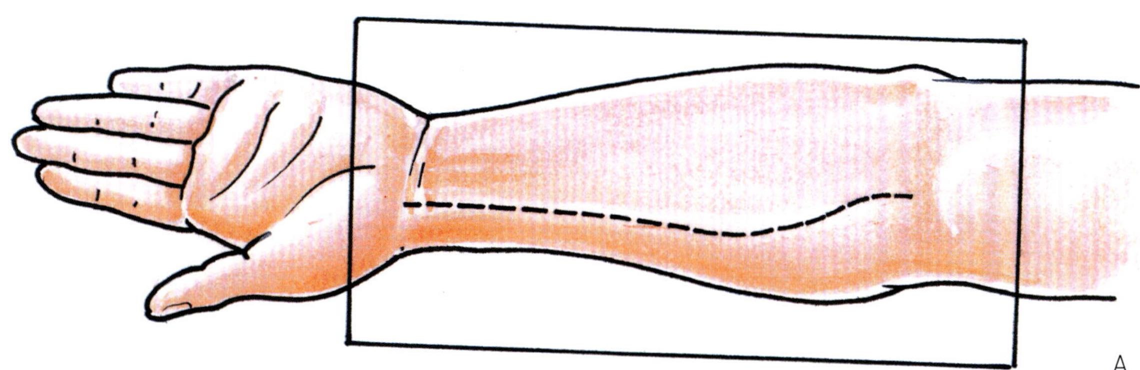

A. 沿桡动脉搏动处和肱桡肌缘从肘关节至腕关节做一弧形切口。

A. An arc incision is made in the forearm from the elbow to the wrist along the radial pulse and the belly of the brachioradialis muscle margin.

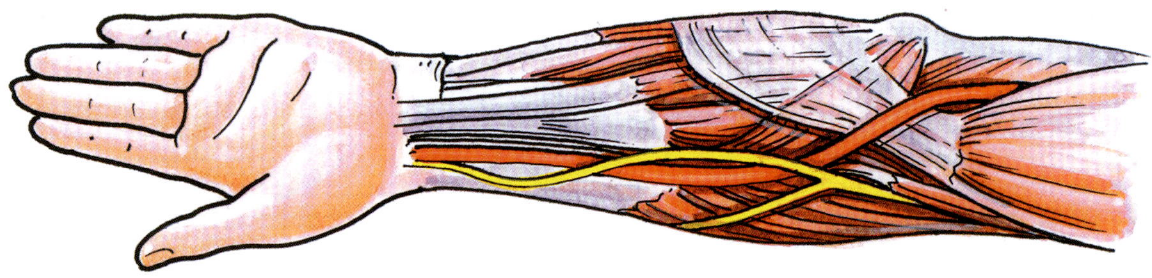

B

B. 逐步分离出桡动脉，结扎其分支。血管外膜尽量保留，甚至连同伴行静脉一并以血管蒂的形式分离下来，有利于保护桡动脉内膜和减少桡动脉痉挛。

B. Gradually dissociate the radial artery and ligate its branches. The outer vascular membrane should be preserved to the greatest extent, and even the accompanying veins should be retained with the vascular pedicle during the dissection, which can protect the radial artery intima and reduce the radial artery spasm.

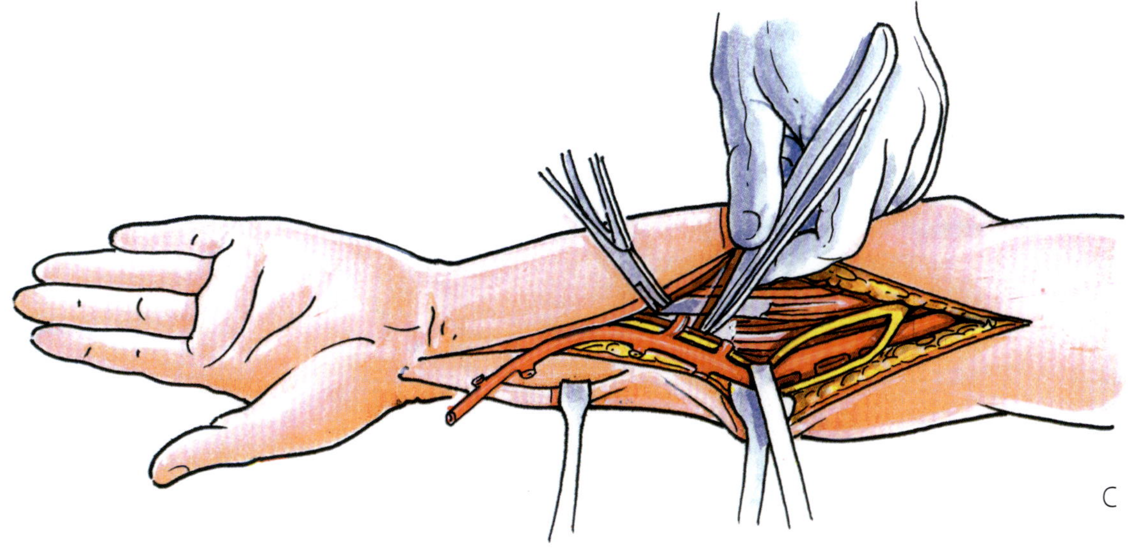

C. 注意避免损伤桡动脉外侧的桡神经。
C. Care should be taken to avoid damaging the radial nerve on the lateral side of the radial artery.

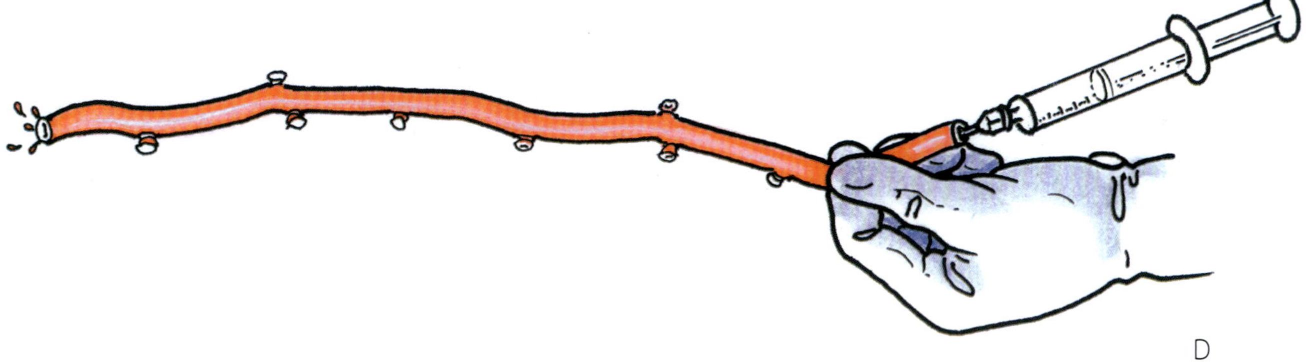

D. 两端切下后用含肝素的生理盐水冲洗桡动脉。
D. After the two ends are cut, the harvested radial artery is irrigated with heparinized saline.

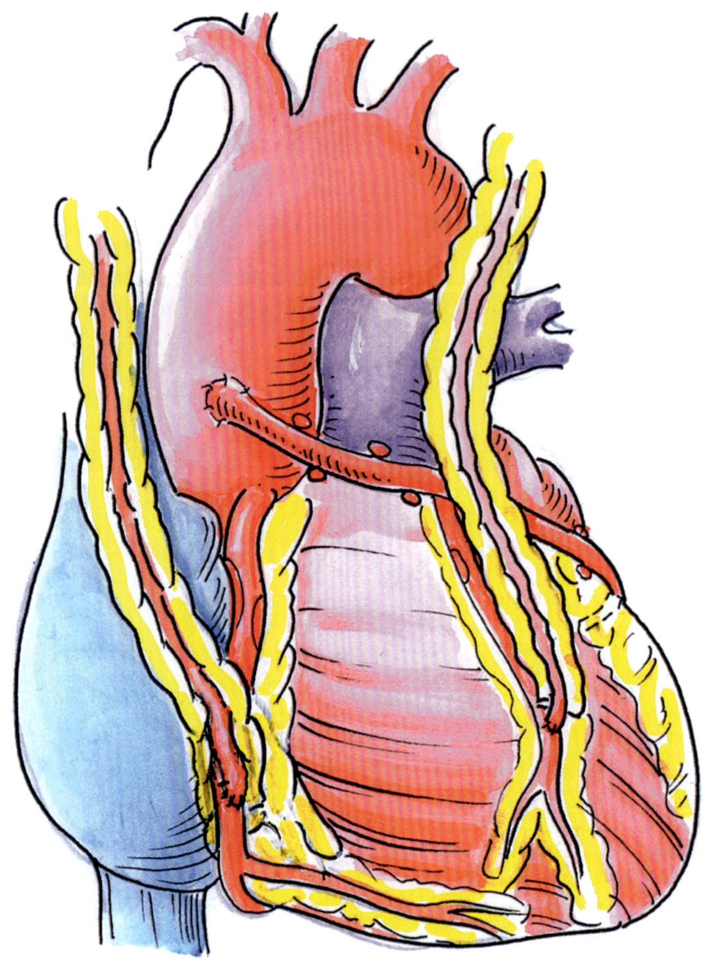

E. 桡动脉远端与钝缘支端侧吻合，近端与升主动脉端侧吻合。左胸廓内动脉与前降支端侧吻合。右胸廓内动脉与右冠状动脉远端做端侧吻合。桡动脉和双侧胸廓内动脉的全动脉冠状动脉旁路移植术完成。

E. The distal side of the radial artery is anastomosed end-to-side to the obtuse marginal artery and the proximal side to the ascending aorta. The left ITA is anastomosed end-to-side to the anterior descending side, and the right ITA is anastomosed end-to-side to the distal end of the right coronary artery. Total arterial CABG with radial artery and bilateral ITAs is completed.

第三节 非体外循环冠状动脉旁路移植术

Section 3 Off-Pump Coronary Artery Bypass Grafting

非体外循环冠状动脉旁路移植术亦称不停跳搭桥术，除巨大左心室外，适用于冠状动脉各支病变，包括多支病变。尤其适用于有体外循环禁忌的病例。

Off-pump coronary artery bypass grafting (OPCAB) is also known as CABG on beating heart. In addition to giant left ventricle, it is indicated for diseases in all branches of coronary artery, including multi-vessel disease, and is especially suitable for cases with contraindications of extracorporeal circulation.

图 2-3-1　非体外循环冠状动脉旁路移植术
Figure 2-3-1　Off-pump coronary artery bypass grafting

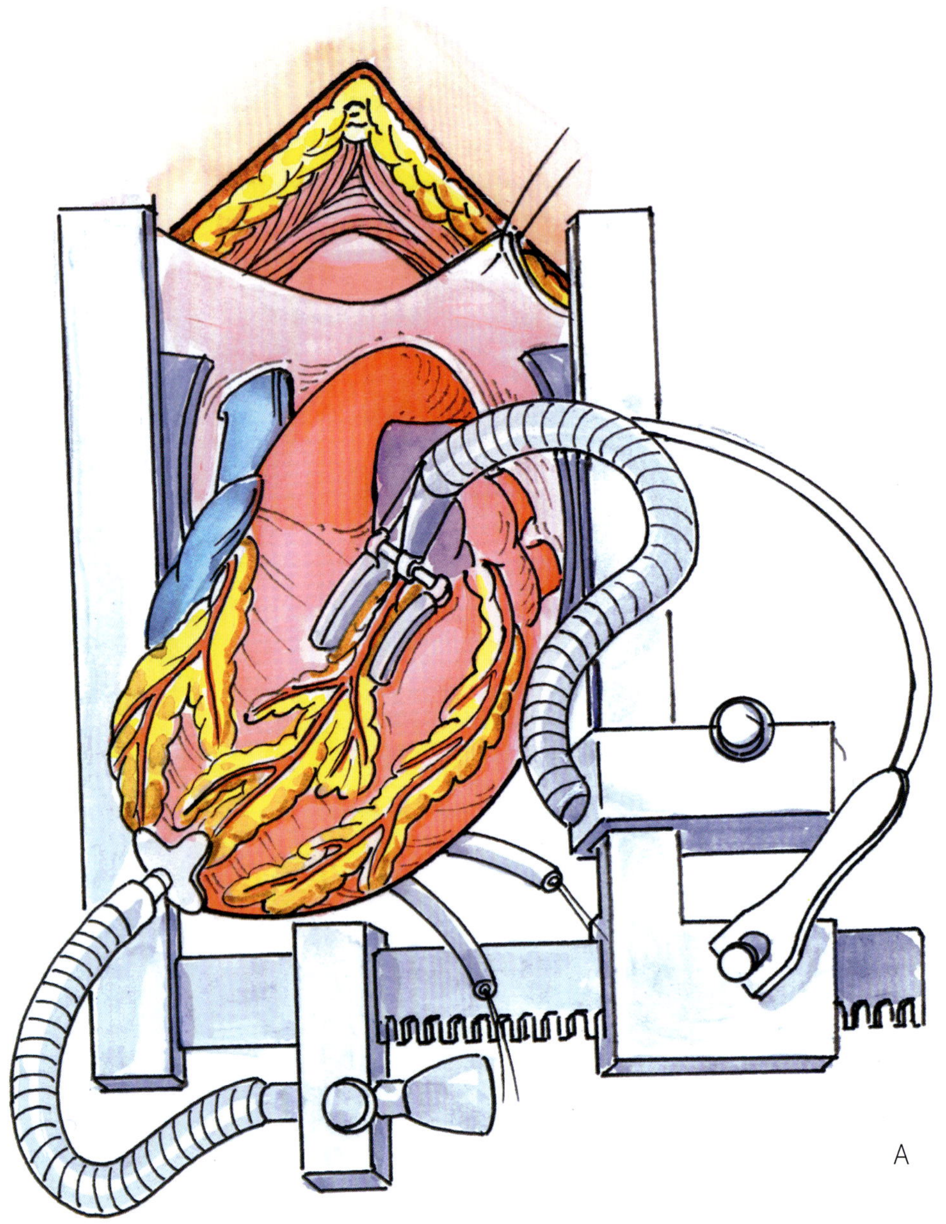

A. 胸骨正中切口，撑开器撑开胸骨，切开心包并悬吊。非体外循环冠状动脉旁路移植术首先做最容易显露的前降支搭桥。右倾位，心包靠近右上、下肺静脉处用粗丝线各悬吊 1 针用作牵引，心尖牵引器将心尖向右上方牵出，稳定器将前降支欲做吻合口处局部固定。

A. A sternotomy is made, and the sternum is opened by a rib spreader. Cut the pericardium and suspend it. OPCAB is begun with the bypass of the anterior descending branch, which can be exposed most easily. In a right-tilted position, the pericardium is suspended by heavy sutures near the right superior and inferior pulmonary veins for traction. A heart apical retractor is used to pull the cardiac apex out to the upper right, and the stabilizer to partially fix the segment of the anterior descending branch to be grafted.

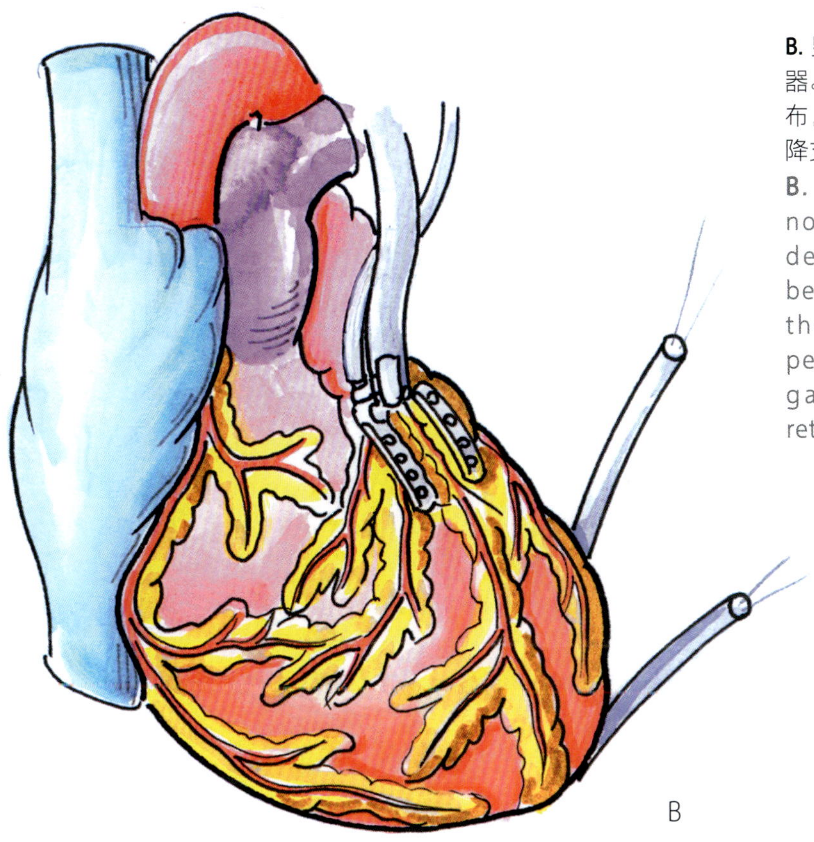

B. 显露前降支也可不用心尖牵引器。托出心尖，心包内垫以温盐水纱布，拉紧牵引线，亦能良好地显露前降支。

B. A heart apical retractor is not a necessity. The anterior descending branch can also be well exposed by displacing the cardiac apex, lining the pericardium with warm saline gauze, and tightening the retracting sutures.

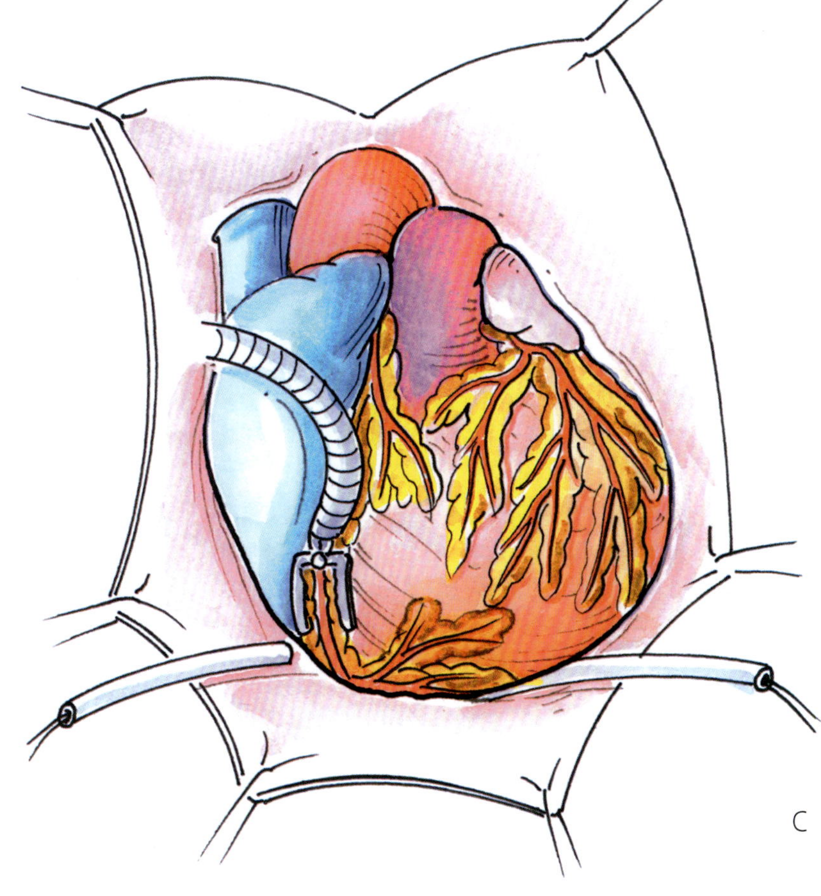

C. 头低脚高位，膈面心包和下腔静脉外侧心包牵引，可显露右冠状动脉远段。

C. In the Trendelenburg position, the distal segment of the right coronary artery can be exposed by retracting the pericardium of the diaphragmatic surface and the lateral aspect of the inferior vena cava.

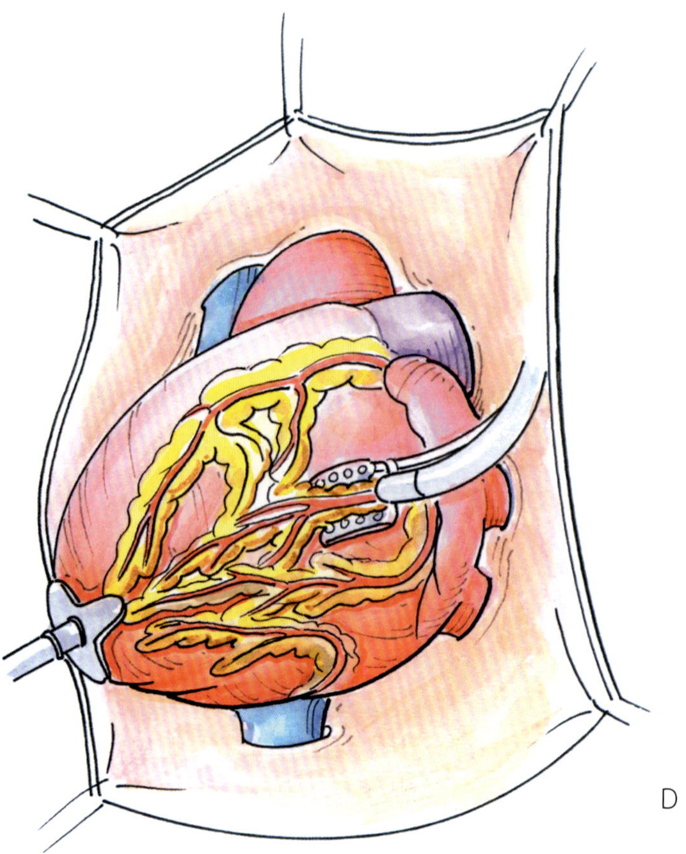

D. 头低脚高位，心尖牵引器将心尖向右上方牵出，显露钝缘支。
D. In the Trendelenburg position, the obtuse marginal artery can be exposed by pulling the cardiac apex out to the upper right with a heart apical retractor.

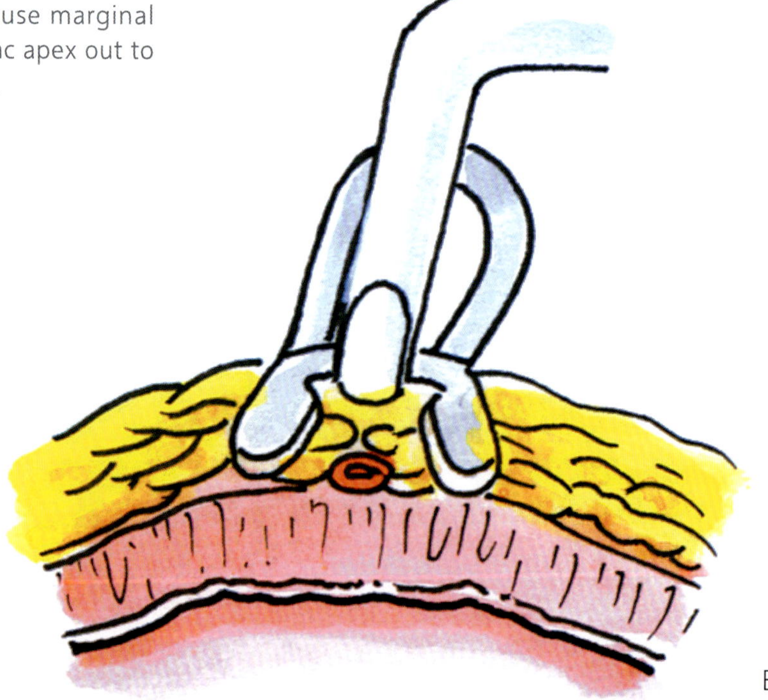

E. 稳定器将吻合口处局部固定，以利吻合操作。
E. The stabilizer can partially fix the anastomotic stoma to facilitate anastomosis.

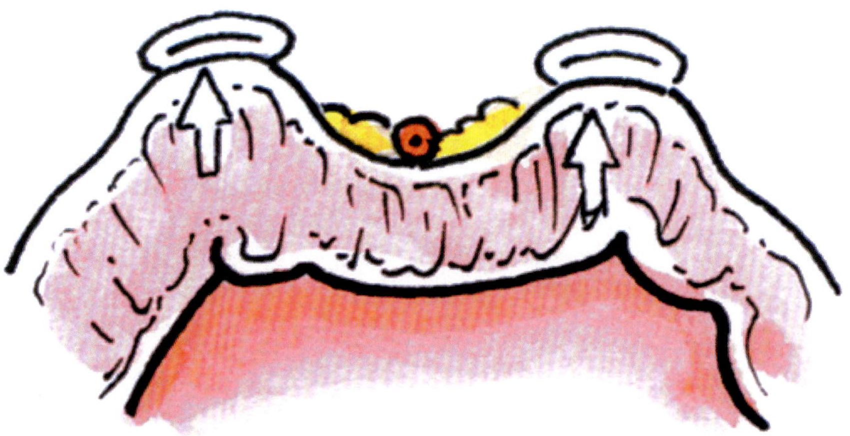

F. 稳定器通过负压吸附心脏壁而限制吻合口局部的心脏活动，对心脏的压迫有限。

F. The stabilizer partially limits the cardiac activity at the anastomotic stoma by absorbing the heart wall with negative pressure, which is limited to the compression of the heart.

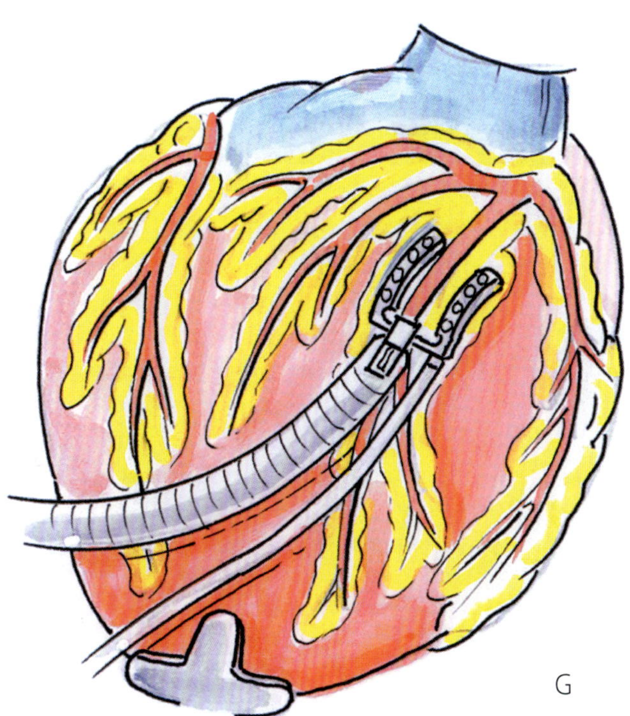

G. 显露钝缘支时空间狭小，有时需倒置稳定器，以利稳定器置入和吻合操作。

G. After the obtuse marginal artery is exposed, if the space is narrow, sometimes the stabilizer needs to be inverted to facilitate the stabilization and anastomosis.

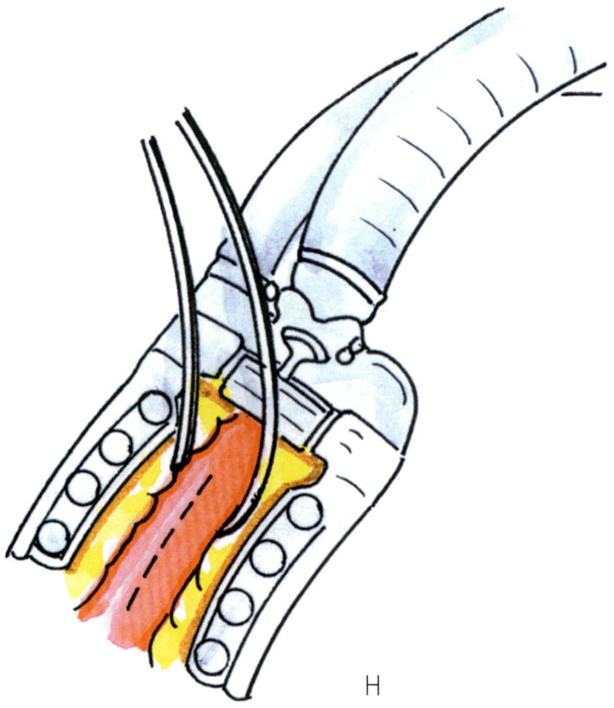

H. 确定并显露固定靶血管欲做吻合口处，切开心外膜，暴露冠状动脉，吻合口近端缝钝头针阻断带。若用 4-0 Prolene 代替专用阻断带，则进针和出针须离开冠状动脉一些，利用心肌的隔垫，避免缝线切割损伤冠状动脉。阻断冠状动脉后切开。

H. The segment of the target vessel is identified for the anastomotic stoma. The epicardium is cut, the coronary artery is exposed, and a blocking band with a blunt needle is placed at the coronary artery near the proximal end of the anastomotic stoma. If a 4-0 Prolene is used instead, the sutures should be extended to the myocardium away from the coronary artery, for the damages to the coronary artery can be avoided with the myocardium as the pledget. After the block, the coronary artery can be dissected.

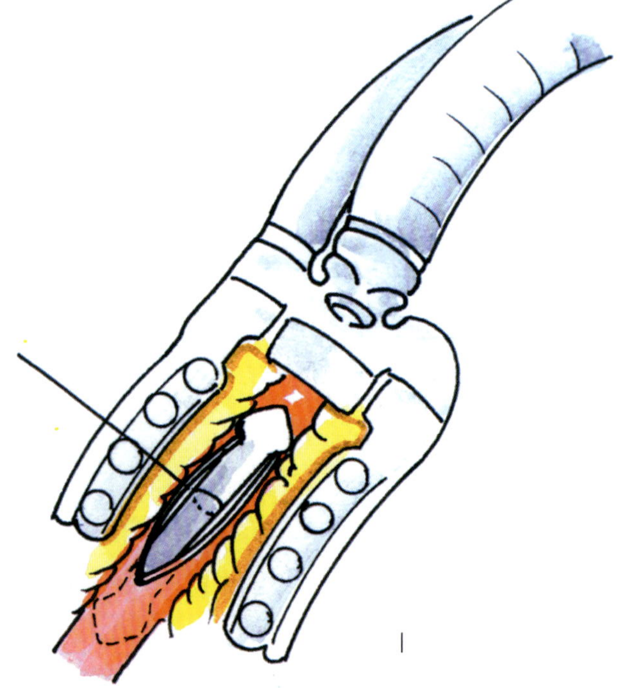

I. 冠状动脉腔内置入口径匹配的分流栓，松开阻断带。

I. Put a caliber-matched intracoronary shunt in the coronary artery and release the blocking band.

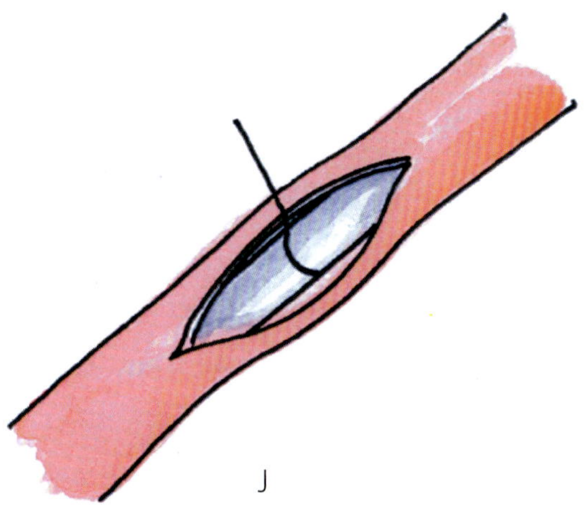

J. 分流栓是中空结构，由吻合口置入冠状动脉后，其远端的冠状动脉继续得到血供，而吻合口基本没有血液涌出。

J. After the intracoronary shunt (a hollow structure) is placed into the coronary artery through the anastomotic stoma, it can provide sufficient blood flow to the distal coronary artery, nearly with no blood oozing from the anastomotic stoma.

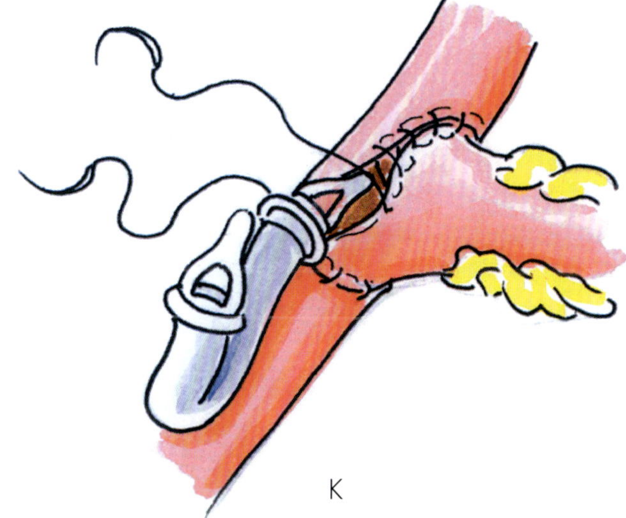

K. 吻合口缝合接近完成时，取出分流栓，然后完成吻合。

K. When the anastomosis is nearly completed, the intracoronary shunt is removed, and the anastomosis is finished.

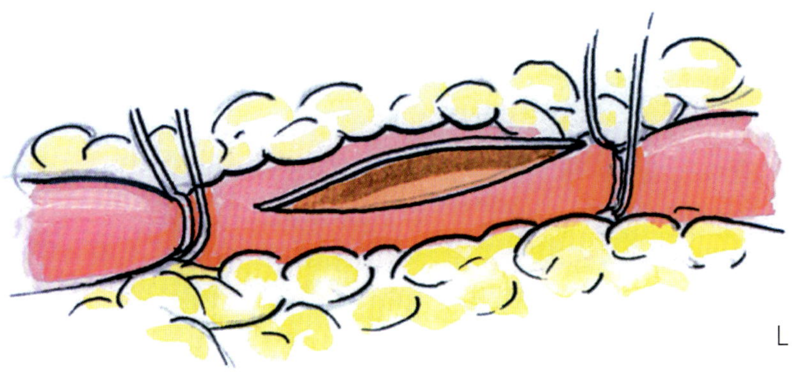

L. 如果没有合适的分流栓，也可以将冠状动脉吻合口两端阻断，切开冠状动脉后直接吻合。

L. If a suitable intracoronary shunt is not available, the coronary artery anastomotic stoma can also be blocked at both ends and then directly anastomosed after the dissection of the coronary artery.

第四节　左心室室壁瘤切除术

Section 4　Resection of Left Ventricular Aneurysm

急性心肌梗死后的最常见机械并发症是室壁瘤。室壁瘤由心肌梗死部位心肌坏死后的瘢痕组织形成，该部位的心肌丧失收缩功能，它的矛盾运动导致心室射血功能下降。室壁瘤切除后的缺损修复，较小者可用经典的“三明治”法直接缝闭，较大者用补片法修复，以维持心室的几何形态及容量。

The ventricular aneurysm is the most common mechanical complication of acute myocardial infarction (AMI). Formed by the scar tissue caused by myocardial necrosis at the site of myocardial infarction where the cardiac muscle loses its systolic function and its contradiction movement usually leads to a lower ventricular ejection function. For a smaller defect after the resection of ventricular aneurysm, a direct suture and closure can be made by the classic sandwich technique, and for a larger one, patch repair is made to maintain the geometric shape and capacity of the ventricle.

图 2-4-1　左心室前壁室壁瘤切除术

Figure 2-4-1　Resection of anterior left ventricular aneurysm

A. 体外循环下室壁瘤向心内塌陷，扪诊该处心室壁较薄。由此沿前降支左侧纵行切开室壁瘤，清除血栓。心腔内看到较薄、没有肌小梁的部位就是室壁瘤的范围。切除部分室壁瘤壁，靠正常心肌处保留一圈约 1cm 宽瘤壁供缝合。较小的左心室室壁瘤用"三明治"法修复，切口两侧覆以毡片条间断水平褥式缝闭。

A. The ventricular aneurysm collapses inward under extracorporeal circulation, and a thin ventricular wall can be felt in palpation. First, longitudinally incise the ventricular aneurysm along the left side of the anterior descending branch from the thinner site, and then remove the thrombus. The range of ventricular aneurysm involves all the thinner parts without trabecular muscles. Remove part of the ventricular aneurysm wall, and reserve a circle of aneurysm wall (about 1 cm wide) near the non-infarcted myocardium for suture. For the smaller left ventricular aneurysm, the sandwich technique is used: two sides of the incision area are covered with felt strips, and the interrupted horizontal mattress sutures are performed.

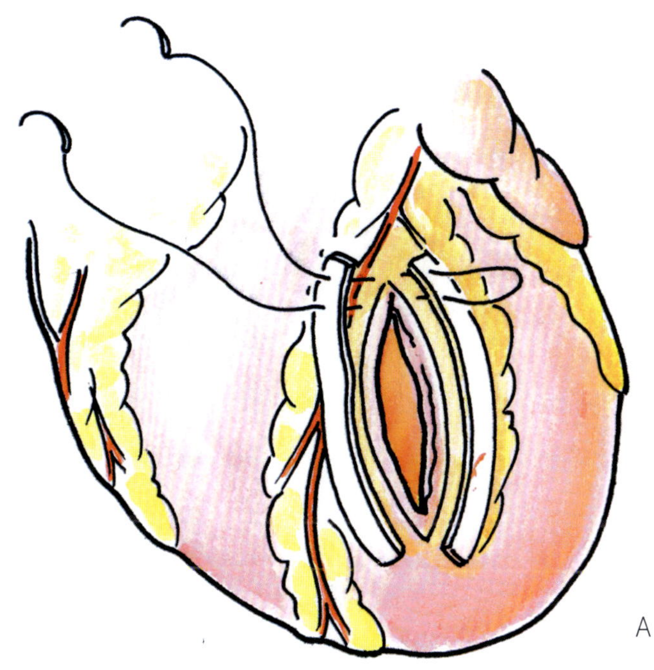

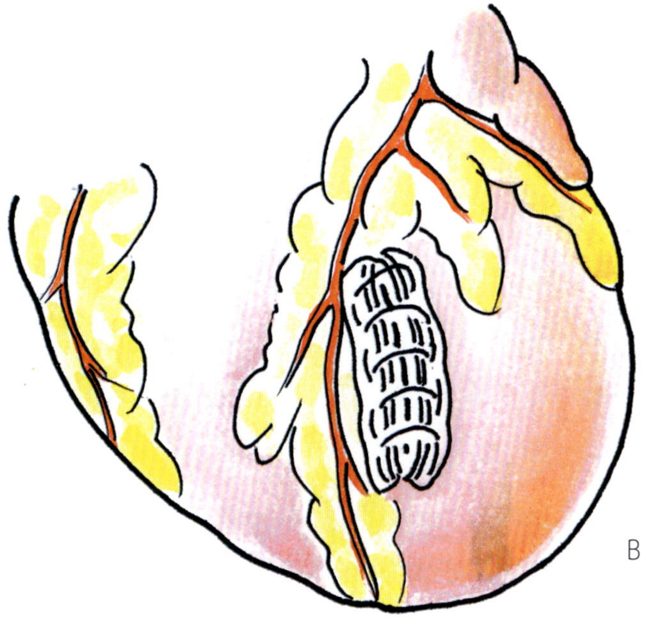

B. 结扎后再做一层单纯连续缝合。

B. Additionally, make simple continuous suture after ligation.

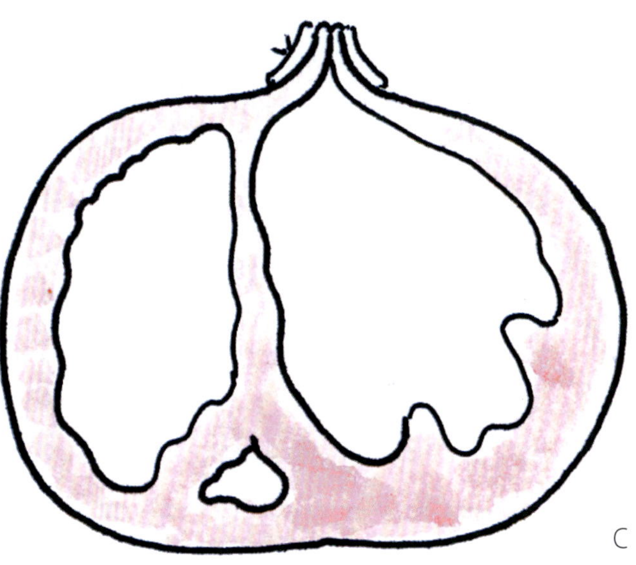

C. 修补完毕示意图。

C. The schematic diagram after the repair.

图 2-4-2　Dor 氏手术
Figure 2-4-2　Dor procedure

Dor 氏手术是一种治疗室壁瘤的左心室重建技术，亦称心室内环缩补片成形术。该术式对左心室的几何形态和容量有着更好的保护，成为现在治疗左心室室壁瘤的常用方式。

The Dor procedure, also known as endoventricular circular patch plasty (EVCPP), is a left ventricular reconstruction technique for the treatment of a ventricular aneurysm. This procedure has become a common treatment for the left ventricular aneurysm, for it can provide better protection for the geometry and capacity of the left ventricle.

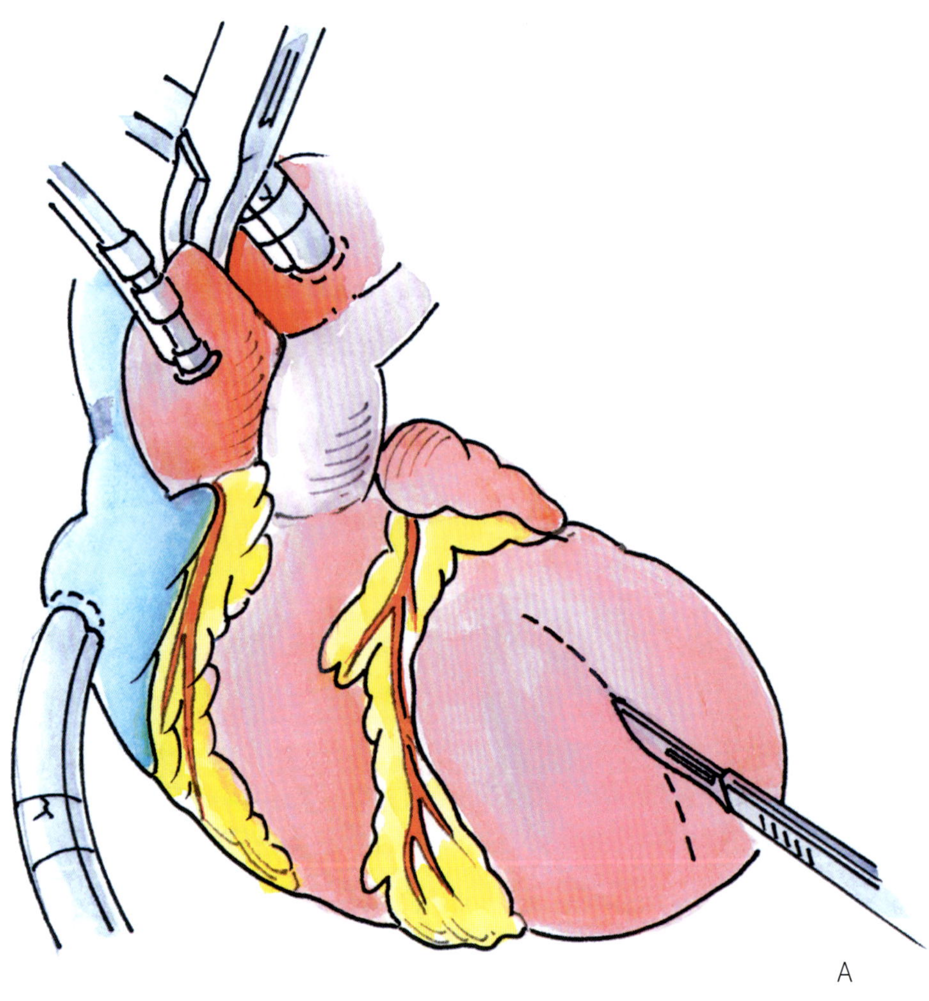

A. 体外循环心脏停搏下纵行切开室壁瘤。

A. A vertical incision is performed on the ventricular aneurysm under the extracorporeal circulation and cardiac arrest.

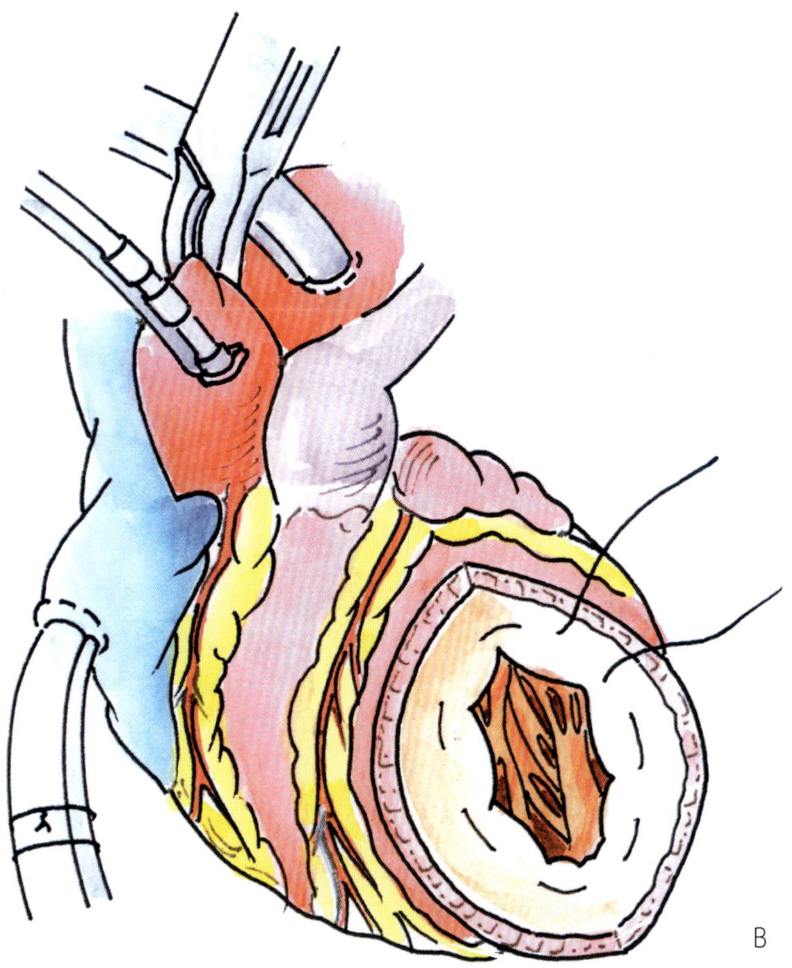

B. 在室壁瘤和正常心肌交界处荷包缝合，将室壁瘤颈部缩小，使左心室的大小恢复到心肌梗死前的状态。

B. A purse-string suture is performed at the junction of the aneurysm and non-infarcted myocardium. During the suture, the neck of the aneurysm is reduced to resume the shape of the left ventricle to its pre-infarction state.

C. 裁剪一椭圆形补片，在缩小的室壁瘤颈部修补左心室壁，单纯连续缝合。该补片还可以向左心室内深入缝至室间隔，以修补前间隔缺损或将反常活动的前间隔隔离。

C. Cut an oval patch. Put the patch on the neck of the reduced ventricular aneurysm to repair the left ventricular wall and perform the simple continuous sutures. The patch can also be sutured deeply into the interventricular septum from the left ventricle to repair the anterior septal defect or isolate the anomalous anterior septum.

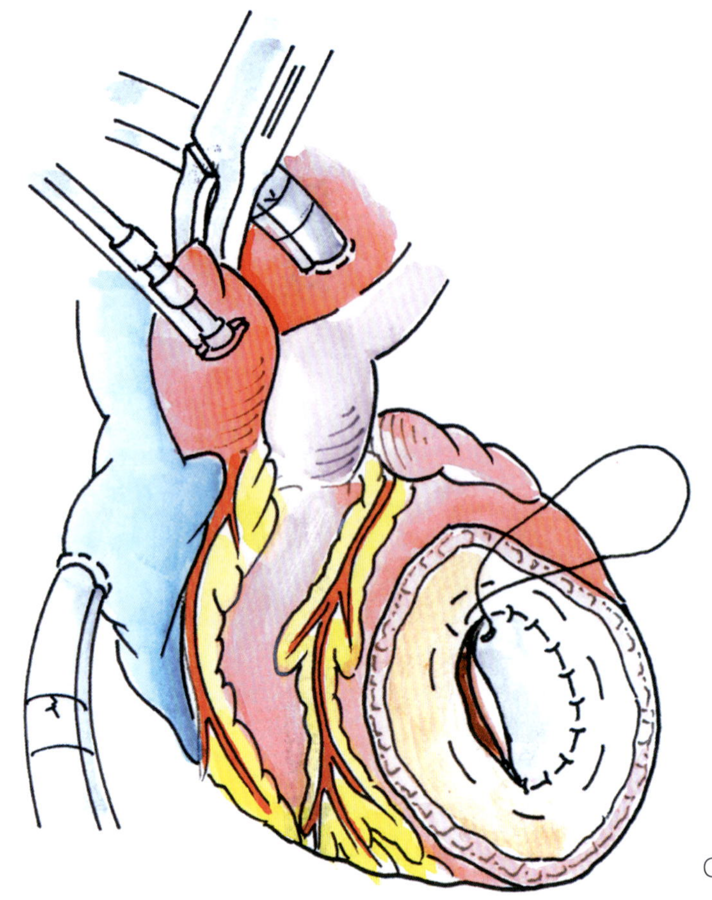

C

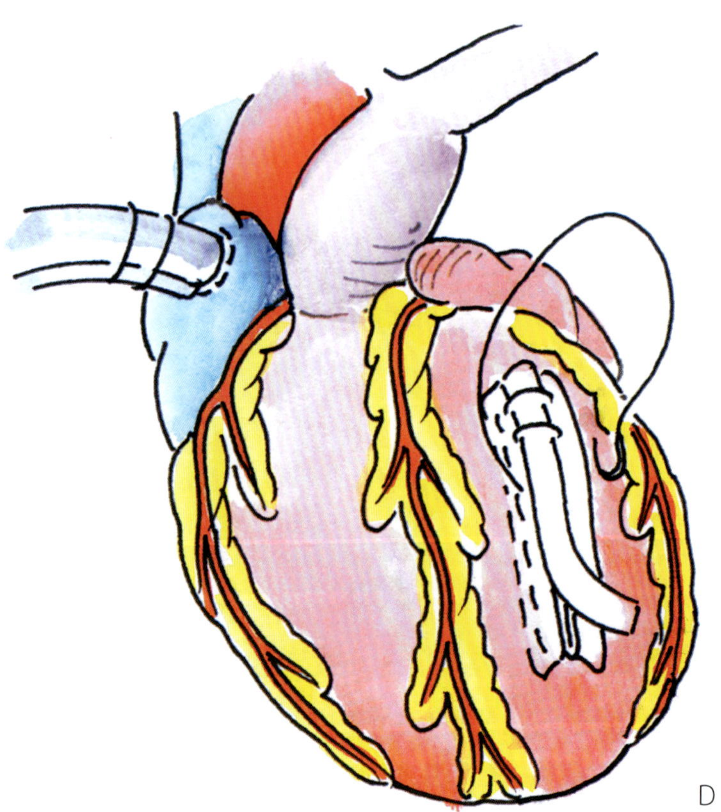

D

D. 切除多余的室壁瘤，缝闭室壁瘤覆盖补片，使补片成为所谓的“心内补片”。室壁瘤切口两侧覆以毡片条，连续褥式外翻缝合，结扎后再做一层单纯连续缝合。

D. Remove the redundant ventricular aneurysm and repair the aneurysm with the patch, making the patch a so-called “internal patch”. Both sides of the ventricular aneurysm incision are covered with felt strips, and continuous exstrophy mattress sutures are performed. After ligation, another layer of simple continuous suture is performed.

第五节 心肌梗死后室间隔穿孔修补术

Section 5 Repair of Postinfarction Ventricular Septal Perforation

心肌梗死后室间隔穿孔亦称心肌梗死后室间隔缺损，是急性心肌梗死的严重并发症。心肌梗死后室间隔缺损患者多因心脏低心排血量进而发展为多脏器功能衰竭而不治，死亡率极高。除少数不伴有血流动力学障碍的小穿孔，积极外科手术是挽救生命的有效方法。

Postinfarction ventricular septal perforation, also known as postinfarction ventricular septal defect (VSD), is a significant complication of AMI. Patients with postinfarction VSD often develop into multiple organ failure due to low cardiac output, and the mortality rate is very high. Surgery is an effective way to save patients' lives, except for those with small perforations without hemodynamic disorders.

心肌梗死后室间隔缺损与先天性室间隔缺损不同，其实际缺血性坏死范围大于术中所见之穿孔，缺损周围组织脆弱，其纤维化通常要在两周以后。因此修补时缝针要离开缺损缘一些，尽量缝到正常心肌，并用带垫片缝合。

Postinfarction VSD is different from congenital VSD. The actual range of ischemic necrosis is larger than that of intraoperative perforation, the tissues around the VSD are fragile, and fibrosis is usually formed two weeks later. So, a pledget is needed, and it is also better to extend the sutures to the non-infarcted myocardium away from the edge of the defect.

图 2-5-1　心肌梗死后室间隔缺损缝合修补术
Figure 2-5-1　Direct closure of postinfarction ventricular septal defect

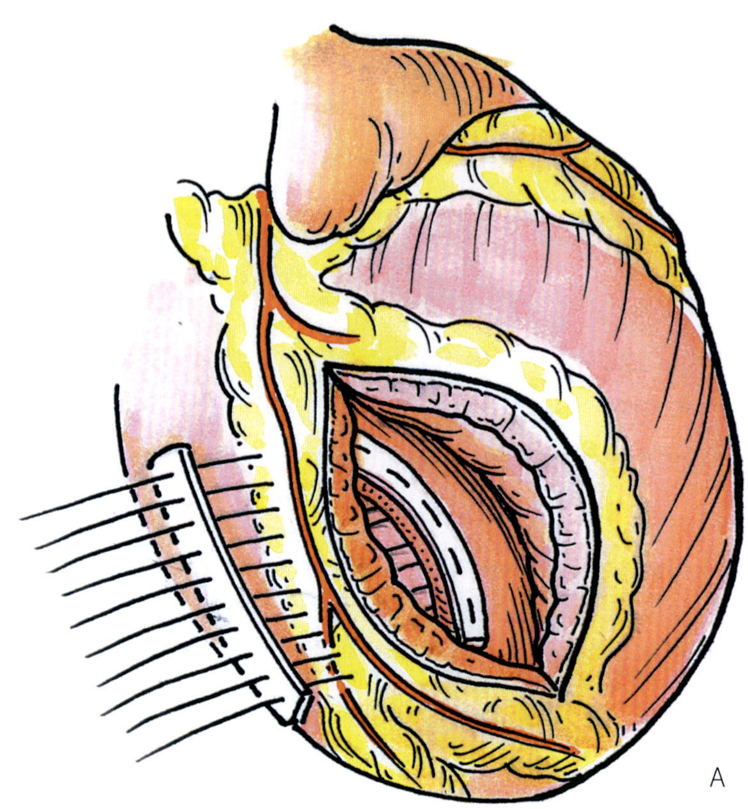

A. 前间隔缺损时于左心室前壁下部沿前降支左侧 1~2cm 纵行切开左心室。心内探查，若有血栓予以清除，辨明室间隔缺损的位置。小的室间隔缺损且边缘有纤维化者，可以直接缝闭。室间隔缺损后缘垫以毡片条，置间断水平褥式缝针，室间隔左心室侧进针贯穿室间隔，再贯穿心室壁由前降支右侧出针，再从另一毡片条穿出。

A. An incision is longitudinally made in the left ventricle parallel to and 1-2 cm away from the left side of the anterior descending branch from the lower part of the anterior wall of the left ventricle when there is an anterior septal defect. If there is a thrombus after the intracardiac examination, clear the thrombus and identify the location of the VSD first. For small ventricular septal defects with edge fibrosis, a direct suture can be used. Felt strips are placed at the posterior edge of the VSD, and the interrupted horizontal mattress suture is used. Laterally pass the suture from the first patch at the left ventricular septum, and then pass the needle transmurally through the ventricular septum and ventricular wall in the right side of the anterior descending branch, and then pass the needle through the second felt strip.

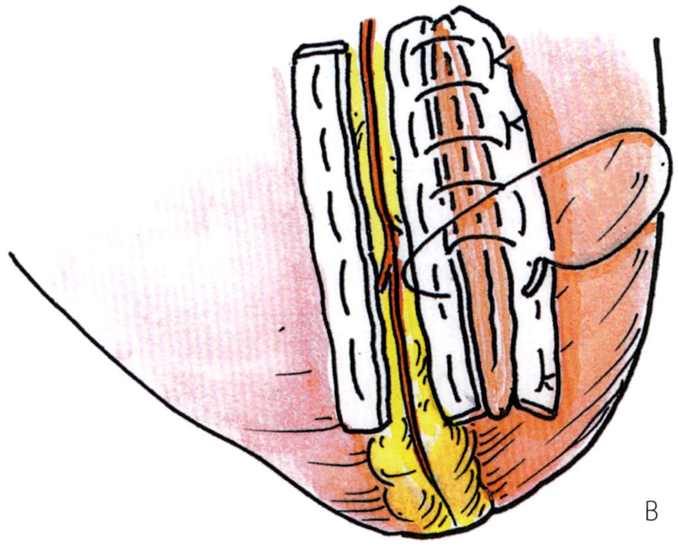

B. 全部缝线安置完成后结扎闭合室间隔缺损。左心室切口两侧覆以毡片条，连续褥式外翻缝合，结扎后再做一层单纯连续缝合。

B. All the sutures are tied to close the VSD. Both sides of the left ventricular incision are covered with felt strips, followed by continuous exstrophy mattress suture. After ligation, a simple continuous suture is added.

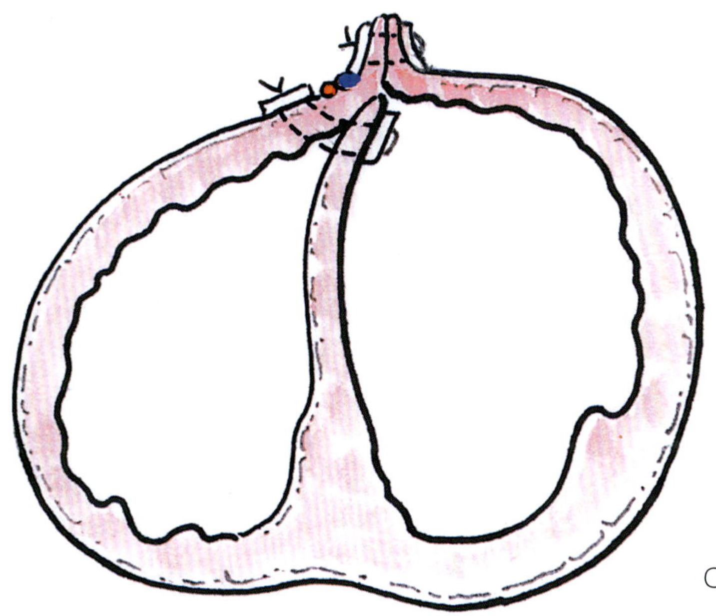

C. 修补完毕示意图。

C. The schematic diagram after the repair.

图 2-5-2 心肌梗死后室间隔缺损补片修补术
Figure 2-5-2 Patch closure of postinfarction ventricular septal defect

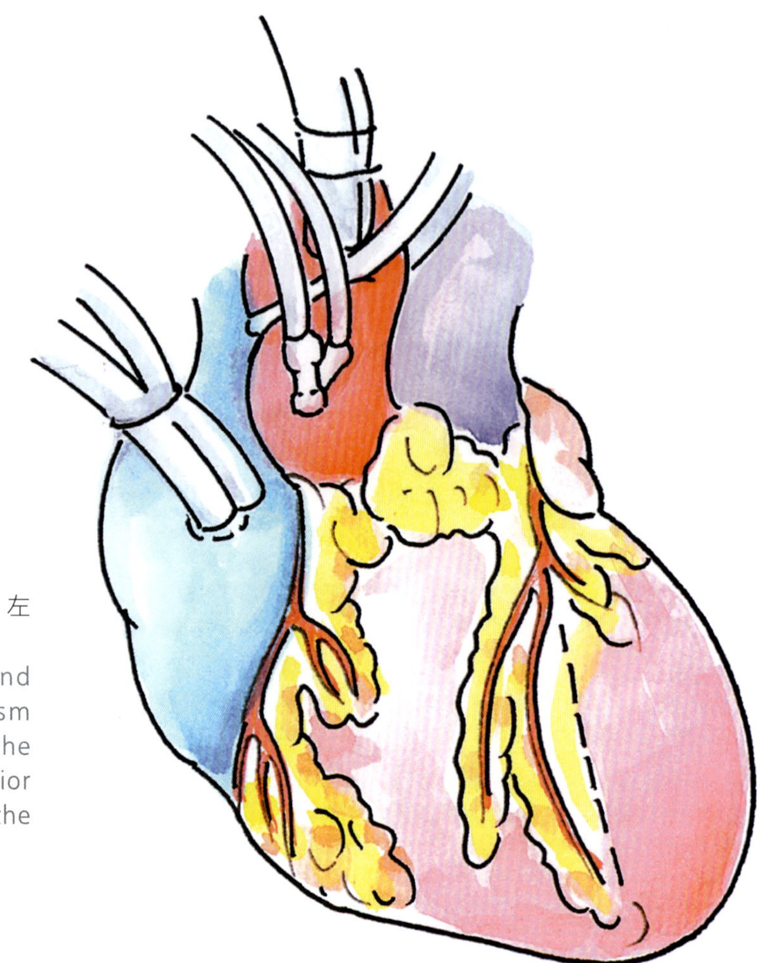

A. 建立体外循环，心脏停搏后确定室壁瘤的范围。左心室前壁下部沿前降支左侧纵行切开室壁瘤。

A. Establish extracorporeal circulation, and identify the area of ventricular aneurysm after cardiac arrest. Longitudinally incise the ventricular aneurysm parallel to the anterior descending branch from the lower part of the anterior wall of the left ventricle.

B. 切开室壁瘤后心内探查，若有室间隔缺损，通常采用补片修补，以降低缝合张力，防止复发。用带垫片缝针将室间隔缺损的室间隔缘与补片间断褥式缝合，缝线由右心室侧进针左心室侧出针，再缝到补片上。

B. Perform intracardiac detection after ventricular aneurysm is incised. If there is VSD, use patch repair to reduce suture tension and prevent a recurrence. The patch is sewn into the edge of VSD with pledget-supported interrupted mattress sutures. The suture is laterally passed from the right ventricle to the left ventricle, and then through the patch.

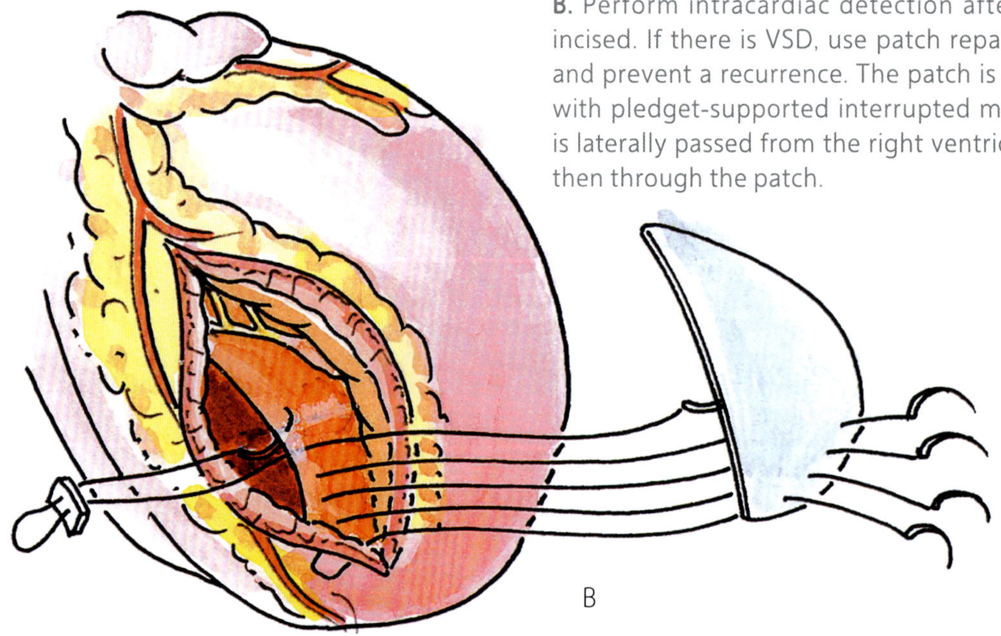

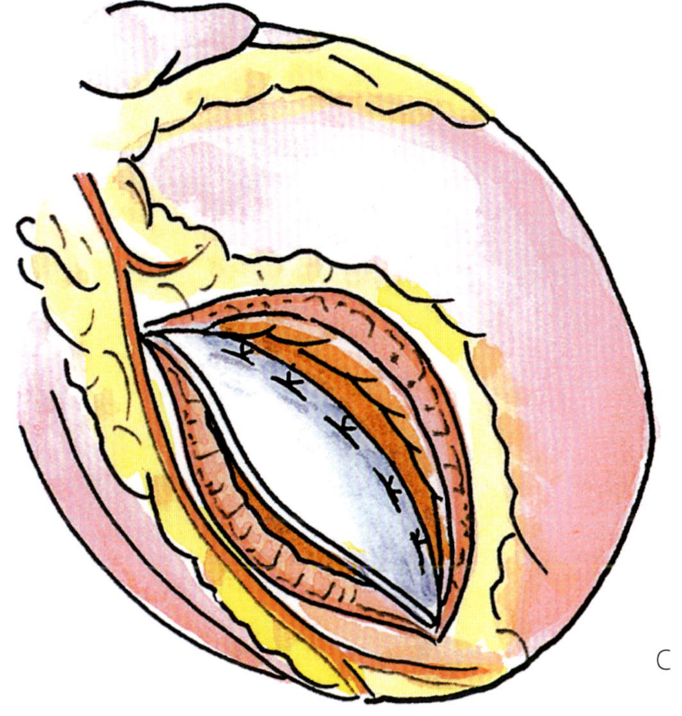

C. 推下补片逐一结扎缝线。

C. Push the patch down and ligate the sutures one by one.

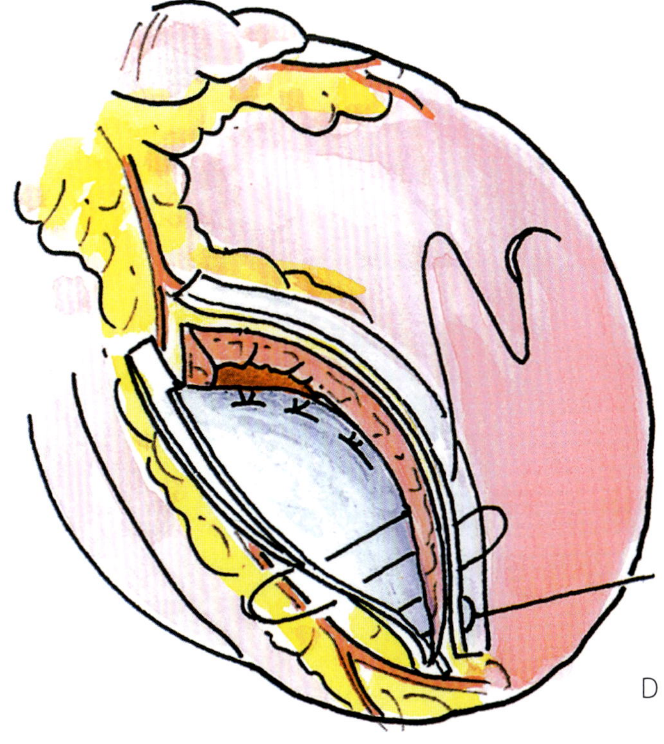

D. 左心室切口两侧垫以毡片条，将毡片条、左心室切口两缘和补片连续水平褥式缝合，使左心室切口外翻。

D. Place felt strips on both sides of the left ventricular incision. Horizontal mattress suture is performed to suture the felt strips (or Teflon felts), the two edges of the left ventricular incision, and the patch. Make the left ventricular incision everted.

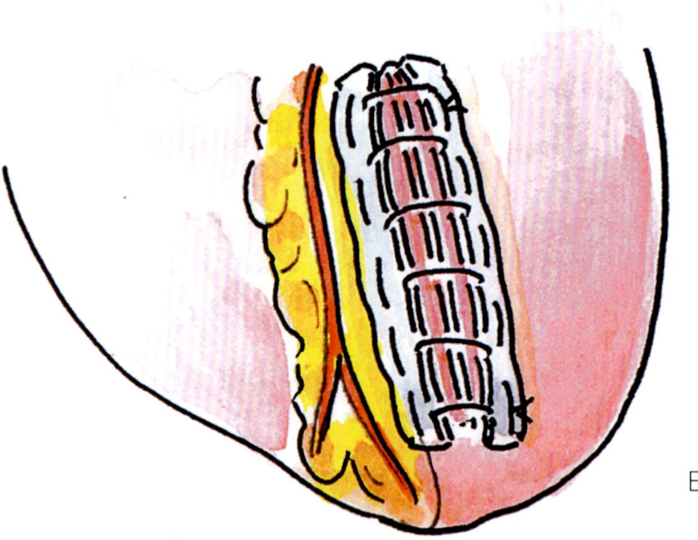

E. 左心室切口再加一层单纯连续缝合。

E. Apply simple running sutures to the left ventricular incision again.

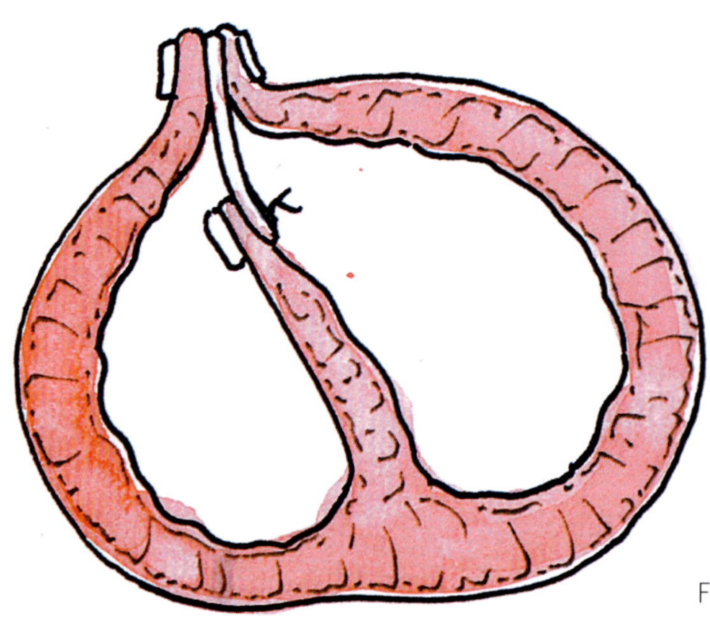

F. 修补完毕示意图。

F. The schematic diagram after the repair.

图 2-5-3 心室前壁重建术
Figure 2-5-3 Anterior ventricular restoration

左心室前壁大面积的室壁瘤合并室间隔穿孔要用补片修复室间隔和左心室壁。

For VSD combined with a large left ventricular aneurysm, the interventricular septum and left ventricular wall should be repaired with a patch.

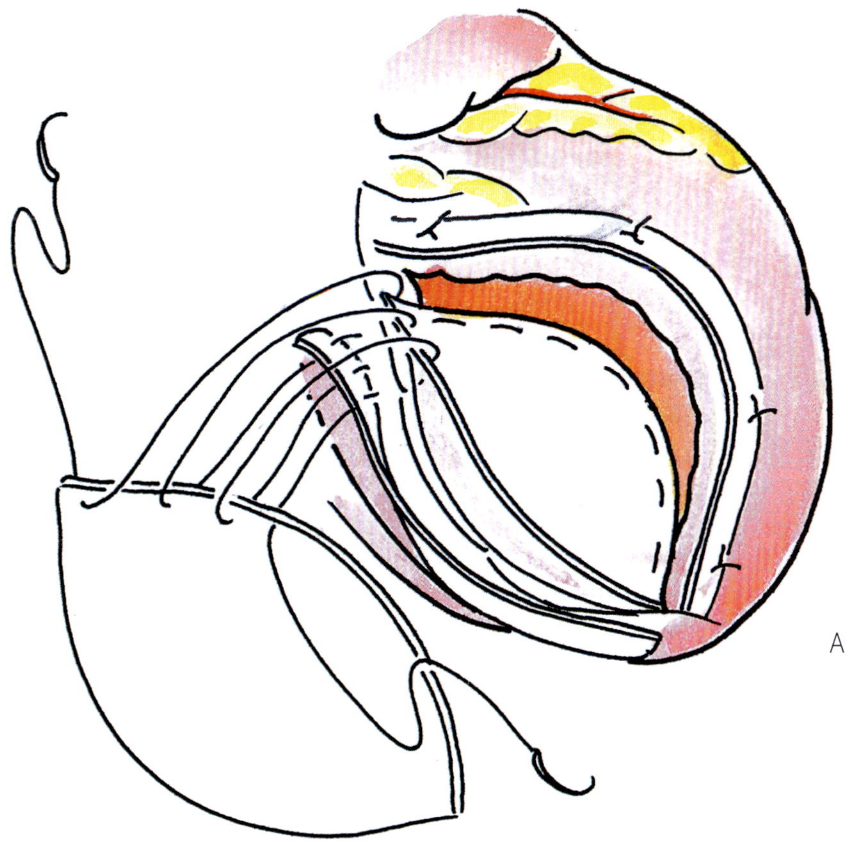

A. 左心室前壁下部沿前降支左侧纵行切开室壁瘤。先在室间隔缺损的室间隔缘缝入一补片。带垫片水平间断缝合。推下补片逐一结扎缝线。裁剪另一补片修补左心室切口。缝针依次穿过室间隔补片、左心室切口右缘、毡片条和左心室切口补片，单纯连续缝合。

A. An incision is made on the ventricular aneurysm longitudinally from the lower part of the anterior wall of the left ventricle parallel to the anterior descending branch at the left side. A patch is sewn into the ventricular septum edge of the VSD first. An interrupted horizontal suture is made with pledgets. Push the patch down and ligate the sutures one by one. Take another patch to repair the left ventricular incision. Pass the needle transmurally through the interventricular septum patch, the right edge of the left ventricular incision, the medical felt strip, and the left ventricular incision patch with simple running sutures.

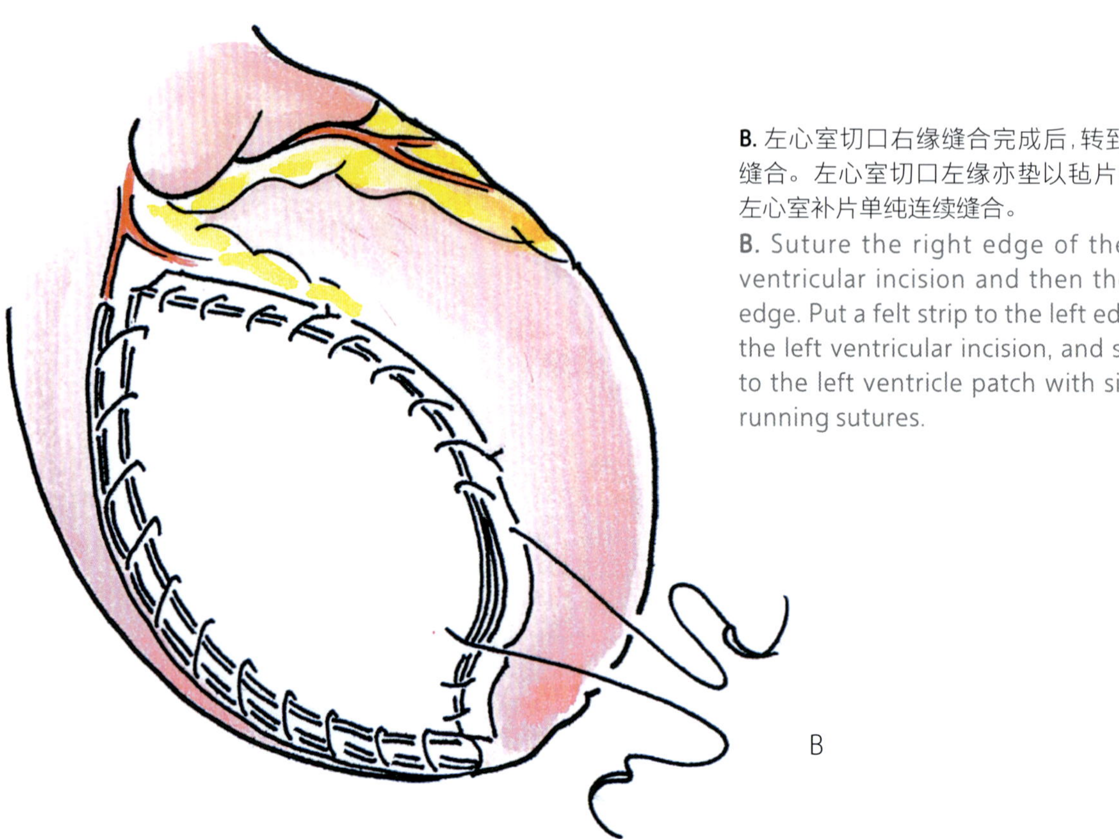

B. 左心室切口右缘缝合完成后，转到左缘缝合。左心室切口左缘亦垫以毡片条，与左心室补片单纯连续缝合。

B. Suture the right edge of the left ventricular incision and then the left edge. Put a felt strip to the left edge of the left ventricular incision, and sew it to the left ventricle patch with simple running sutures.

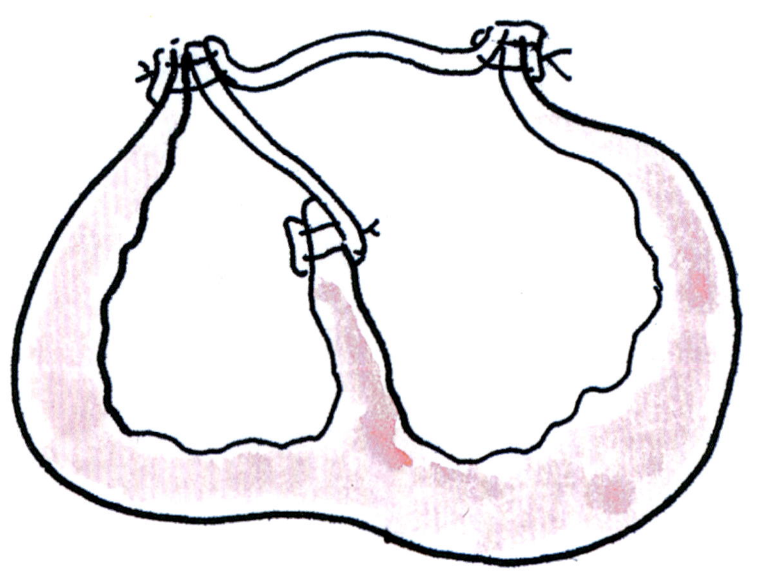

C. 修补完毕示意图。

C. The schematic diagram after the repair.

图 2-5-4　心尖修补术

Figure 2-5-4　Repair of apical ventricular septal defect

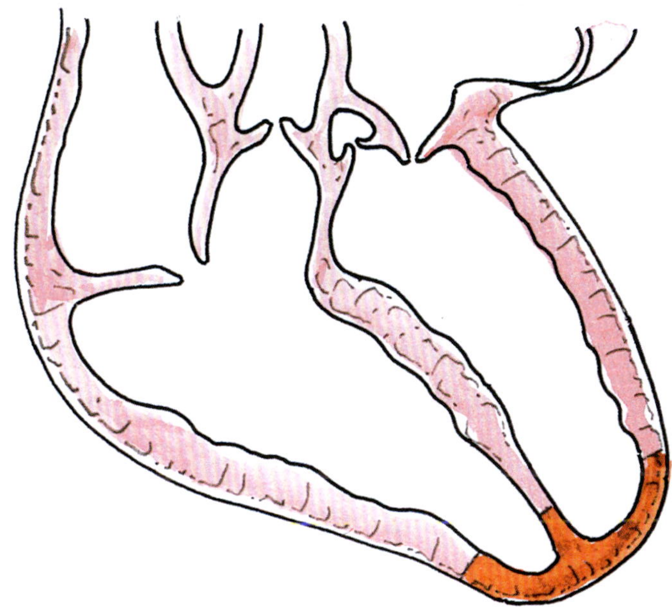

A. 心尖部心肌梗死累及左、右心室和室间隔。

A. Apical myocardial infarction usually influences the left and right ventricles and ventricular septum.

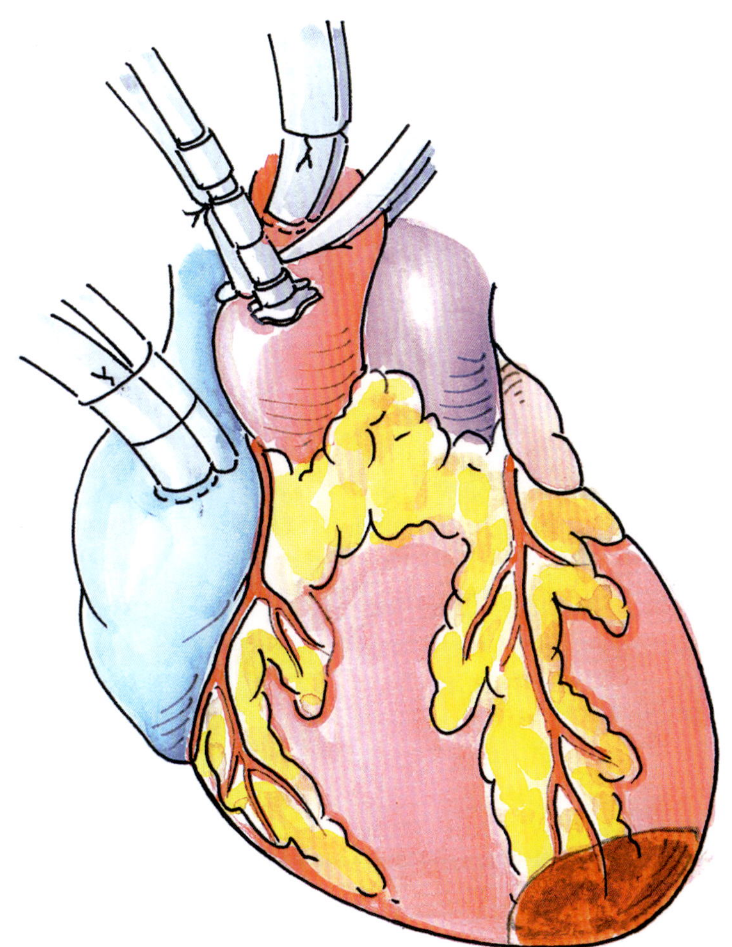

B. 建立体外循环，心脏停搏后确定室壁瘤的范围。

B. Establish extracorporeal circulation and identify the area of ventricular aneurysm after cardiac arrest.

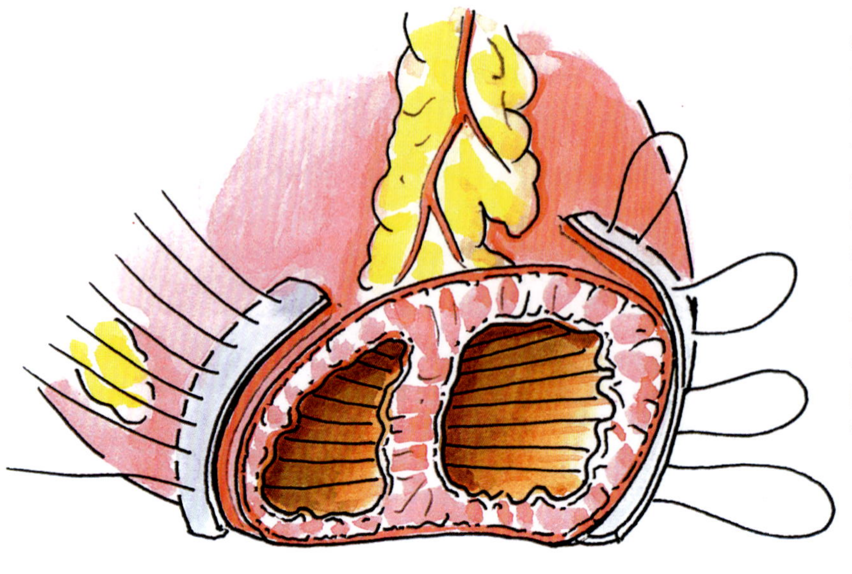

C. 切除部分心尖梗死区域，包括室间隔缺损两侧的左、右心室。左、右心室切口分别垫以毡片条，间断褥式缝合，将室间隔切缘亦一并缝入。

C. Excise some parts of apical myocardial infarction, including the left and right ventricles on both sides of the VSD. Place the felt strips separately on the left and right ventricular incisions. An interrupted mattress suture is performed with a ventricular septal edge.

D

D. 结扎褥式缝线，在毡片条上再加一层连续缝合。

D. The sutures are tied, and additional running sutures are performed on the felt strips.

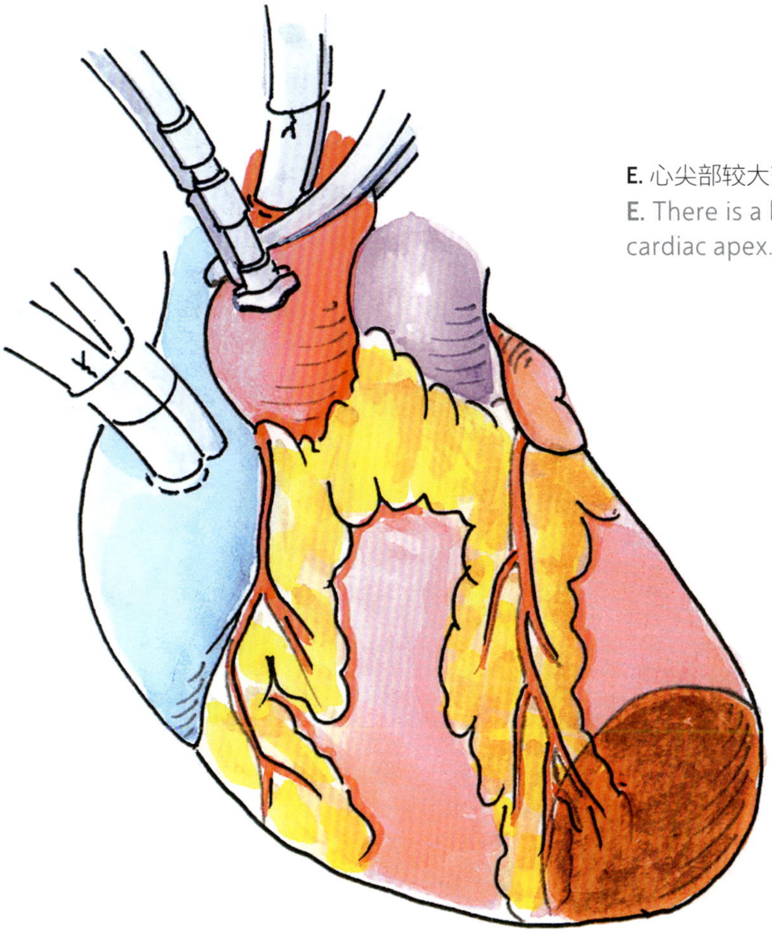

E. 心尖部较大范围的心肌梗死。

E. There is a large area of myocardial infarction at the cardiac apex.

E

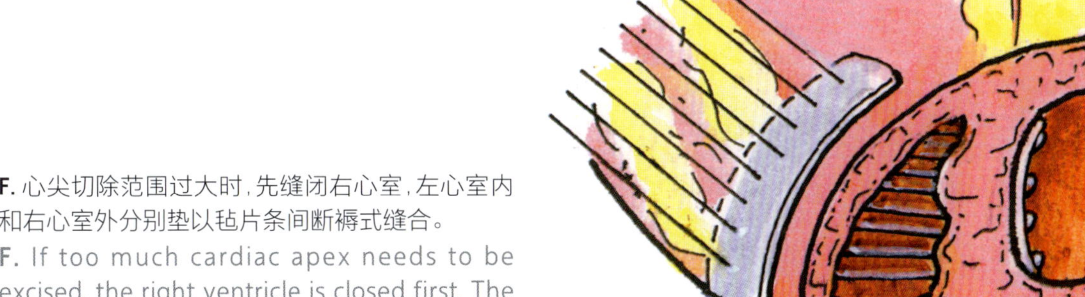

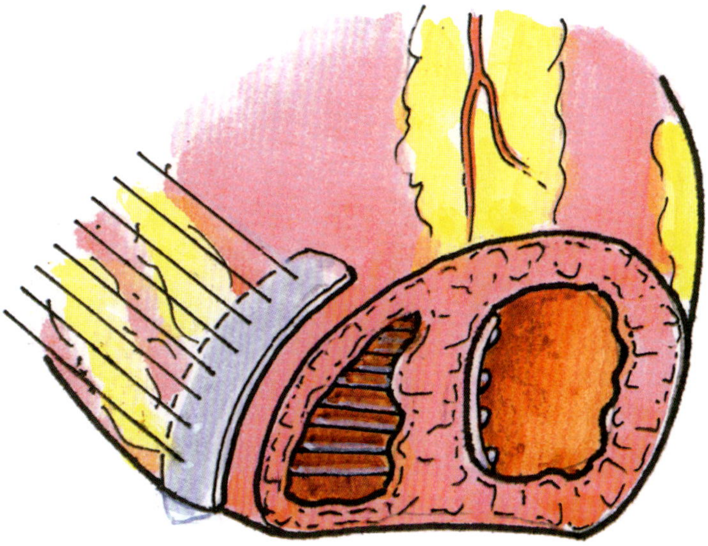

F. 心尖切除范围过大时，先缝闭右心室，左心室内和右心室外分别垫以毡片条间断褥式缝合。

F. If too much cardiac apex needs to be excised, the right ventricle is closed first. The inside of the left ventricle and the outside of the right ventricle can be sewn up by interrupted mattress sutures with the felt strips respectively.

F

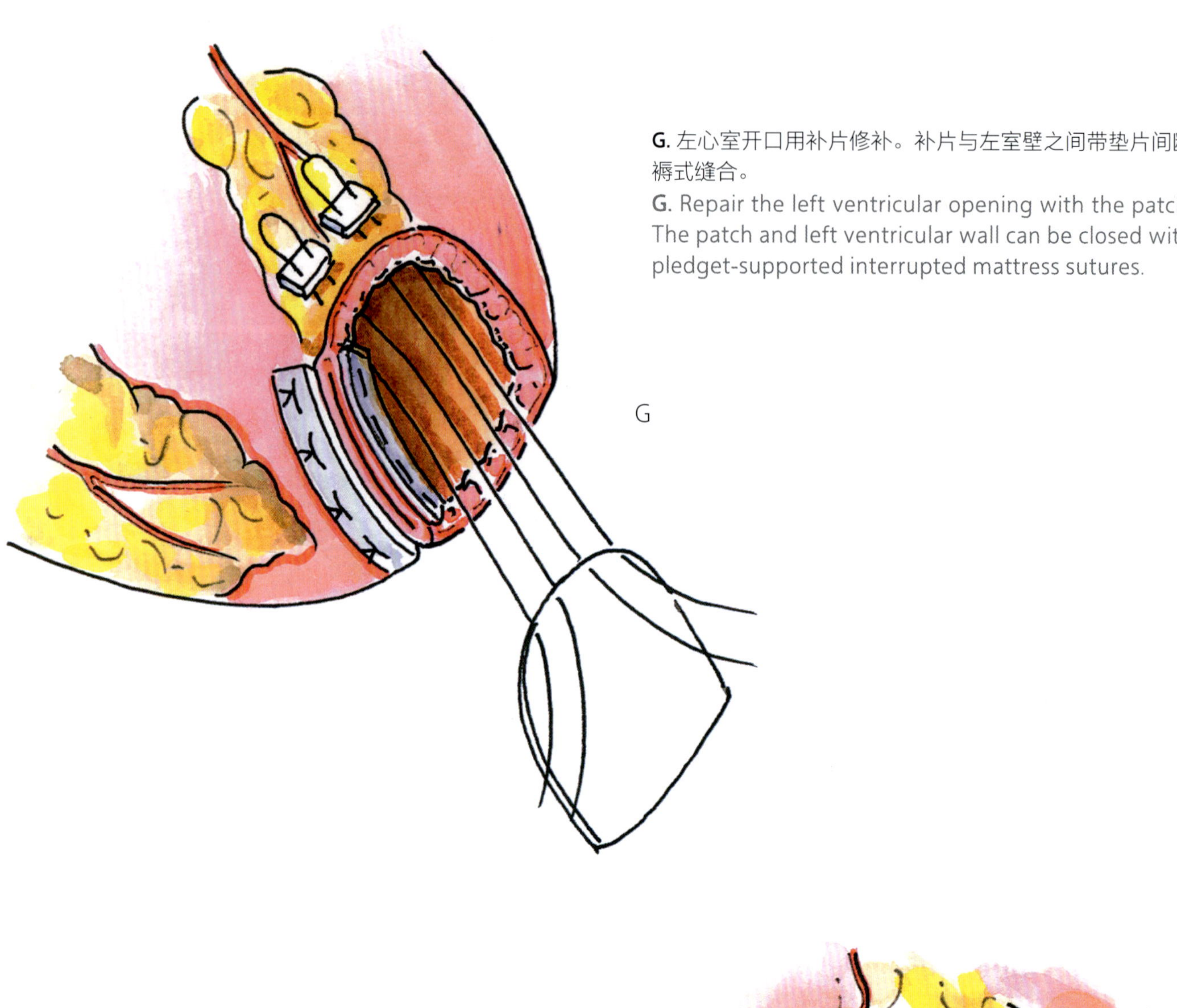

G. 左心室开口用补片修补。补片与左室壁之间带垫片间断褥式缝合。

G. Repair the left ventricular opening with the patch. The patch and left ventricular wall can be closed with pledget-supported interrupted mattress sutures.

H. 补片再连续缝合至右室和室间隔缝合处。

H. The patch is sutured between the right ventricle and the interventricular septum with running sutures.

H

图 2-5-5　心室下壁重建术

Figure 2-5-5　Inferior ventricular restoration

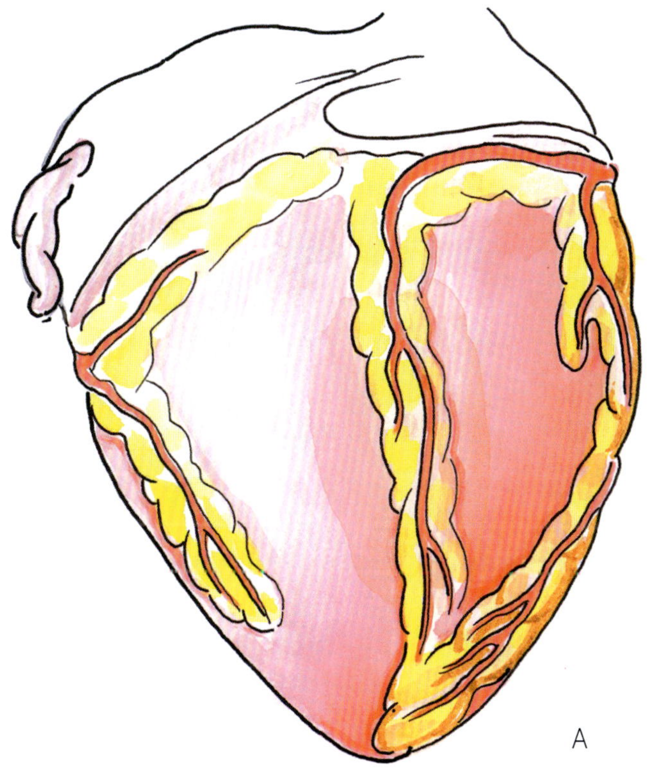

A. 位于后室间沟部位的心室下壁心肌梗死，经室壁瘤沿后降支左心室侧做切口。

A. If myocardial infarction is located in the inferior ventricular wall at the posterior interventricular groove, the incision is performed on the left ventricular side through the ventricular aneurysm and along the posterior descending branch.

B. 后间隔缺损组织更为薄弱用补片修补为宜，以减少张力。将补片与室间隔缘带垫片间断褥式缝合，垫片放在右心室侧，补片放到左心室侧。再将左心室切口两侧垫以毡片条，将毡片条、左心室切口两缘和室间隔补片连续水平褥式缝合，使左室切口外翻。

B. Posterior ventricular septal defect tissue is weaker and should be repaired with a patch to reduce tension. The patch is attached to the ventricular septal edge by a pledget-supported interrupted mattress suture, with the pledget being placed on the right ventricle and the patch on the left ventricle. Both sides of the left ventricle incision are padded with felt strips, and the running horizontal mattress suture is performed on the felt strips, two edges of the left ventricular incision, and the ventricular septal patch to make the left ventricular incision everted.

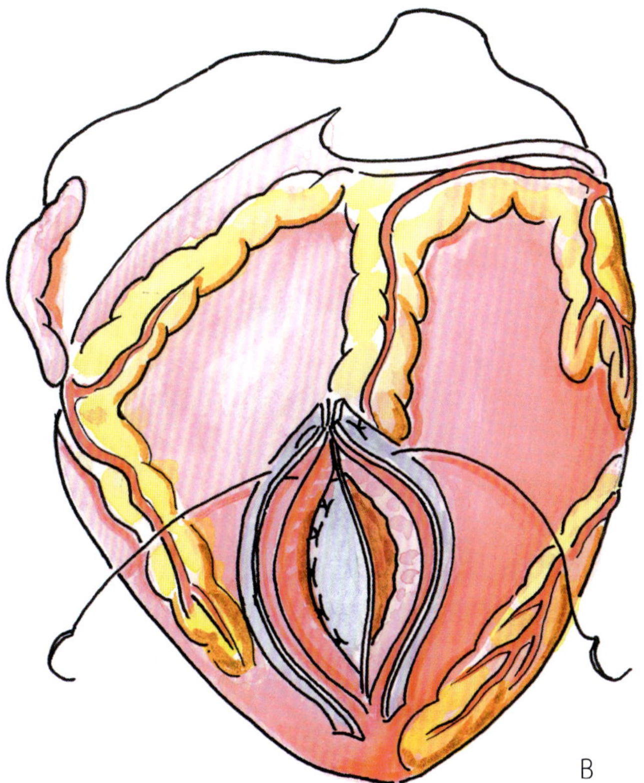

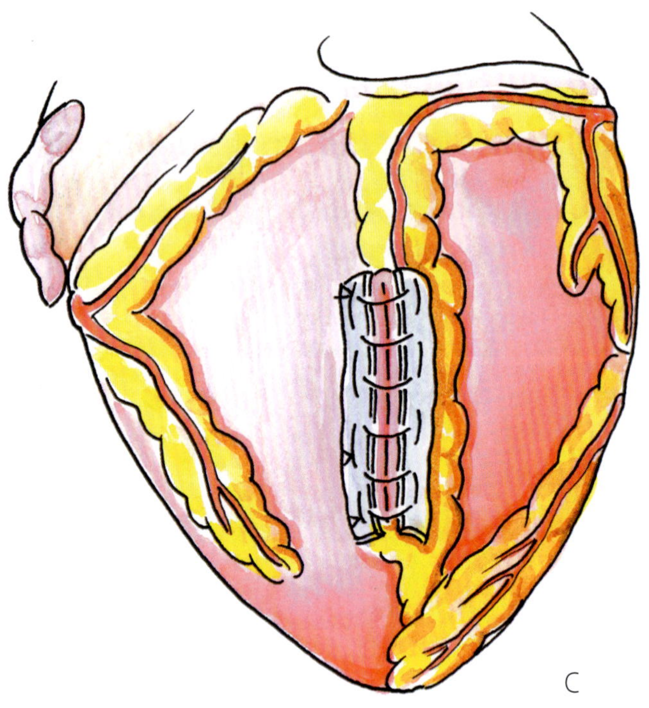

C. 毡片条上再做一层单纯连续缝合。

C. Simple running suture is additionally performed on the felt strips.

D. 小的室间隔缺损也可直接缝闭。室间隔游离缘左心室侧垫以毡片条，置间断水平褥式缝针，室间隔左心室侧进针，心室壁后降支右心室侧出针，再由另一毡片条穿出。

D. Small VSD can also be closed by direct suture. The left ventricular side of the ventricular septal free edge is padded with a felt strip and an interrupted horizontal mattress suture is performed. The needle passes from the left ventricle of the ventricular septum to the right ventricle at the posterior descending branch of the ventricular wall and then goes through another felt strip.

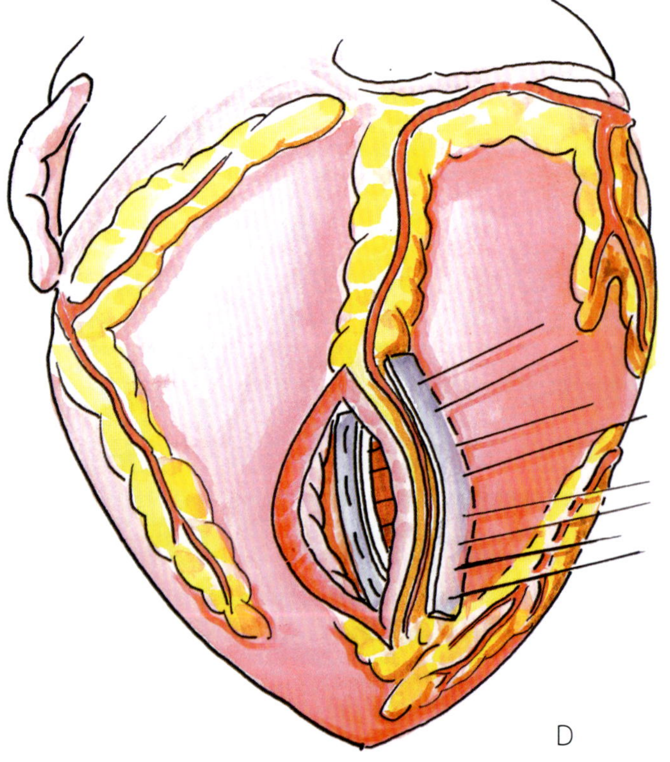

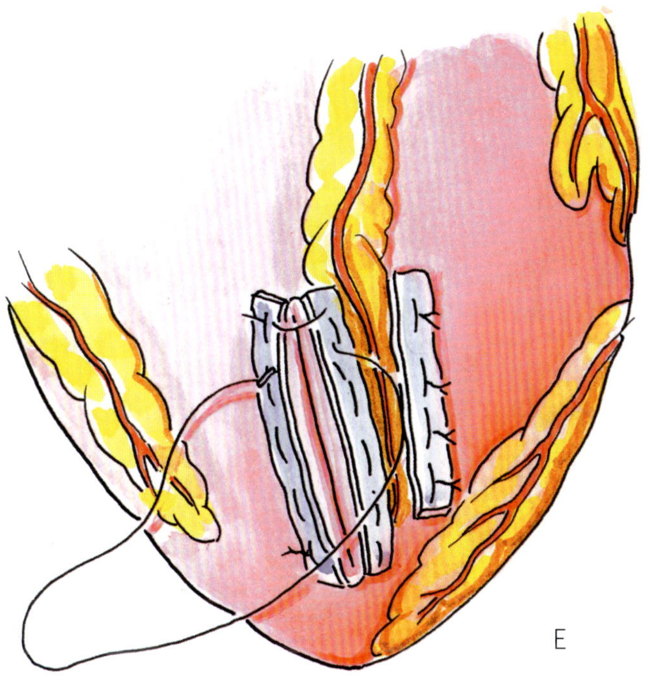

E. 全部缝线安置完成后结扎闭合室间隔缺损。左心室切口两侧覆以毡片条，连续褥式外翻缝合，结扎后再做一层单纯连续缝合。

E. Ligate and close VSD after all sutures are finished. Both sides of the left ventricular incision are covered with felt strips. Perform the running exstrophy mattress suture, and after the ligation, a layer of the simple running suture is added.

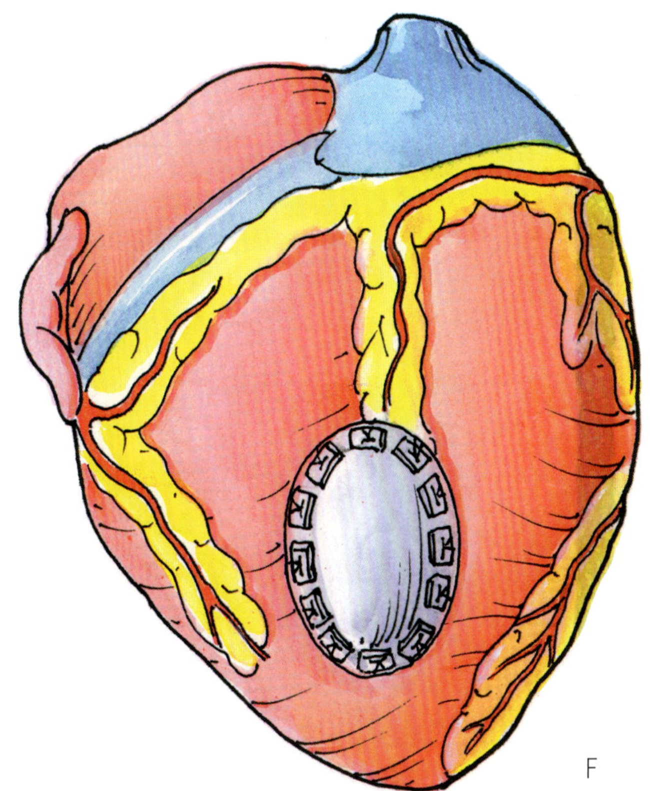

F. 较大的下壁室壁瘤通常用补片修补左心室壁，以避免左心室变形。补片用带垫片间断褥式缝合。

F. For a larger inferior ventricular aneurysm, the left ventricular wall is to be repaired with a patch to avoid its deformation. The patch shall be sutured by an interrupted mattress suture with a pledget.

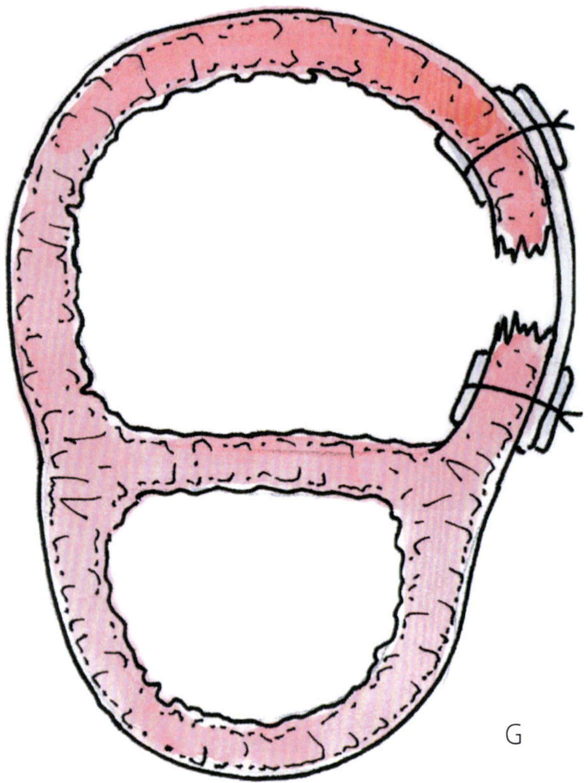

G. 修补完毕示意图。

G. The schematic diagram after the repair.

第六节　干细胞应用

Section 6　Stem Cell Application

人脐带间充质干细胞混悬剂5ml，细胞含量1×10^7个，在冠状动脉旁路移植术桥血管远端吻合完成后于心肌缺血部位周围进行20个点位注射，针头与心外膜成15°角，每个注射点位注射0.25ml细胞混悬液，并在注射完成后使用生物胶水覆盖注射点位。注射前10分钟，给予甲泼尼龙80mg静脉输注预处理，以预防过敏和非溶血反应。术后持续监测生命体征。

After the anastomosis at the bridge vessel's distal end in coronary artery bypass grafting (CABG), 5 ml human umbilical cord mesenchymal stem cell suspension with a cell content of 1×10^7 is injected at 20 sites around the myocardial ischemia site, with 0.25 ml per site. During the injection, the needle should remain at a 15-degree angle to the epicardium. After the injection, the sites are to be covered with biological glue. Make sure that 80 mg methylprednisolone is administered intravenously as a pretreatment to avoid allergic and nonhemolytic reactions 10 minutes before the injection, and that vital signs should be monitored continuously after the surgery.

图 2-6-1 **干细胞注射**

Figure 2-6-1 **Stem cell delivery**

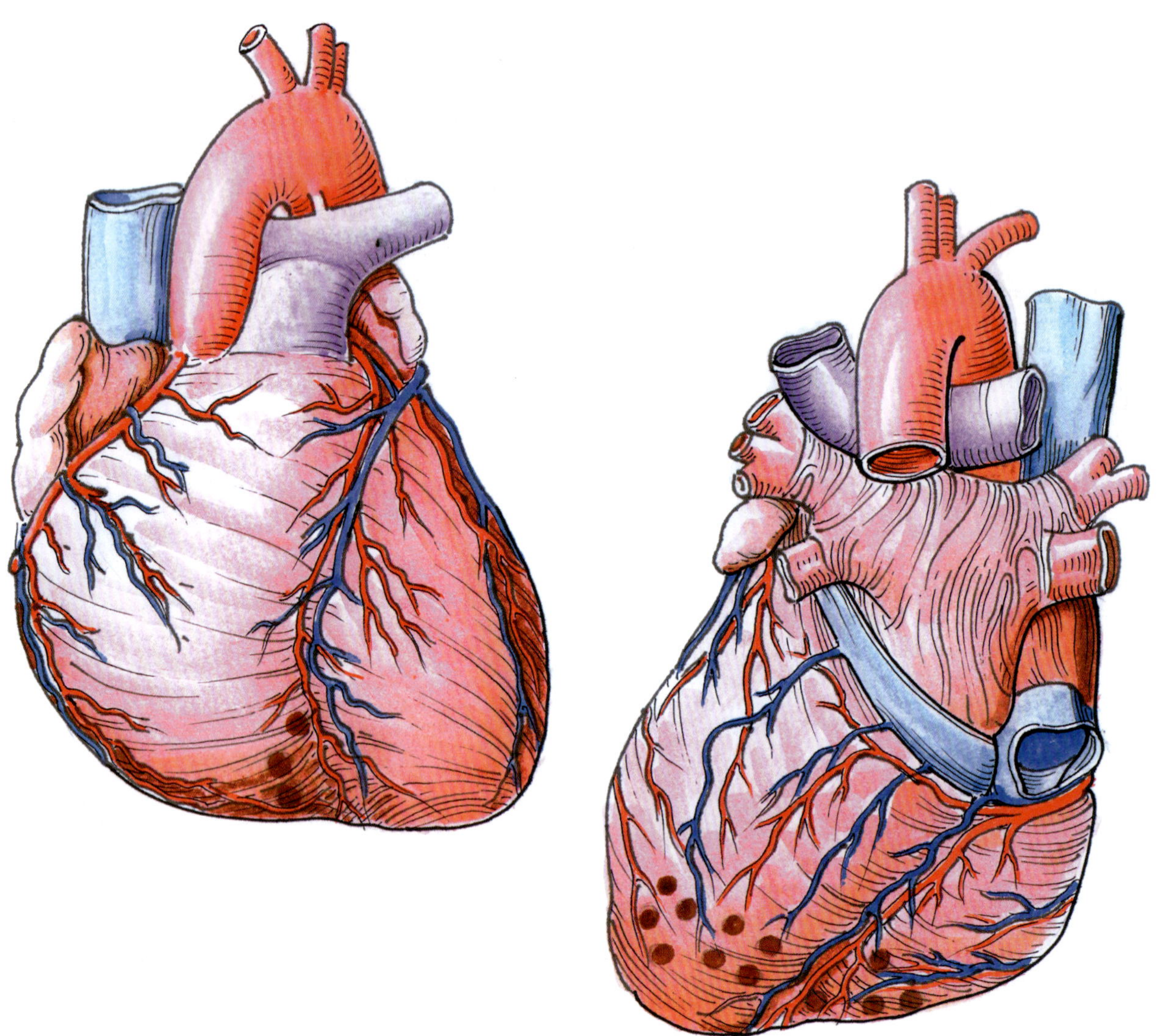

心尖区心肌梗死，心肌注射点位如图示意。

Schematic diagram of myocardial injection sites with apical myocardial infarction is shown in the figure.

第三章

成人心脏瓣膜疾病

Chapter 3

Adult Valvular Heart Disease

第 一 节　二尖瓣手术

Section 1　Surgery for Mitral Valve Disease

图 3-1-1　经左心房二尖瓣入路

Figure 3-1-1　Left atrium approach to mitral valve

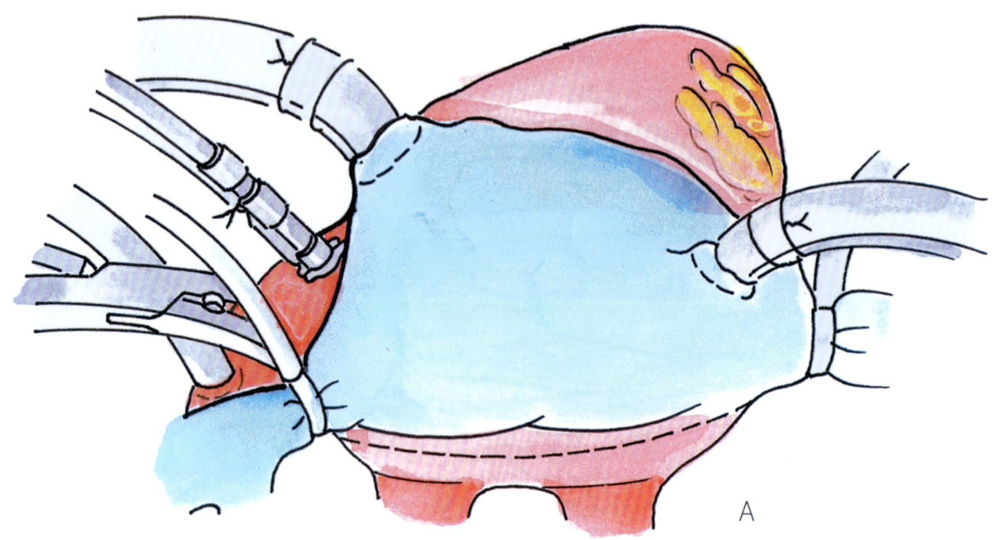

A. 房间沟入路。建立体外循环，在房间沟处剪开心外膜和其下的脂肪组织，在解剖开的房间沟内纵行切开左心房。

A. The interatrial groove approach. Under extracorporeal circulation, dissect the epicardium and adipose tissues at the interatrial groove, and longitudinally incise the left atrium.

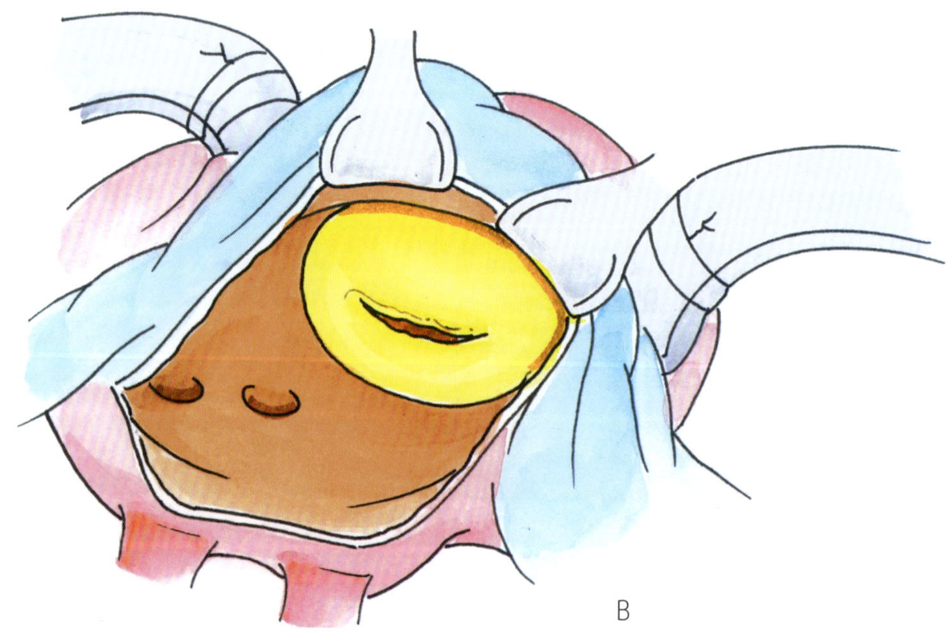

B. 用拉钩或牵引器向上牵开右心房，显露二尖瓣。

B. Retract the right atrium upwards with a hook or retractor to expose the mitral valve.

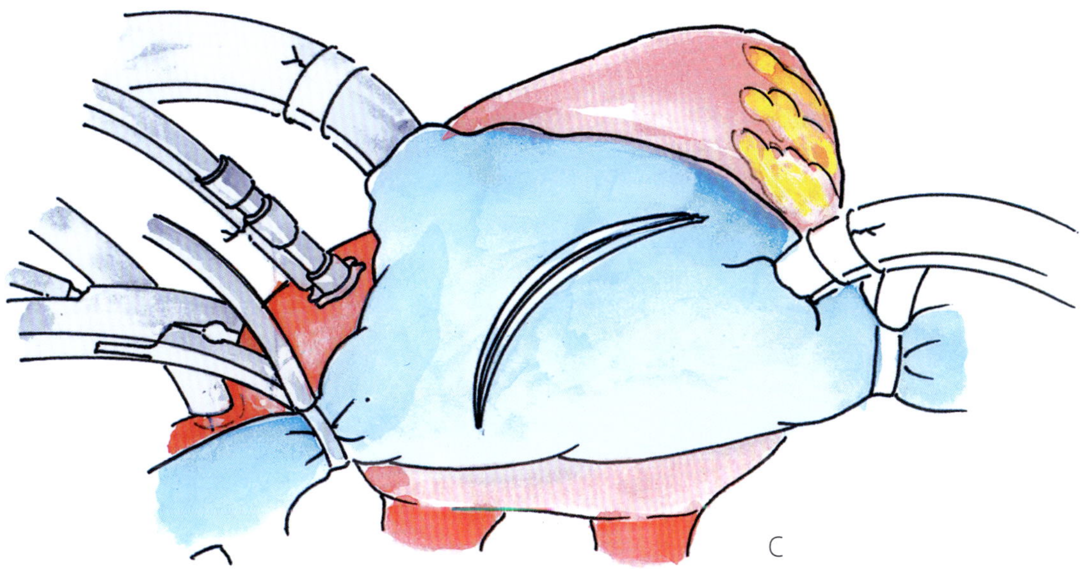

C. 右心房 - 房间隔入路。体外循环下切开右心房。

C. Right atrium-atrial septal approach. Open the right atrium under extracorporeal circulation.

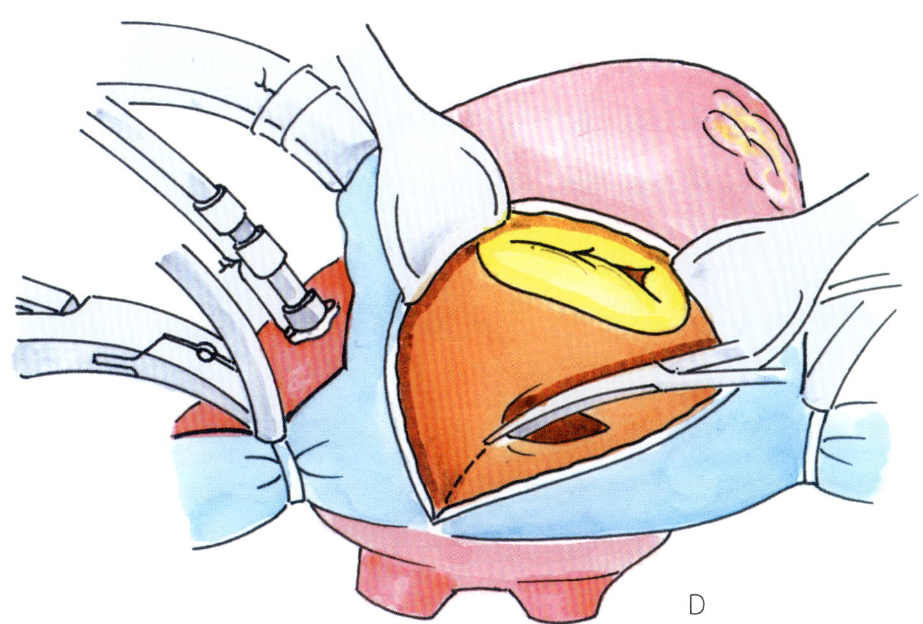

D. 切开卵圆窝，分别向上、向下纵行切开房间隔，扩大切口。右心房内可见三尖瓣。

D. Cut open the oval fossa, make a vertical incision inferiorly and superiorly, and enlarge the incision. Tricuspid valves are seen in the right atrium.

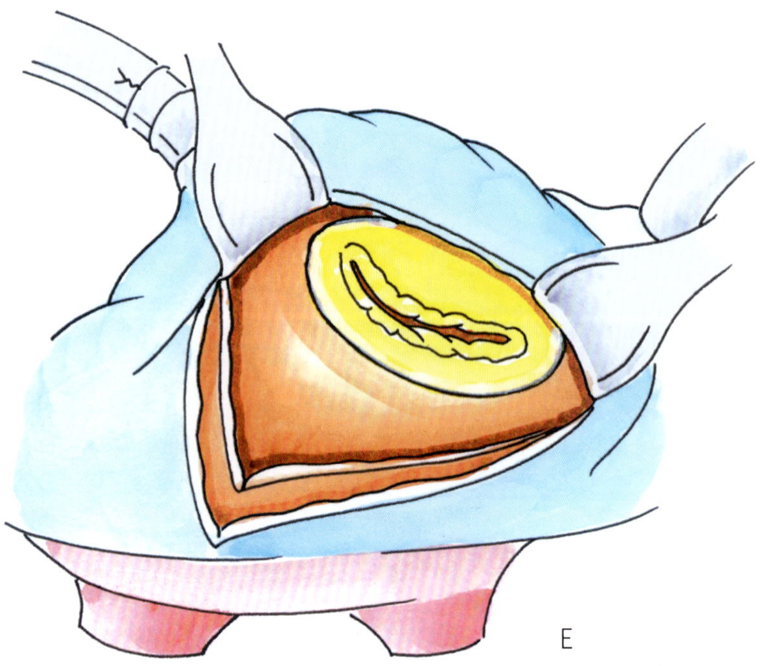

E. 用拉钩或牵引器牵开房间隔，显露二尖瓣。

E. Retract the atrial septum with a hook or retractor to expose the mitral valve.

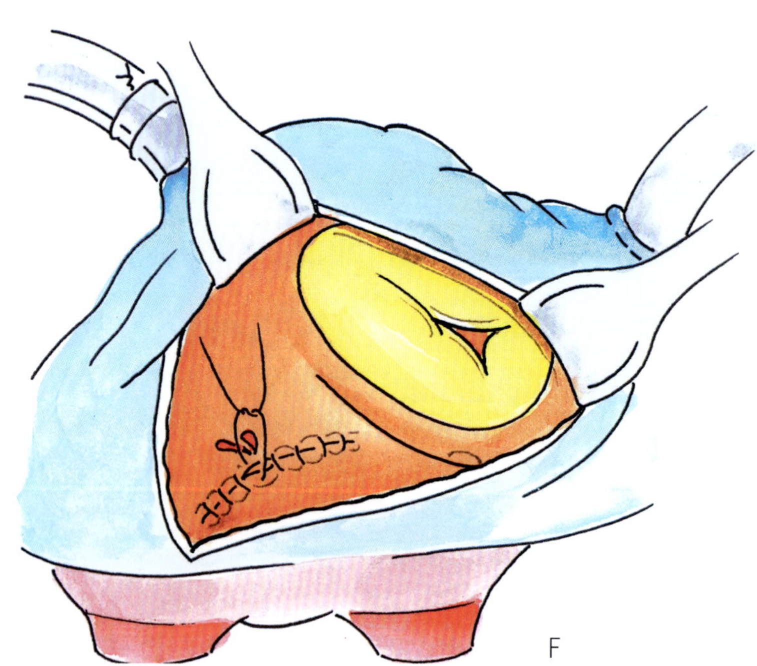

F. 术毕缝合房间隔切口，缝线结扎前左心房排气。

F. After the operation, the left atrial venting is conducted before the closure of the atrial septal incision.

图 3-1-2 直视二尖瓣狭窄交界分离术
Figure 3-1-2 Open commissurotomy for mitral stenosis

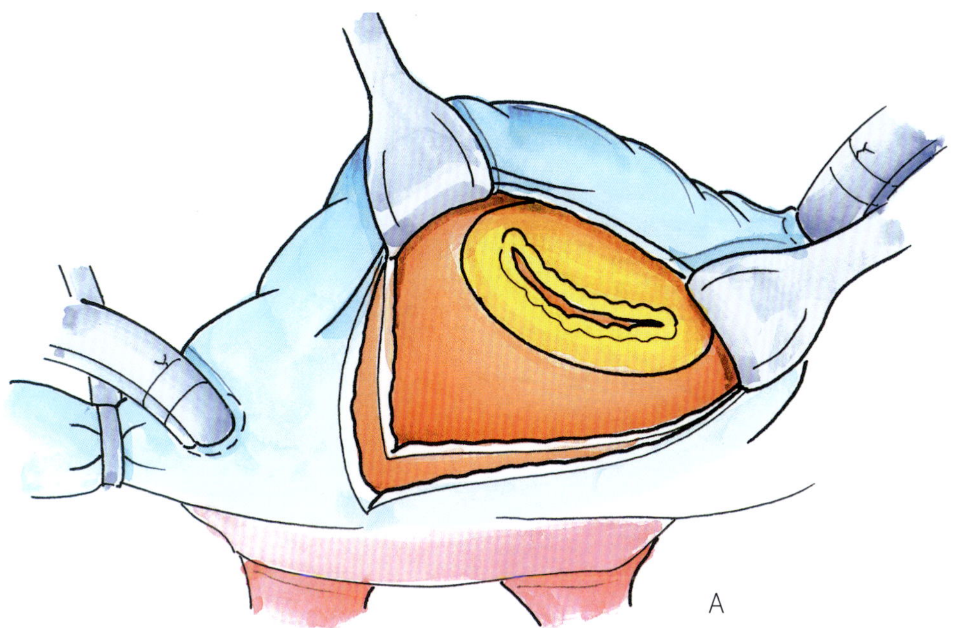

A. 胸骨正中切口，建立体外循环。经右心房 - 房间隔入路打开左心房，显露二尖瓣。

A. Exposure is through a median sternotomy, and extracorporeal circulation is established. Open the left atrium through the right atrial-atrial septal approach to expose the mitral valve.

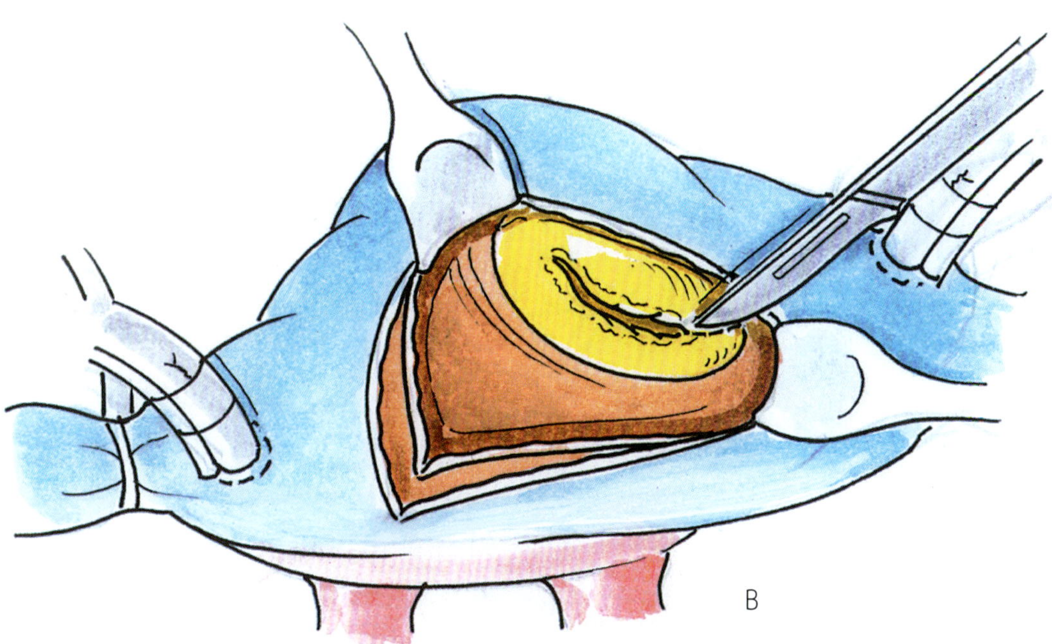

B. 用尖头刀循二尖瓣交界切开粘连至二尖瓣环。

B. Dissect the fused commissures along the mitral junction to the mitral annulus with a sharp blade.

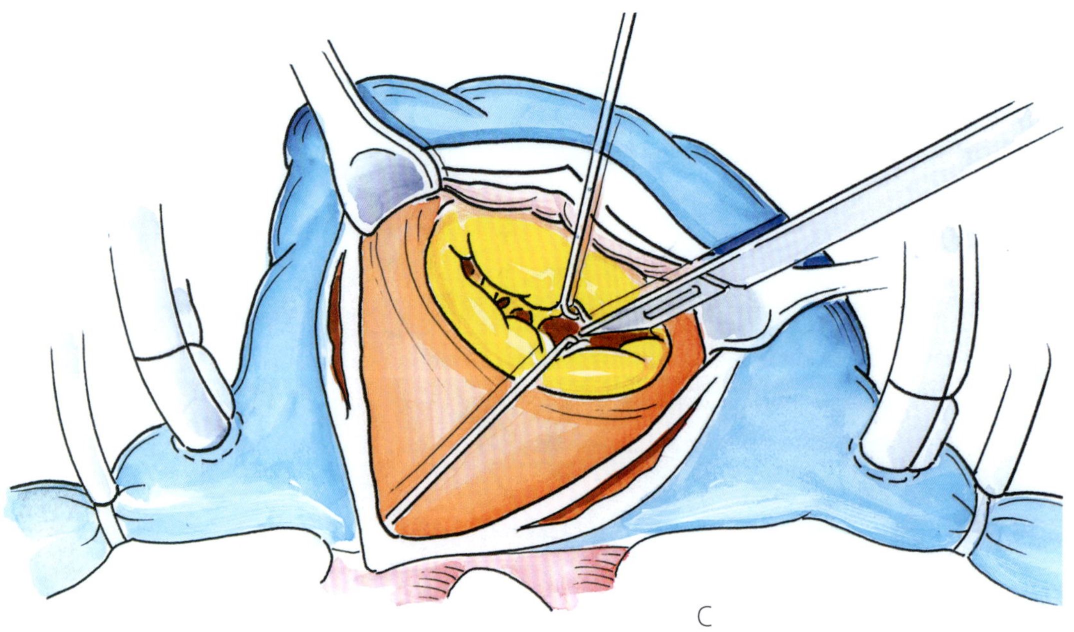

C. 牵开二尖瓣叶，把融合的乳头肌切开。
C. Retract the mitral valve leaflets, and dissect the fused papillary muscles.

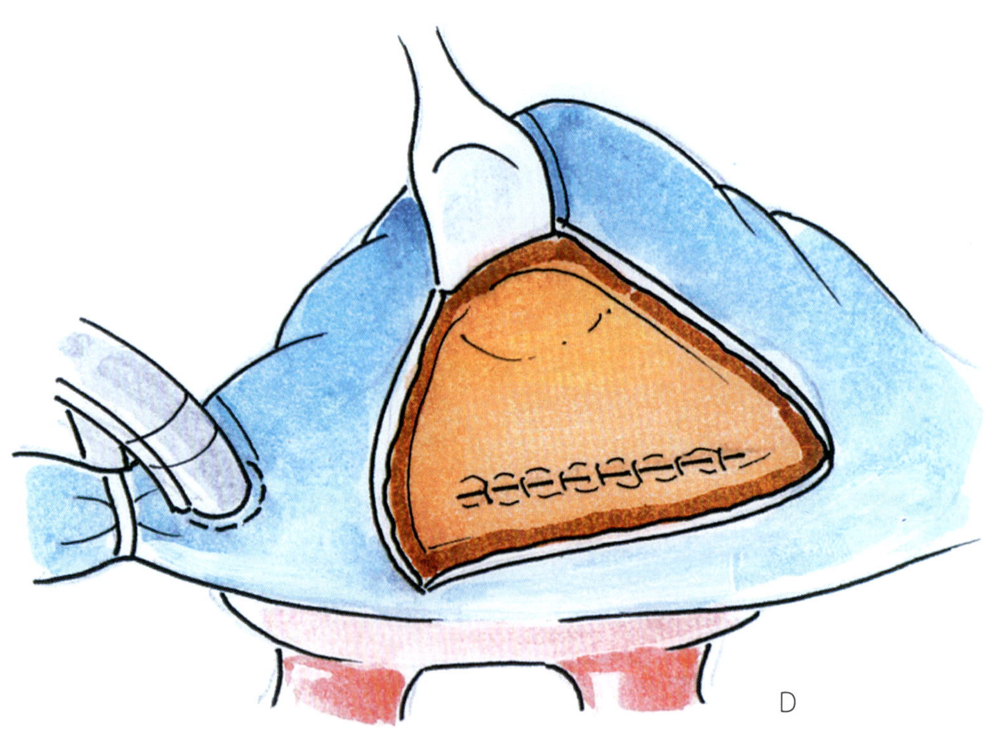

D. 缝合房间隔切口，结扎前鼓肺将左心房气体排出。
D. Close the atrial septal incision and place positive pressure on the lung to express air from the left atrium before ligation.

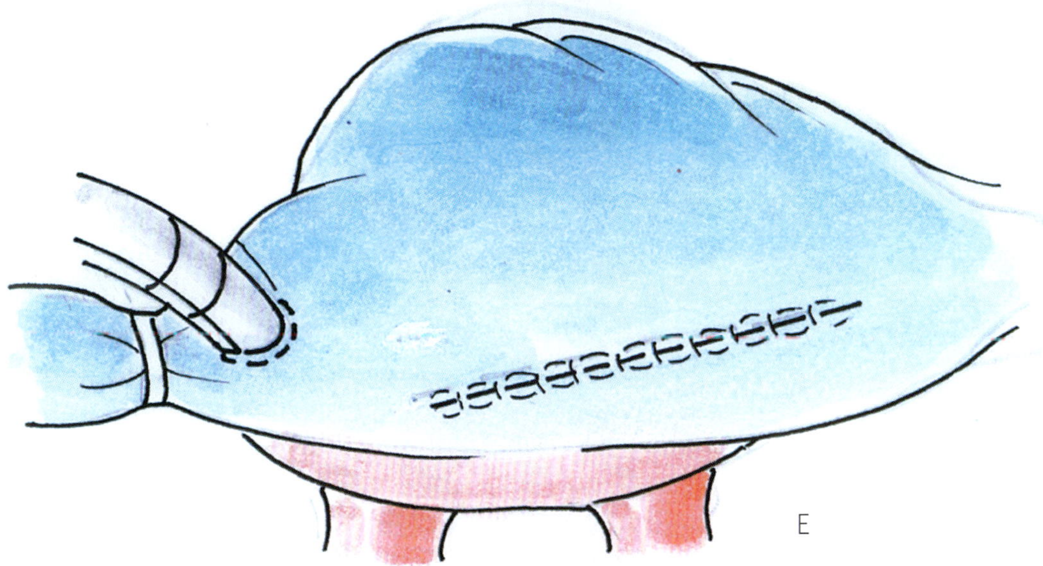

E. 缝合右心房切口。

E. Close the right atrial incision.

图 3-1-3　心包条瓣环成形术（Hetzer Ⅰ式）
Figure 3-1-3　Annuloplasty with pericardial strip (Hetzer approach Ⅰ)

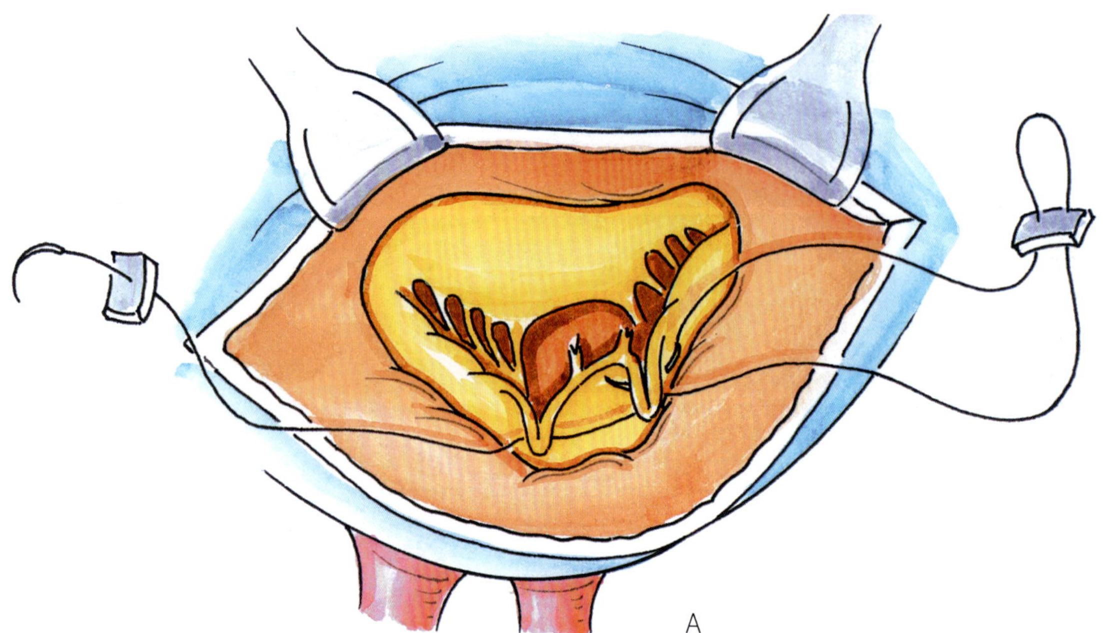

A. 二尖瓣后瓣脱垂病例，用带垫片间断褥式折叠缝合二尖瓣后叶脱垂处。

A. In the case of posterior mitral valve prolapse, the posterior leaflet prolapse is plicated and sutured with pledgeted interrupted mattress sutures.

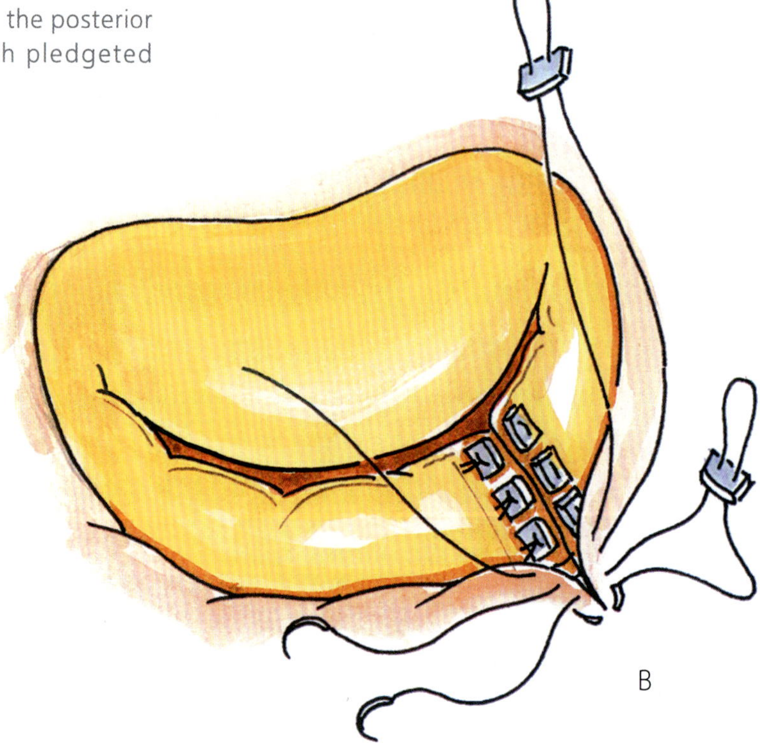

B. 继续将折叠缝合二尖瓣后叶对应处左心房间断褥式折叠缝合 2 针。

B. Two interrupted mattress sutures are made at left atrium in correspondence to the plicated and sutured posterior leaflet of the mitral valve.

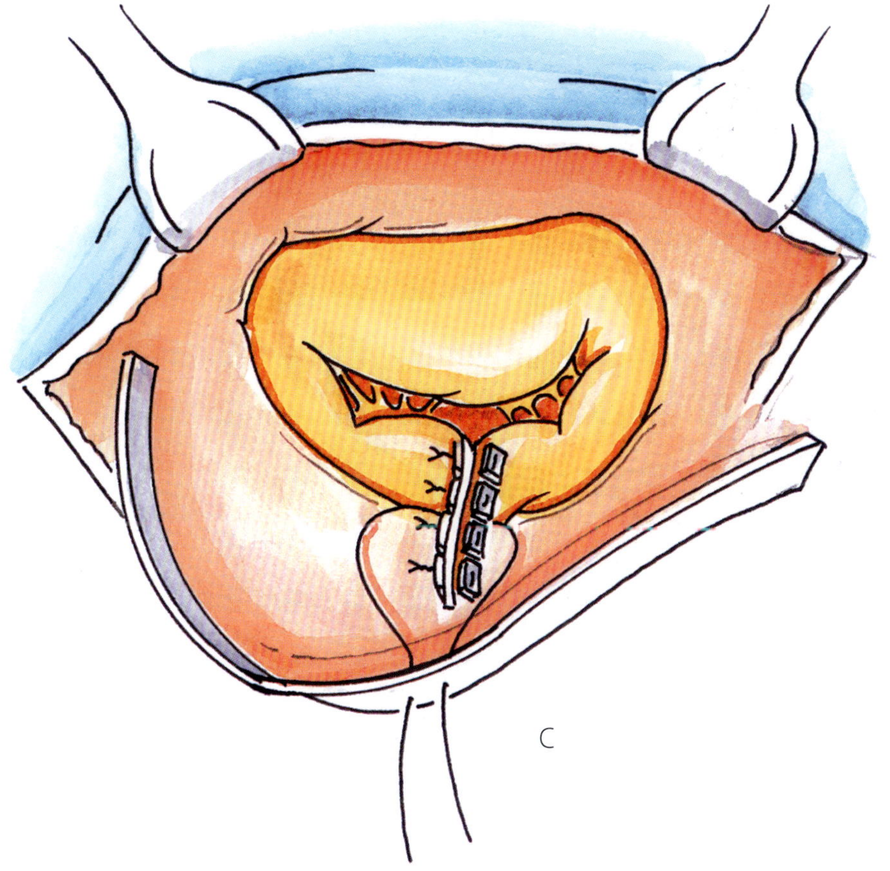

C. 裁剪一心包条，在二尖瓣后瓣环折叠缝合处先褥式缝合 1 针。

C. A pericardial strip is prepared, and one mattress suture is made over the plicated and sutured posterior mitral annulus first.

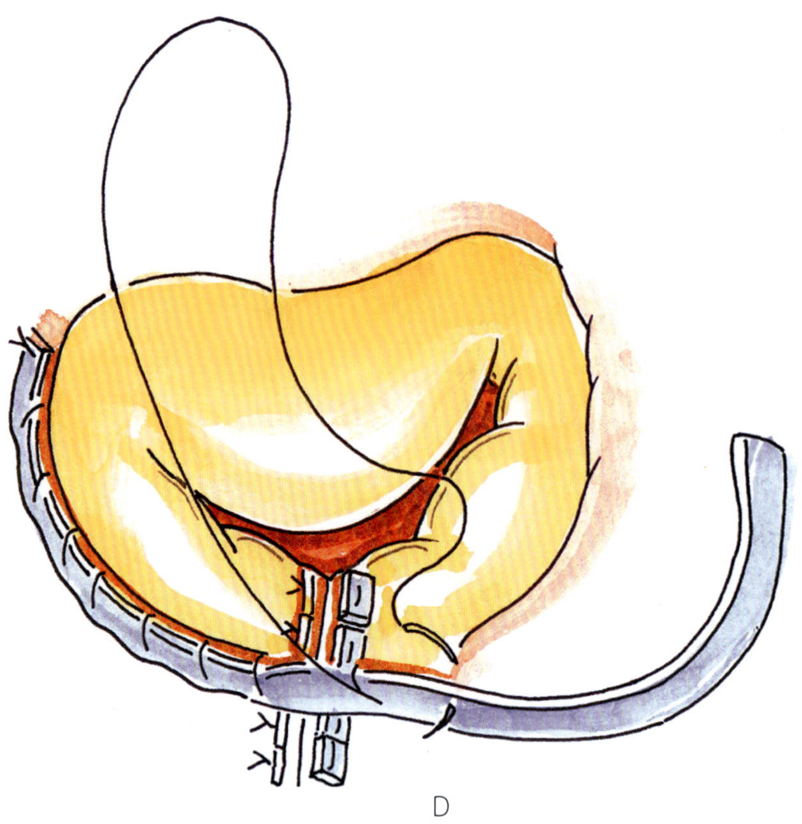

D. 推下心包条结扎，将心包条与二尖瓣后瓣环连续缝合，两端超过二尖瓣交界。

D. The pericardial strip is pushed down and ligated. Sew the pericardial strip to the posterior leaflet of the mitral annulus by using running sutures with both ends beyond the mitral junction.

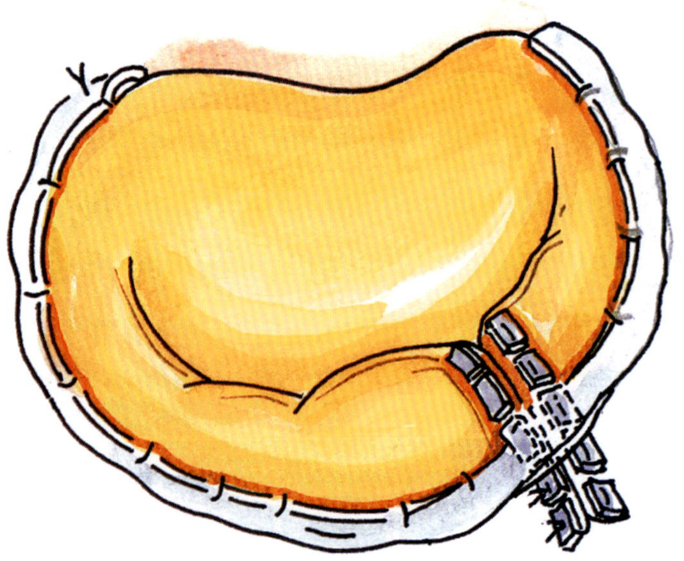

E. 二尖瓣成形完成。

E. Mitral valvuloplasty is completed.

图 3-1-4　交界折叠术
Figure 3-1-4　Commissural plication

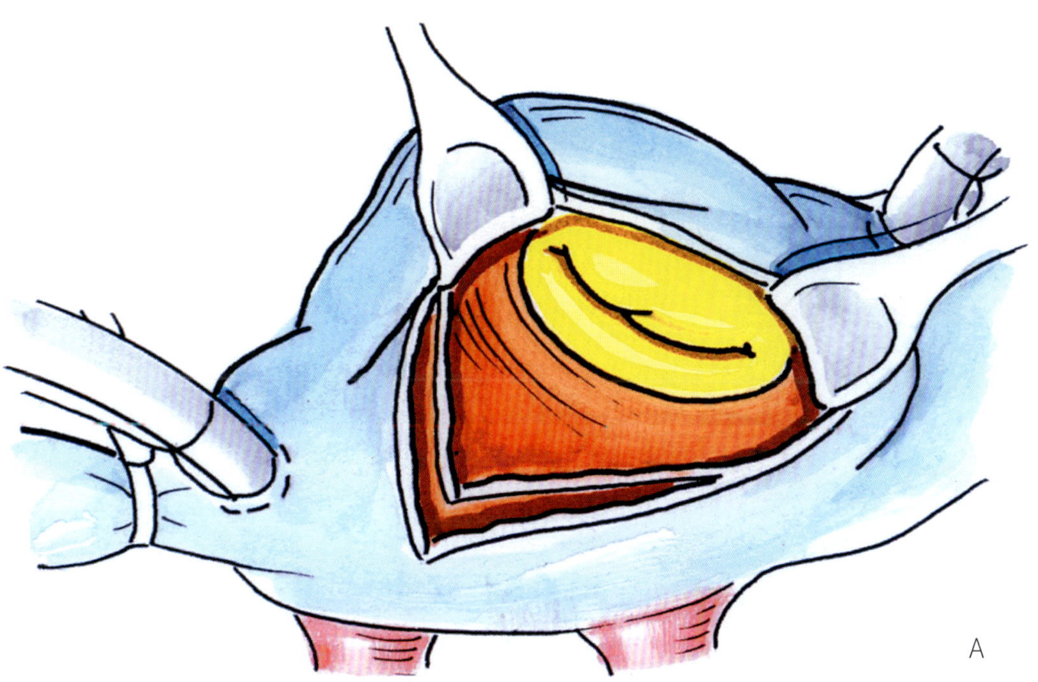

A. 经右心房 - 房间隔切口进入左心房，显露二尖瓣。

A. The left atrium is accessed via a right atrial-atrial septal incision, and the mitral valve is exposed.

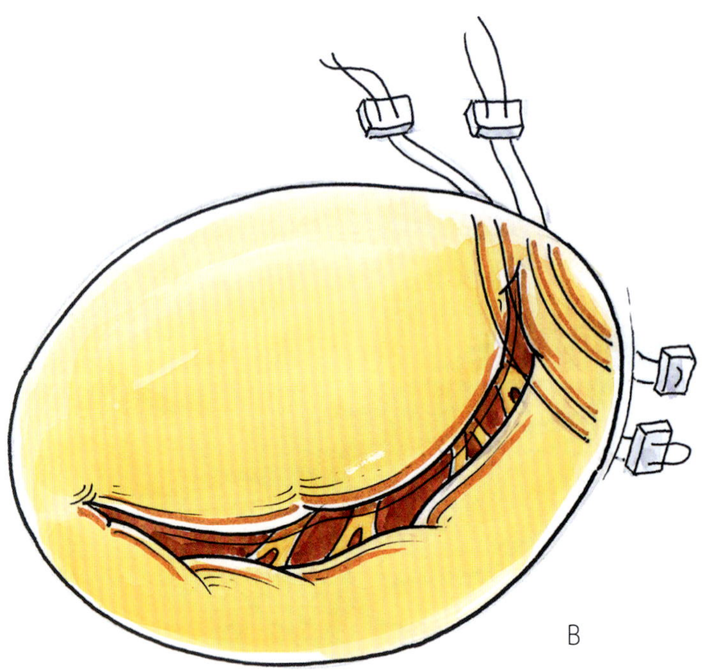

B. 在后内交界二尖瓣环上做 1~3 个褥式缝合，后瓣环的针距略大于前瓣环。

B. 1-3 mattress sutures are placed on the junction between the posterior and anterior mitral annulus with the needle gauge on the posterior annulus slightly greater than that on the anterior annulus.

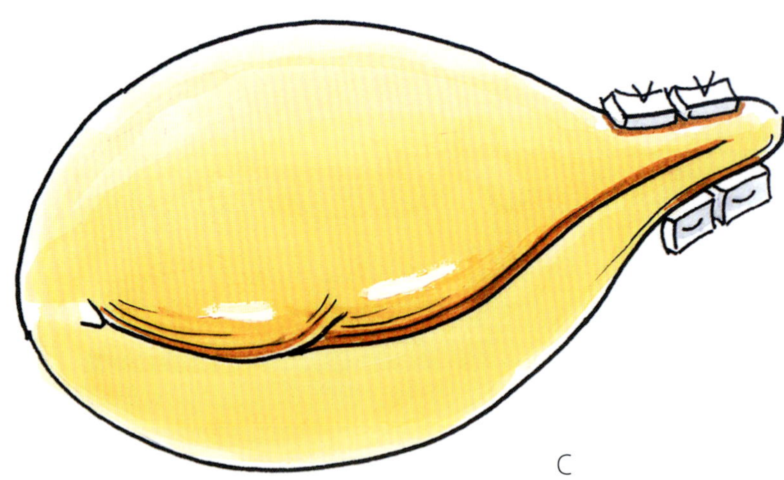

C. 结扎后局部反流消失。

C. Local regurgitation disappears after ligation.

图 3-1-5 缘对缘技术用于 Barlow 氏病

Figure 3-1-5 Edge-to-edge technique for Barlow's disease

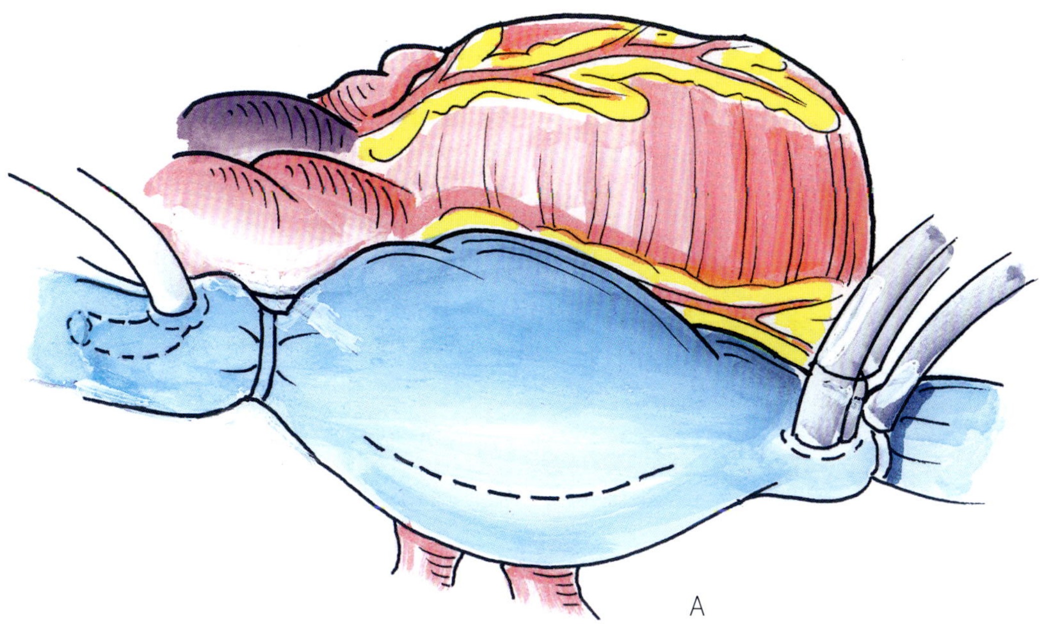

A. 体外循环下经右心房 - 房间隔切口进入左心房。

A. Under extracorporeal circulation, the left atrium is accessed through a right atrial-transseptal incision.

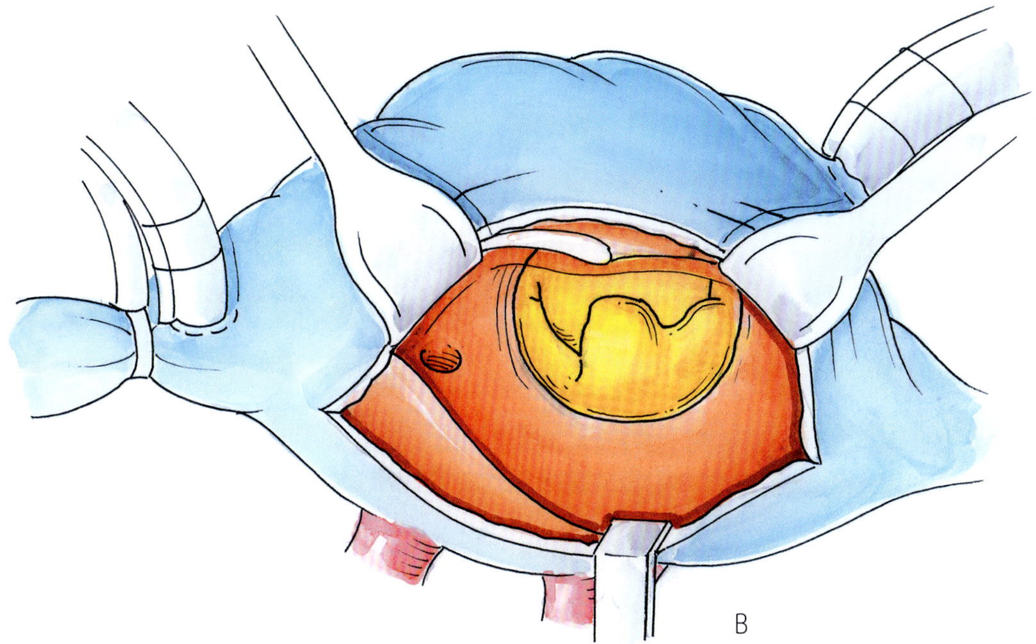

B. 显露二尖瓣，见二尖瓣后叶冗长脱垂。

B. The mitral valve is exposed, and the prolapsed and elongated posterior mitral leaflet is identified.

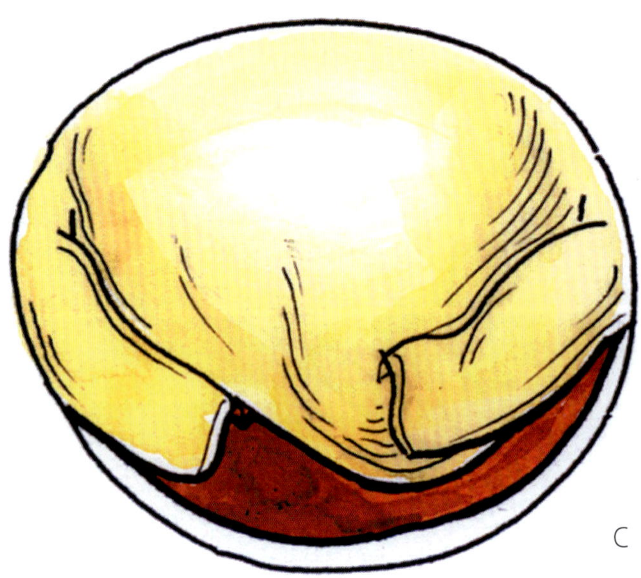

C. 矩形切除二尖瓣后叶脱垂的部分。

C. A rectangular resection of the prolapsed section of the posterior leaflet is done.

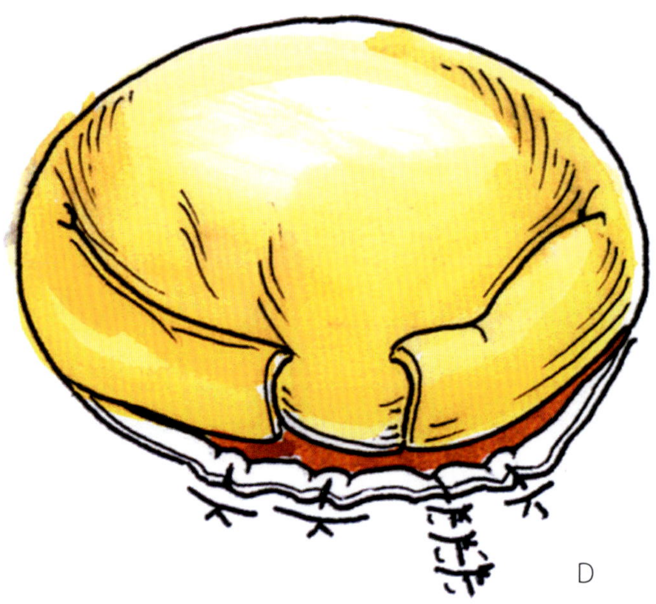

D. Barlow 氏病二尖瓣后叶通常须切除较多部分，先将二尖瓣后瓣环做几个折叠缝合，缩小后瓣环的长度。

D. In Barlow's disease, much of the posterior mitral valve leaflet is usually to be excised, and several plication sutures are placed on the posterior annulus to shorten its length.

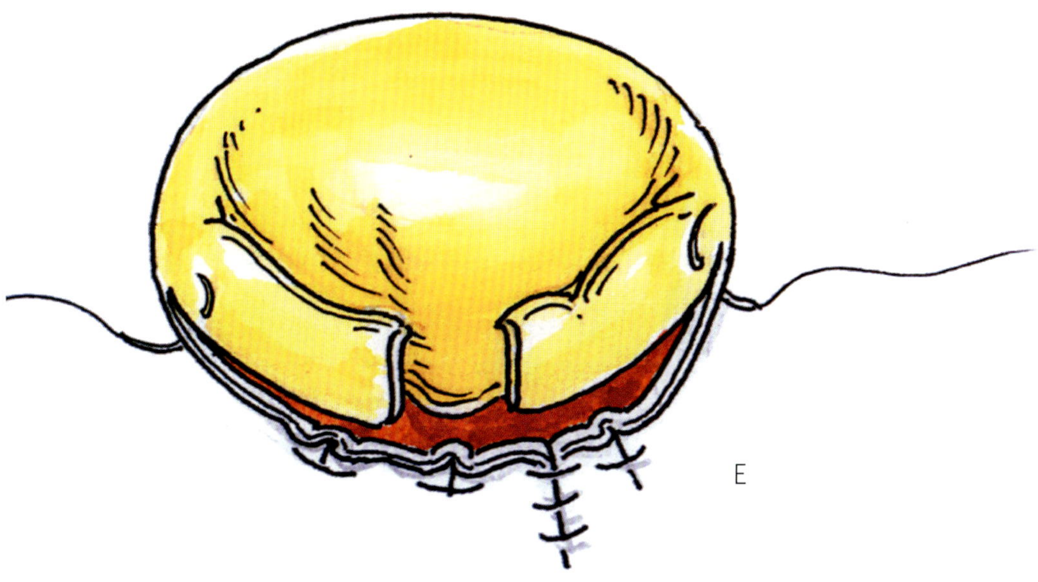

E. 再应用瓣叶滑行技术修复二尖瓣后叶。将切开的后叶与瓣环单纯连续缝合，把二尖瓣后叶逐渐向中间移行，使两断端对拢缝合。

E. The posterior mitral leaflet is then repaired by the sliding leaflet technique. The incised posterior leaflet and annulus are sutured with simple running sutures, and the posterior leaflet is moved centrally little by little to allow the anastomosis of two cut edges of leaflets.

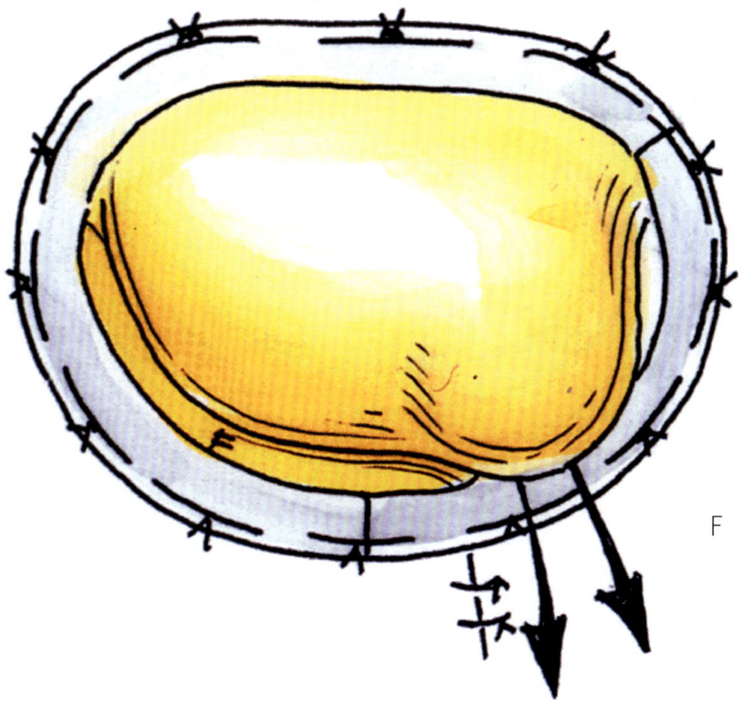

F. 植入人工瓣环，见二尖瓣前叶脱垂。

F. An annulus prosthesis is implanted, and the anterior mitral leaflet prolapse is visualized.

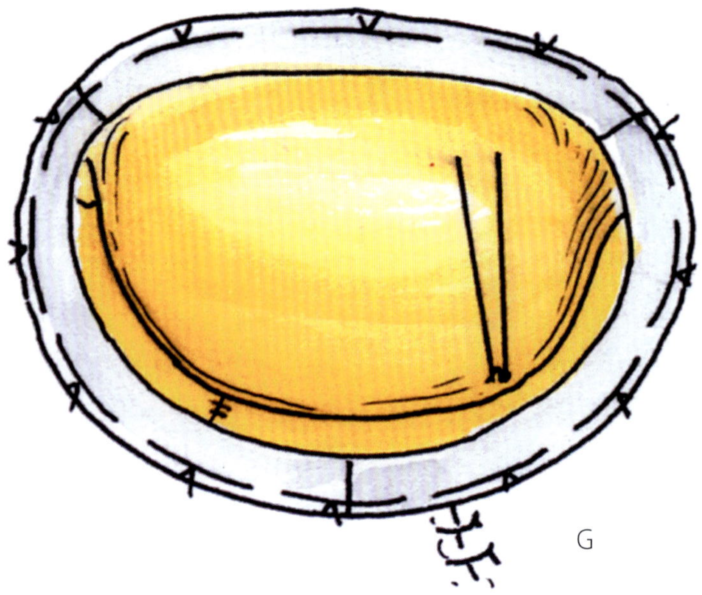
G

G. 二尖瓣前叶脱垂处用缘对缘技术纠正。将二尖瓣后叶缘与二尖瓣前叶脱垂对应处做缘对缘缝合，单纯缝合，贯穿全层，二尖瓣形成两孔开口。缘对缘技术较腱索成形简便，通过降低前、后叶对合缘，能有效地预防收缩期前向活动现象。

G. Anterior mitral leaflet prolapse is corrected with edge-to-edge technique. The edge of the posterior leaflet is sutured in full-thickness to the corresponding edge of the anterior leaflet prolapse of the mitral valve to create a double-orifice mitral valve. The edge-to-edge technique is more convenient than the chordal plasty, as it may effectively avoid the systolic anterior motion (SAM) by lowering the coapted edges of anterior and posterior leaflets.

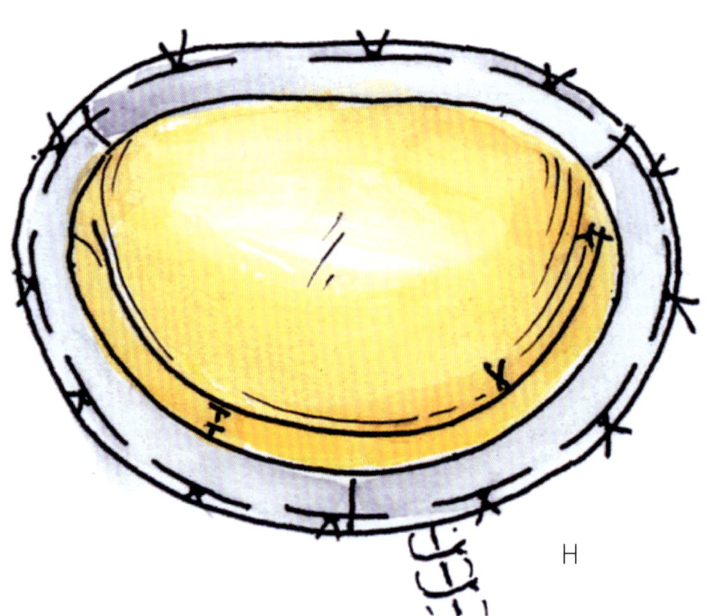
H

H. 手术完成。

H. The surgery is completed.

图 3-1-6 Duran 瓣膜成形环植入术
Figure 3-1-6 Annuloplasty with Duran ring

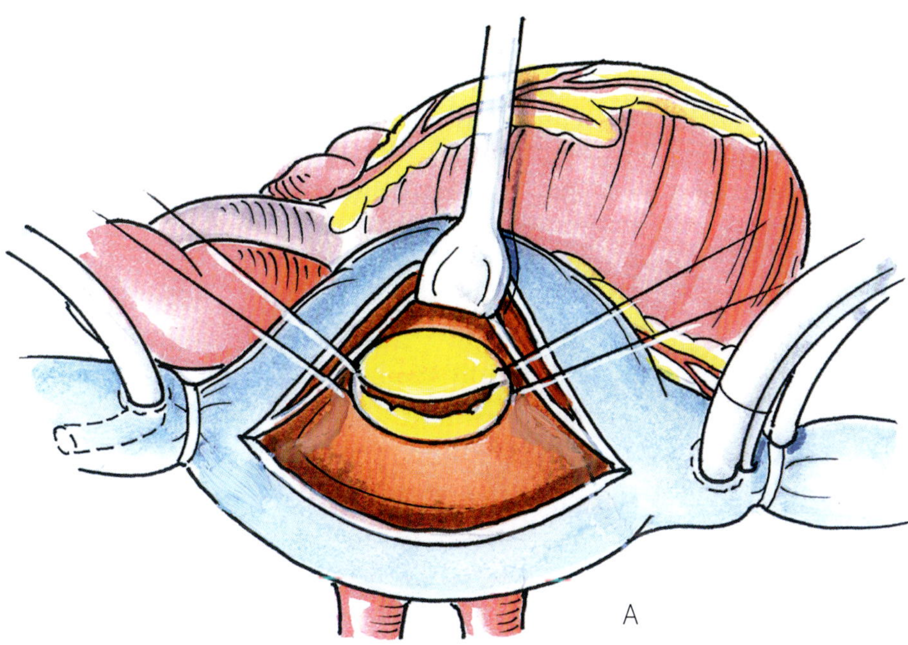

A. 体外循环下切开右心房和房间隔，显露二尖瓣。在左、右纤维三角区的瓣环上各缝 1 针水平褥式缝合作为标记。

A. Right atrium and atrial septum are incised under extracorporeal circulation to expose the mitral valve. One horizontal mattress suture is placed into the annulus of the left and right fibrous triangles respectively as a marker.

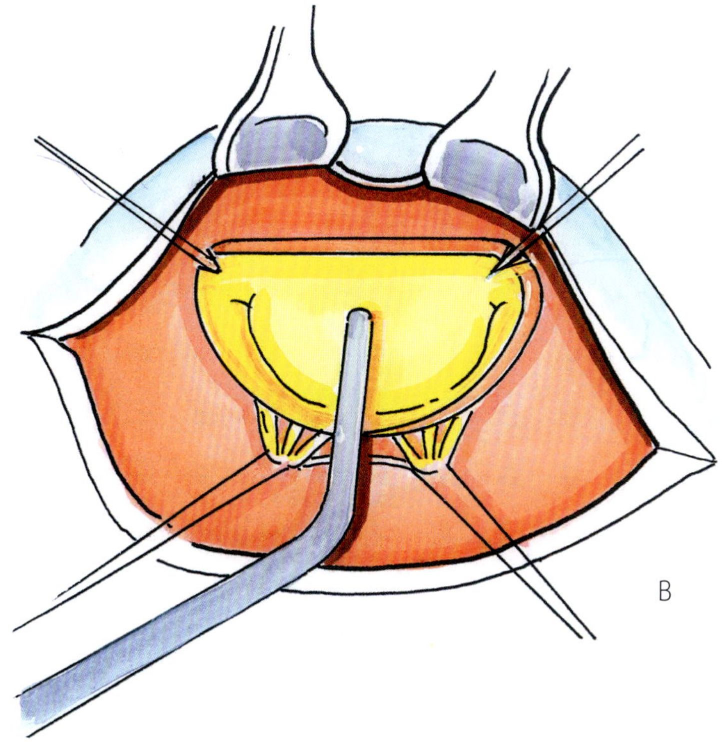

B. 向下牵引前瓣腱索，用测瓣器选择与二尖瓣前瓣面积匹配的瓣膜成形环。

B. Tract the anterior chordae downward and choose an annuloplasty ring in proportion to the anterior mitral valve with a sizer.

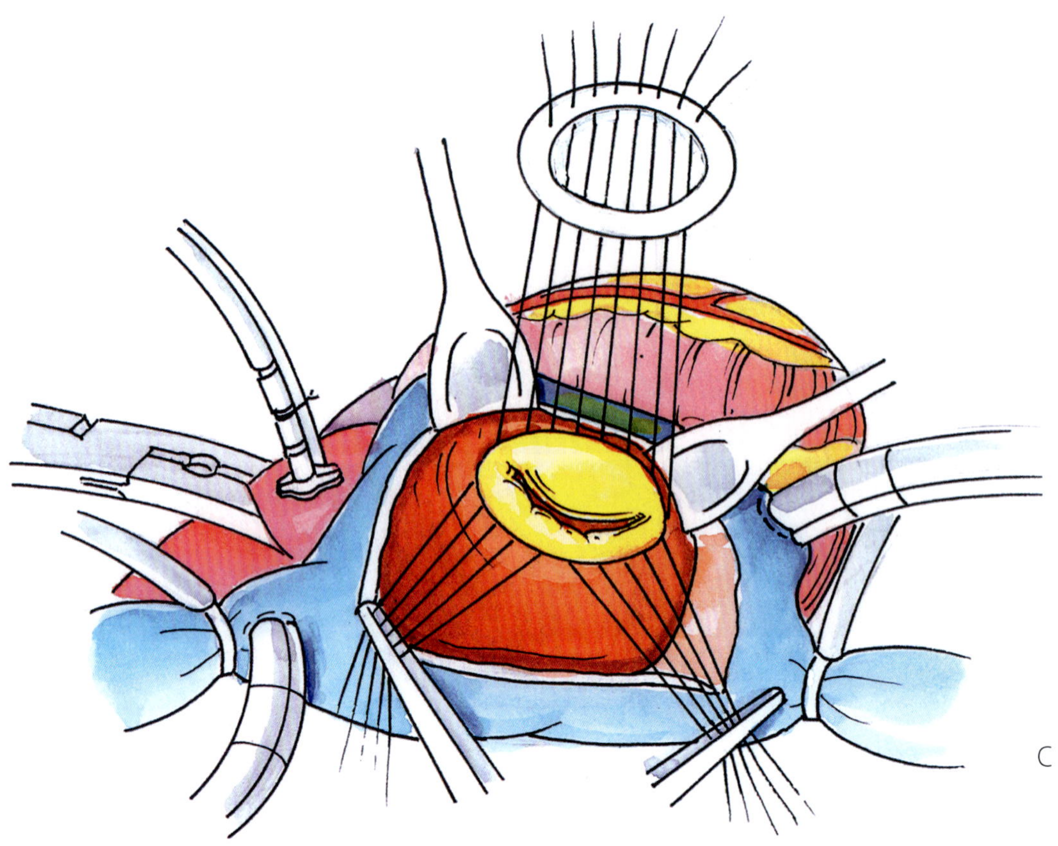

C. 沿二尖瓣环做水平褥式缝合。前瓣环缝 4~6 针，然后缝线穿过对应的瓣膜成形环，瓣膜成形环上的针距应与前瓣环的针距相仿，使二尖瓣前叶保持舒展。后瓣环和两交界处的针距要大于在瓣膜成形环上的针距，从而将该区域的瓣环缩小。

C. Horizontal mattress sutures are placed around the mitral annulus. 4-6 stitches are made in the anterior annulus, and then the needle is passed through the corresponding annuloplasty ring with the needle gauge similar to that on the anterior annulus to keep the anterior mitral leaflet stretched. The needle gauges in the posterior annulus and in the junction are to be larger than that in the annuloplasty ring, so as to narrow the annulus in this area.

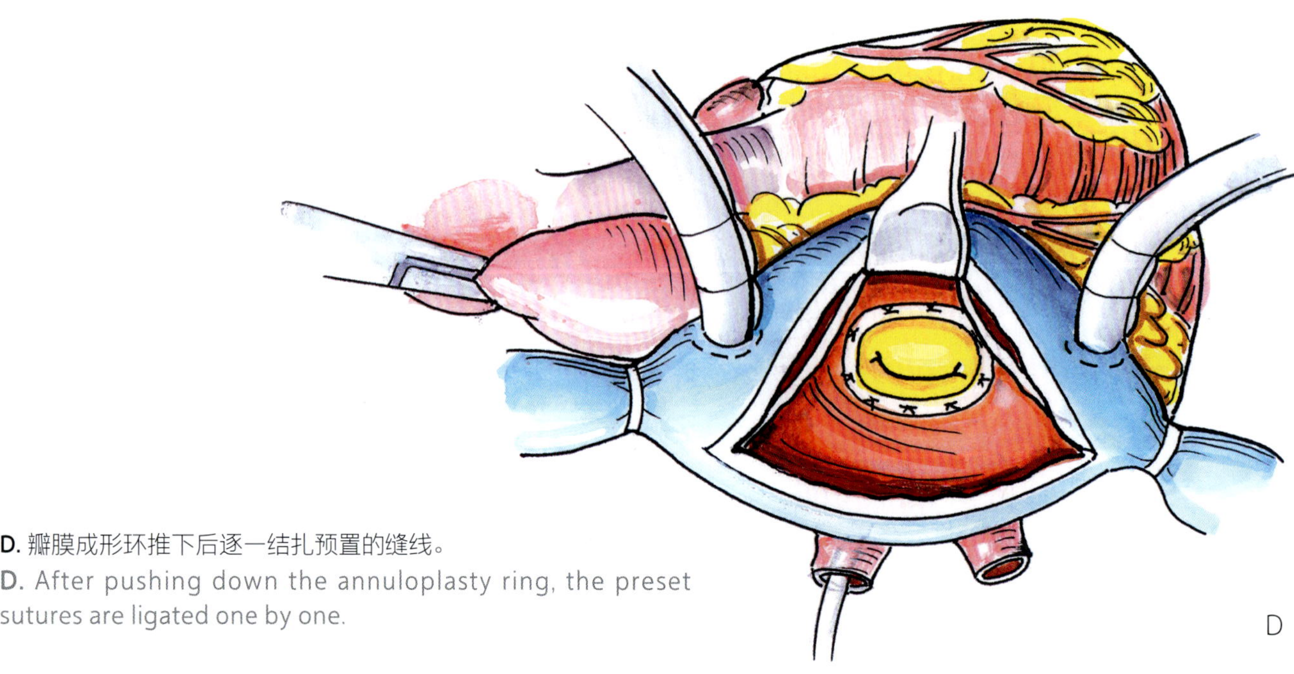

D. 瓣膜成形环推下后逐一结扎预置的缝线。

D. After pushing down the annuloplasty ring, the preset sutures are ligated one by one.

图 3-1-7　二尖瓣后叶矩形切除修补术
Figure 3-1-7　Posterior mitral leaflet rectangular resection and reconstruction

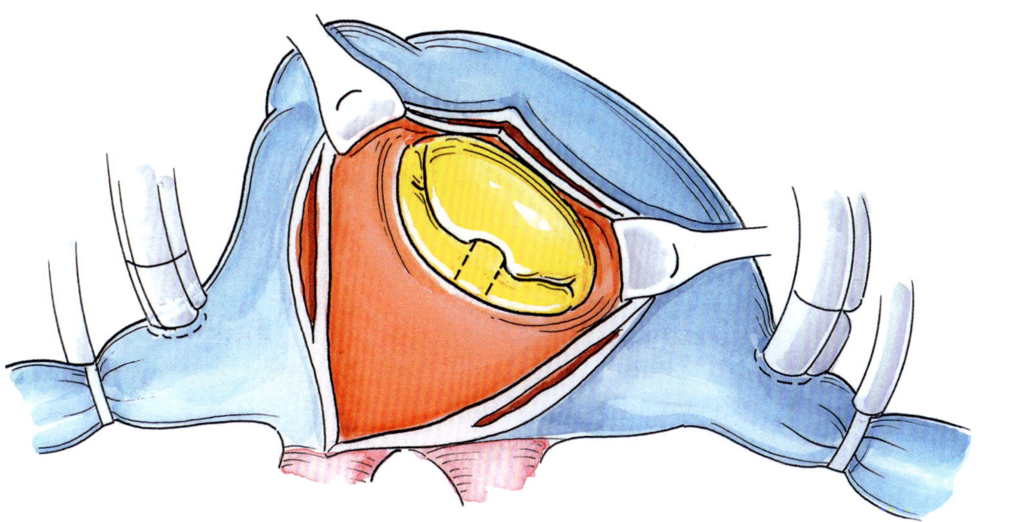

A. 二尖瓣后叶局部脱垂可用矩形切除法矫正。
A. Partial posterior mitral leaflet prolapse can be corrected by rectangular resection.

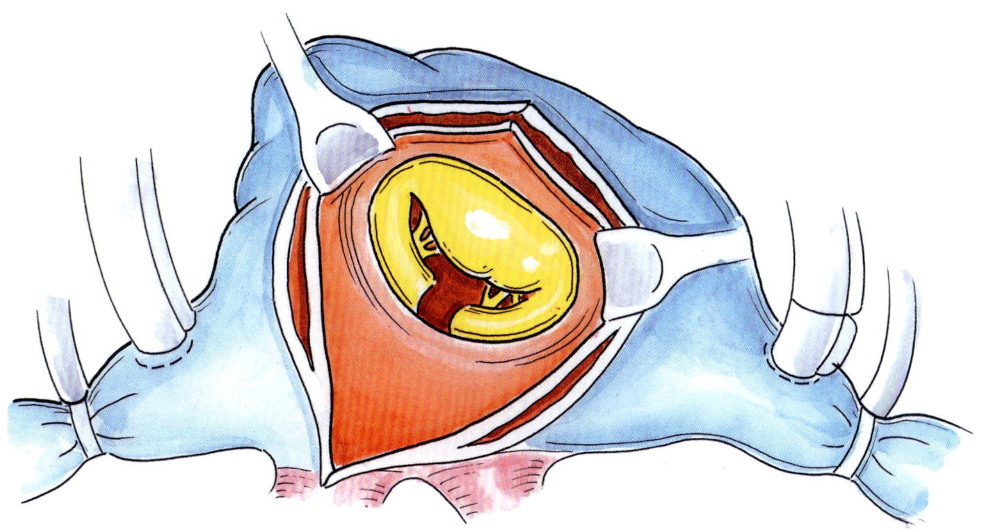

B. 矩形切除脱垂的瓣叶。垂直切向瓣环，勿损伤瓣环。脱垂切除段瓣叶两侧的腱索要尽量保留。
B. A rectangular resection of prolapsed leaflets is done. A vertical incision is made in the annulus, and care must be taken to avoid damage to the annulus. The chordae tendineae on both sides of the resected segment of the prolapsed leaflet should be preserved as much as possible.

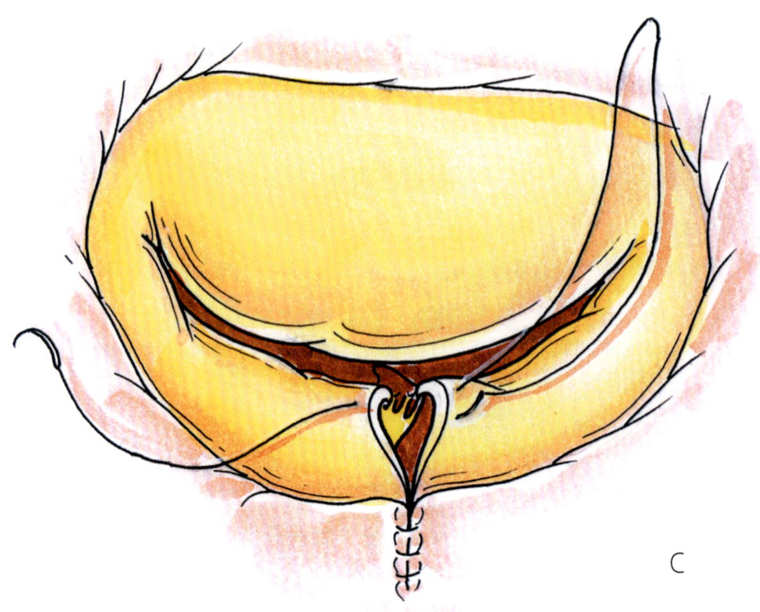

C. 从瓣环起将二尖瓣后叶间断缝合。

C. Interrupted sutures are made on the posterior mitral valve leaflet from the annulus.

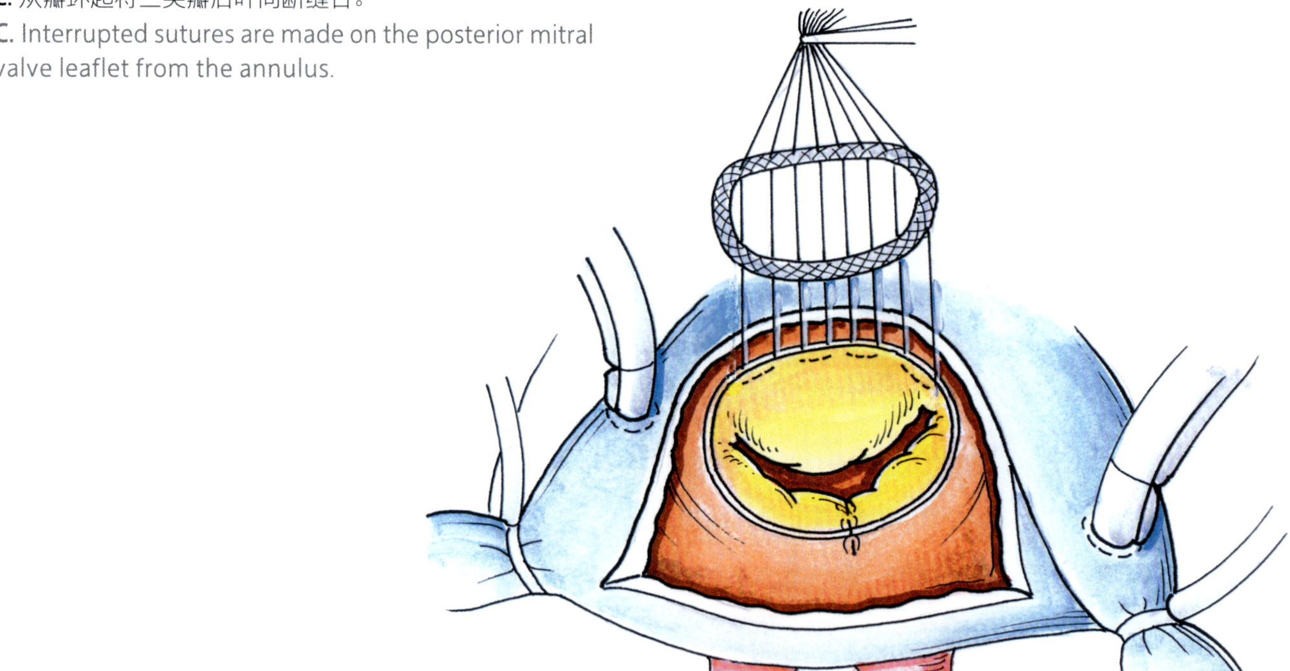

D. 选用合适口径的人工瓣环植入。后叶矩形切除瓣环处的缝针要跨后叶缝合线，以减少该处的张力。

D. An appropriately sized annulus prosthesis is implanted. The sutures at the annulus shall straddle the sutures made in the resected posterior mitral leaflet, with an aim to reduce tension there.

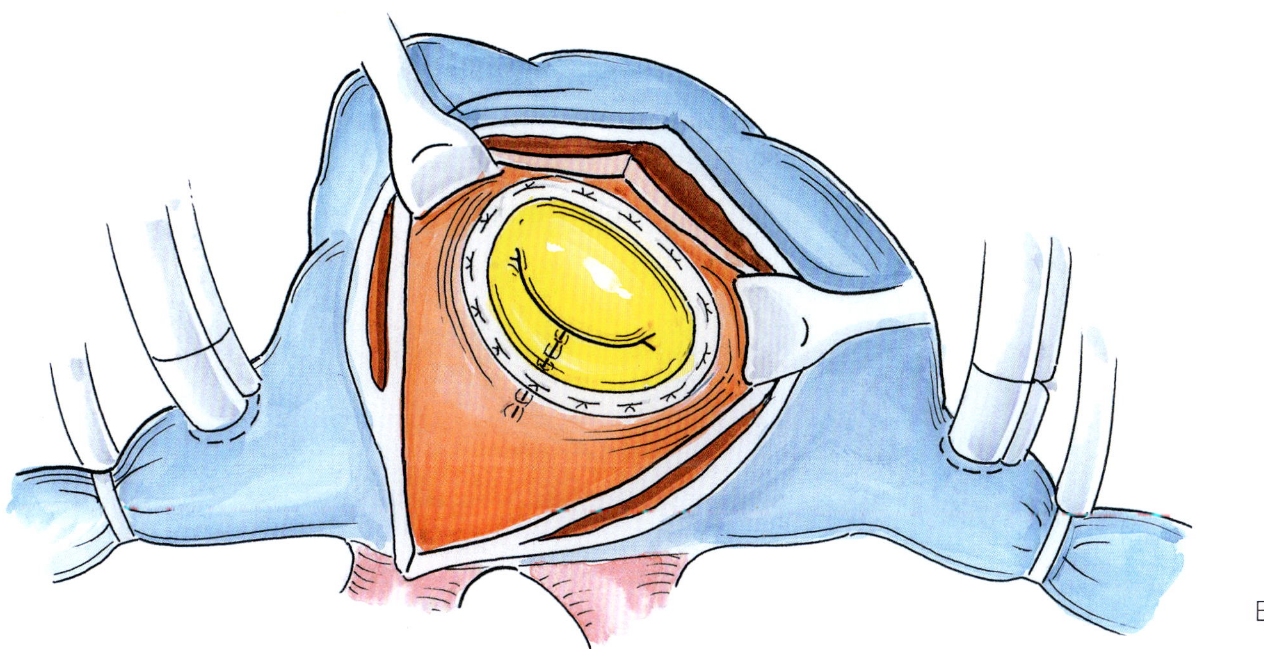

E. 人工瓣环推下打结，修复完成。

E. The annulus prosthesis is pushed down and knotted, and repair is completed.

图 3-1-8　二尖瓣前叶修补术
Figure 3-1-8　Anterior mitral leaflet repair

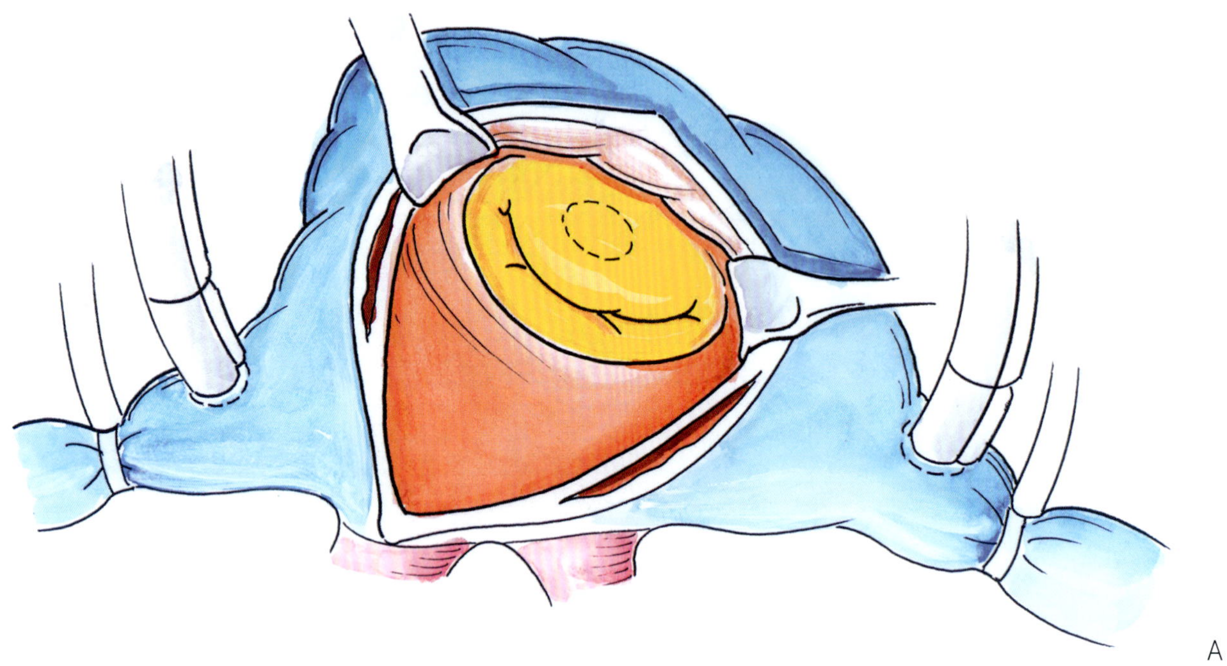

A. 体外循环下经右心房 - 房间隔切口进入左心房，见二尖瓣前叶穿孔。

A. The left atrium is entered through a right atrial-atrial septal incision with extracorporeal circulation, and anterior mitral valve perforations are exposed.

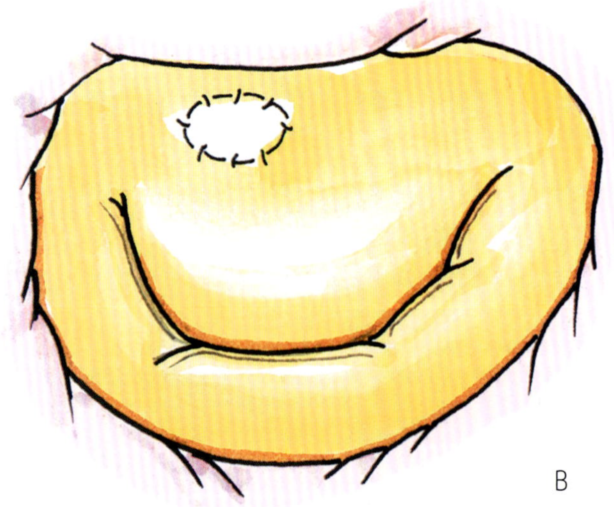

B. 先将穿孔适当修剪。然后裁剪一块自体心包，用 0.5% 戊二醛浸泡处理，单纯连续缝合补片修补瓣叶缺损。

B. Trim the perforation properly first. Cut a piece of the autologous pericardium for a patch and soak it in 0.5% glutaraldehyde. The pericardium patch is then used to repair the leaflet defect by simple running sutures.

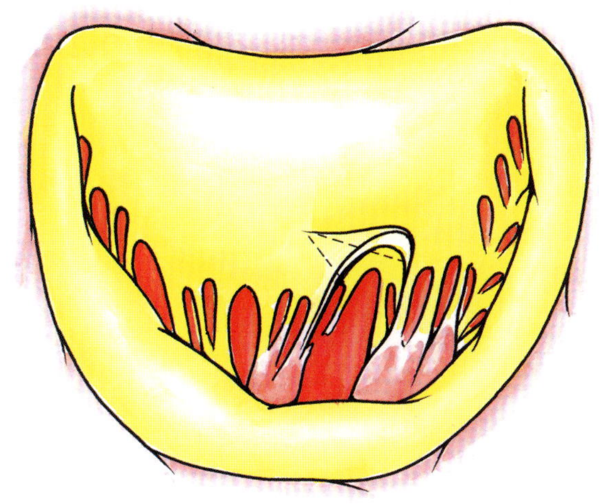

C

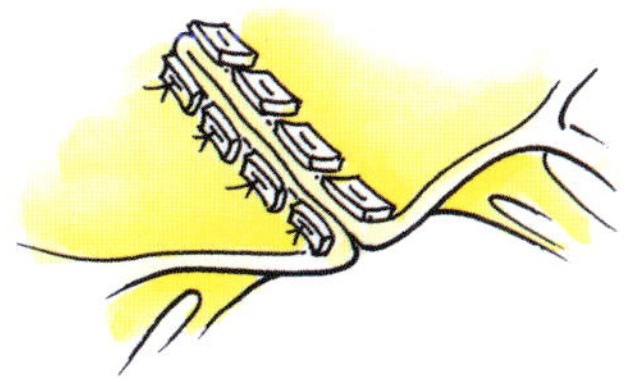

C. 二尖瓣前叶小范围的脱垂可以采取楔形切除后直接缝合修复。

C. Partial prolapse of the anterior mitral leaflet can be repaired by wedge resection of the prolapsed area followed by direct sutures.

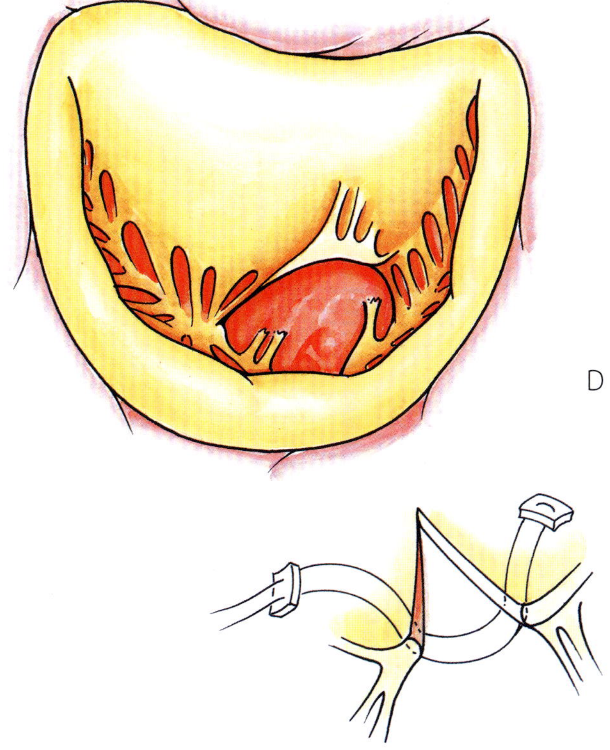

D. 二尖瓣前叶小范围的腱索断裂瓣叶外翻。也可以采取楔形切除后直接缝合修复。

D. If partial rupture of the chordae tendineae and leaflet eversion are present, the anterior mitral leaflet can be repaired by wedge resection followed by direct sutures.

图 3-1-9　二尖瓣人工腱索重建术
Figure 3-1-9　Artificial chordal reconstruction

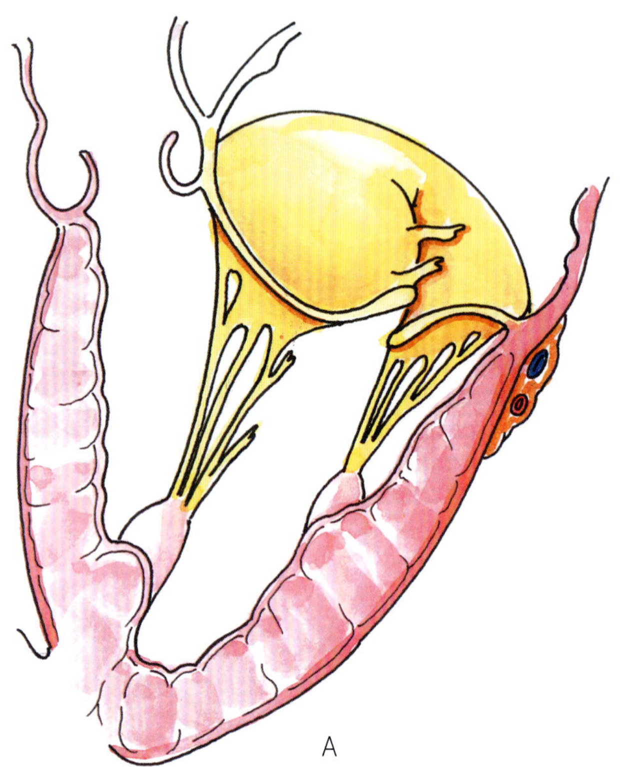

A. 二尖瓣前叶腱索断裂致瓣膜外翻，形成二尖瓣关闭不全。

A. Rupture of the anterior mitral chordae tendineae results in leaflet eversion and hence generates mitral regurgitation.

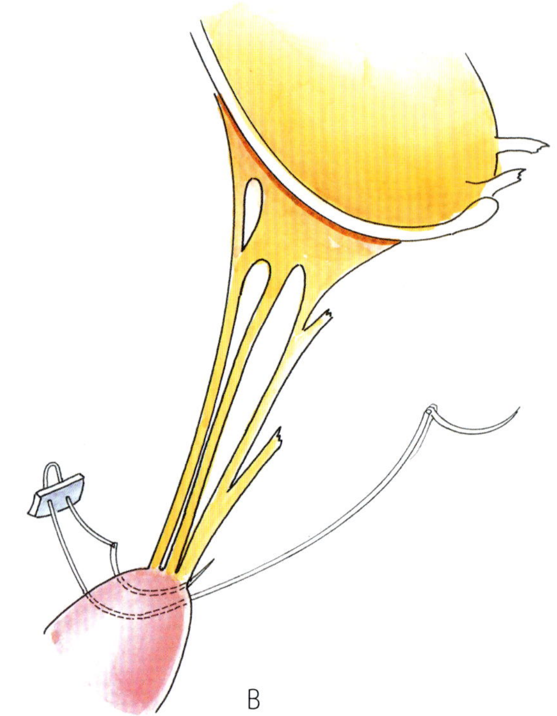

B. 用 4-0 Gore-Tex 缝线做人工腱索替代断裂的腱索。先在断裂腱索的相应乳头肌做带垫片褥式缝合。

B. The ruptured chordae is replaced by an artificial substitute created with 4-0 Gore-Tex sutures. Pledgeted mattress sutures are performed on the corresponding papillary muscle of the broken chordae tendon.

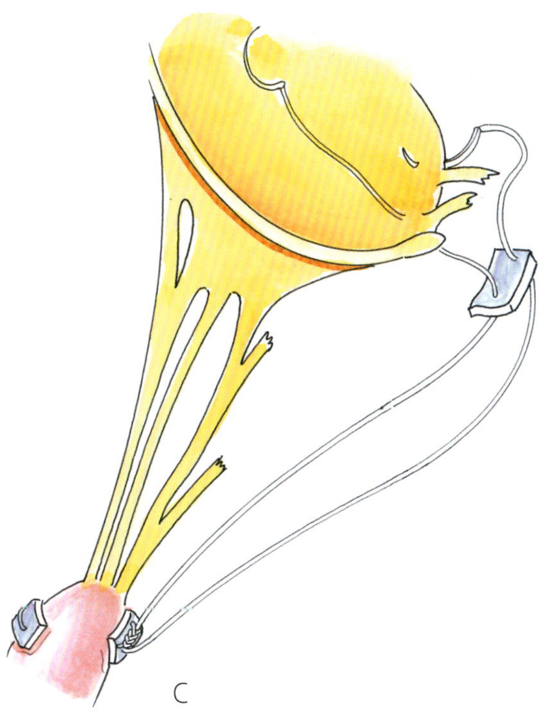

C. 乳头肌端结扎 Gore-Tex 缝线，缝线再缝到外翻的瓣膜缘，心室面进针，心房面出针。

C. The papillary muscle is ligated with the Gore-Tex suture first, and the suture is then passed through the everted leaflet edges from the ventricular to the atrial side.

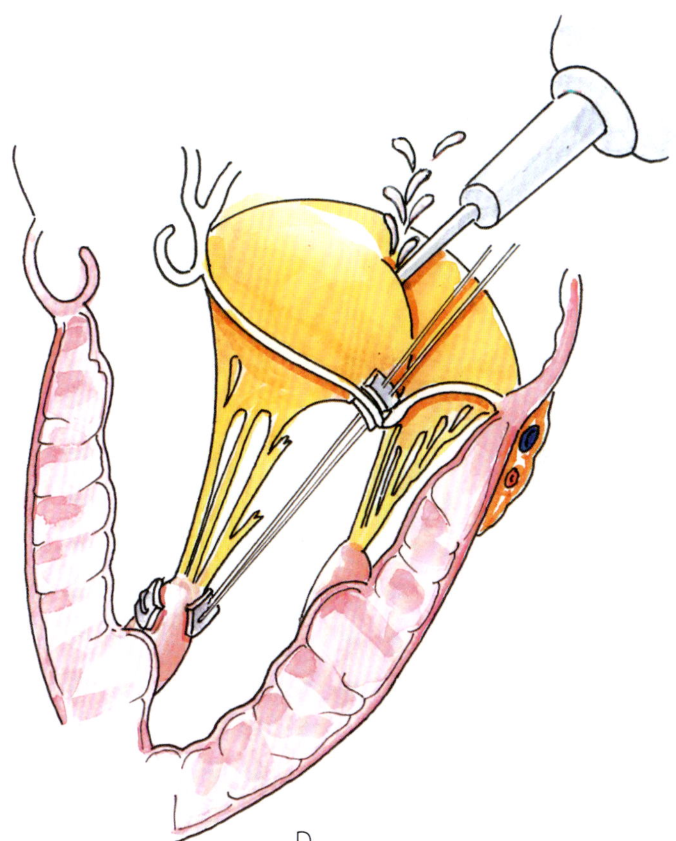

D. 左心室注生理盐水，调节人工腱索的长度，使二尖瓣前瓣缘和后瓣缘贴合完好，二尖瓣反流消失。

D. The left ventricle is infused with normal saline (NS) to adjust the length of the artificial chordae tendineae, allowing the anterior and posterior leaflet edges to fit well for the disappearance of mitral regurgitation.

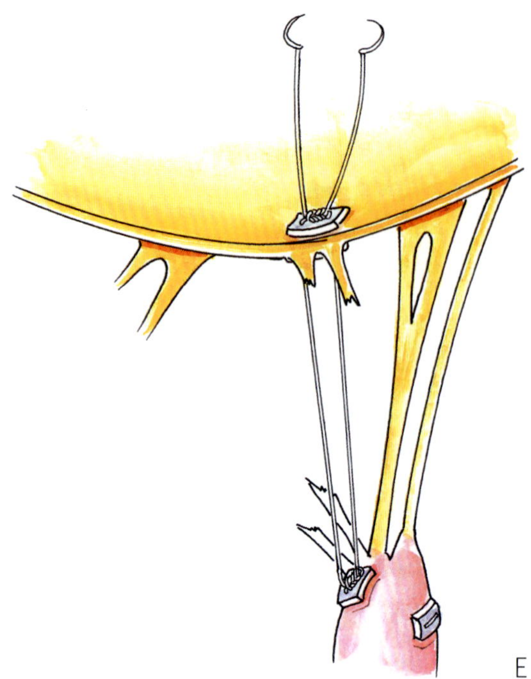

E. 结扎瓣膜侧 Gore-Tex 缝线。

E. Ligate the Gore-Tex suture on the valve side.

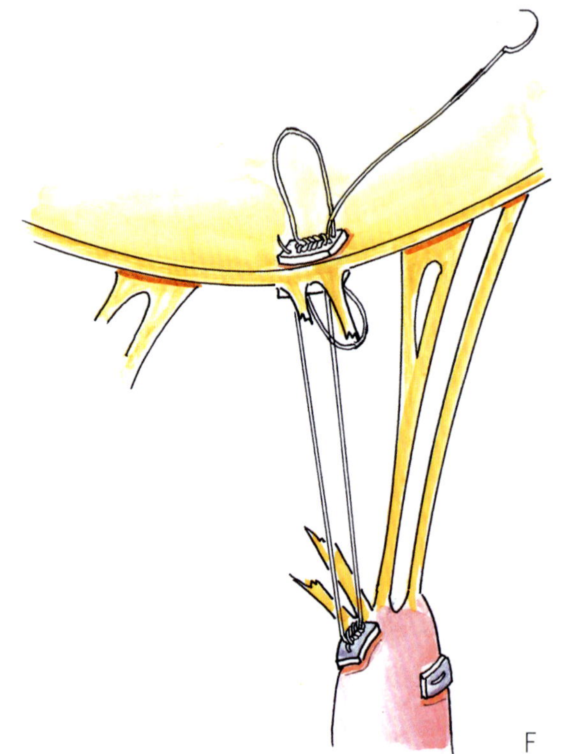

F. 缝线穿过垫片。

F. One arm of the suture then passes through a pledget.

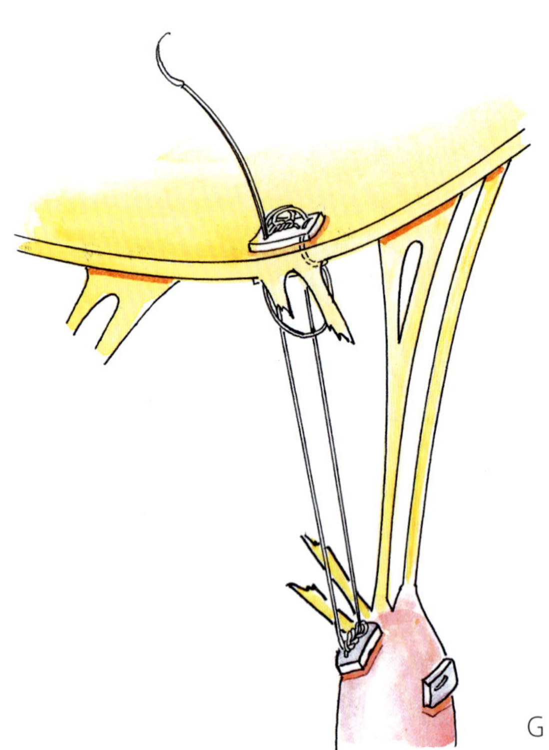

G. 缝线另一头也穿过垫片，再次打结，人工腱索植入完成。

G. The other arm is also passed through the pledget and knotted again, and the implantation of artificial chordae is completed.

图 3-1-10 二尖瓣人工机械瓣置换术
Figure 3-1-10 Mitral valve replacement with mechanical prosthesis

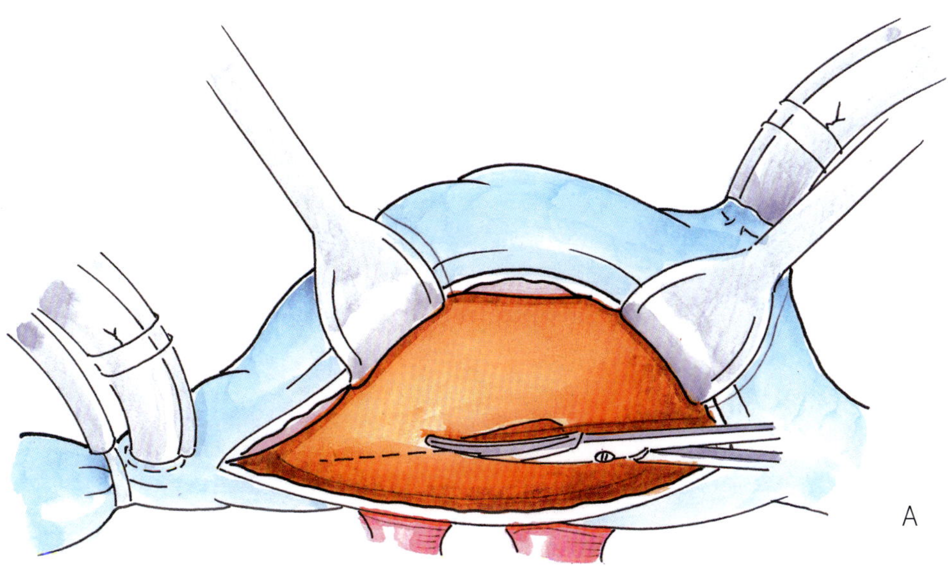

A. 体外循环下纵行切开右心房，切开卵圆窝并延长切口剪开房间隔，进入左心房。
A. The right atrium is opened longitudinally under extracorporeal circulation, and the oval fossa is incised, with the incision extending to the atrial septum, and then into the left atrium.

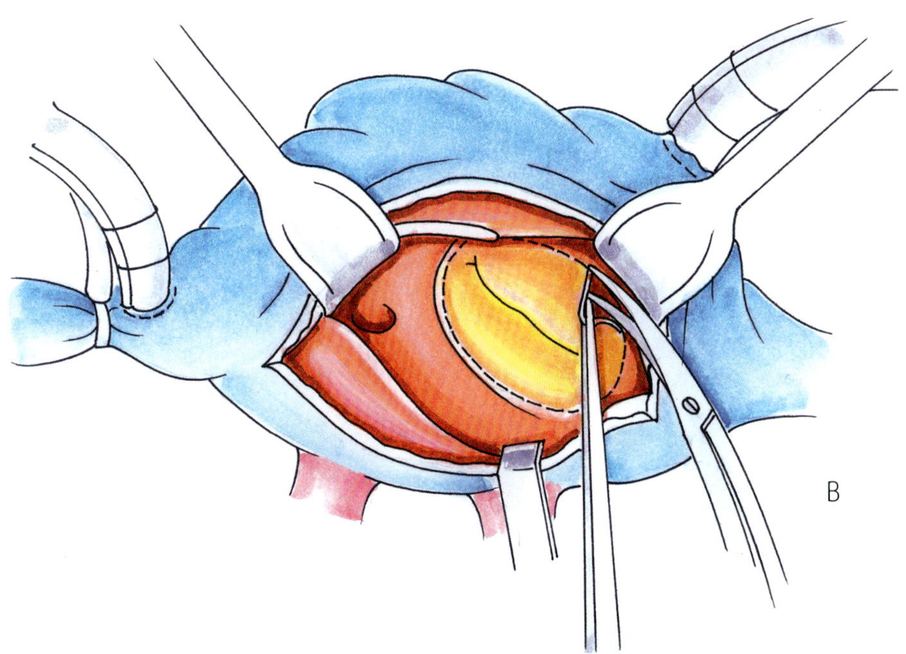

B. 左心房探查，若有血栓予以彻底清除。距二尖瓣环约 2mm 切除二尖瓣瓣叶及其腱索。
B. Left atrial exploration is performed. If present, the thrombus should be cleared completely. Mitral valve leaflets and their chordae tendineae are removed around 2 mm away from the mitral annulus.

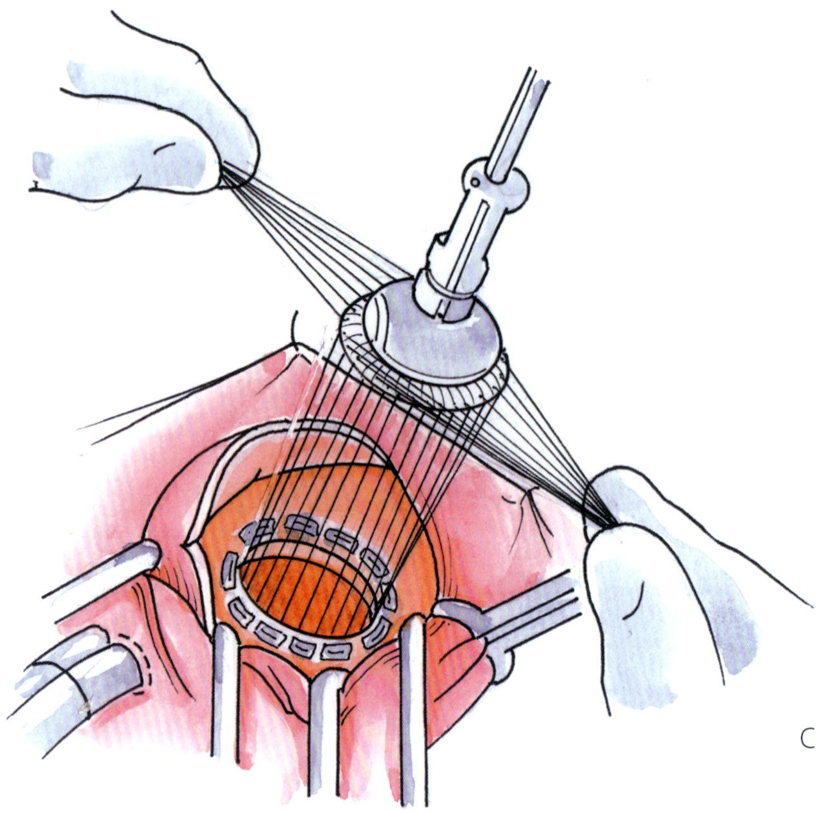

C. 经二尖瓣环用带垫片双头瓣膜缝线缝入。左心房进针垫片留在左心房，二尖瓣环左心室侧出针。进针可缝入少量左心房心肌，出针避免缝到左心室心肌。一圈缝合完成后，将全部缝线再缝到人工机械瓣膜缝合环上。

C. A double-armed pledgeted suture is passed through the mitral annulus from the left atrium side to the left ventricular side, with the pledget left in the left atrium. The suture can bite a small amount of the left atrial myocardium when going inside, but avoid the left ventricular myocardium when going outside. After one loop of suture, all sutures are re-sutured to the mechanical prosthetic valve's sewing ring.

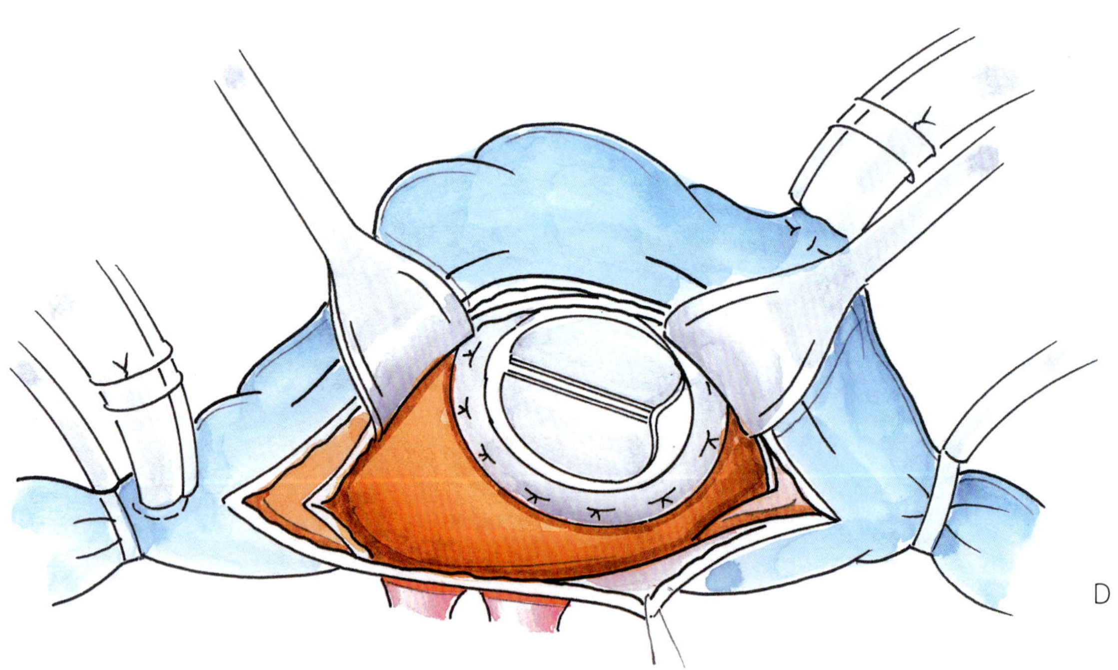

D. 人工机械瓣推下，落位二尖瓣环，逐一打结。

D. The mechanical prosthetic valves are pushed down to the mitral annulus, and all sutures are tied one by one.

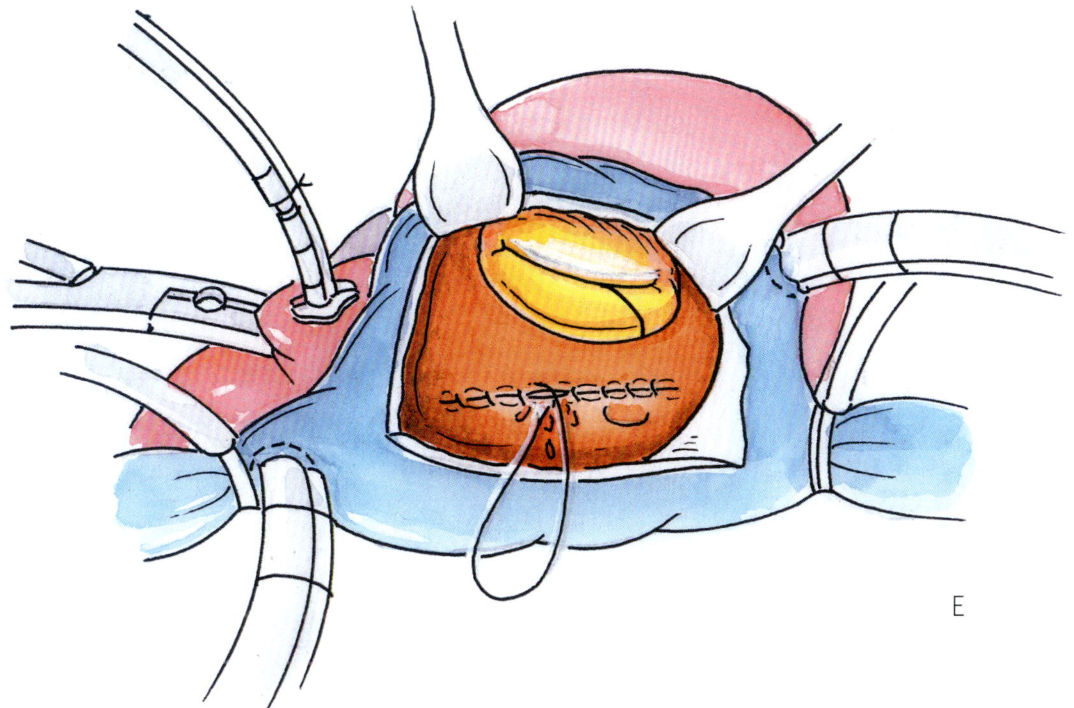

E. 连续缝合房间隔切口，左心房排气后结扎闭合房间隔。

E. The atrial septal incision is closed with running sutures, and the atrial septum is ligated and closed after the left atrial venting.

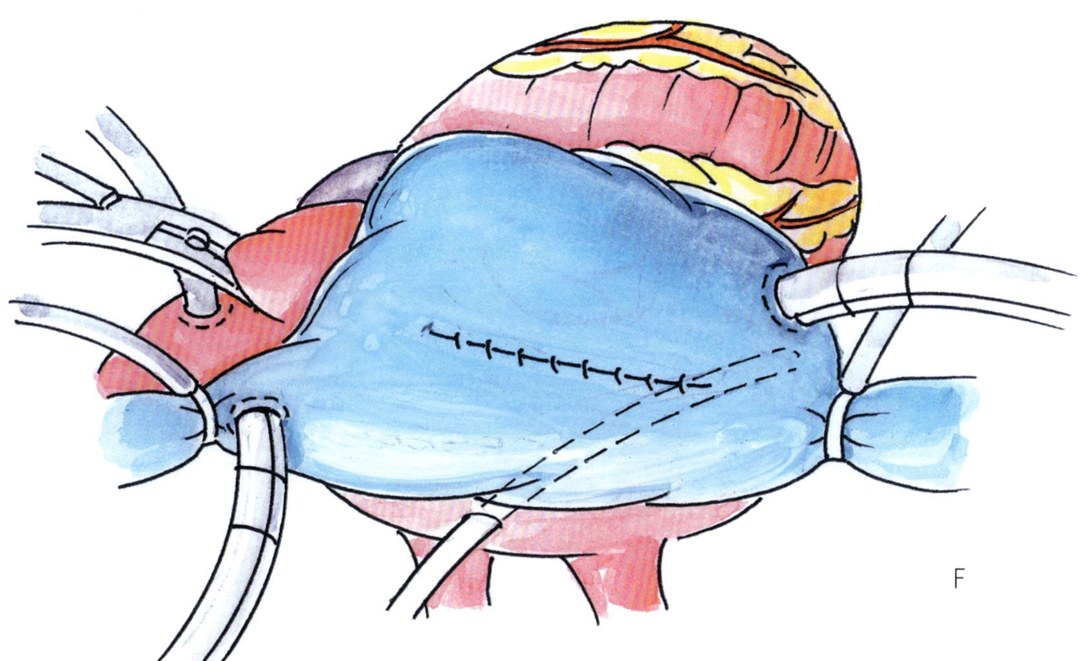

F. 缝合右心房切口。

F. Close the right atrial incision.

图 3-1-11 保留后叶及瓣下结构的二尖瓣置换术

Figure 3-1-11 Mitral valve replacement with preservation of posterior mitral leaflet and subvalvular structure

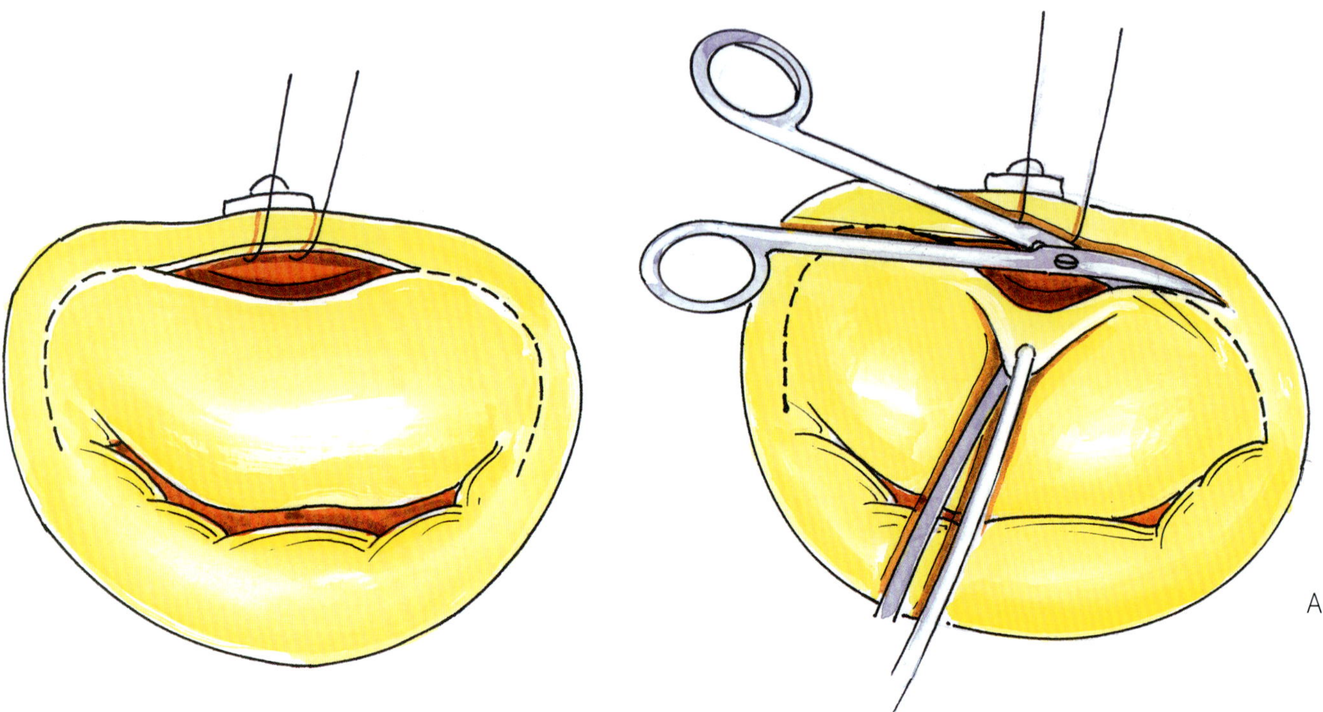

A. 体外循环下经右心房-房间隔路径进入左心房。距二尖瓣环约 2mm 处切开二尖瓣前叶，见其瓣下结构病变严重，腱索融合短缩致无法保留全部瓣下结构。

A. The left atrium is accessed via a right atrial-transseptal approach with extracorporeal circulation. An incision is made on the anterior mitral valve leaflet about 2 mm from the mitral annulus, and a severe anomaly of subvalvular structure can be found. Due to the fusion and shortening of chordae tendineae, the subvalvular structure cannot be fully preserved.

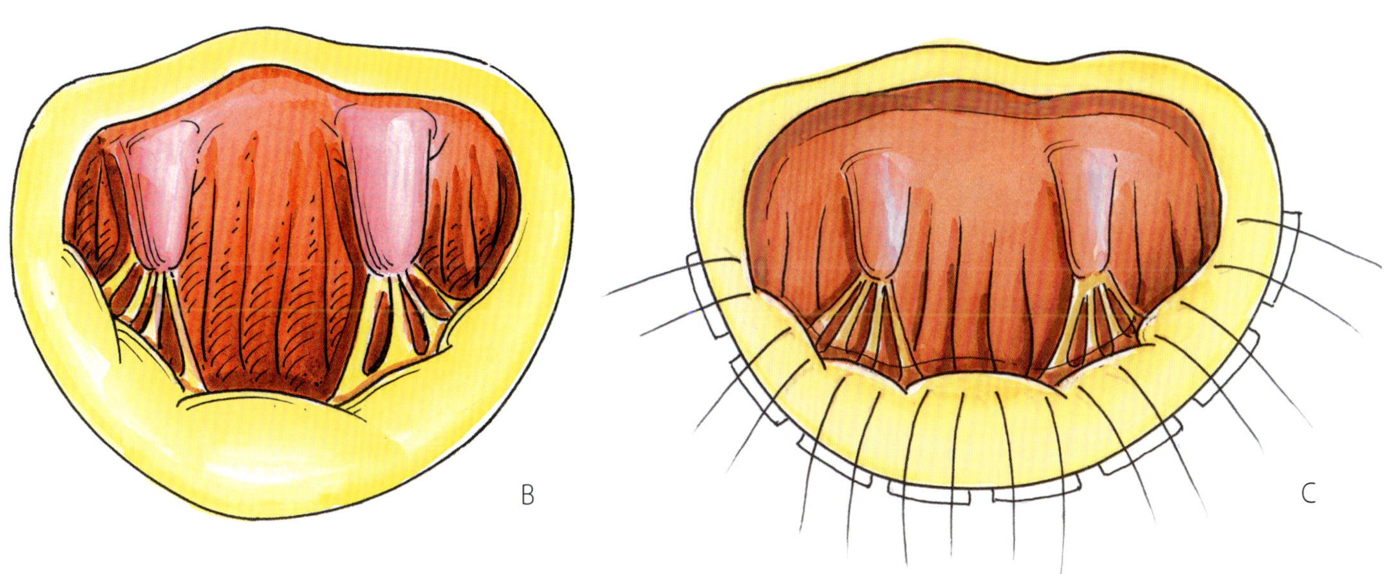

B. 切除二尖瓣前叶及附着其上的腱索，二尖瓣后叶及其瓣下结构予以保留。

B. Resect the anterior mitral valve leaflet and the chordae tendineae attached to the leaflet. Preserve the posterior mitral leaflet and its subvalvular structure.

C. 安置带垫片瓣膜褥式缝线。后叶瓣环处由左心房侧进针，穿过二尖瓣环左心室侧出针，缝针继续穿过后叶，在后叶瓣膜缘心房面出针。前叶瓣环处由左心房侧进针，穿过二尖瓣环左心室侧出针。

C. Pledgeted mattress sutures are performed. Sutures are introduced into the posterior leaflet annulus from the left atrial side and then passed through the mitral annulus to the left ventricle side. The suture sequentially passes through the posterior leaflet and goes out of the atrial surface near the posterior leaflet edge. Other sutures go into the anterior leaflet annulus from the left atrium, pass through the left ventricle of the mitral annulus and go out from the left ventricular side.

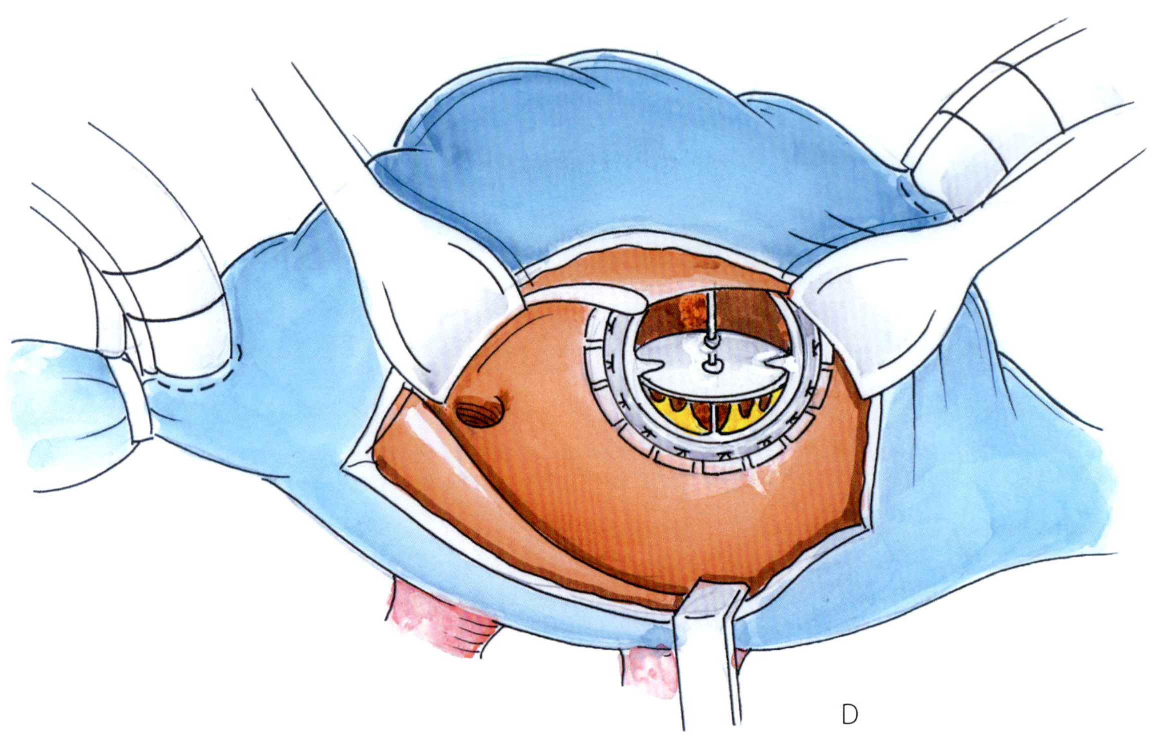

D. 缝线穿过人工心脏瓣膜缝合环，推下瓣膜，逐一结扎缝线。人工心脏瓣膜大开口对二尖瓣前瓣。

D. The sutures are passed through the prosthetic valve sewing ring, and all sutures are ligated after the valve is pushed down. The wider opening of the prosthetic valve aligns with the anterior mitral valve.

图 3-1-12　保留全部瓣下结构的二尖瓣置换术

Figure 3-1-12　Mitral valve replacement with total subvalvular structures preserved

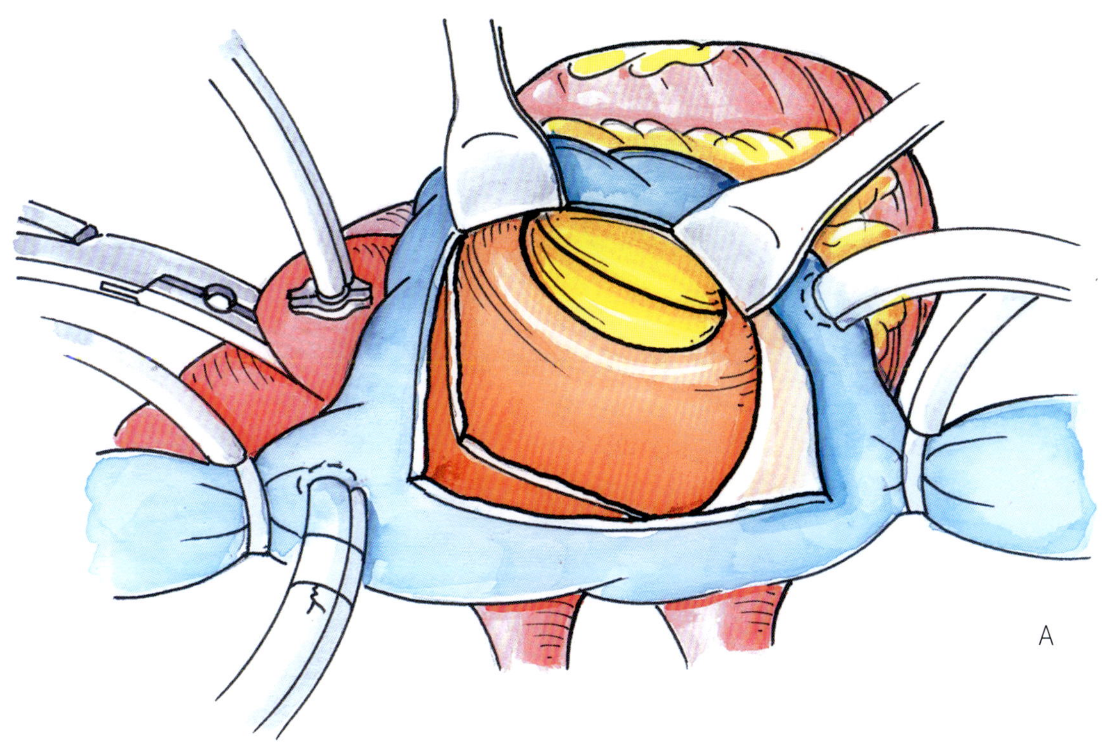

A. 体外循环下经右心房 - 房间隔路径进入左心房，探查左心房和二尖瓣。

A. The left atrium is accessed via a right atrial-transseptal approach under extracorporeal circulation. The left atrium and mitral valve should be inspected.

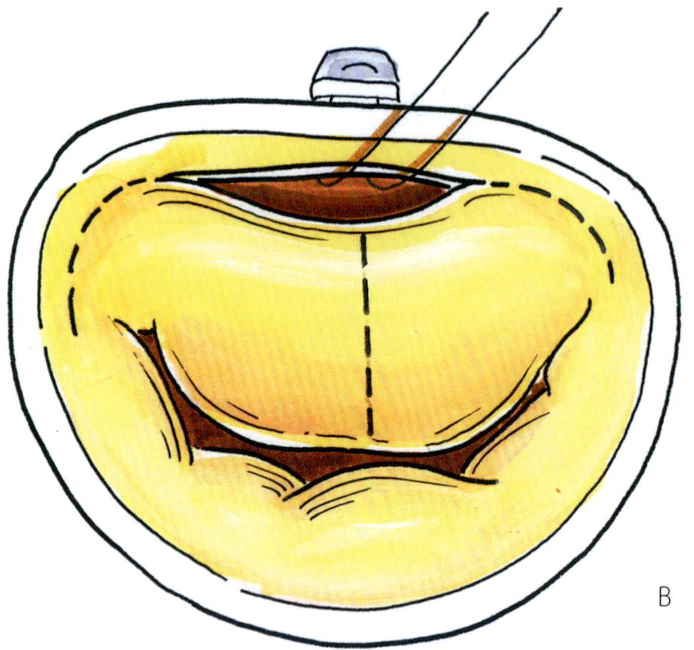

B. 二尖瓣前叶距二尖瓣环约 2mm 处切开，再于二尖瓣前叶中部纵行剪开。

B. An incision is made on the anterior mitral valve leaflet about 2 mm from the mitral annulus, and the midportion of the anterior leaflet is longitudinally separated.

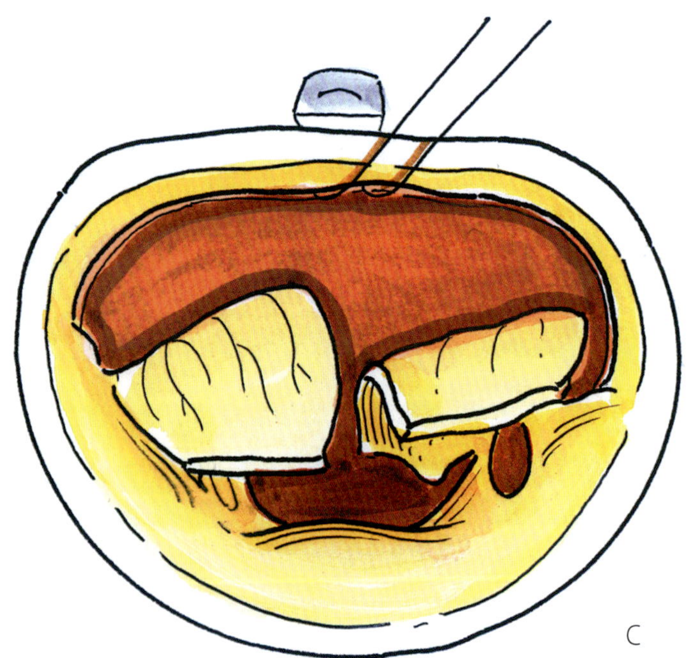

C. 剪去多余的瓣叶组织，把前、后乳头肌腱索附着的前瓣叶剪成为两个游离片。

C. The residual leaflet tissue is cut off, and the anterior mitra leaflet attached to the anterior and posterior papillary chordae tendineae is cut into two free pieces.

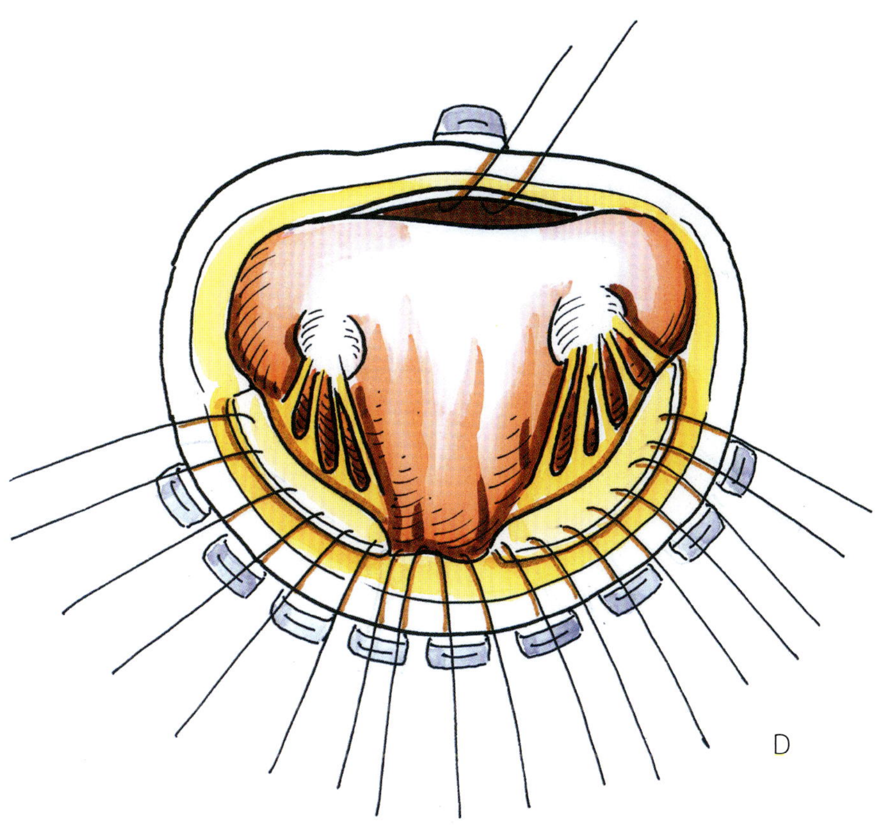

D. 将两个连接腱索的游离片分别翻向二尖瓣后叶瓣环靠近交界处。该处带垫片瓣膜褥式缝线由左心房侧进针，穿过二尖瓣环左心室侧出针，缝针继续穿过后叶瓣膜缘，再将前叶游离片一并缝入。

D. Turn over the two free pieces connecting the chordae and let them towards the posterior mitral annulus near the commissure. A pledgeted mattress suture is passed through the mitral annulus from the left atrial to the left ventricular side and continued to be placed through the posterior leaflet edge, and then the free pieces of the anterior leaflet are sewed together.

E. 其余部分带垫片瓣膜褥式缝线按常规安置，植入人工心脏瓣膜。人工机械心脏瓣膜的大开口朝向前瓣侧，以避免卡瓣。

E. The rest of the pledgeted mattress sutures are routinely placed. The prosthetic valve is implanted, with the wider opening of the prosthetic valve towards the anterior mitral valve to avoid clogging.

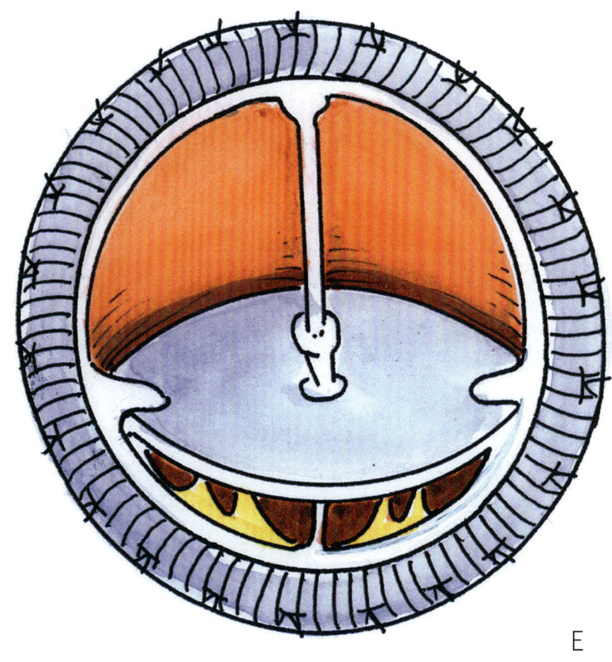

第 二 节　主动脉瓣手术

Section 2　Surgery for Aortic Valve Disease

图 3-2-1　主动脉瓣狭窄交界切开术
Figure 3-2-1　Commissurotomy for aortic valve stenosis

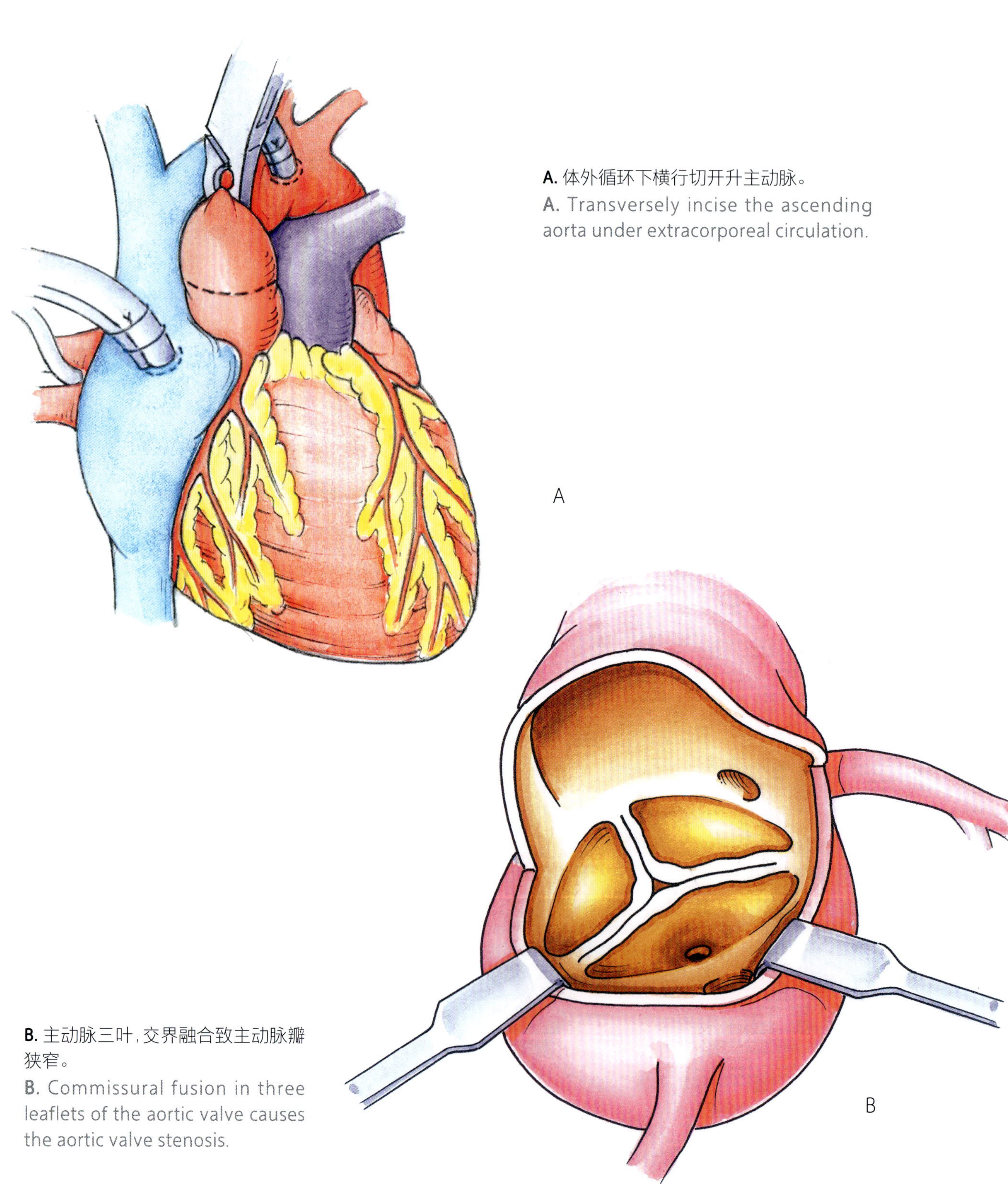

A. 体外循环下横行切开升主动脉。
A. Transversely incise the ascending aorta under extracorporeal circulation.

B. 主动脉三叶，交界融合致主动脉瓣狭窄。
B. Commissural fusion in three leaflets of the aortic valve causes the aortic valve stenosis.

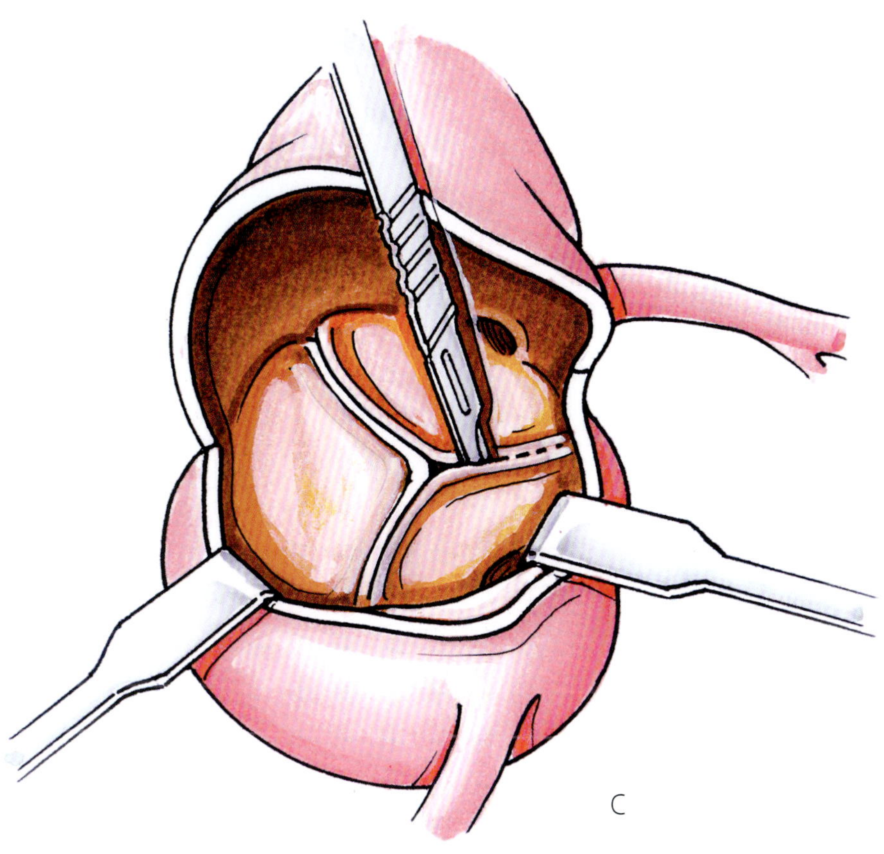

C. 用尖头刀切开融合的交界，从瓣口开始向瓣环方向切，直至距瓣环约 1.5mm 处。

C. An incision is made on the fused commissure with a sharp-pointed scalpel, which is extended from the orifice towards the annulus and stopped at about 1.5 mm from the annulus.

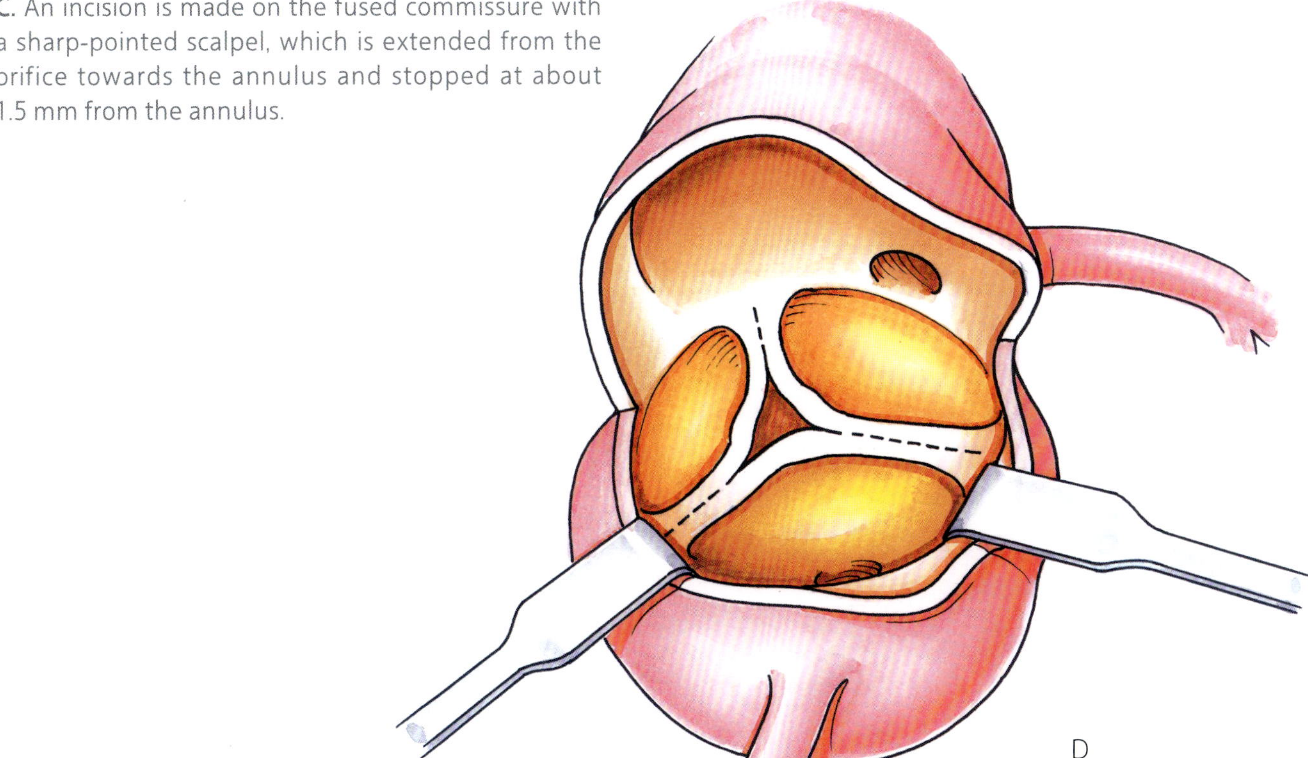

D. 三个交界均予切开。

D. All three commissures are cut open.

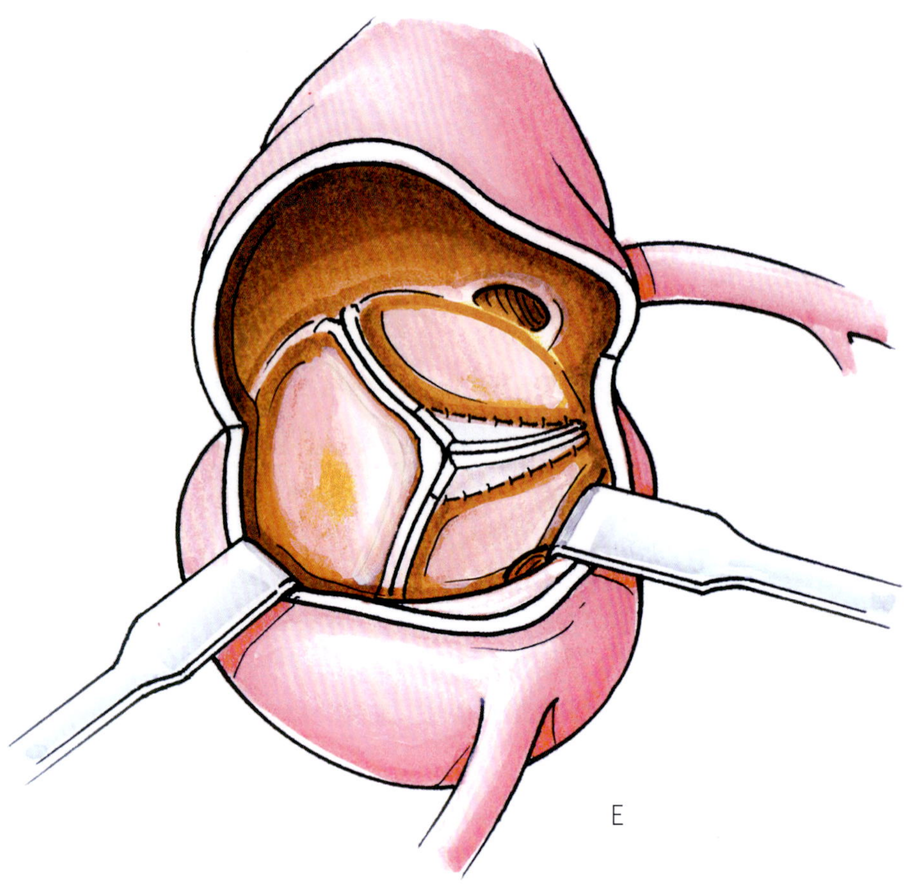

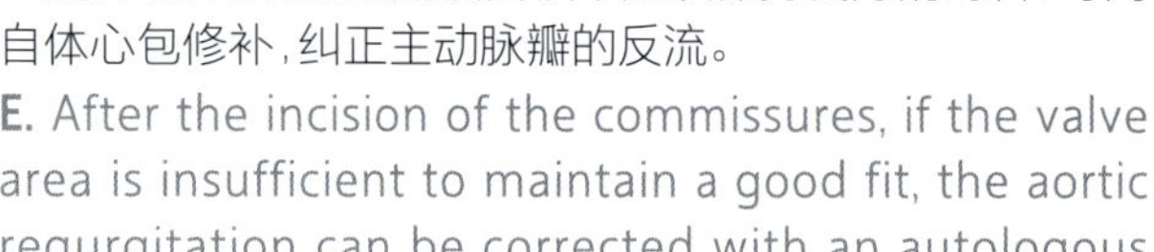

E. 交界切开后，如果瓣膜面积不足以保持良好的对合，可用自体心包修补，纠正主动脉瓣的反流。

E. After the incision of the commissures, if the valve area is insufficient to maintain a good fit, the aortic regurgitation can be corrected with an autologous pericardial patch.

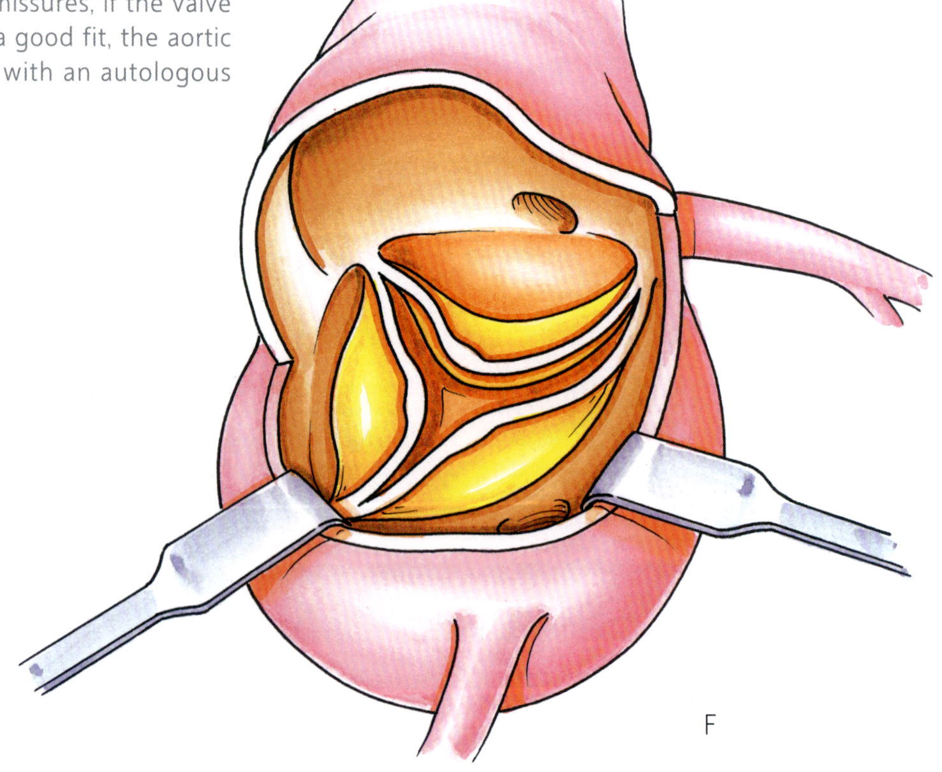

F. 主动脉瓣开放良好，狭窄已解除。

F. The aortic valve is well opened, and the stenosis is relieved.

图 3-2-2 主动脉瓣环环缩术
Figure 3-2-2 Aortic annulus retraction

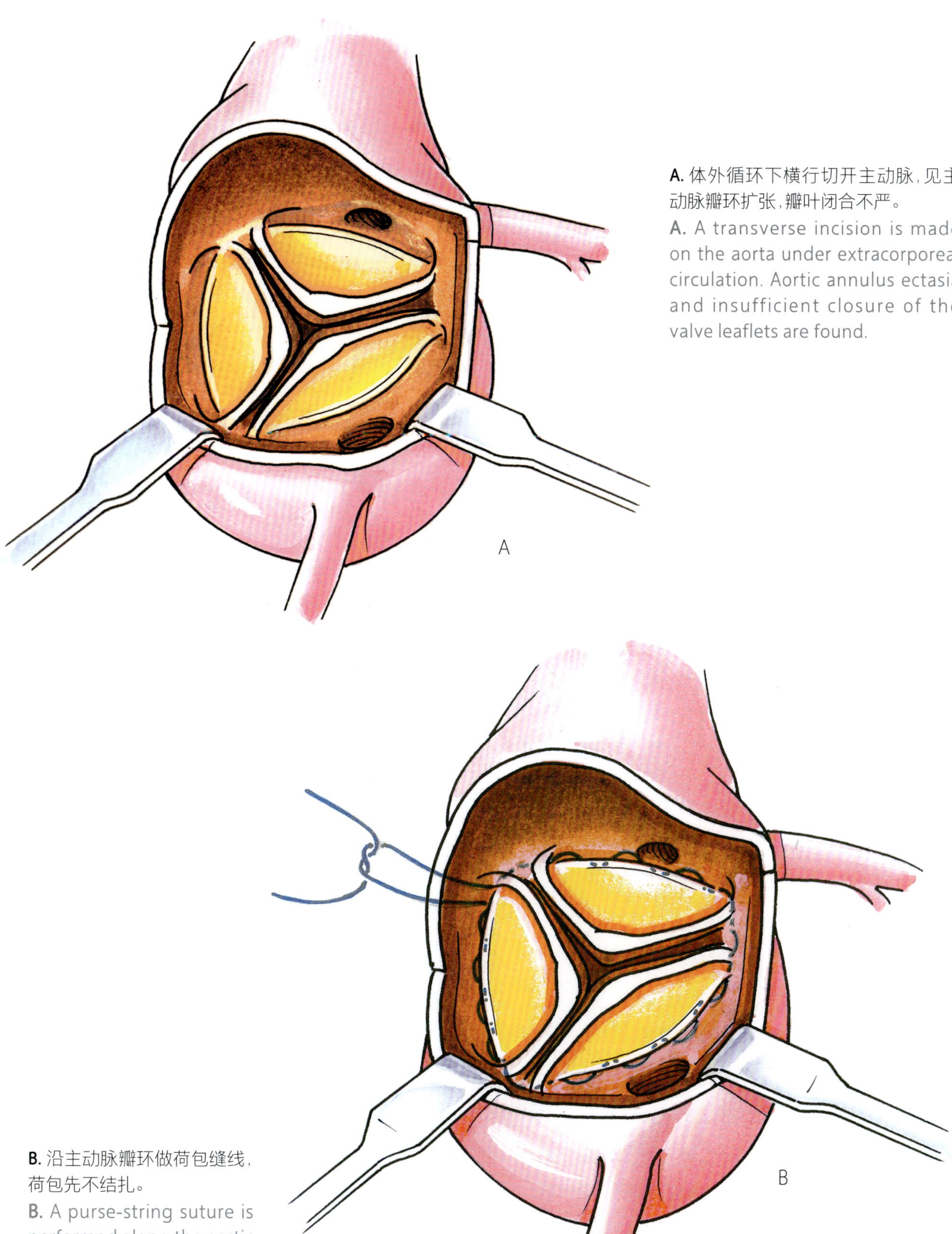

A. 体外循环下横行切开主动脉，见主动脉瓣环扩张，瓣叶闭合不严。

A. A transverse incision is made on the aorta under extracorporeal circulation. Aortic annulus ectasia and insufficient closure of the valve leaflets are found.

B. 沿主动脉瓣环做荷包缝线，荷包先不结扎。

B. A purse-string suture is performed along the aortic annulus without ligation.

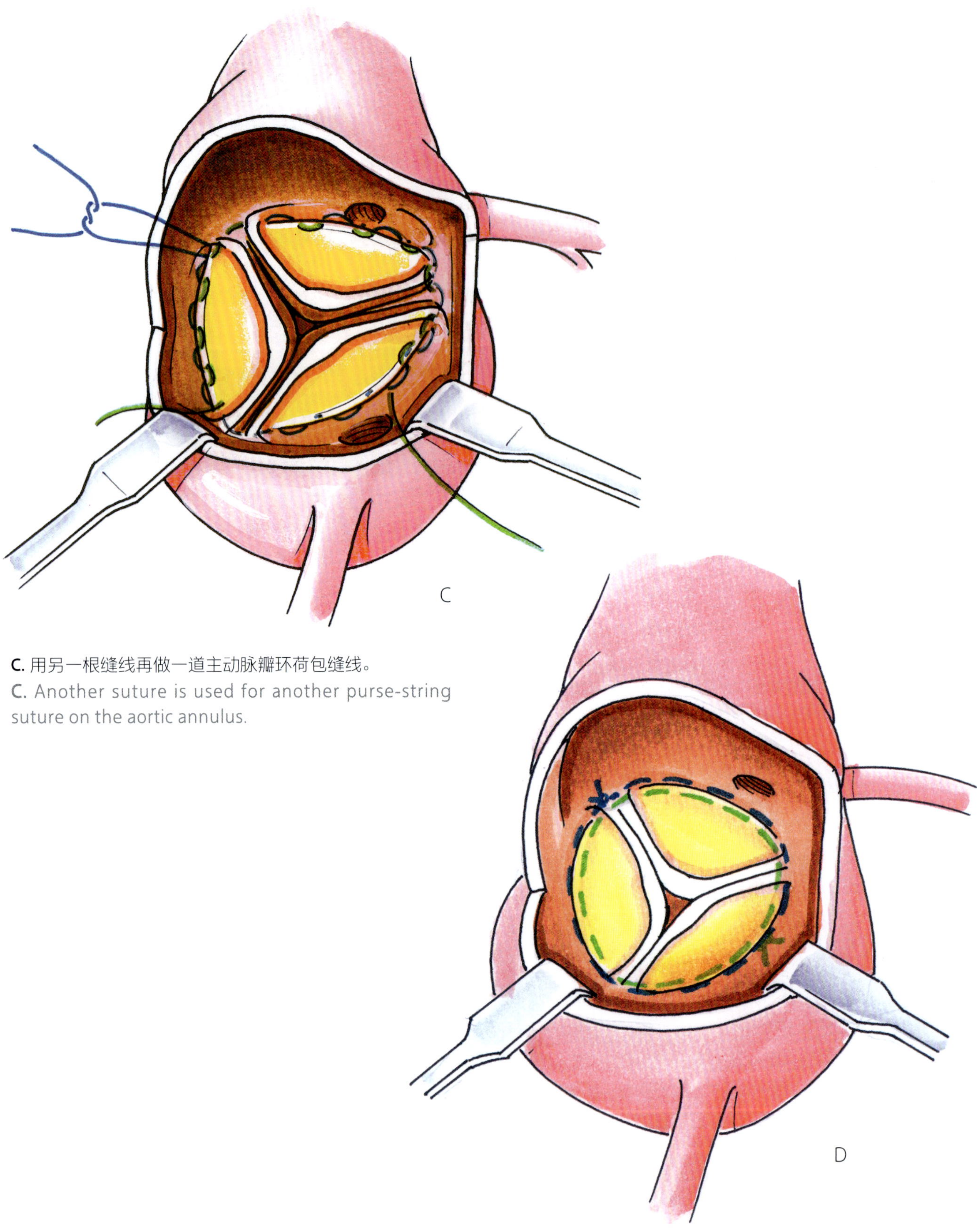

C. 用另一根缝线再做一道主动脉瓣环荷包缝线。

C. Another suture is used for another purse-string suture on the aortic annulus.

D. 收紧荷包缝线，使主动脉瓣环缩小，直至注水试验主动脉反流消失。结扎荷包缝线。

D. Tighten the purse-string sutures to narrow the aortic annulus until aortic regurgitation disappears in the water injection test, and then ligate the purse-string sutures.

图 3-2-3　主动脉瓣叶切除成形术

Figure 3-2-3　Aortic valve leaflet resection and valvuloplasty

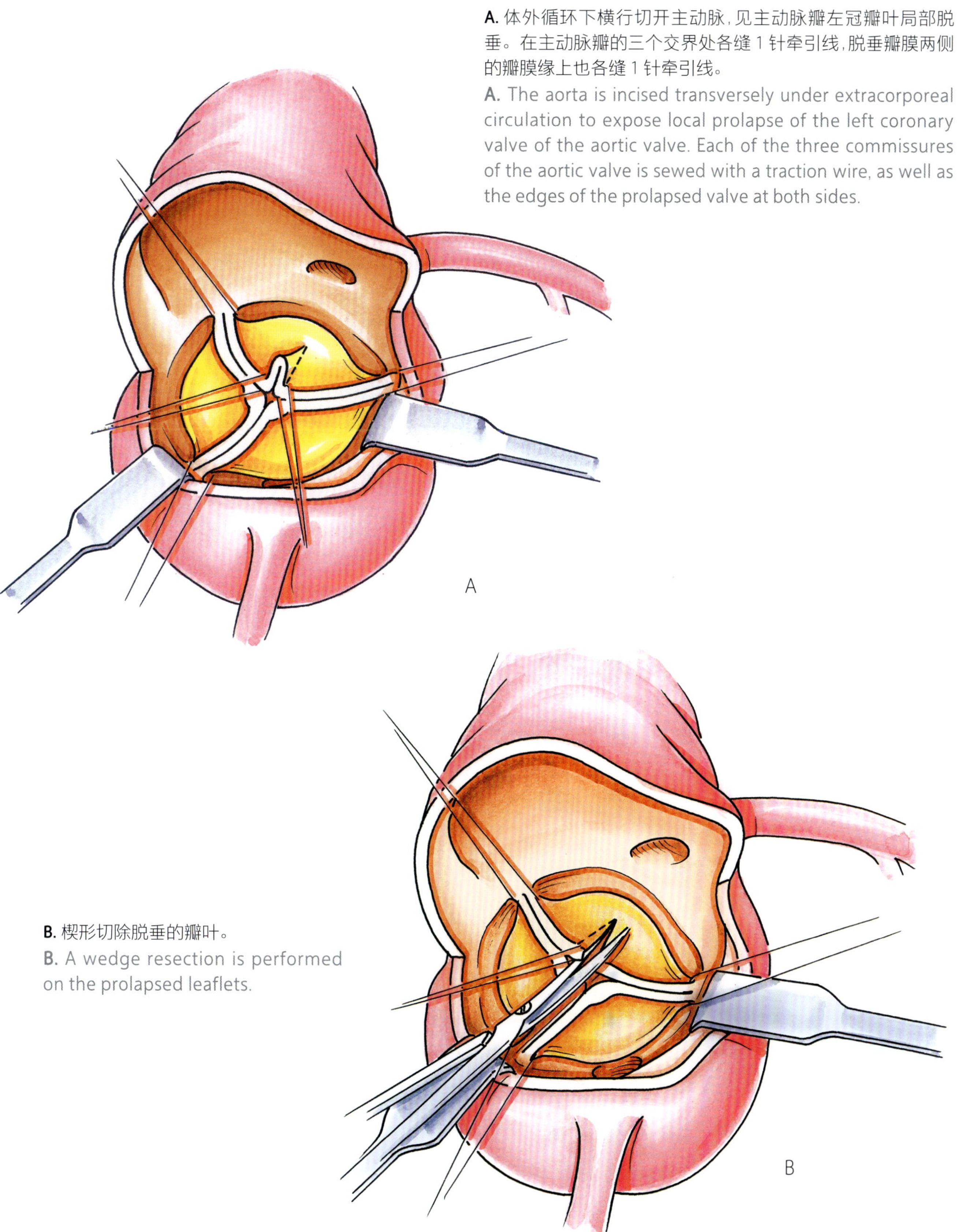

A. 体外循环下横行切开主动脉，见主动脉瓣左冠瓣叶局部脱垂。在主动脉瓣的三个交界处各缝 1 针牵引线，脱垂瓣膜两侧的瓣膜缘上也各缝 1 针牵引线。

A. The aorta is incised transversely under extracorporeal circulation to expose local prolapse of the left coronary valve of the aortic valve. Each of the three commissures of the aortic valve is sewed with a traction wire, as well as the edges of the prolapsed valve at both sides.

B. 楔形切除脱垂的瓣叶。

B. A wedge resection is performed on the prolapsed leaflets.

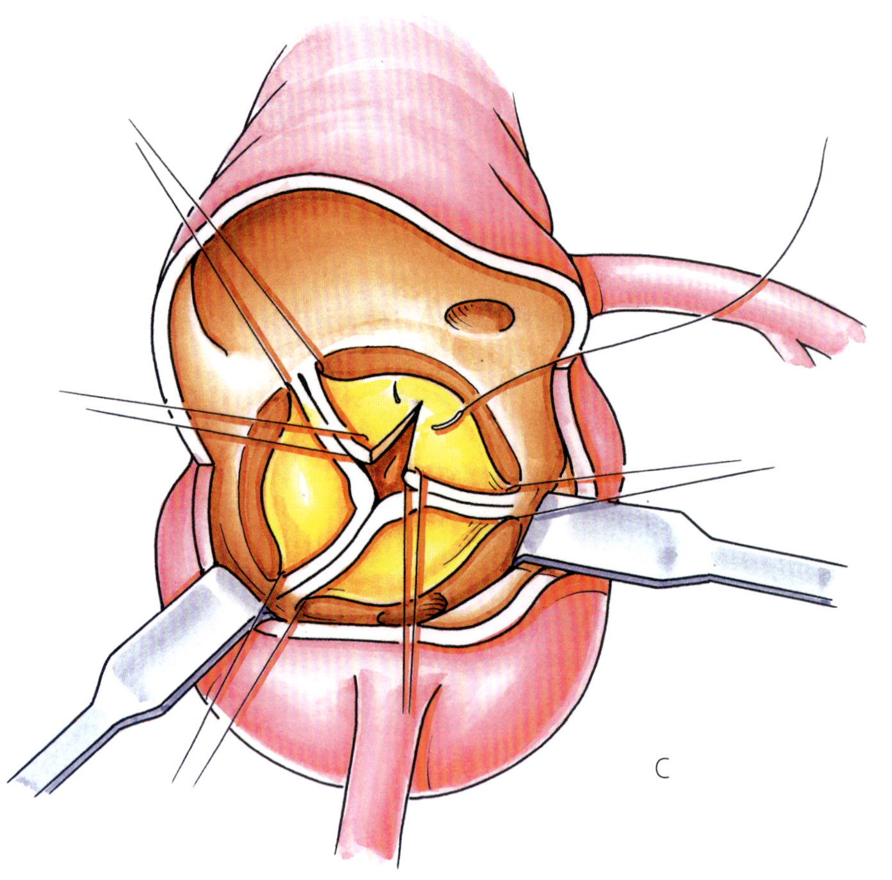

C. 将剪开的瓣叶单纯间断缝合。

C. The incised leaflets are closed with simple interrupted sutures.

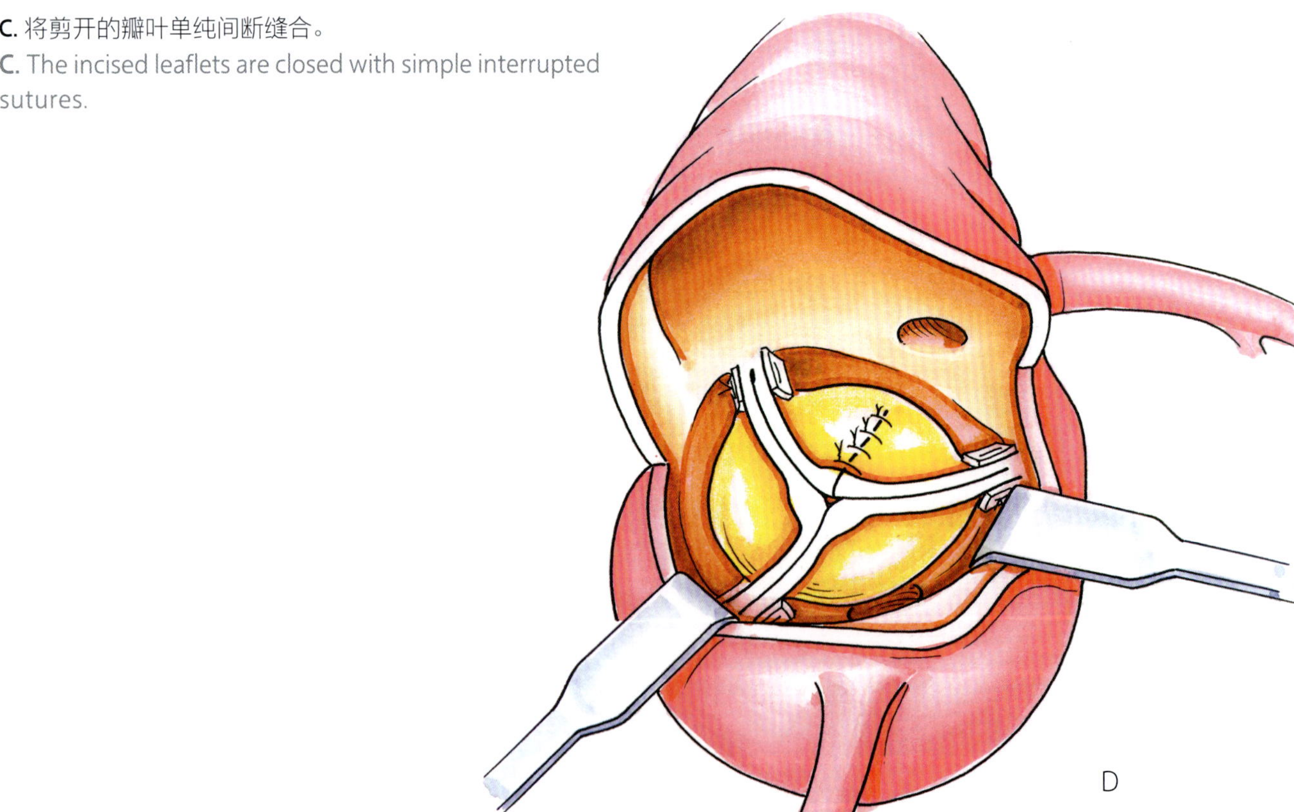

D. 主动脉瓣三个交界处各做一带垫片褥式缝合。

D. A pledgeted mattress suture is placed on each of the three commissures of the aortic valve.

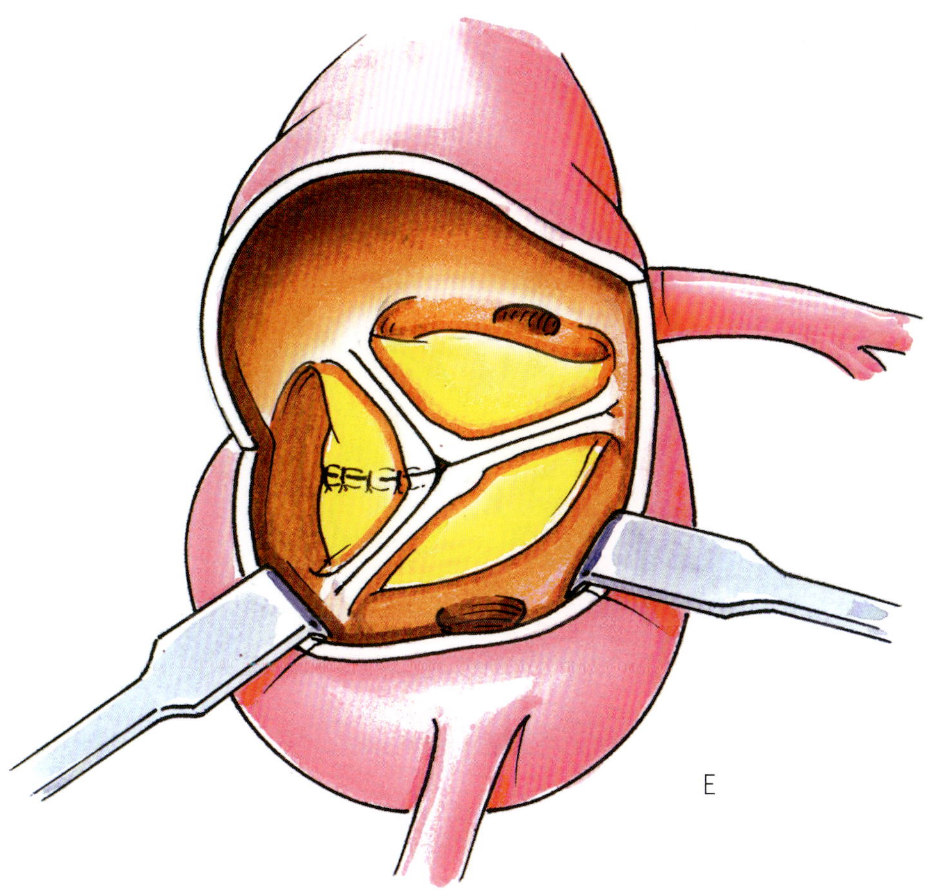

E. 瓣叶切除范围小，切除缝合后没有主动脉瓣反流时，主动脉瓣交界处褥式缝合也可以不做。

E. With a small portion of leaflet resection, the mattress suture at the aortic valve commissure may not be a necessity if there is no aortic regurgitation after resection and sutures.

图 3-2-4　二叶主动脉瓣切除成形术

Figure 3-2-4　Bicuspid aortic valve resection and valvuloplasty

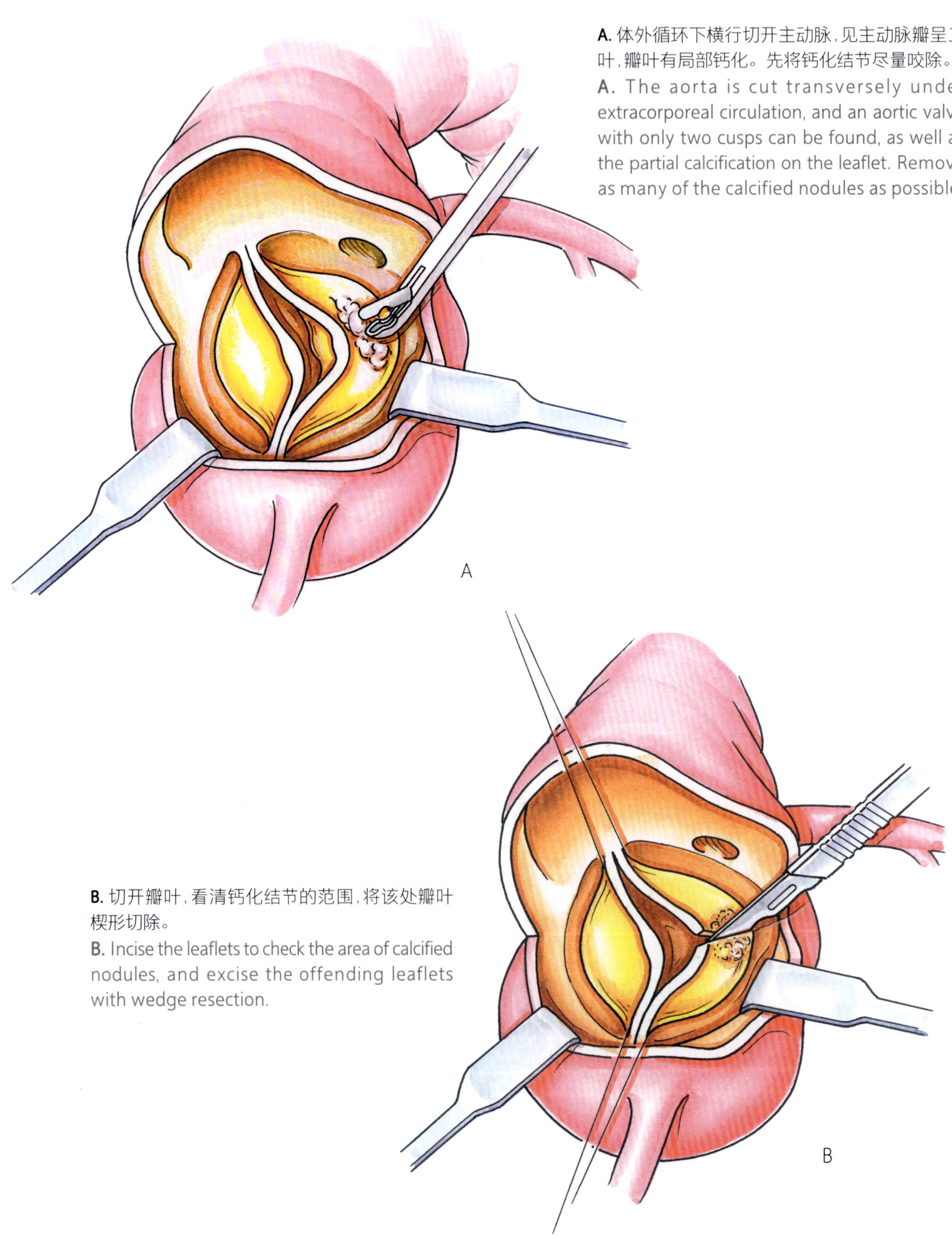

A. 体外循环下横行切开主动脉，见主动脉瓣呈二叶，瓣叶有局部钙化。先将钙化结节尽量咬除。

A. The aorta is cut transversely under extracorporeal circulation, and an aortic valve with only two cusps can be found, as well as the partial calcification on the leaflet. Remove as many of the calcified nodules as possible.

B. 切开瓣叶，看清钙化结节的范围，将该处瓣叶楔形切除。

B. Incise the leaflets to check the area of calcified nodules, and excise the offending leaflets with wedge resection.

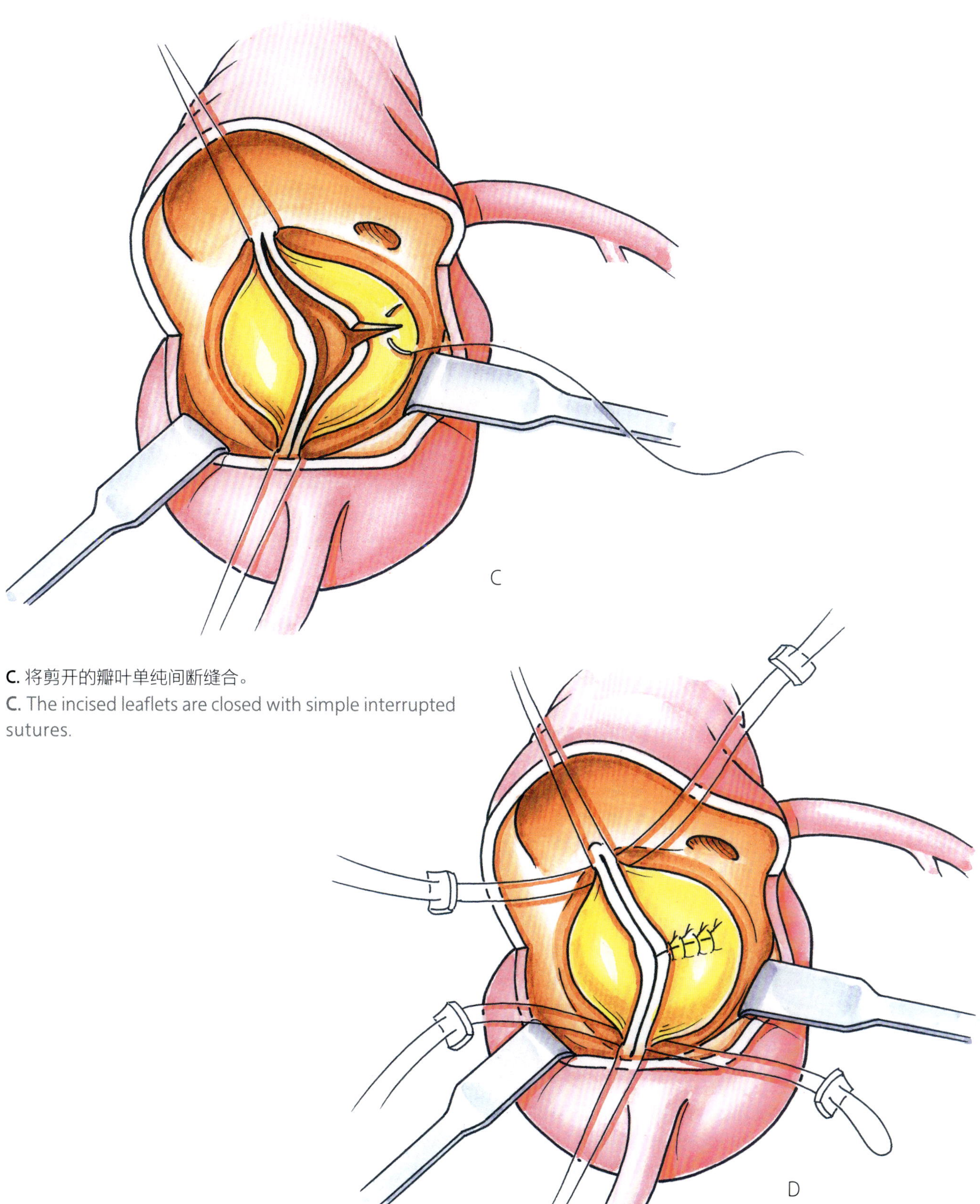

C. 将剪开的瓣叶单纯间断缝合。

C. The incised leaflets are closed with simple interrupted sutures.

D. 主动脉瓣两个交界处各做一带垫片褥式缝合。

D. A pledgeted mattress suture is placed at each of the two commissure sites of the aortic valve.

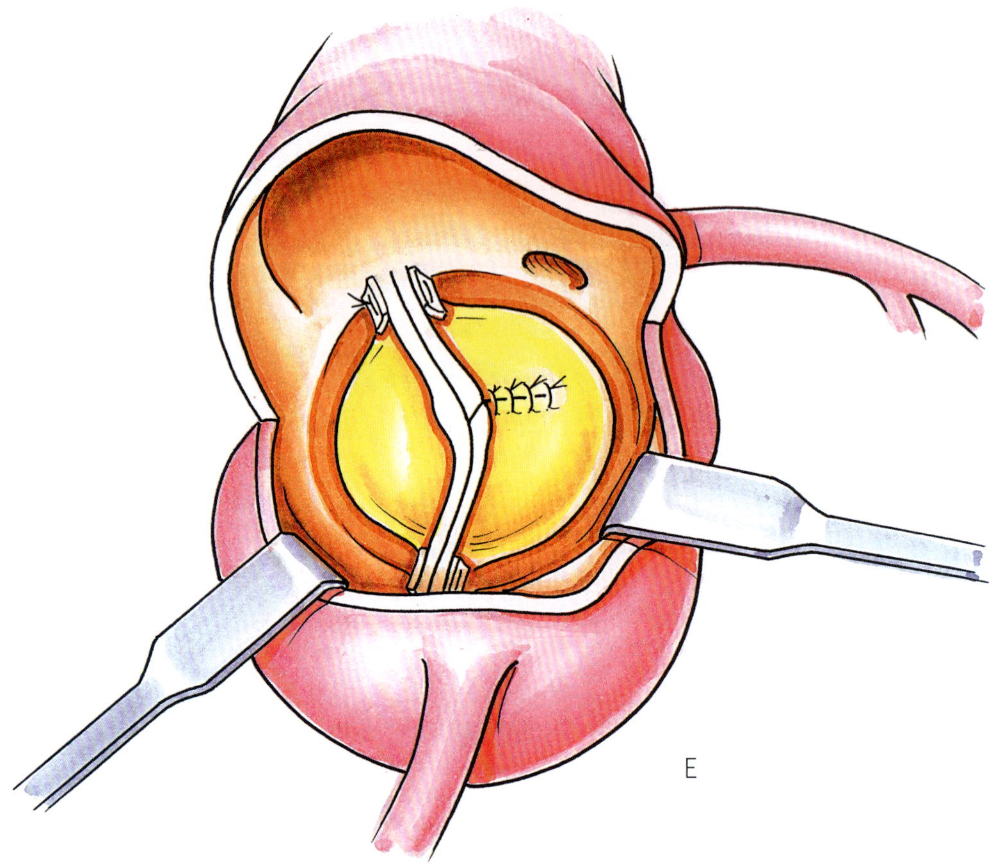

E. 结扎褥式缝合，主动脉瓣修补完成。

E. The mattress suture is tied, and aortic valve repair is completed.

图 3-2-5　主动脉瓣叶补片修补术

Figure 3-2-5　Patch repair of aortic leaflet

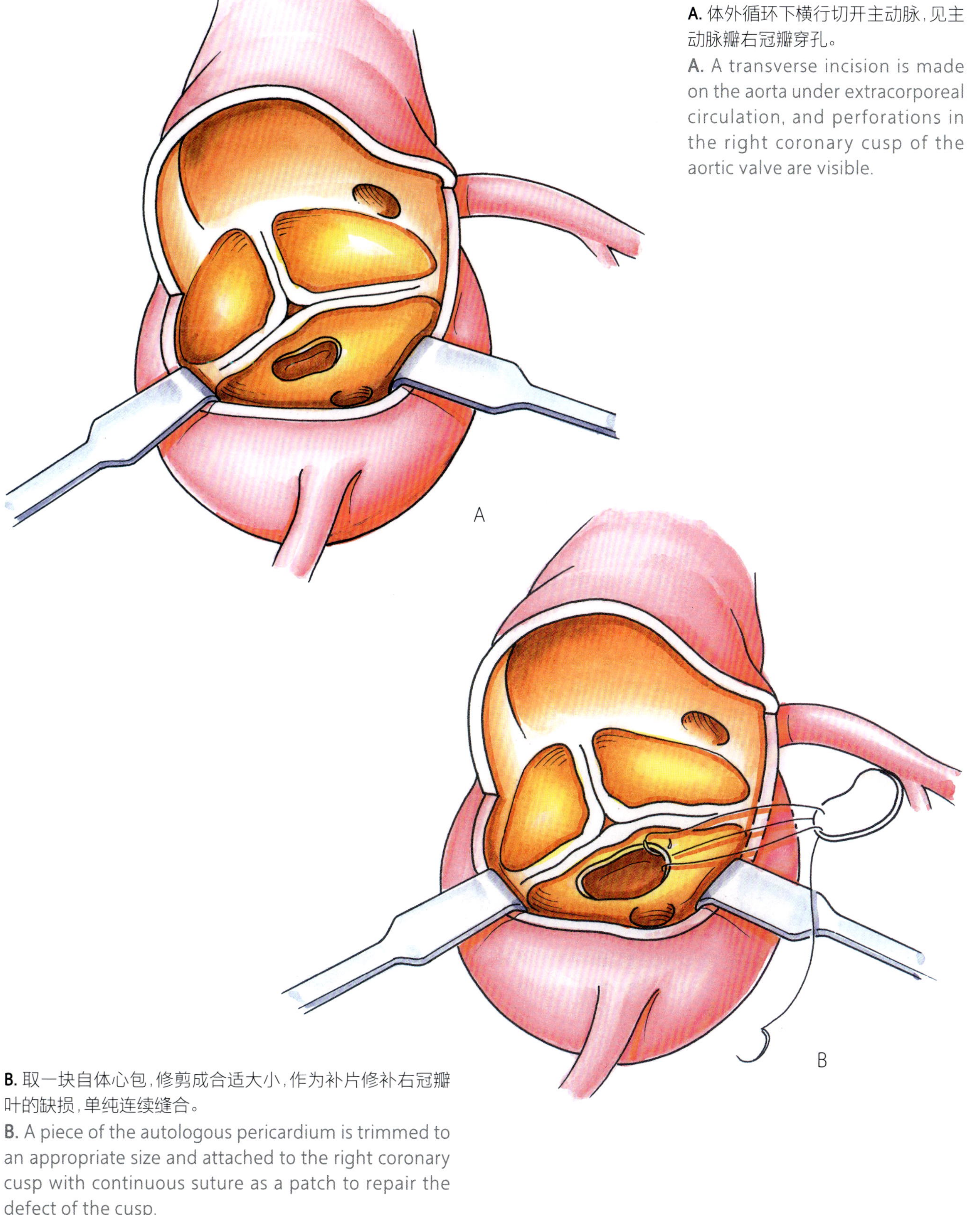

A. 体外循环下横行切开主动脉，见主动脉瓣右冠瓣穿孔。

A. A transverse incision is made on the aorta under extracorporeal circulation, and perforations in the right coronary cusp of the aortic valve are visible.

B. 取一块自体心包，修剪成合适大小，作为补片修补右冠瓣叶的缺损，单纯连续缝合。

B. A piece of the autologous pericardium is trimmed to an appropriate size and attached to the right coronary cusp with continuous suture as a patch to repair the defect of the cusp.

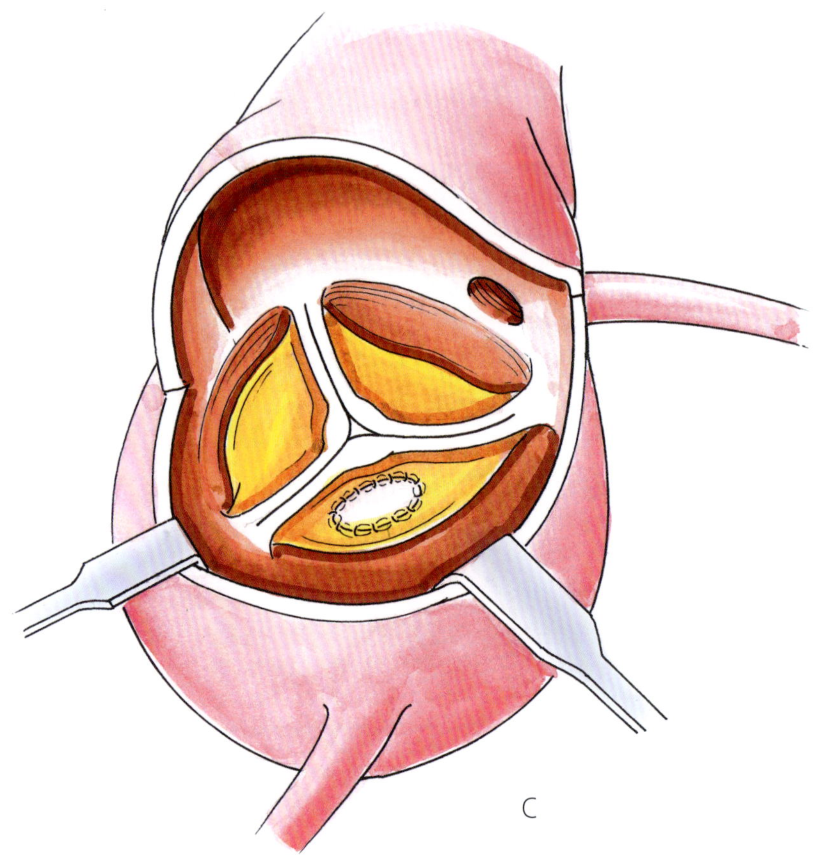

C. 瓣叶缺损修补毕。

C. Leaflet defect repair is completed.

图 3-2-6　**主动脉瓣叶心包加宽术**

Figure 3-2-6　**Enlargement of aortic leaflet with pericardial patch**

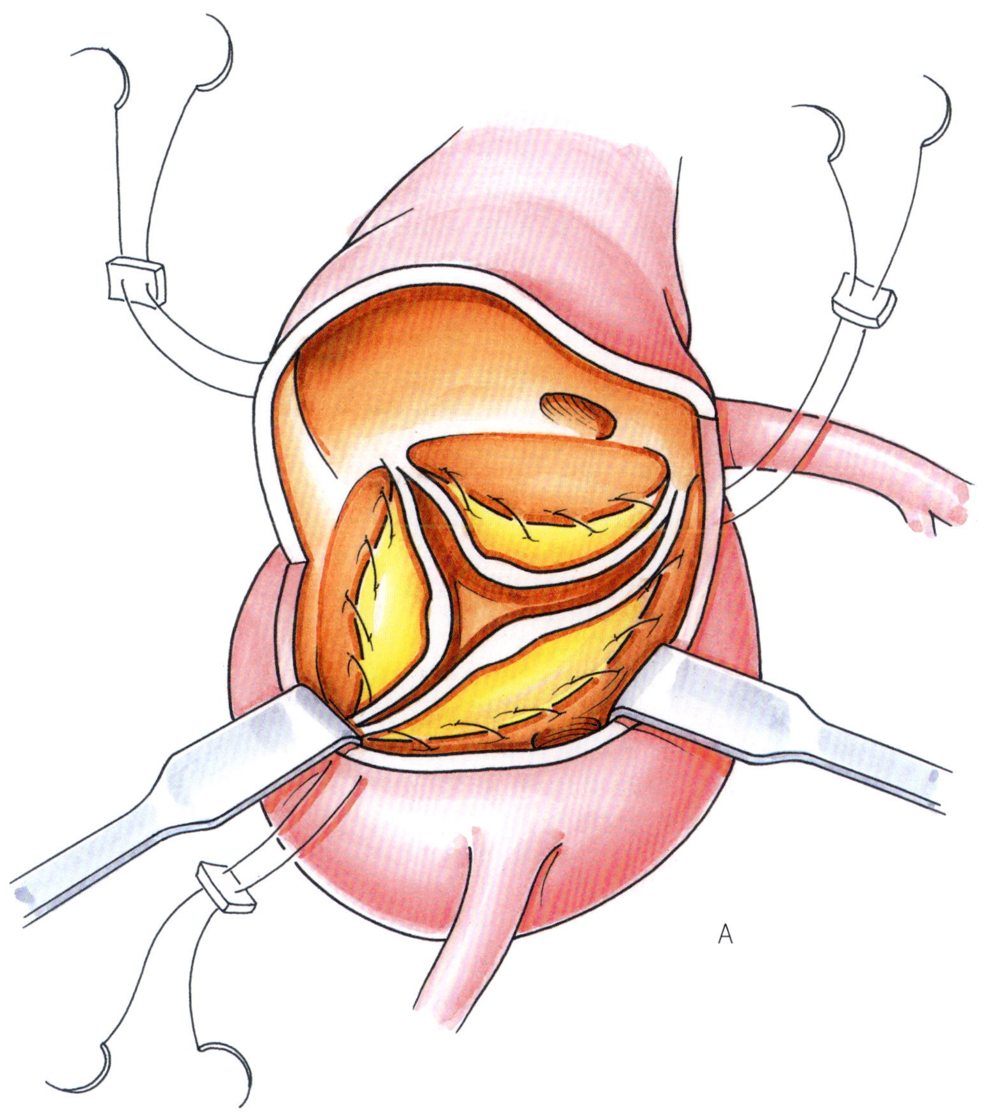

A. 主动脉瓣叶缘因瓣叶挛缩或因病变剪除后，瓣叶高度不够，致瓣叶闭合不好，主动脉瓣反流。用自体心包补片加宽瓣叶做瓣叶成形。自体心包先用 0.5% 戊二醛浸泡处理 5~15 分钟，裁剪成适当大小和形状，与瓣叶单纯连续缝合。缝线在交界处穿到主动脉外加垫片结扎。

A. The excision of aortic leaflet margin due to contracture of the valve leaflet or the presence of lesions may make the leaflet height inadequate for complete leaflet closure, and then cause aortic regurgitation. Then, the leaflet can be augmented with an autologous pericardial patch. Having been soaked in 0.5% glutaraldehyde for 5-15 minutes, the autologous pericardial patch is cut into proper size and shape, and sewn to the leaflets with simple running sutures. The sutures are passed through the commissure point to the outside of the aorta and tied there with pledgets.

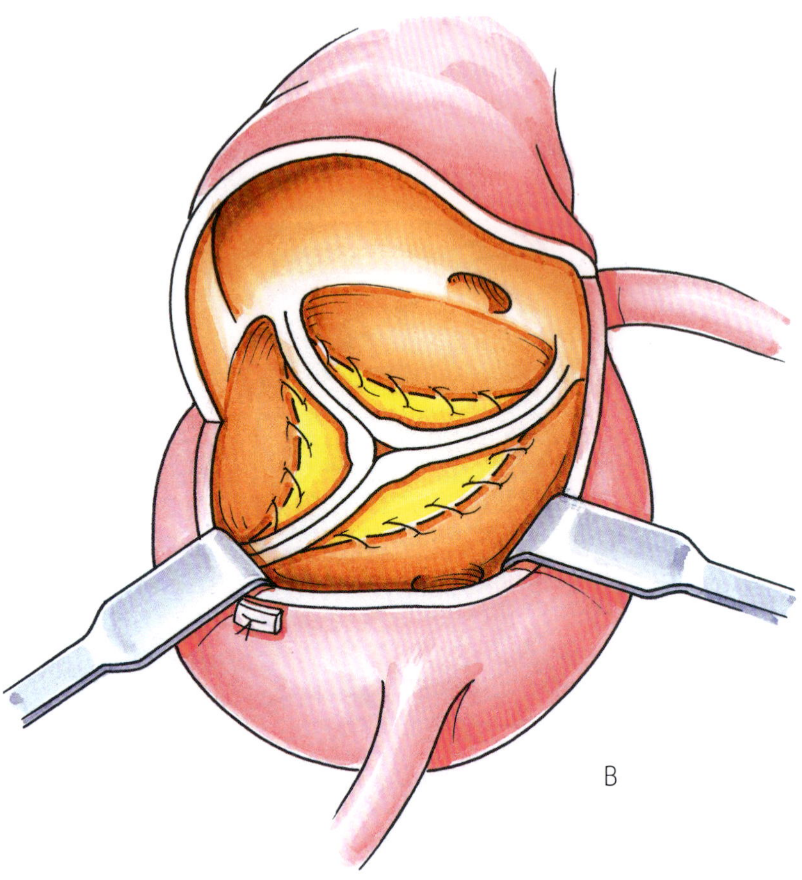

B. 主动脉三个瓣叶成形完毕。

B. Valvuloplasty of the three aortic valve leaflets is completed.

图 3-2-7　主动脉瓣交界缩缝术

Figure 3-2-7　Aortic valve commissure constriction by compression suture

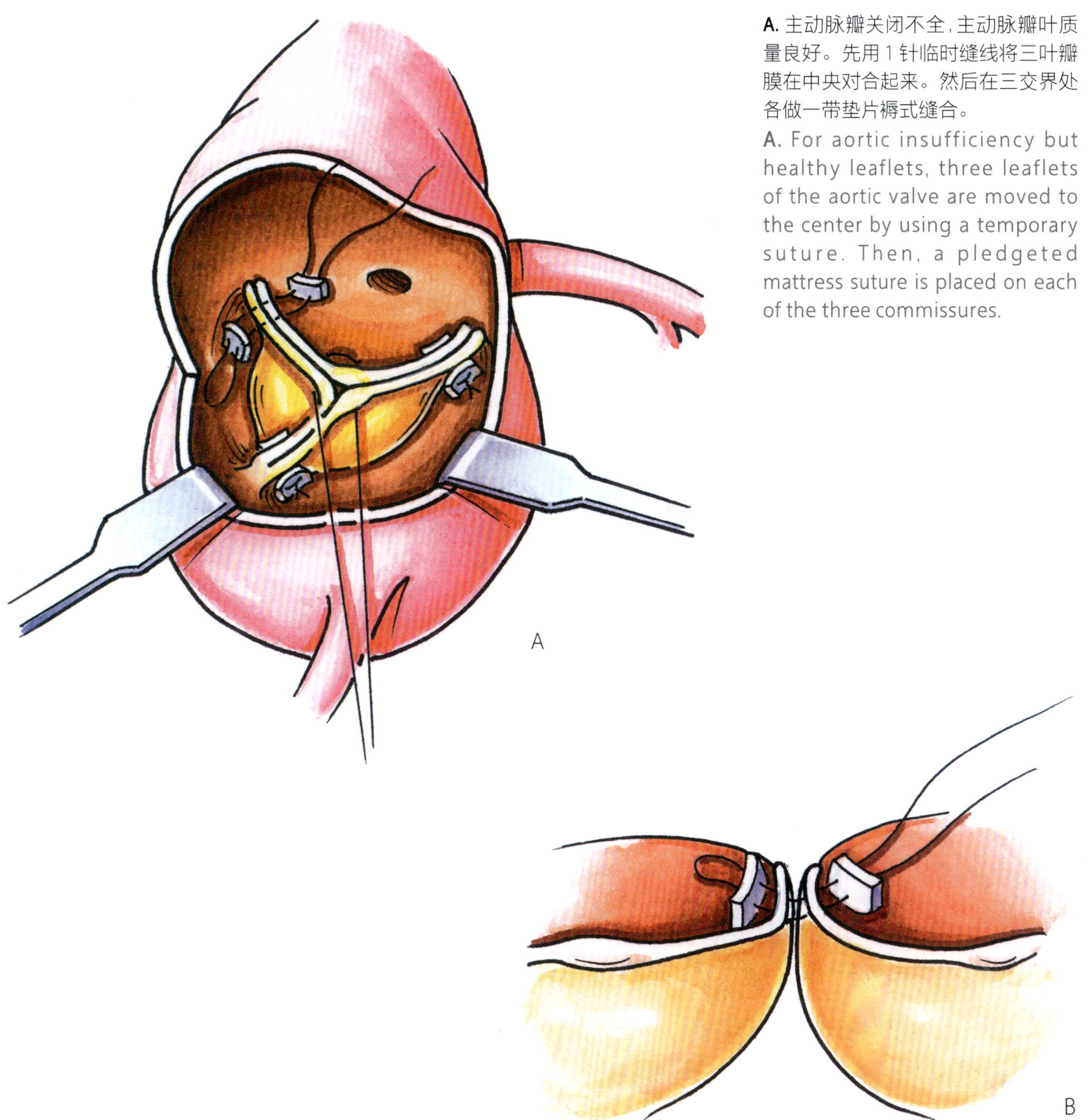

A. 主动脉瓣关闭不全，主动脉瓣叶质量良好。先用 1 针临时缝线将三叶瓣膜在中央对合起来。然后在三交界处各做一带垫片褥式缝合。

A. For aortic insufficiency but healthy leaflets, three leaflets of the aortic valve are moved to the center by using a temporary suture. Then, a pledgeted mattress suture is placed on each of the three commissures.

B. 交界的缝线做在瓣膜上，使主动脉瓣口缩小。

B. Those sutures are placed on the valve to narrow the aortic orifice.

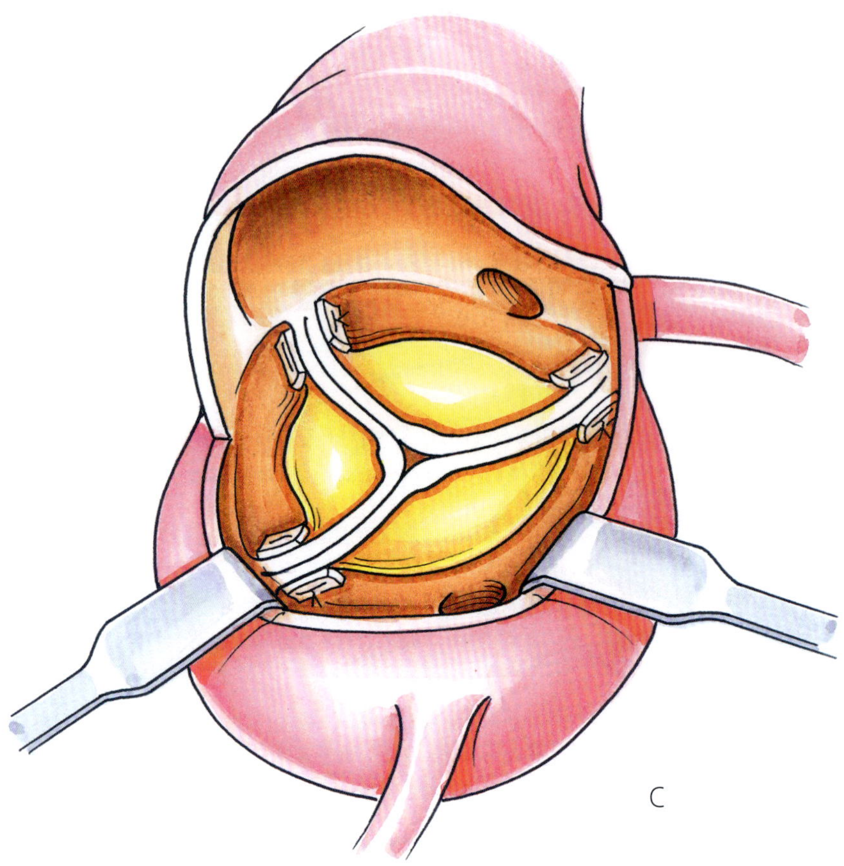

C. 推下垫片，结扎缝线。抽去临时缝线，纠治完成。

C. Push down the pledget and tie the sutures. The temporary suture is removed and the correction is completed.

图 3-2-8 主动脉瓣折叠成形术
Figure 3-2-8 Aortic valve folding plasty

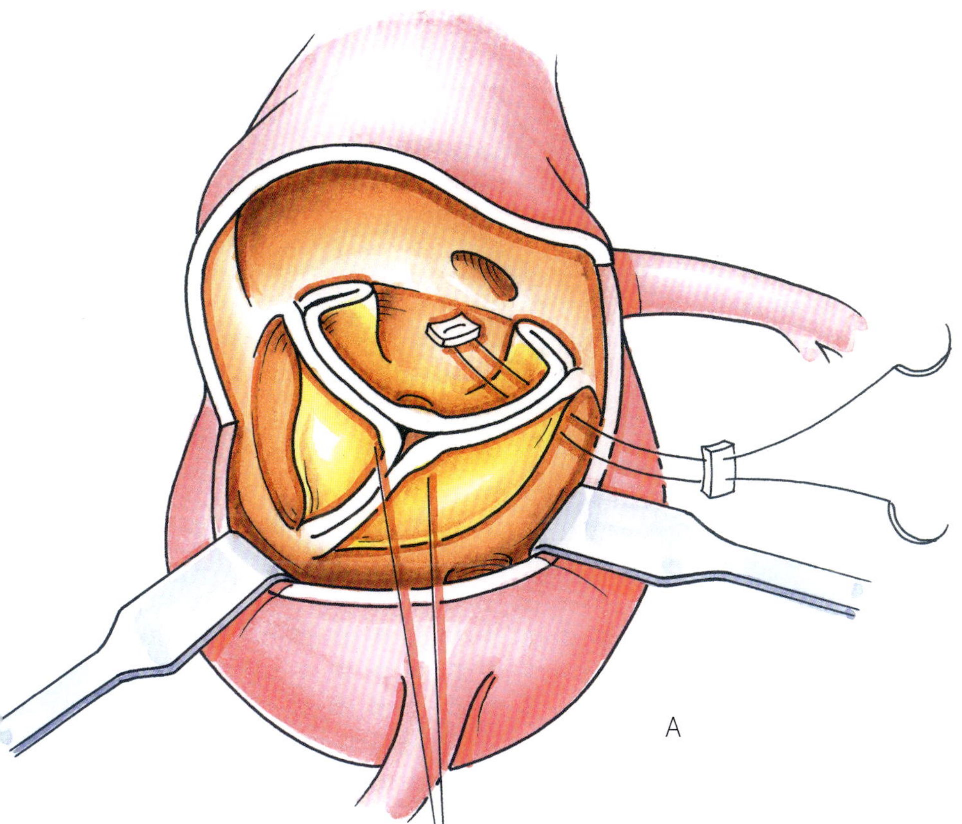

A. 主动脉左冠瓣冗长脱垂致主动脉瓣反流。先用 1 针临时缝线将三叶瓣膜在中央对合起来，以此为基准点将左冠瓣与相邻的瓣叶对比，确定要折叠的范围。然后做一带垫片褥式缝合固定左冠瓣保留的长度，再将多余的左冠瓣叶在两端交界处折叠。

A. For aortic regurgitation induced by the prolapsed and elongated left coronary valve of the aortic valve, the three leaflets of the aortic valve are coapted in the center with a temporary suture at first. Compare the left coronary valve with the adjacent leaflets and determine the length to be plicated. A pledgeted mattress suture is then used to fix the reserved left coronary valve, and the excessive part is folded at the two commissures.

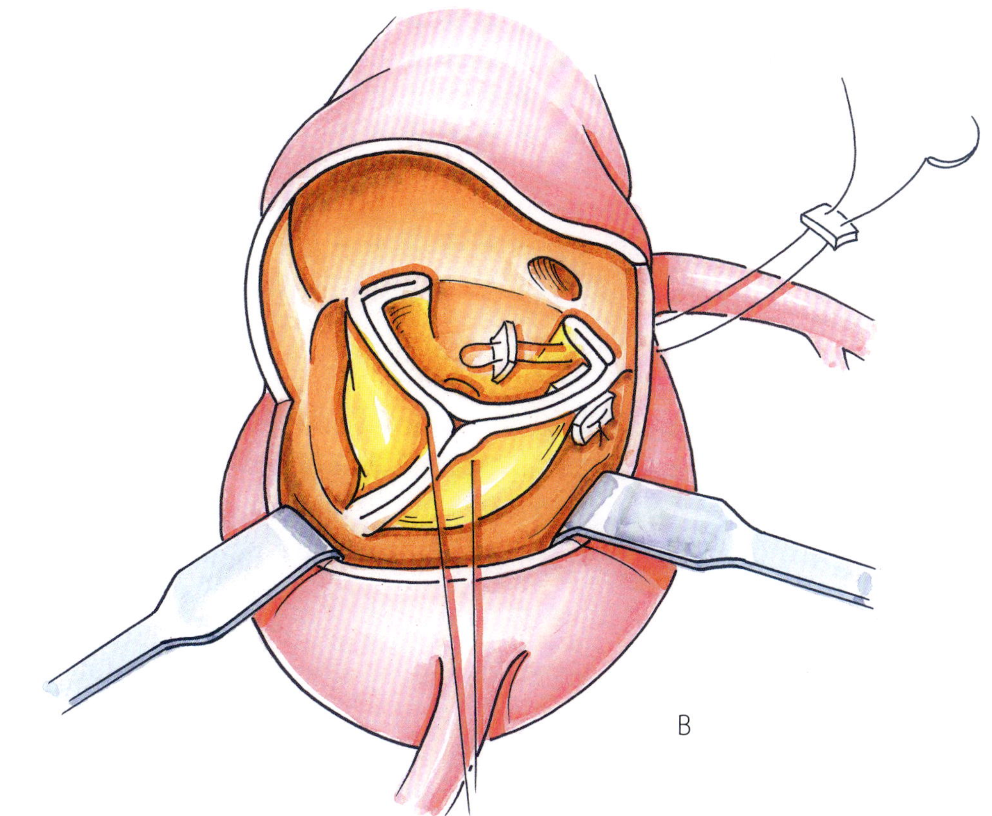

B. 带垫片褥式缝合把折叠的瓣叶与相邻的主动脉壁缝合。

B. The folded leaflet is attached to the adjacent aortic wall with pledgeted mattress sutures.

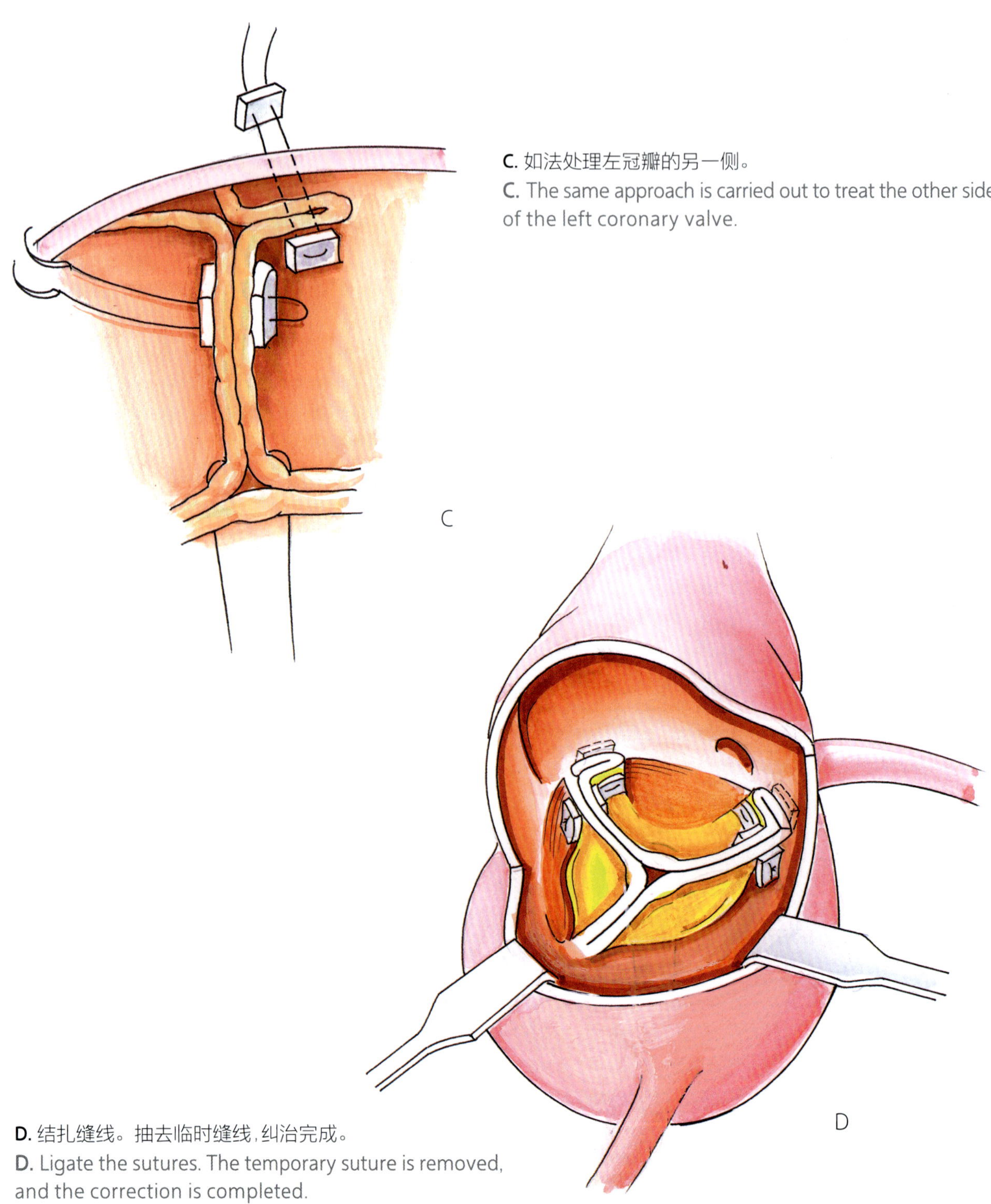

C. 如法处理左冠瓣的另一侧。

C. The same approach is carried out to treat the other side of the left coronary valve.

D. 结扎缝线。抽去临时缝线，纠治完成。

D. Ligate the sutures. The temporary suture is removed, and the correction is completed.

图 3-2-9 主动脉瓣置换术
Figure 3-2-9 Aortic valve replacement

A. 建立体外循环。升主动脉切口有三种。

A. Establish extracorporeal circulation.There are three types of ascending aortic incisions。

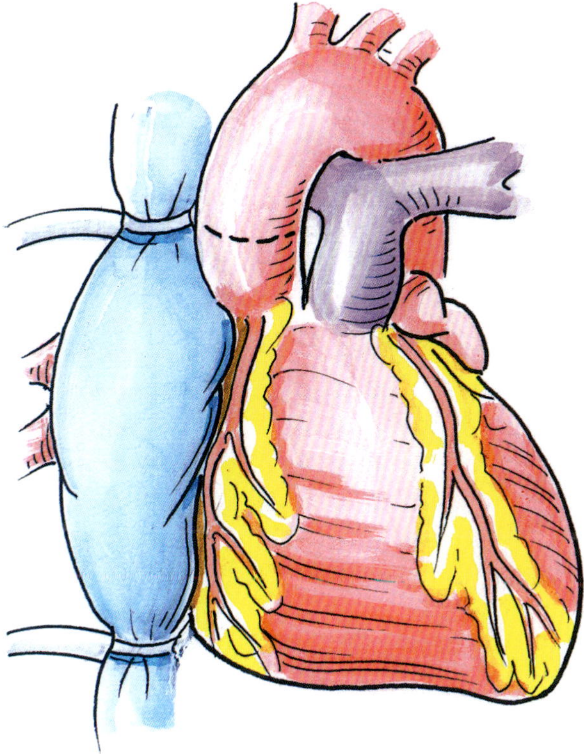

1. 横切口，在右冠状动脉开口上方 1.5~2cm 切开升主动脉前壁，切口长度视手术显露需要向两侧延长，通常需切开升主动脉周径的三分之二，必要时可横断升主动脉。

1. Transverse incision. An incision is made on the anterior wall of the ascending aorta 1.5-2 cm above the ostium of the right coronary artery, and is to be extended on both sides depending on the surgical exposure. Usually, two-thirds of the ascending aorta circumference needs to be incised, and if necessary, the ascending aorta can be transected.

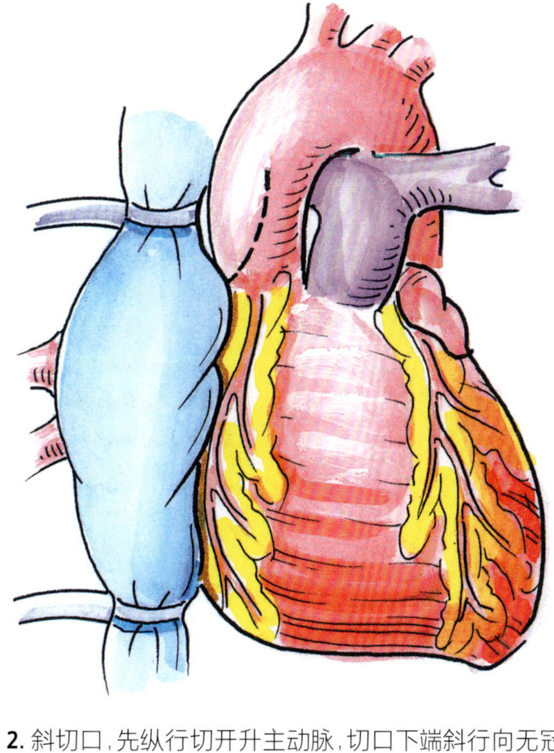

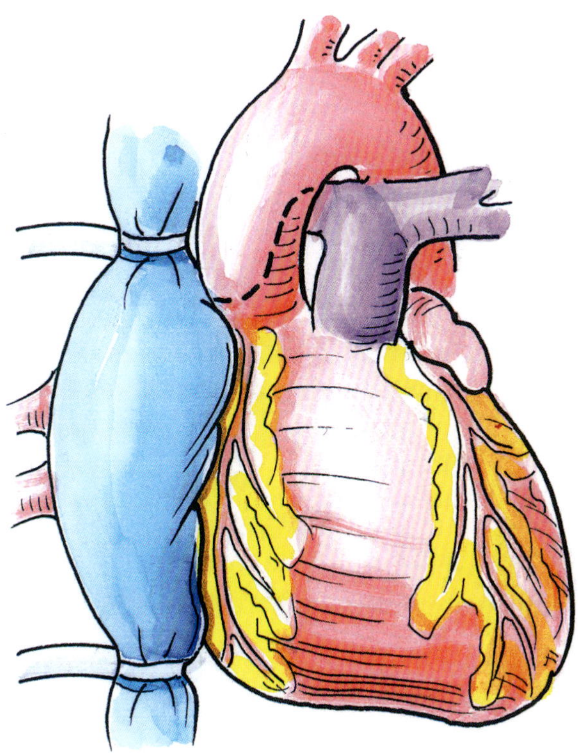

2. 斜切口，先纵行切开升主动脉，切口下端斜行向无冠瓣和左冠瓣交界方向延长。该切口有利于同时做主动脉瓣环扩大成形和 / 或升主动脉成形。

2. Oblique incision. A longitudinal incision is made on the ascending aorta and is obliquely extended to the commissure of the left and the noncoronary cusps. This incision is preferred if the aortic annuloplasty and/or ascending aortoplasty are required simultaneously.

3. 曲棍形切口，在斜切口的基础上，切口上端向左上方延长。

3. A hockey stick incision is performed on the base of the oblique incision with its upper end extended to the upper left.

A

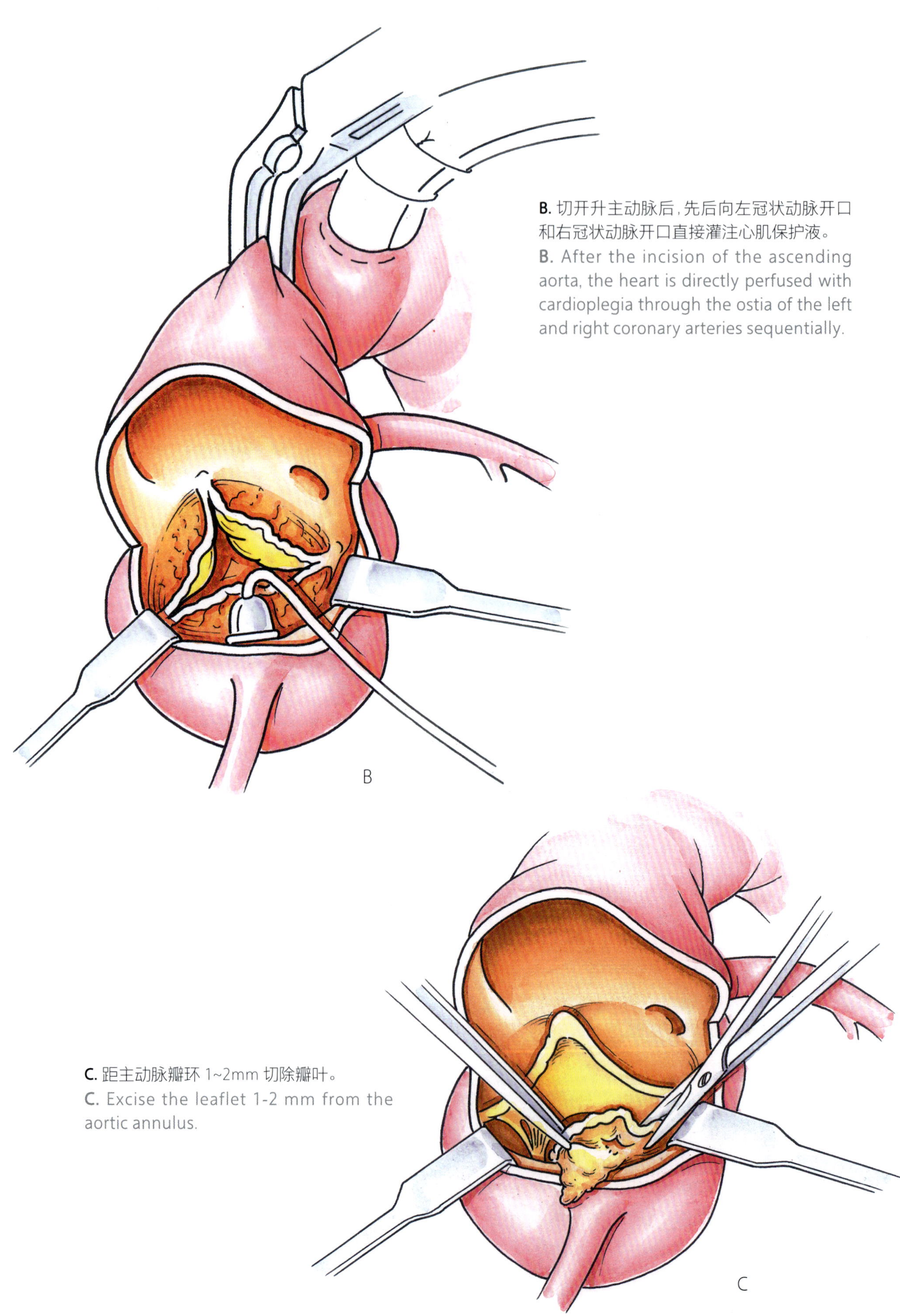

B. 切开升主动脉后，先后向左冠状动脉开口和右冠状动脉开口直接灌注心肌保护液。

B. After the incision of the ascending aorta, the heart is directly perfused with cardioplegia through the ostia of the left and right coronary arteries sequentially.

C. 距主动脉瓣环 1~2mm 切除瓣叶。

C. Excise the leaflet 1-2 mm from the aortic annulus.

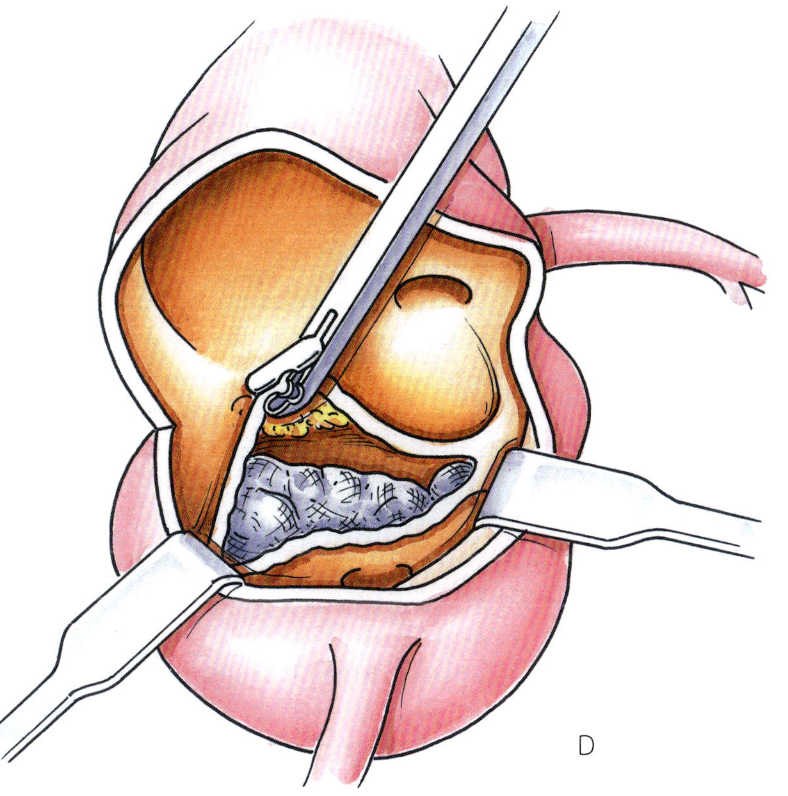

D. 瓣环处的钙化块夹碎后逐一咬除，保留主动脉瓣环的完整性。清除钙化前左心室内置入纱布，避免碎屑落入左心室肌小梁的间隙中而难以清除。

D. Remove the calcified masses at the annulus, while preserving the integrity of the aortic annulus. Before removal of the calcifications, gauze is placed in the left ventricle to prevent debris from falling into the trabecular space in the left ventricle, for debris is difficult to remove.

E. 褥式缝入瓣膜缝线。从瓣环上方紧邻的主动脉组织入针，穿过主动脉瓣环由左心室侧出针，不要缝到左心室心肌。如果主动脉瓣环较小，可用环上置瓣的方法缝入褥式缝线，即从左心室侧缝入主动脉瓣环，由主动脉瓣环上方紧邻的主动脉组织出针。

E. Mattress sutures are passed through the aortic annulus from its adjoining aortic tissues above the annulus to the left ventricular side, keeping away from the left ventricular myocardium. In cases of the small aortic annulus, the valve prosthesis is implanted above the aortic annulus (supra-annular), i.e., the needle is passed from the left ventricular side of the annulus to the adjoining aortic tissue above the aortic annulus.

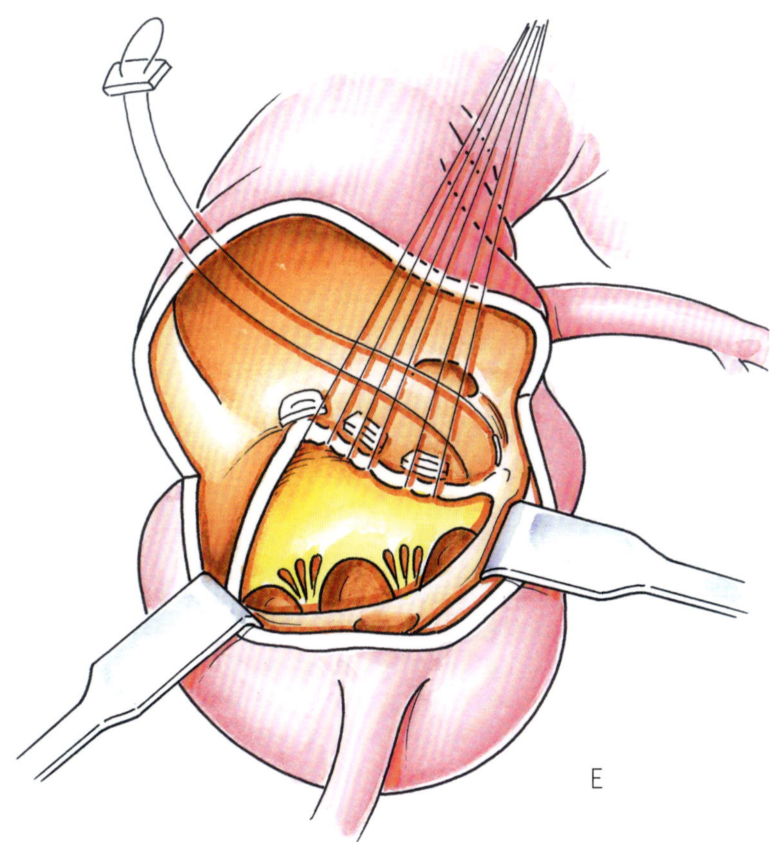

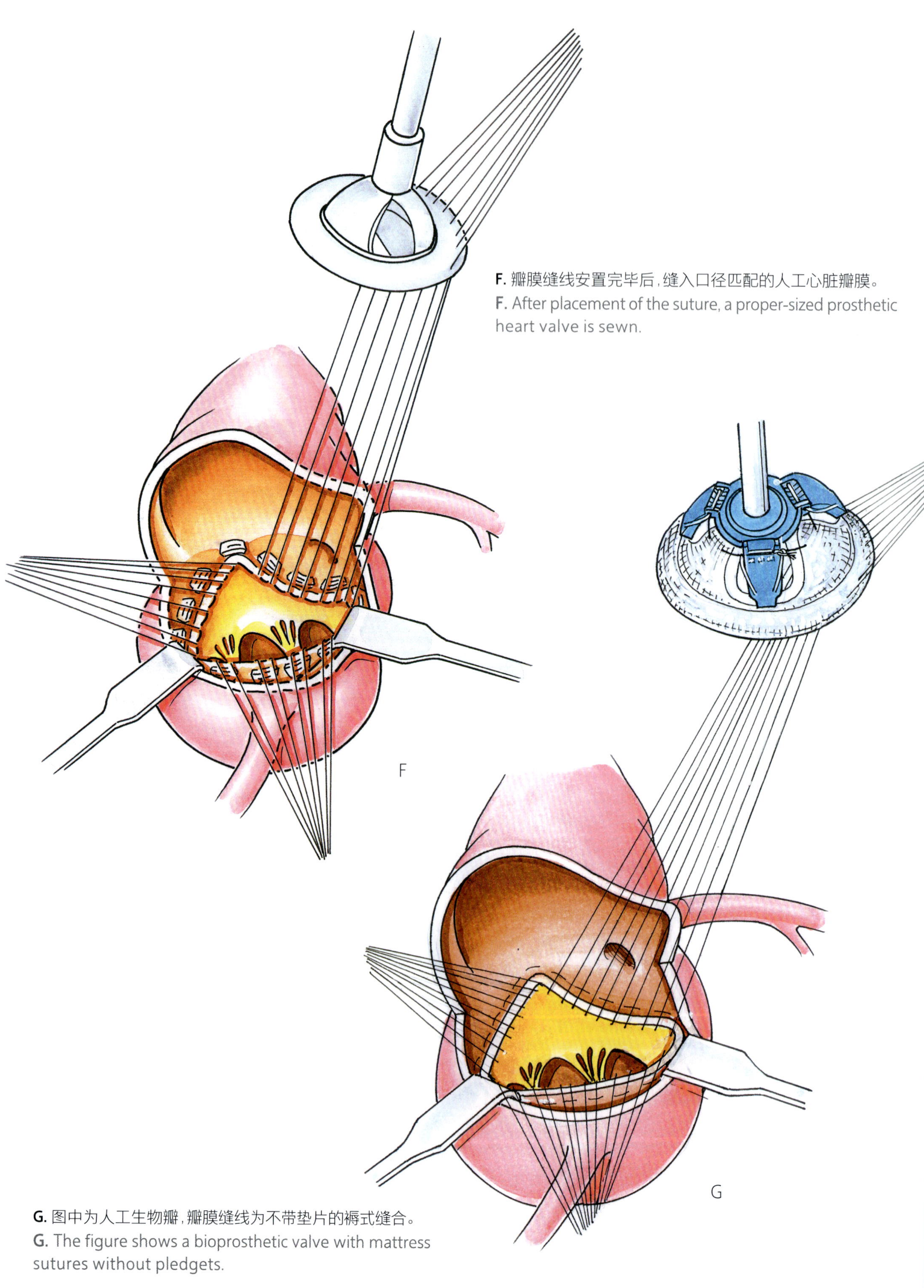

F. 瓣膜缝线安置完毕后，缝入口径匹配的人工心脏瓣膜。

F. After placement of the suture, a proper-sized prosthetic heart valve is sewn.

G. 图中为人工生物瓣，瓣膜缝线为不带垫片的褥式缝合。

G. The figure shows a bioprosthetic valve with mattress sutures without pledgets.

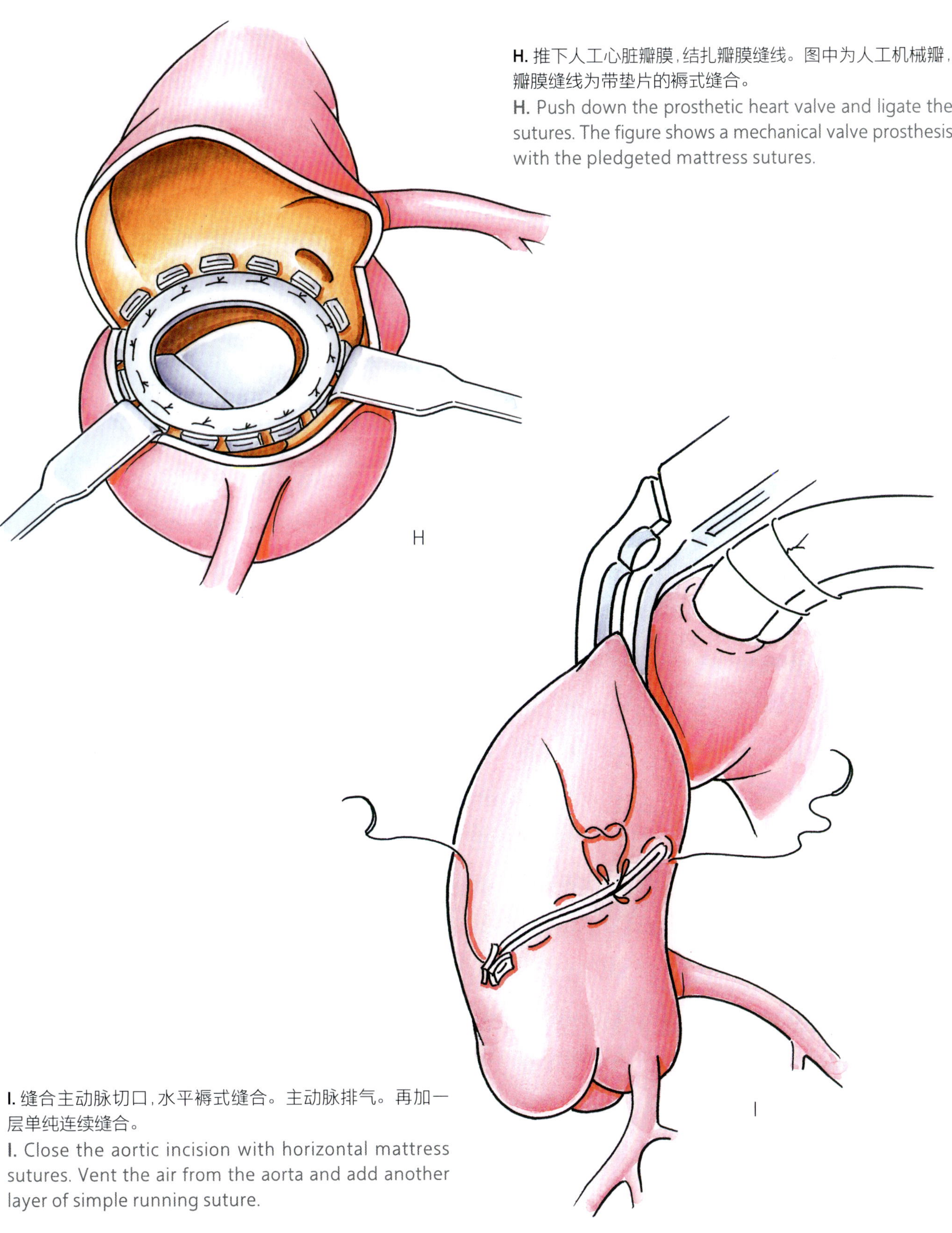

H. 推下人工心脏瓣膜，结扎瓣膜缝线。图中为人工机械瓣，瓣膜缝线为带垫片的褥式缝合。

H. Push down the prosthetic heart valve and ligate the sutures. The figure shows a mechanical valve prosthesis with the pledgeted mattress sutures.

I. 缝合主动脉切口，水平褥式缝合。主动脉排气。再加一层单纯连续缝合。

I. Close the aortic incision with horizontal mattress sutures. Vent the air from the aorta and add another layer of simple running suture.

图 3-2-10 Freestyle 无支架生物瓣置换术
Figure 3-2-10 Aortic valve replacement with the Freestyle stentless bioprosthesis

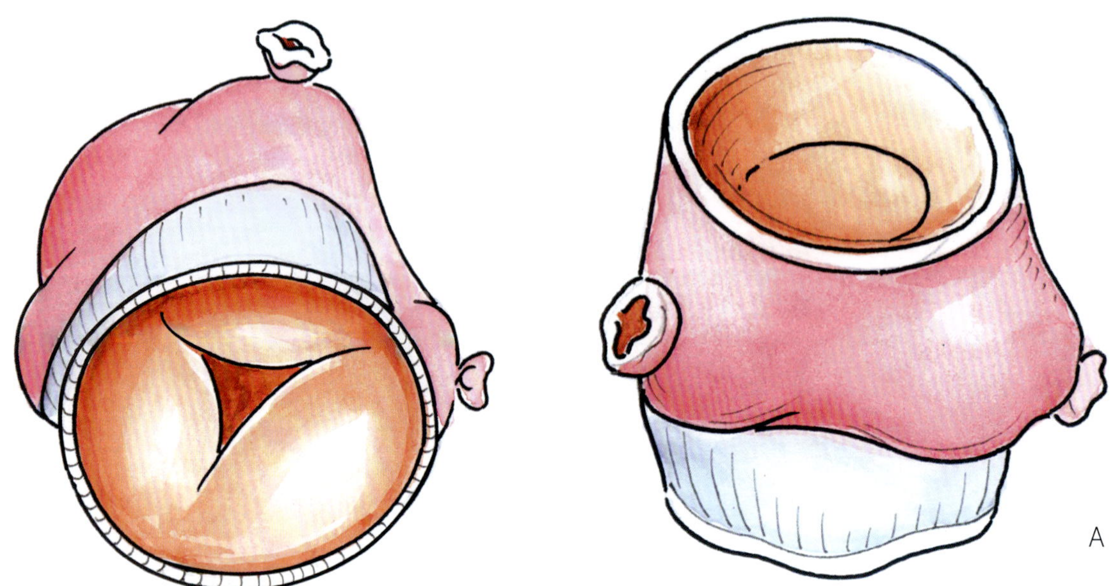

A. Freestyle 无支架生物瓣是由猪主动脉根部制成，其内包含主动脉瓣，其下端加入了一段织物缝合环。

A. The Freestyle stentless bioprosthesis is made from a porcine aortic root, which contains an aortic valve with a fabric suture ring attached to its lower end.

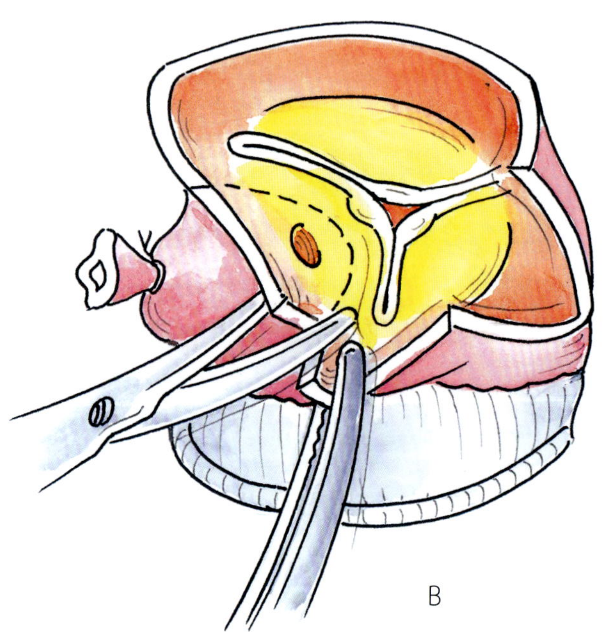

B. 修剪无支架生物瓣的主动脉窦。剪去左冠窦和右冠窦的主动脉壁，无冠窦壁予以保留。

B. Trim the aortic sinus of the stentless bioprosthesis, and cut off the aortic wall of the left and right coronary sinuses, preserving the noncoronary aortic cusp.

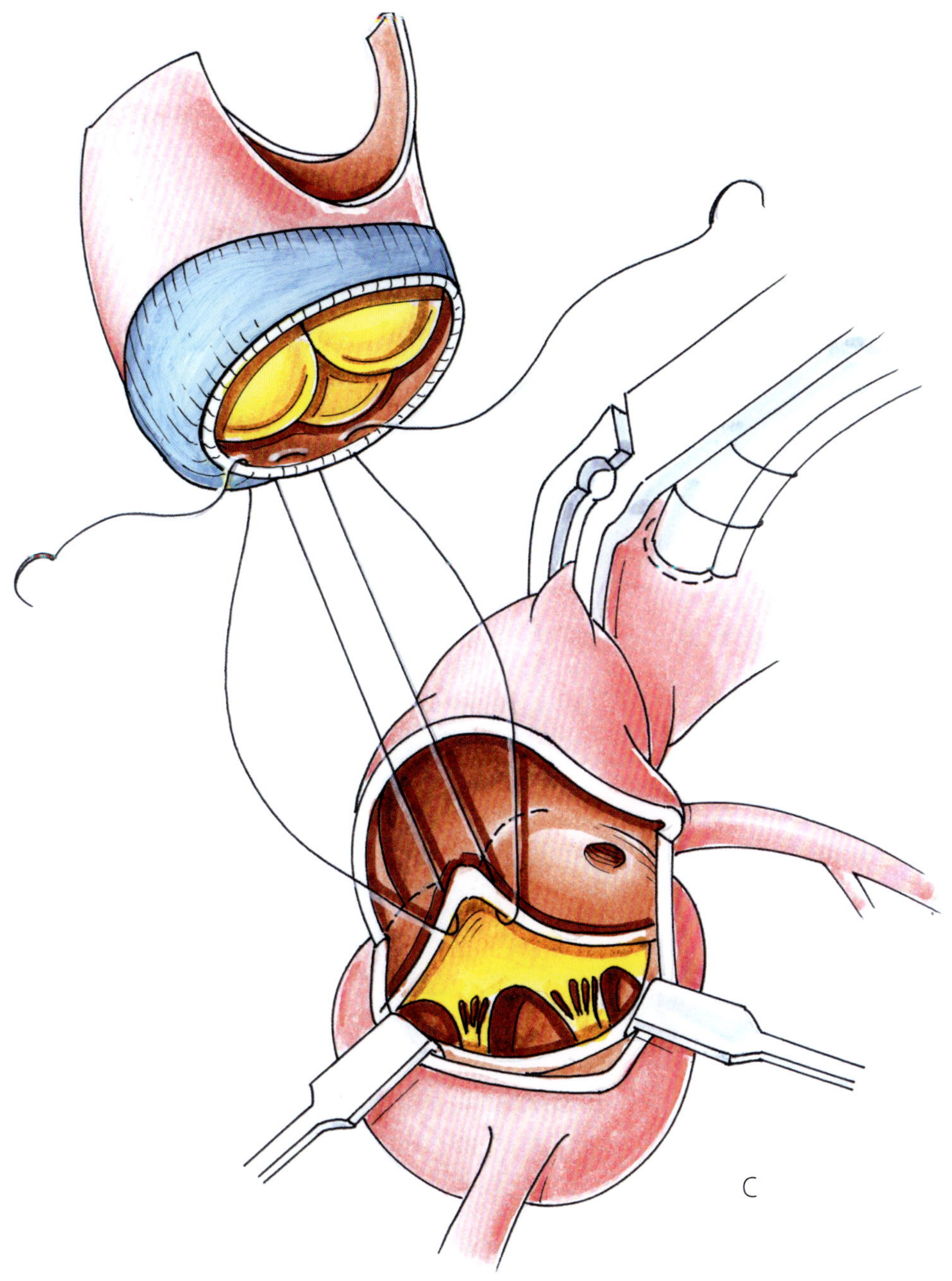

C. 体外循环下在窦管交界远端 0.5~1cm 横行切开升主动脉，距主动脉瓣环 2~3mm 剪除主动脉瓣叶。从左冠窦和无冠窦交界处开始缝入无支架生物瓣。

C. Under extracorporeal circulation, a transverse incision is made on the ascending aorta 0.5-1 cm from the sinotubular junction, and the aortic leaflets are resected at 2-3 mm from the aortic annulus. The suture of stentless bioprosthesis starts at the commissure of the left coronary and noncoronary sinus.

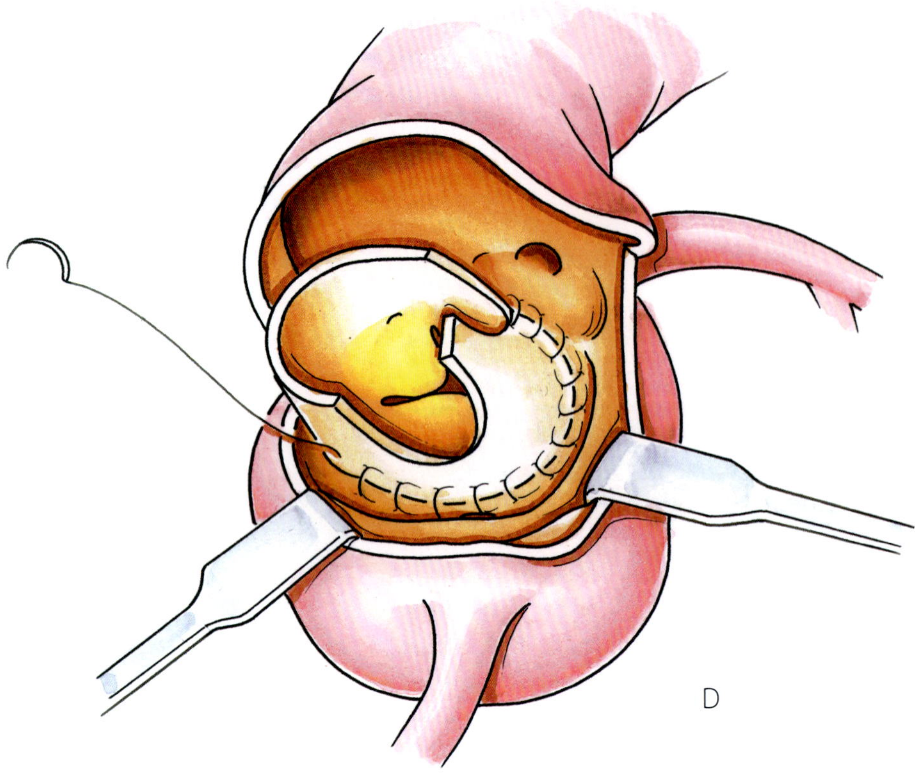

D. 单纯连续缝合将无支架生物瓣的缝合环与主动脉瓣环缝合。

D. The inflow sewing ring of stentless bioprosthesis is attached to the aortic valve annulus with simple running sutures.

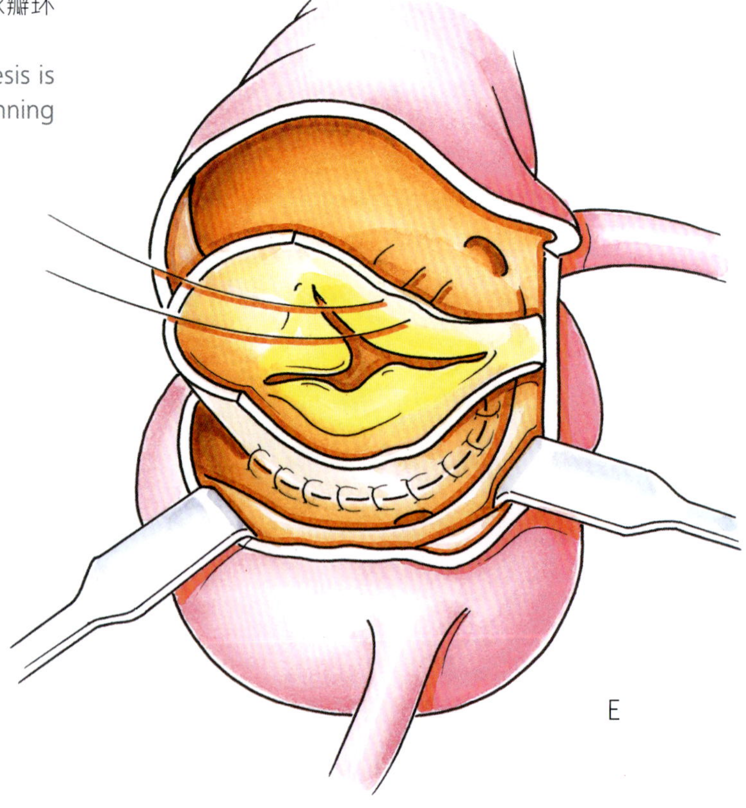

E. 将无支架生物瓣主动脉缘与主动脉缝合。从左冠窦开始，单纯连续缝合。

E. The aortic edge of the stentless bioprosthesis is sutured to the aorta with simple running sutures, which start from the left coronary sinus.

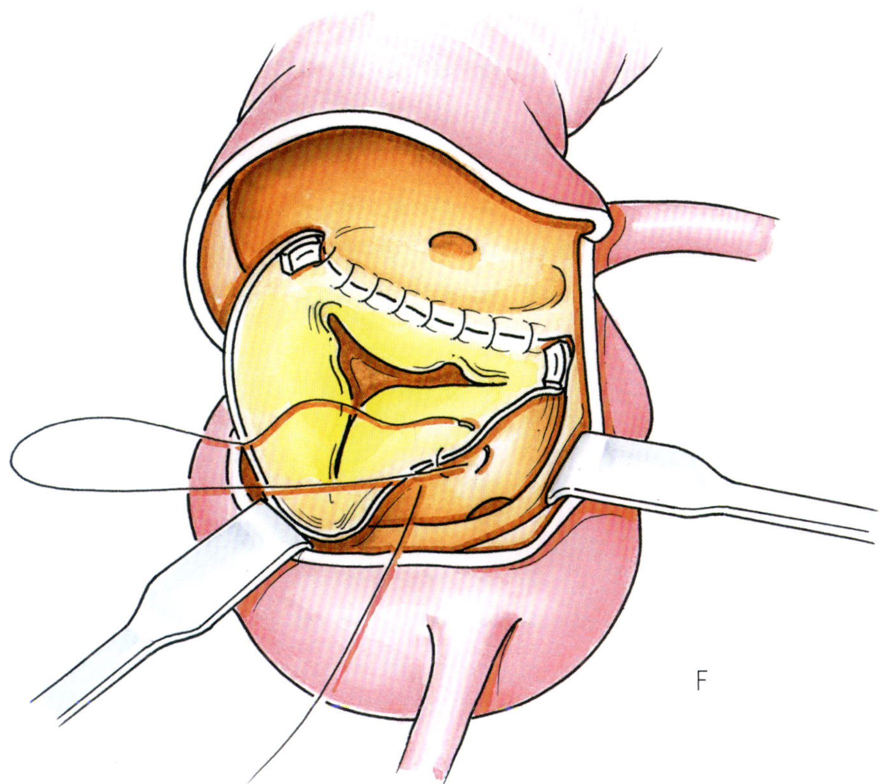

F. 瓣膜交界处带垫片褥式缝合，缝线穿出主动脉，在主动脉外加垫片结扎。继续将无支架生物瓣的主动脉缘与主动脉缝合，注意保持左、右冠状动脉开口的通畅。

F. The valve commissure is sutured by a pledgeted mattress suture which is passed through the aorta and ligated with another pledget outside the aorta. The rest of the aortic edge of the stentless bioprosthesis will continue to be sutured to the aorta, with care being taken to maintain the patency of the left and right coronary ostia.

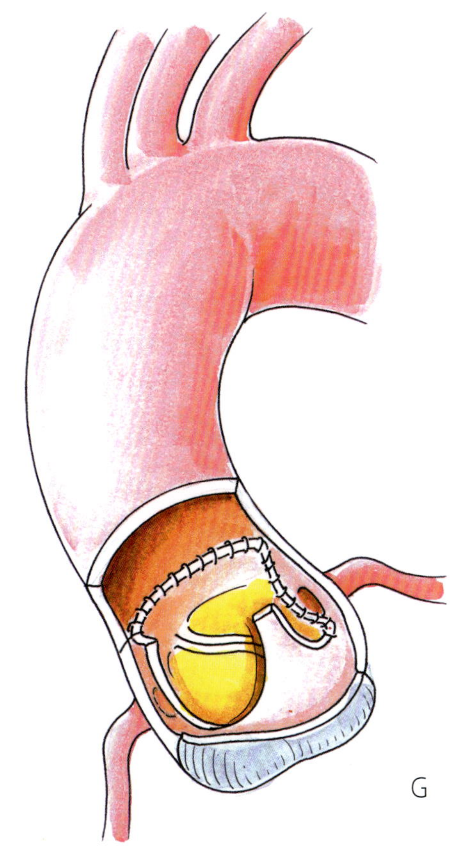

G. 无支架生物瓣植入完成。

G. Stentless bioprosthesis implantation is completed.

图 3-2-11　小主动脉瓣环的主动脉瓣置换术（Konno 法）
Figure 3-2-11　Aortic valve replacement in small aortic annulus (Konno procedure)

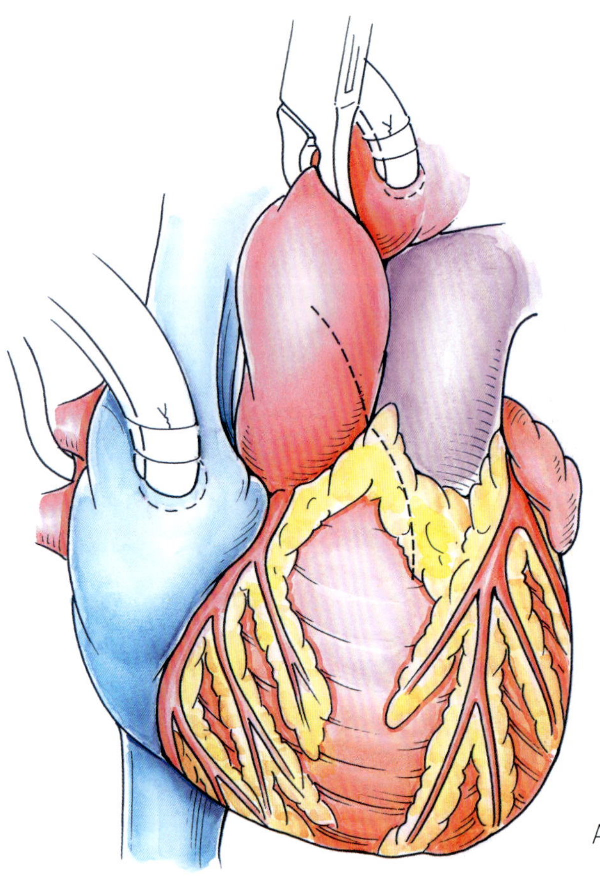

A

A. 小主动脉瓣环伴左心室流出道狭窄时须用 Konno 法扩大主动脉瓣环和左心室流出道。

A. In cases of the small aortic annulus with left ventricular outflow tract stenosis, the Konno procedure is introduced to enlarge the aortic annulus and left ventricular outflow tract.

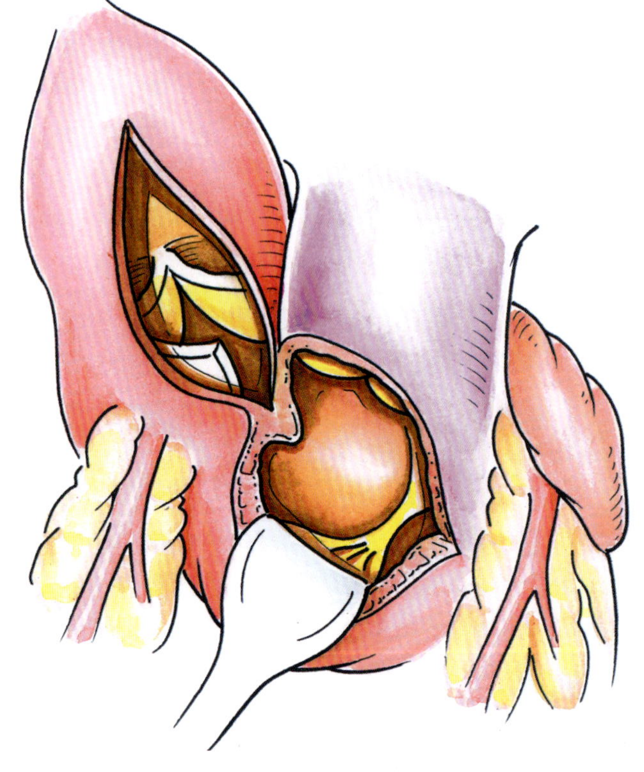

B

B. 在右冠状动脉开口左侧纵行切开升主动脉及主动脉瓣环，切口向左下延伸，切开右心室流出道。

B. A longitudinally incision is made on the ascending aorta and aortic annulus on the left side of the right coronary ostium and extended to the bottom left, and the right ventricular outflow tract can be incised.

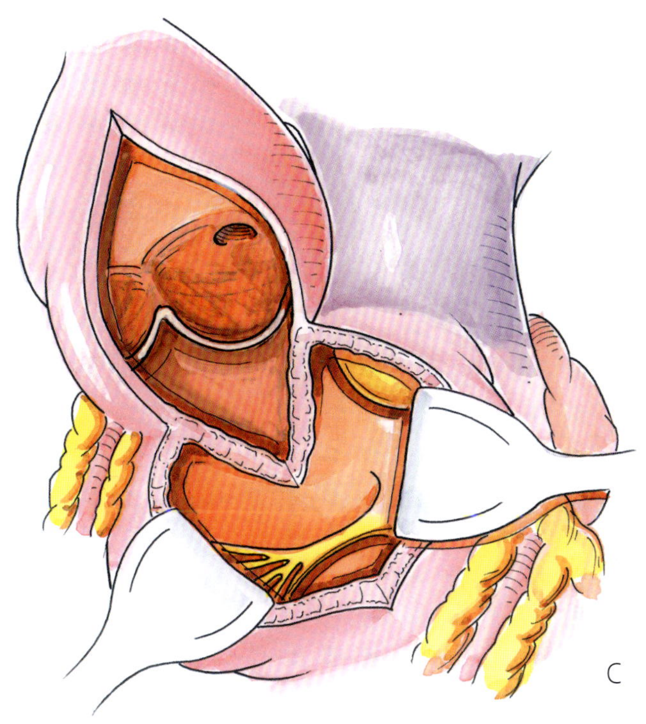

C. 继而切开室间隔，切开的长度取决于左心室流出道狭窄的长度。切除主动脉瓣叶。

C. Then an incision is made on the ventricular septum, and the length depends on the length of left ventricular outflow tract stenosis. Aortic leaflets are removed.

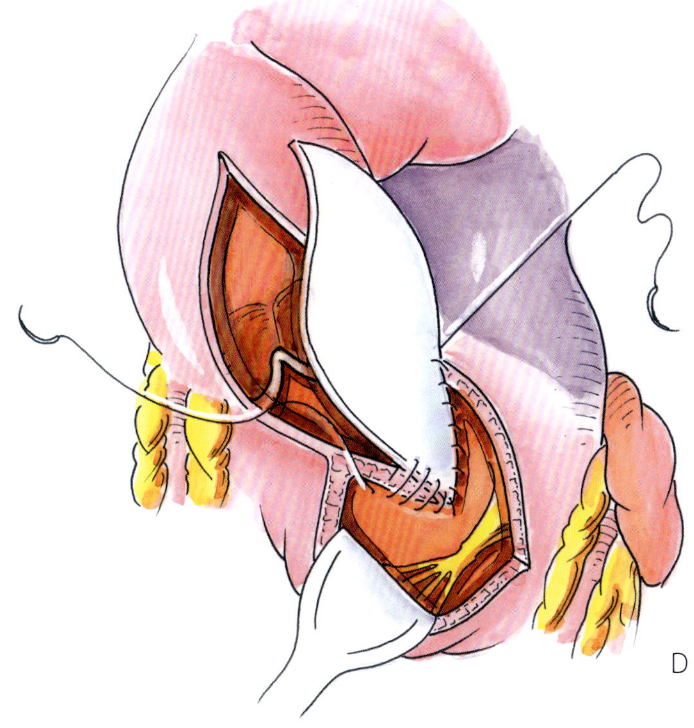

D. 室间隔切口与一片梭形补片单纯连续缝合，加宽左心室流出道和主动脉瓣环。

D. A fusiform patch is sutured to the ventricular septal incision with simple continuous sutures. The left ventricular outflow tract and aortic annulus are to be widened.

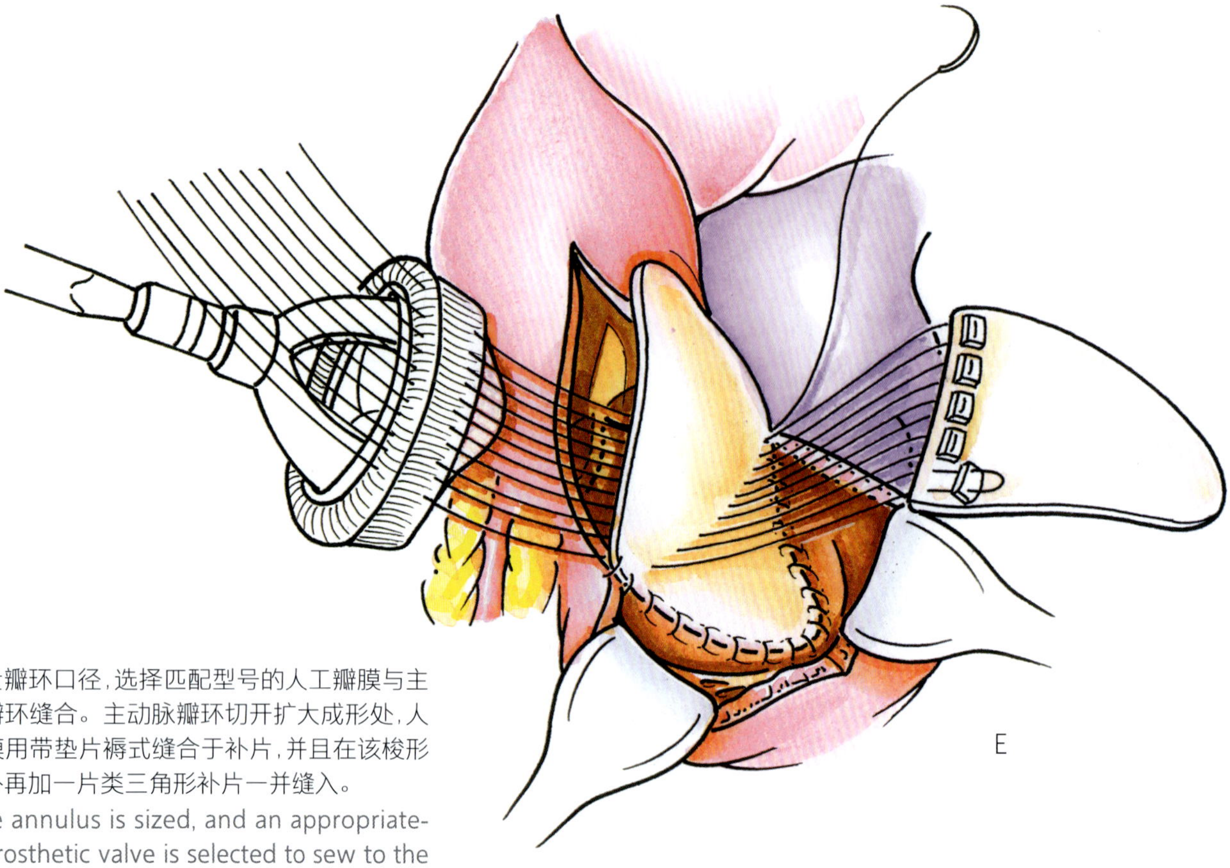

E. 测量瓣环口径，选择匹配型号的人工瓣膜与主动脉瓣环缝合。主动脉瓣环切开扩大成形处，人工瓣膜用带垫片褥式缝合于补片，并且在该梭形补片外再加一片类三角形补片一并缝入。

E. The annulus is sized, and an appropriate-size prosthetic valve is selected to sew to the aortic annulus. Where the aortic annuloplasty and enlargement is performed, the prosthetic valve is sewn to the fusiform patch with pledgeted mattress sutures, and a triangular-like patch is added to the fusiform patch and sewed into the annulus together.

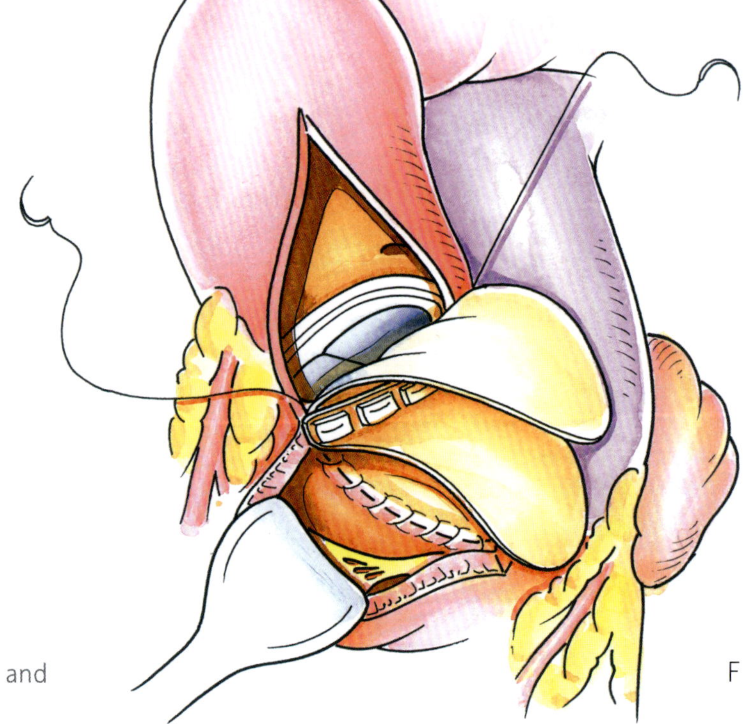

F. 人工瓣膜推下打结。

F. The prosthetic valve is pushed down and the sutures are knotted.

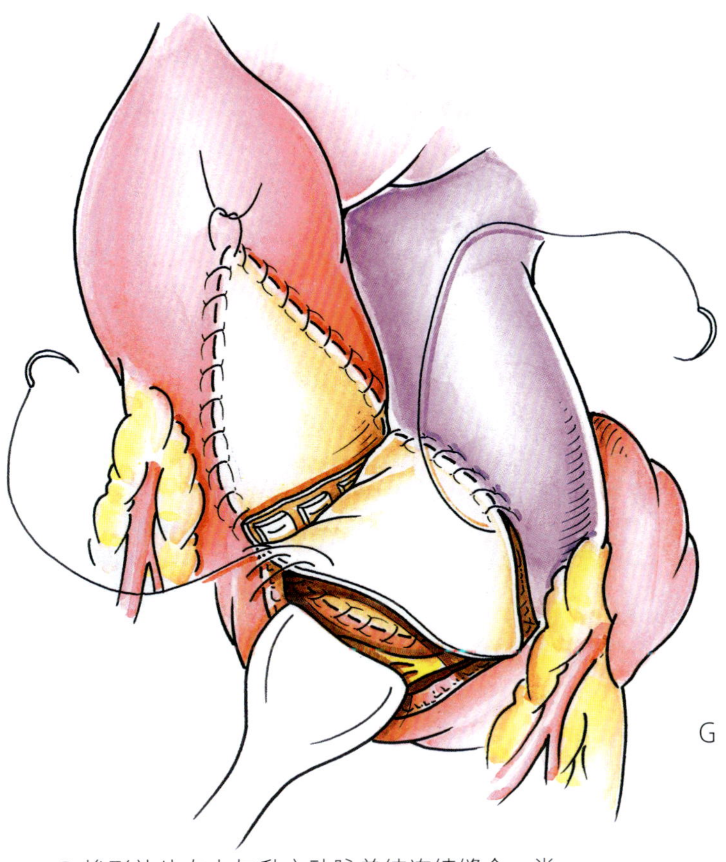

G. 梭形补片向上与升主动脉单纯连续缝合。类三角形补片向下与右心室壁切开处缝合，扩大成形右心室流出道。

G. The fusiform patch is sutured up to the ascending aorta with simple running sutures. The triangular-like patch is sutured down to the right ventricular wall, enlarging the shaped right ventricular outflow tract.

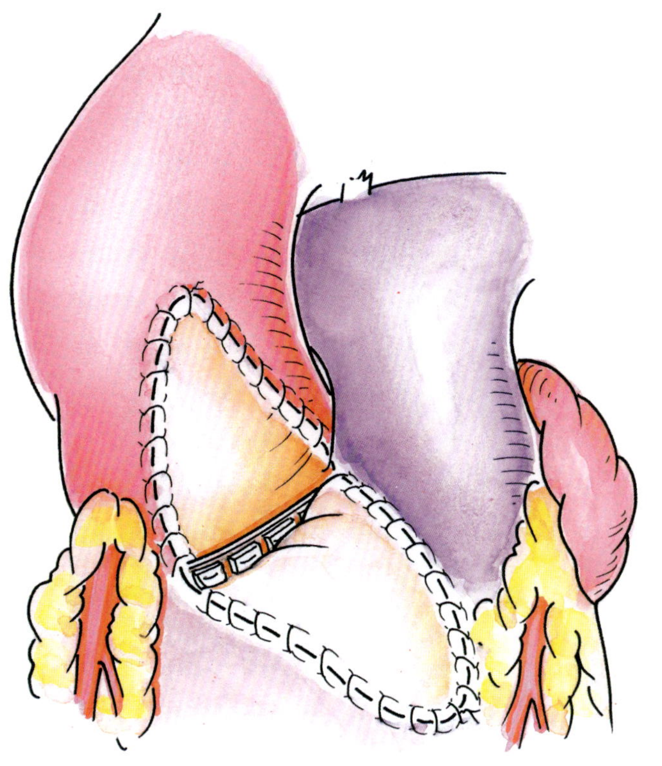

H. 缝合毕。

H. Suture is completed.

图 3-2-12 同种瓣膜移植术

Figure 3-2-12 Aortic valve replacement with homograft

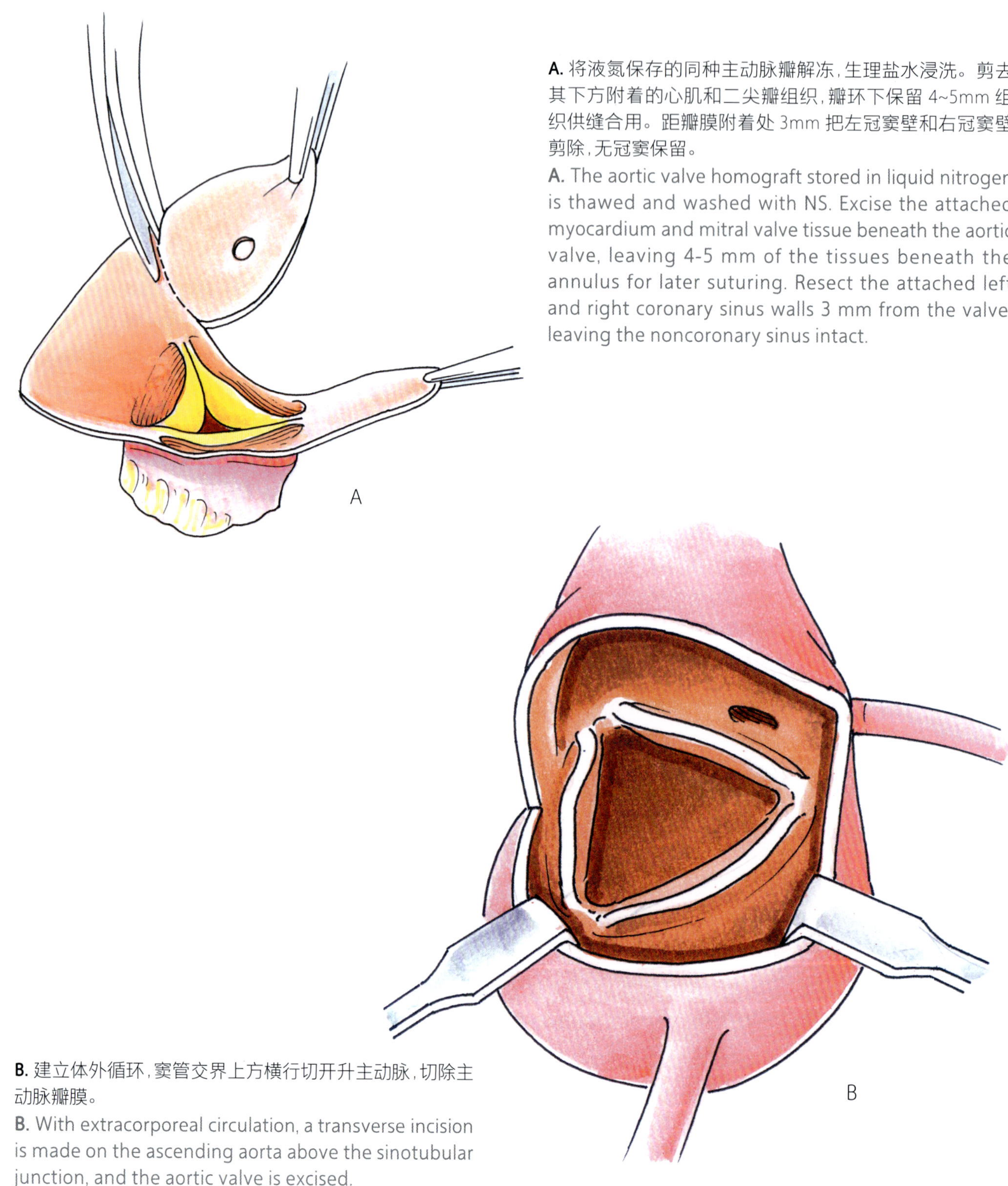

A. 将液氮保存的同种主动脉瓣解冻，生理盐水浸洗。剪去其下方附着的心肌和二尖瓣组织，瓣环下保留 4~5mm 组织供缝合用。距瓣膜附着处 3mm 把左冠窦壁和右冠窦壁剪除，无冠窦保留。

A. The aortic valve homograft stored in liquid nitrogen is thawed and washed with NS. Excise the attached myocardium and mitral valve tissue beneath the aortic valve, leaving 4-5 mm of the tissues beneath the annulus for later suturing. Resect the attached left and right coronary sinus walls 3 mm from the valve, leaving the noncoronary sinus intact.

B. 建立体外循环，窦管交界上方横行切开升主动脉，切除主动脉瓣膜。

B. With extracorporeal circulation, a transverse incision is made on the ascending aorta above the sinotubular junction, and the aortic valve is excised.

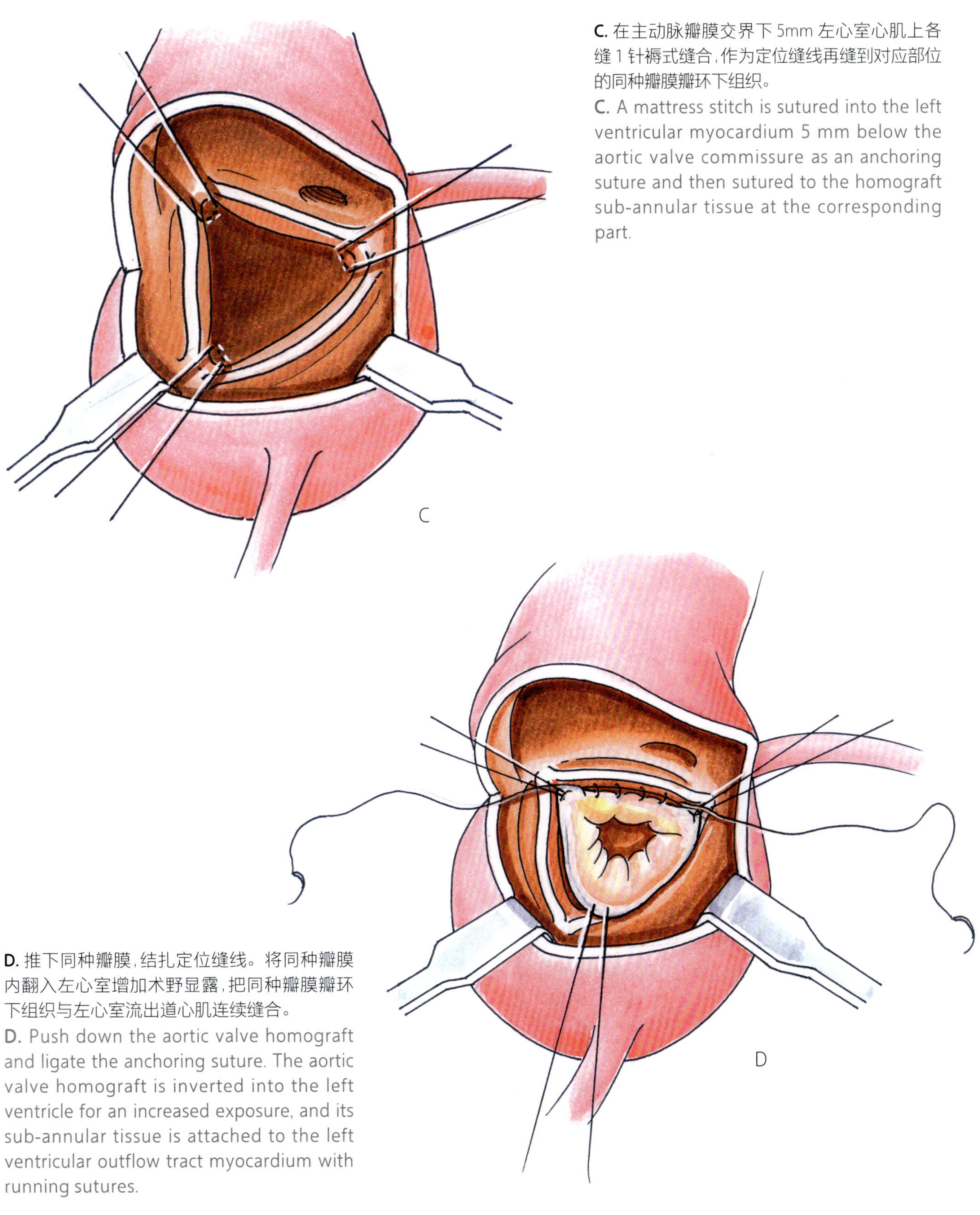

C. 在主动脉瓣膜交界下 5mm 左心室心肌上各缝 1 针褥式缝合，作为定位缝线再缝到对应部位的同种瓣膜瓣环下组织。

C. A mattress stitch is sutured into the left ventricular myocardium 5 mm below the aortic valve commissure as an anchoring suture and then sutured to the homograft sub-annular tissue at the corresponding part.

D. 推下同种瓣膜，结扎定位缝线。将同种瓣膜内翻入左心室增加术野显露，把同种瓣膜瓣环下组织与左心室流出道心肌连续缝合。

D. Push down the aortic valve homograft and ligate the anchoring suture. The aortic valve homograft is inverted into the left ventricle for an increased exposure, and its sub-annular tissue is attached to the left ventricular outflow tract myocardium with running sutures.

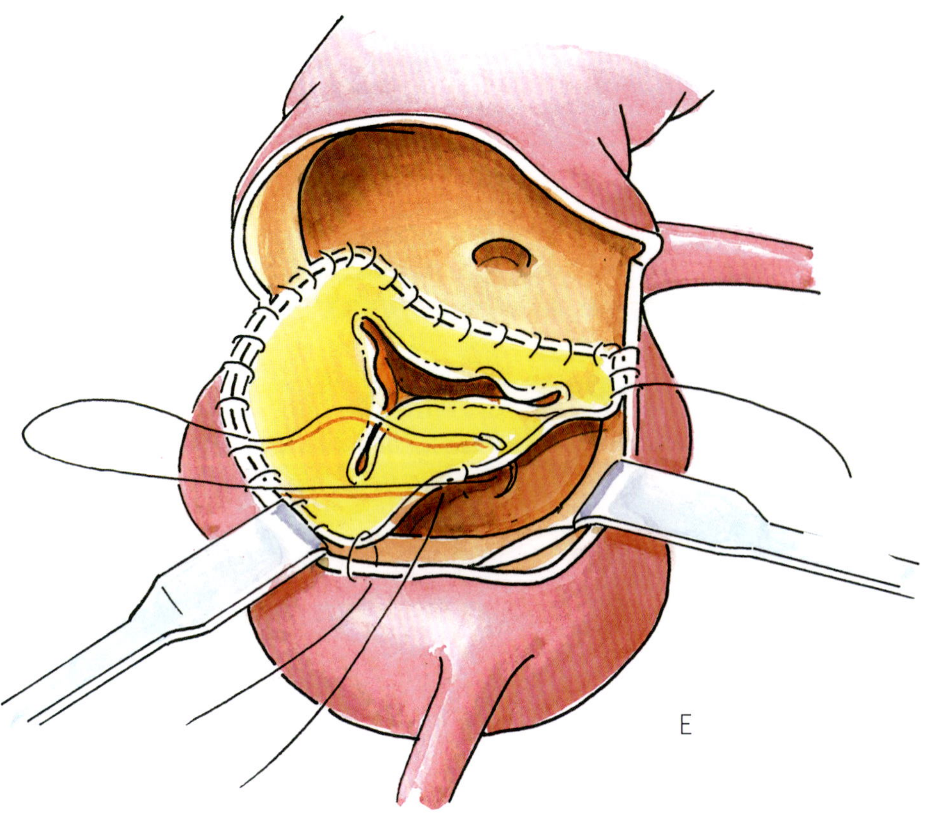

E. 同种瓣膜下缘缝合完成后，把同种瓣膜从左心室内翻回到主动脉内，交界顶端分别缝到主动脉壁，缝线不结扎调整位置务使同种瓣膜的瓣叶对合良好。将同种瓣膜的上缘与主动脉缝合。

E. After the closure of the lower margin of the aortic valve homograft, the homograft is inverted from the left ventricle back into the aorta, and the top of the commissures are sutured to the aortic wall respectively. Sutures proceed but without ligation, so that the location of the valves can be adjusted to ensure the leaflets of aortic valve homograft are well coapted. The upper margin of the allograft is sewn to the aorta.

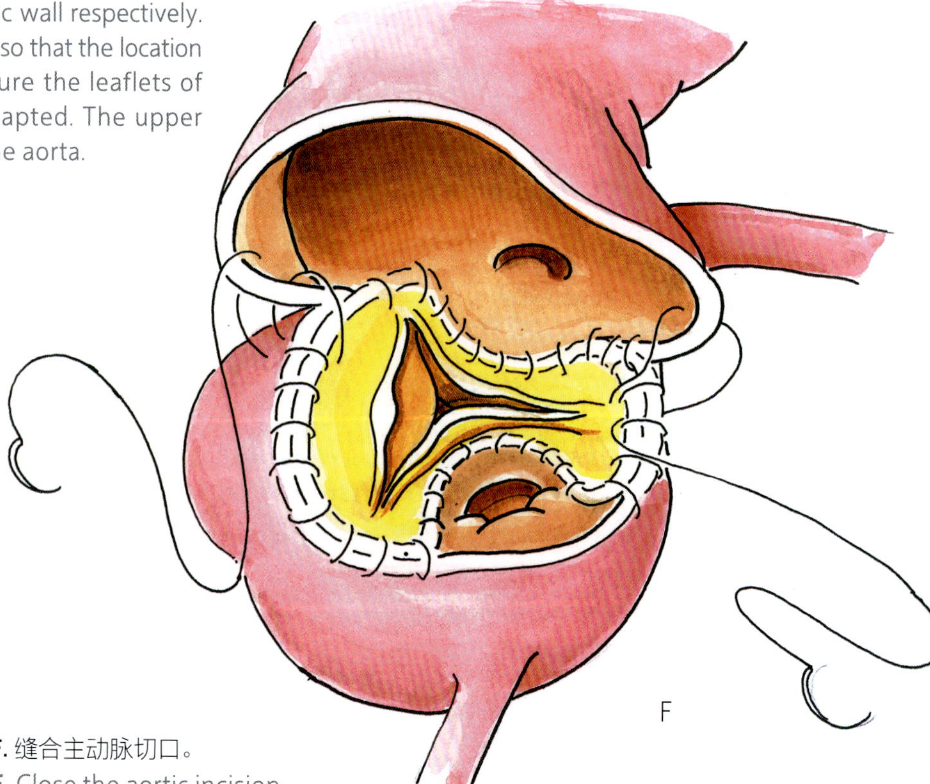

F. 缝合主动脉切口。

F. Close the aortic incision.

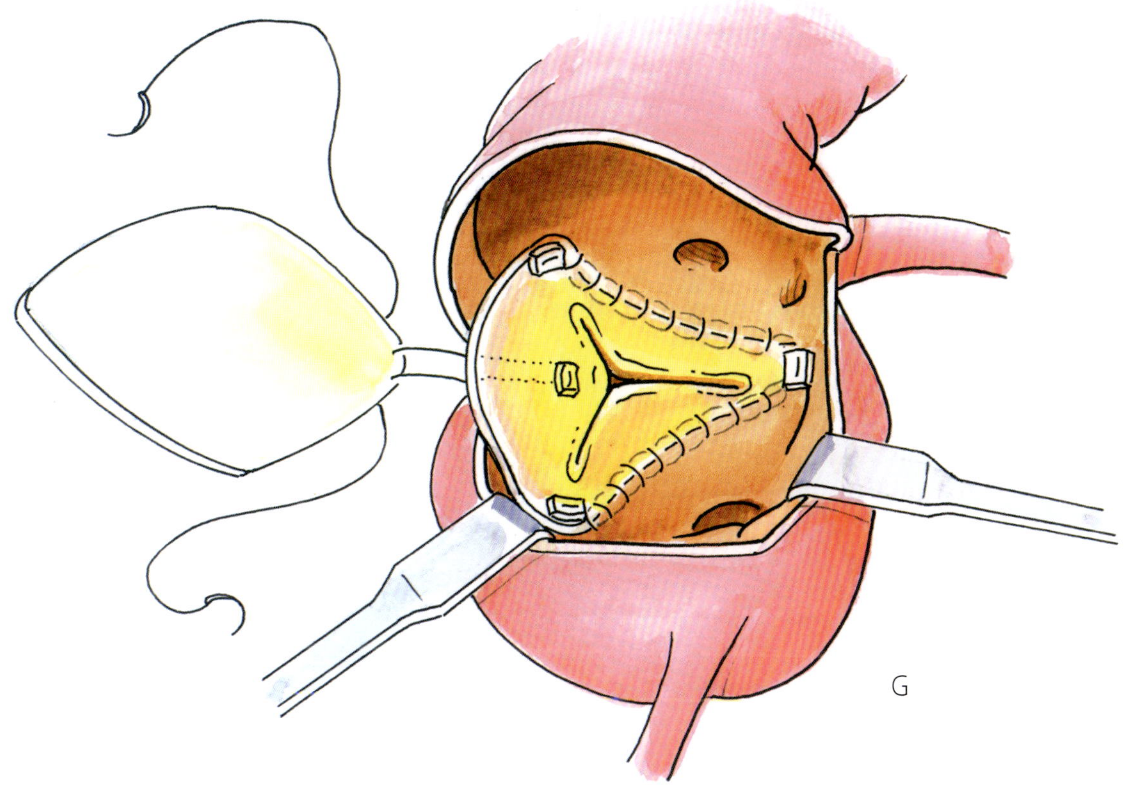

G. 如果主动脉窦部偏小，可将主动脉切口向右下延长，加一块心包补片拓宽主动脉窦。

G. In the case of small aortic sinus, the aortic incision can be extended to the low right, and a pericardial patch can be added to widen the aortic sinus.

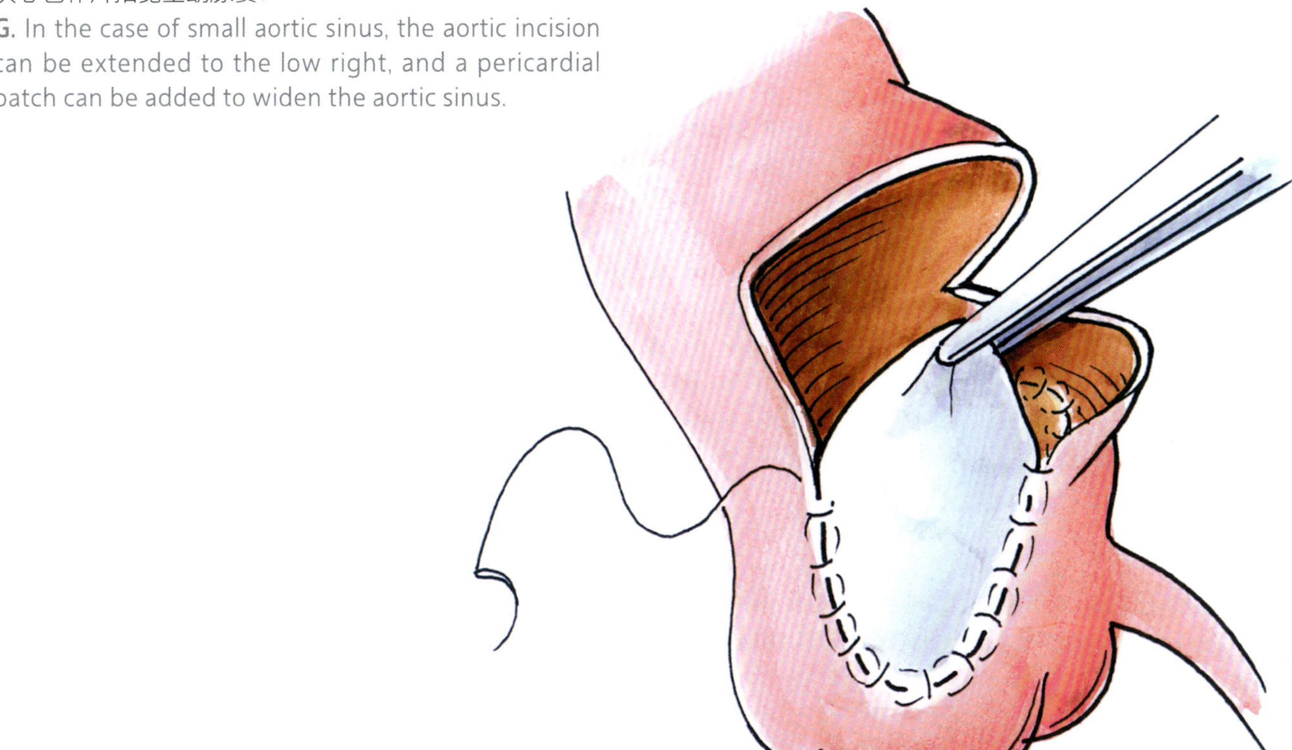

H. 心包补片与剪开的无冠窦壁单纯连续缝合。

H. The pericardial patch is sewn to the open noncoronary sinus wall with running sutures.

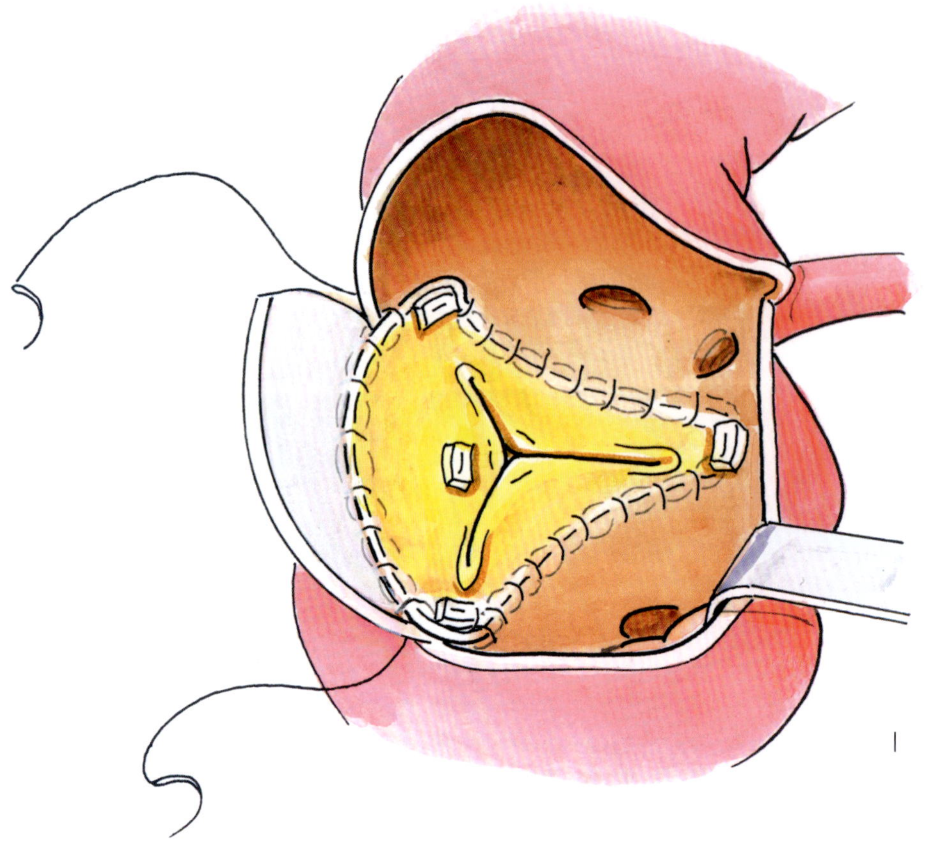

I. 同种瓣膜的无冠窦上缘缝到心包补片上。

I. The superior edge of the noncoronary sinus of homograft is sutured to the pericardial patch.

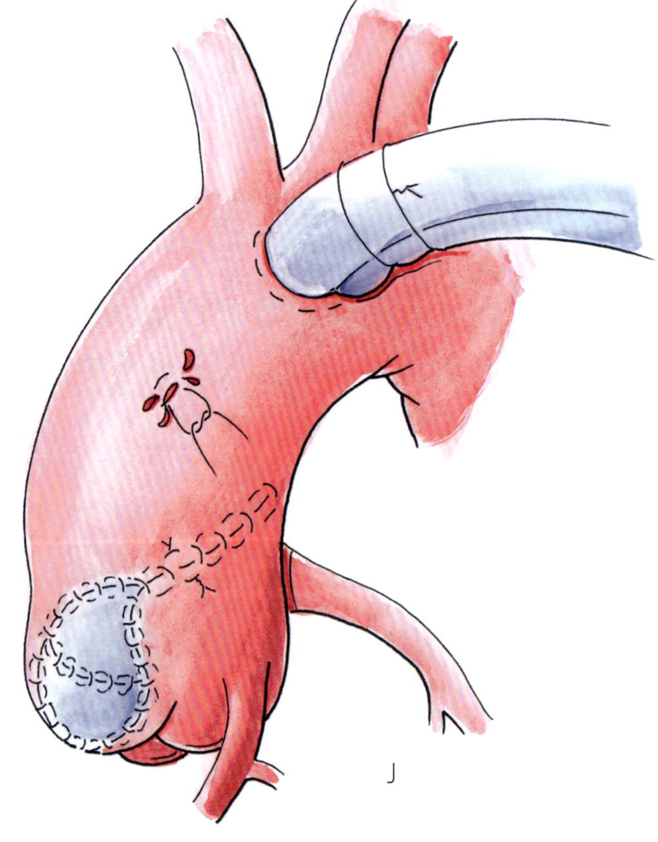

J. 关闭主动脉切口。主动脉排气。

J. Close the aortic incision. Vent the aorta.

图 3-2-13　经心尖主动脉瓣植入术
Figure 3-2-13　Transapical aortic valve implantation

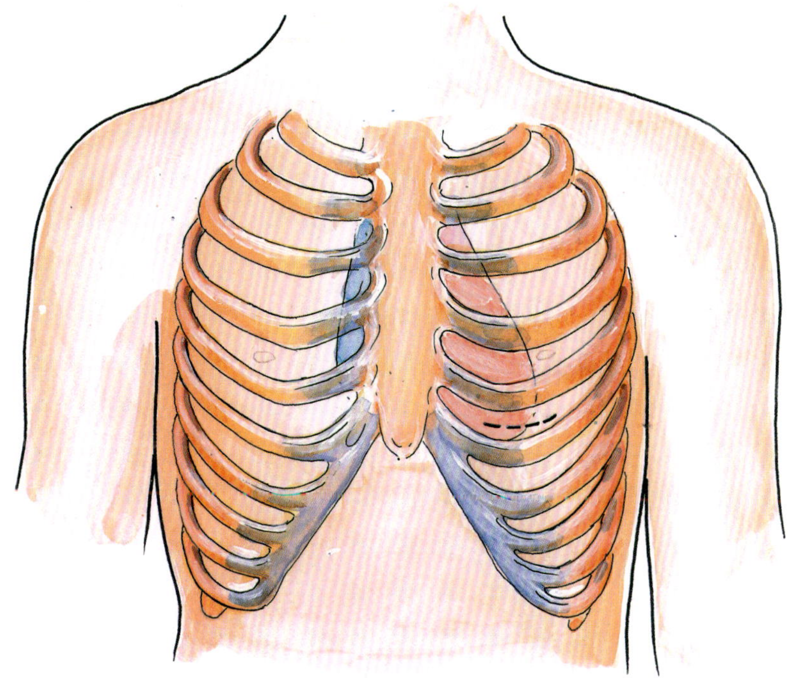

A. 经心尖主动脉瓣植入术要在杂交手术室进行，用 X 线检查和经食管超声心动图检查做引导。左胸第 5 肋间锁骨中线做约 5cm 切口。

A. Transapical aortic valve implantation is performed in a hybrid operative theater under the guidance of X-ray and transesophageal echocardiography (TEE). An approximately 5 cm incision is made in the fifth intercostal space at the left midclavicular line.

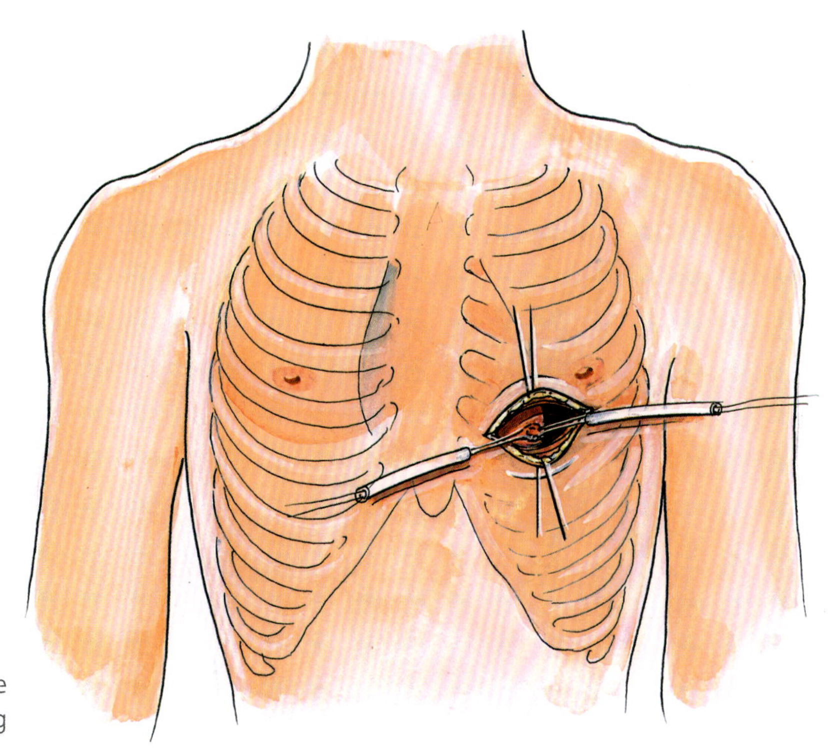

B. 切开心包显露心尖，做两个荷包缝合。

B. Open the pericardium to expose the apex and make two purse-string sutures.

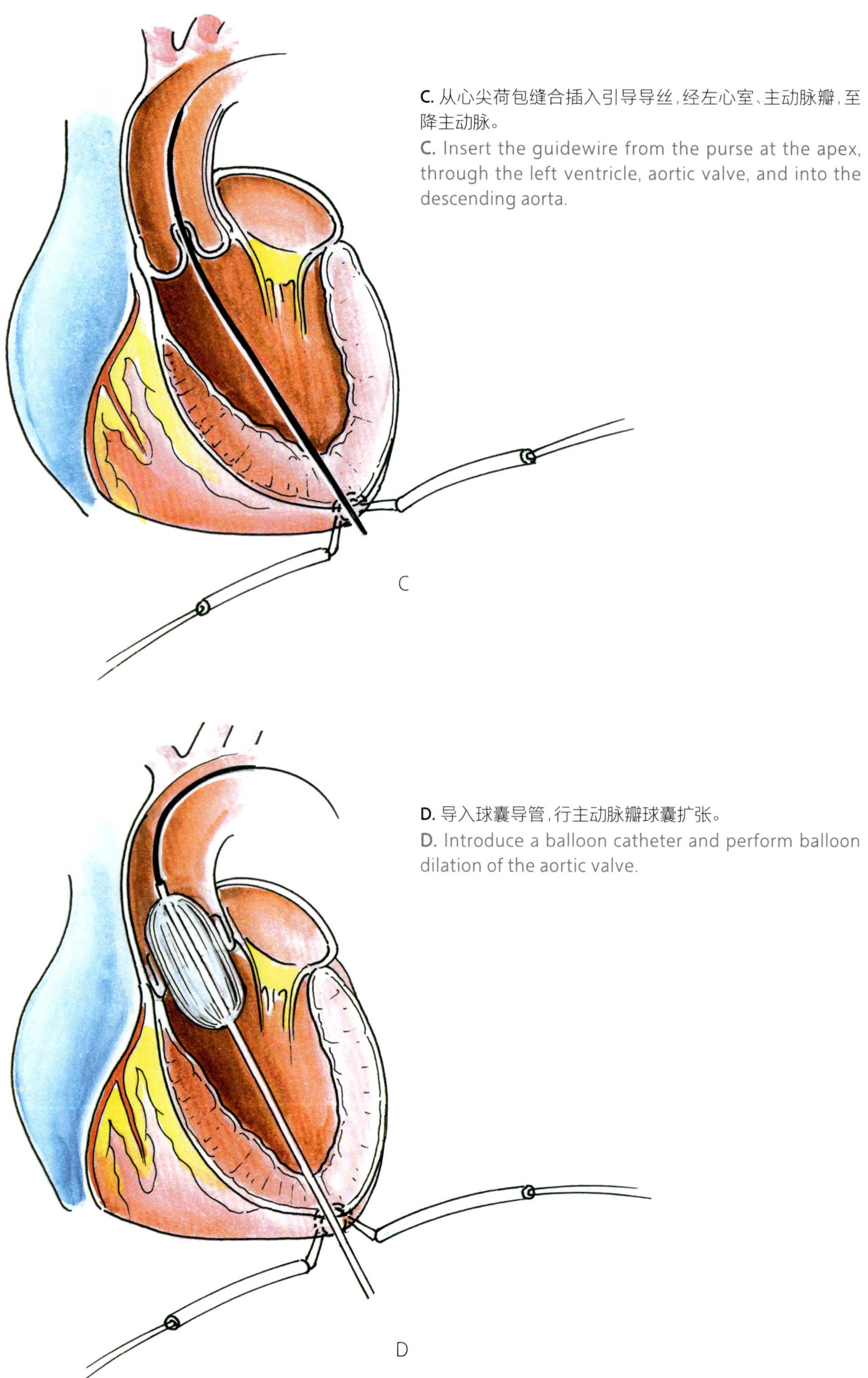

C. 从心尖荷包缝合插入引导导丝，经左心室、主动脉瓣，至降主动脉。

C. Insert the guidewire from the purse at the apex, through the left ventricle, aortic valve, and into the descending aorta.

D. 导入球囊导管，行主动脉瓣球囊扩张。

D. Introduce a balloon catheter and perform balloon dilation of the aortic valve.

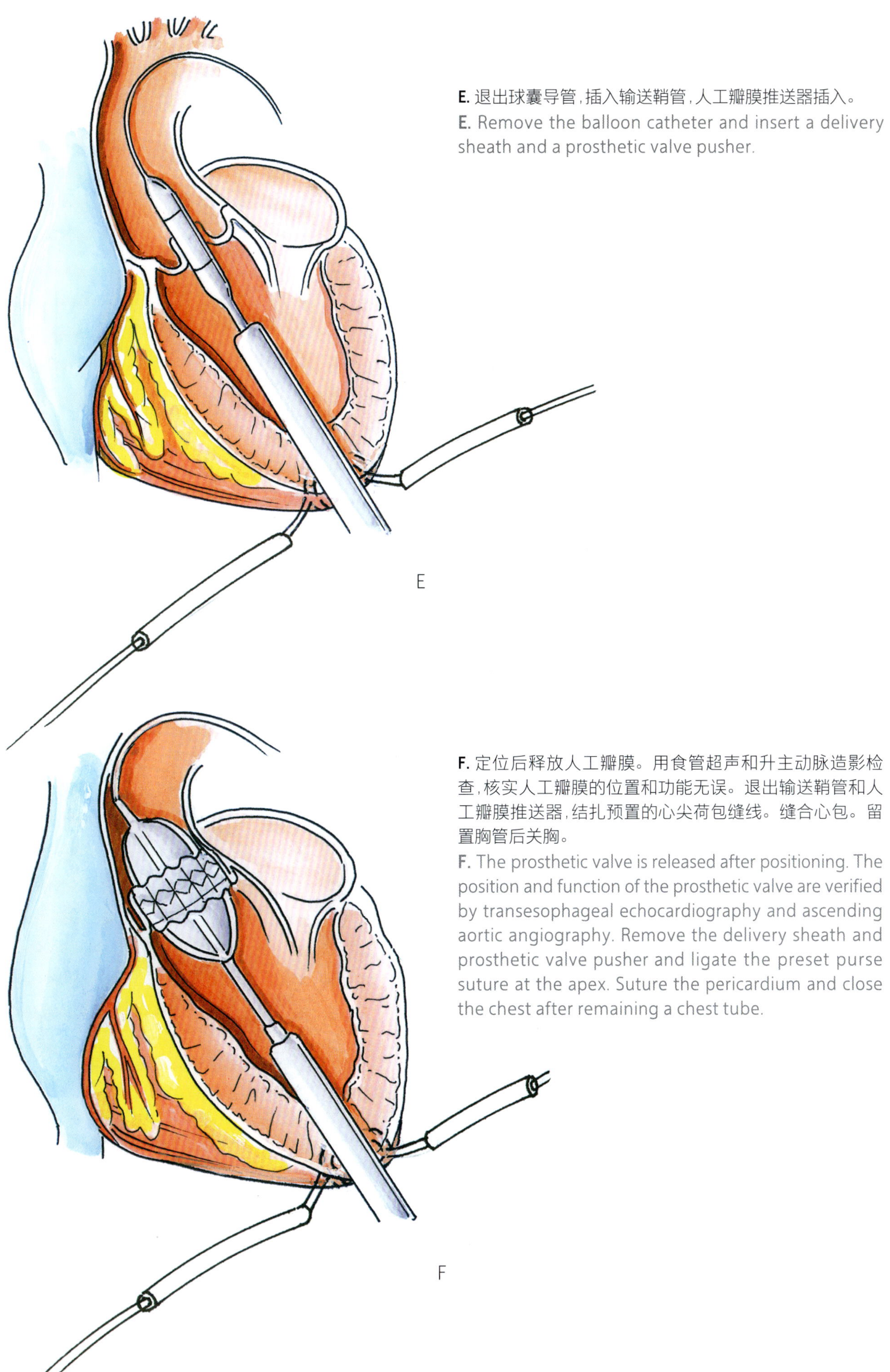

E. 退出球囊导管，插入输送鞘管，人工瓣膜推送器插入。

E. Remove the balloon catheter and insert a delivery sheath and a prosthetic valve pusher.

F. 定位后释放人工瓣膜。用食管超声和升主动脉造影检查，核实人工瓣膜的位置和功能无误。退出输送鞘管和人工瓣膜推送器，结扎预置的心尖荷包缝线。缝合心包。留置胸管后关胸。

F. The prosthetic valve is released after positioning. The position and function of the prosthetic valve are verified by transesophageal echocardiography and ascending aortic angiography. Remove the delivery sheath and prosthetic valve pusher and ligate the preset purse suture at the apex. Suture the pericardium and close the chest after remaining a chest tube.

图 3-2-14 经皮介入主动脉瓣植入术

Figure 3-2-14 Percutaneous aortic valve implantation

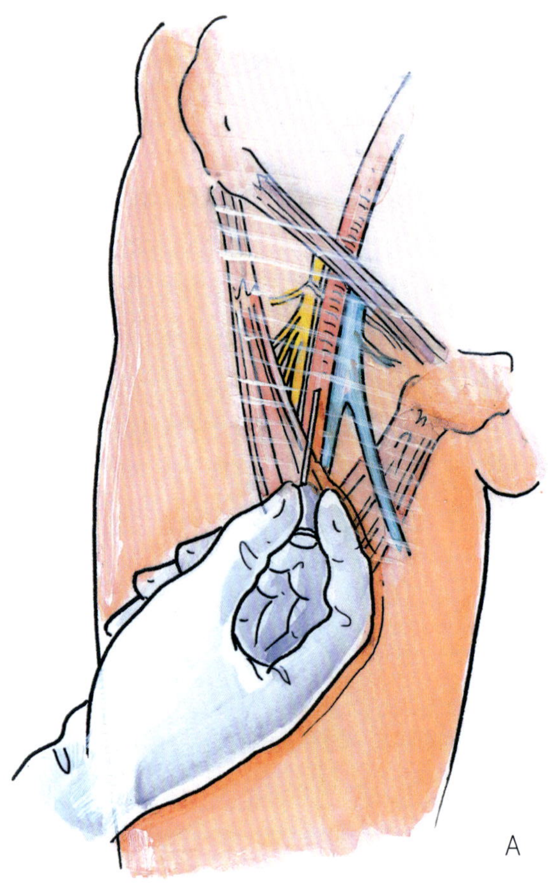

A. 全身麻醉或局部麻醉，经皮穿刺股动脉。

A. Under general or local anesthesia, a percutaneous puncture of the femoral artery is performed.

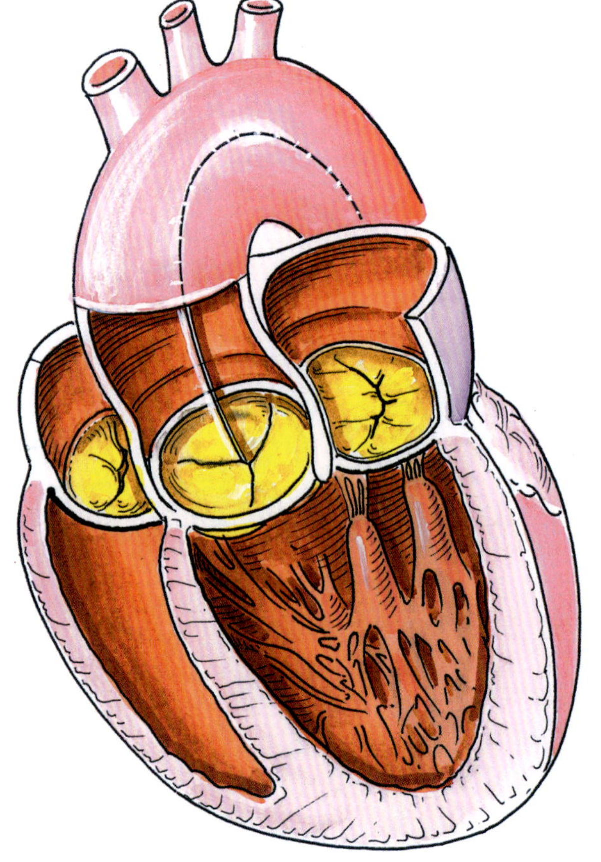

B. 在造影导管的引导下，将直头钢丝逆向穿过严重狭窄的主动脉瓣进入左心室，经猪尾导管将直头钢丝换成强支撑硬钢丝。

B. Under the guidance of a contrast catheter, a straight wire is passed back across the severely narrowed aortic valve and advanced into the left ventricle, and it is replaced by a stiff wire through a pigtail catheter.

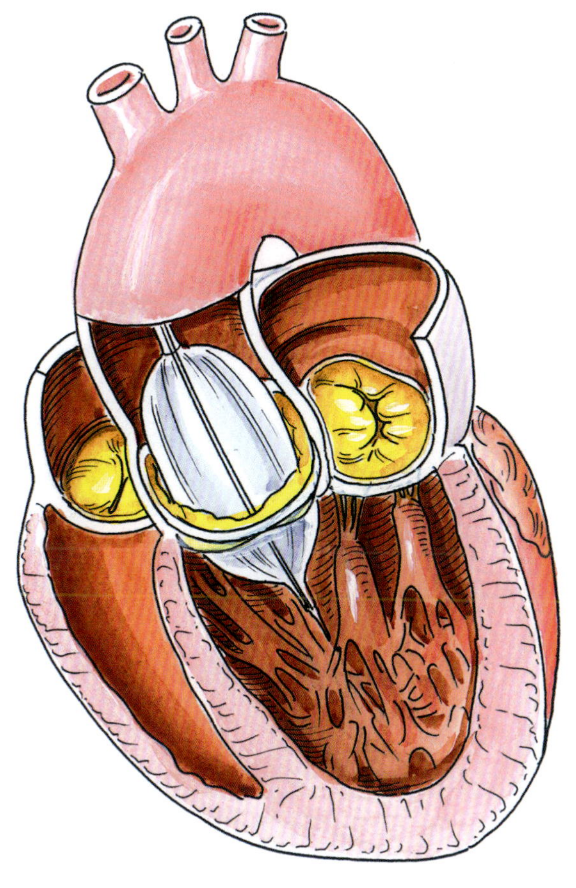

C. 将瓣膜扩张球囊沿钢丝推送至主动脉瓣狭窄处，快速起搏，手动加压扩张主动脉瓣狭窄。行升主动脉造影，以球囊直径为参考选择瓣膜大小，并撤出扩张球囊。

C. Push the valve balloon along the wire to the aortic stenosis site with rapid pacing and manual compression to augment the aortic stenosis. Perform ascending aortography, decide the size of the aortic valve based on the balloon diameter, and remove the balloon.

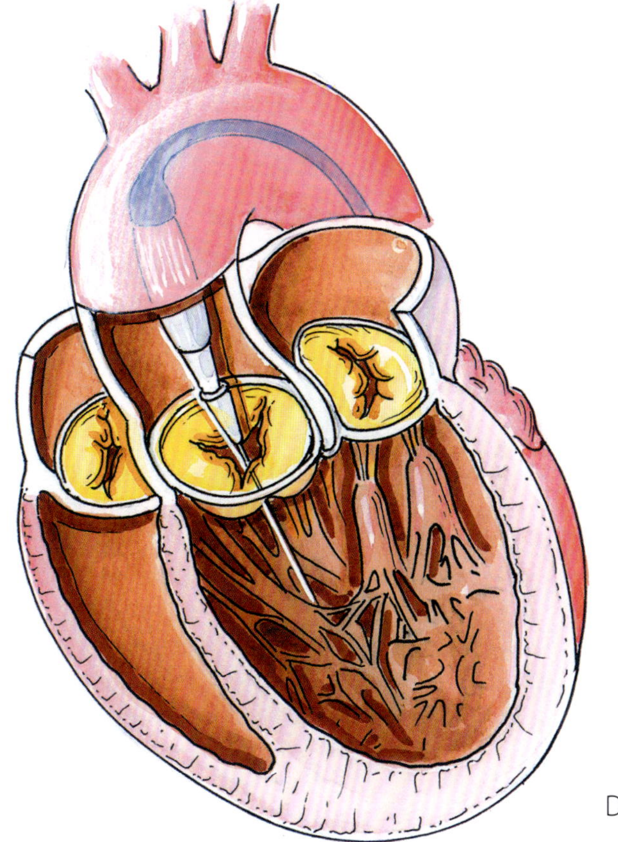

D. 将人工主动脉瓣膜通过输送导管送到自体主动脉瓣的位置。

D. Place a prosthetic aortic valve to the native aortic valve position through a delivery catheter.

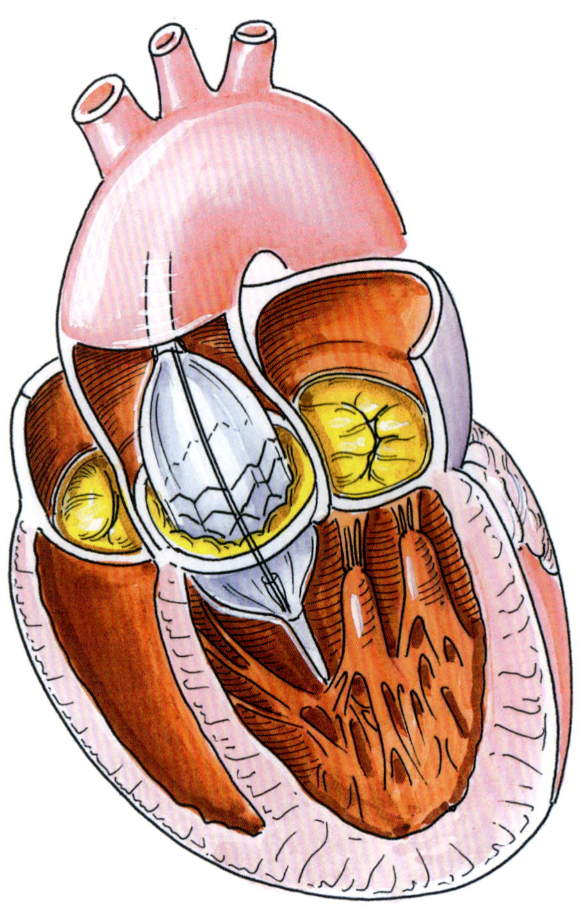

E. 将人工瓣膜推送通过主动脉瓣后，依据升主动脉造影下右冠状动脉窦最低水平来定位瓣膜的准确位置并释放人工瓣膜。释放瓣膜时，应在右心室快速起搏，使左心室压力下降到 60mmHg（1mmHg=0.133kPa）以下，扩张球囊植入人工瓣膜。

E. While pushing the prosthetic valve through the aortic valve, the exact position of the valve is to be decided and the valve is to be released according to the lowest level of the right coronary sinus under ascending aortic angiography. Rapid right ventricular pacing should be performed to reduce left ventricular pressure below 60 mmHg (1 mmHg=0.133 kPa), and the balloon is to be inflated for implantation of the prosthetic valve.

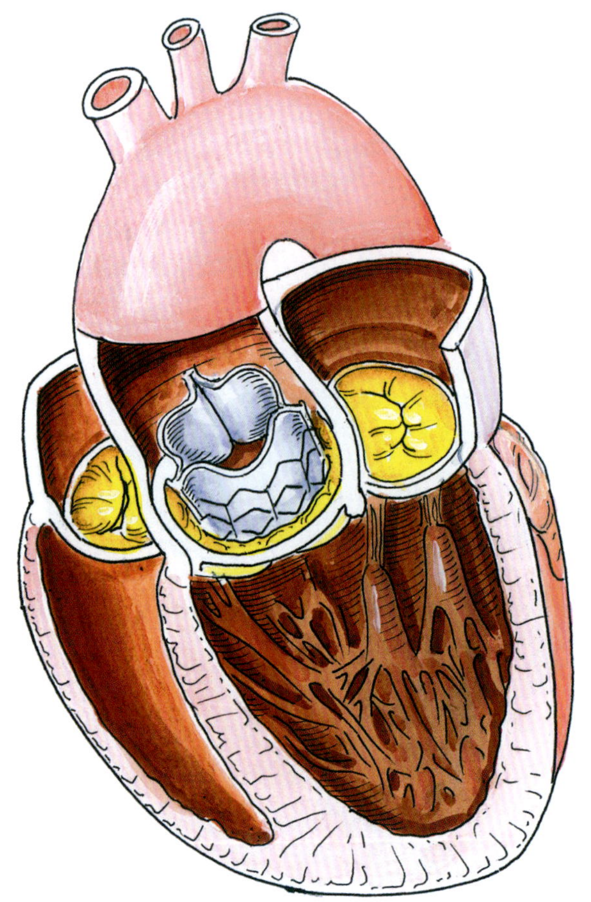

F. 球囊排气、停止起搏并撤出球囊，人工主动脉瓣植入完成。

F. The balloon is deflated, with pacing stopped and the balloon withdrawn, and the implantation of the prosthetic aortic valve is completed.

第 三 节　三尖瓣手术

Section 3　Surgery for Tricuspid Valve Disease

图 3-3-1　两孔技术三尖瓣修复术

Figure 3-3-1　Repair for tricuspid valve with double-orifice technique

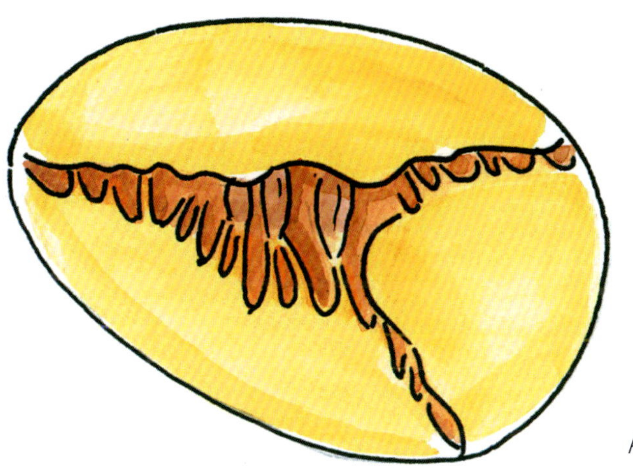

A

A. 三尖瓣关闭不全，见三尖瓣口反流。

A. Tricuspid insufficiency is featured by tricuspid regurgitation.

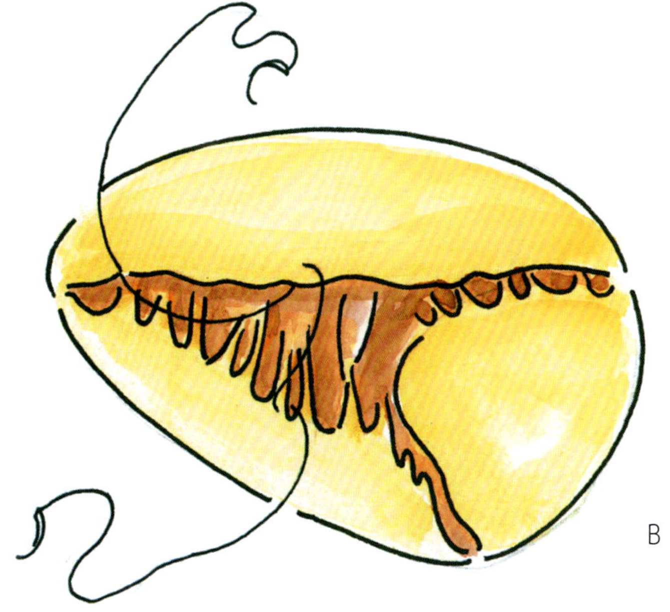

B

B. 将三尖瓣前瓣叶和隔瓣叶对应处缝合。

B. Sew the corresponding sites of the anterior and septal leaflets of the tricuspid valve.

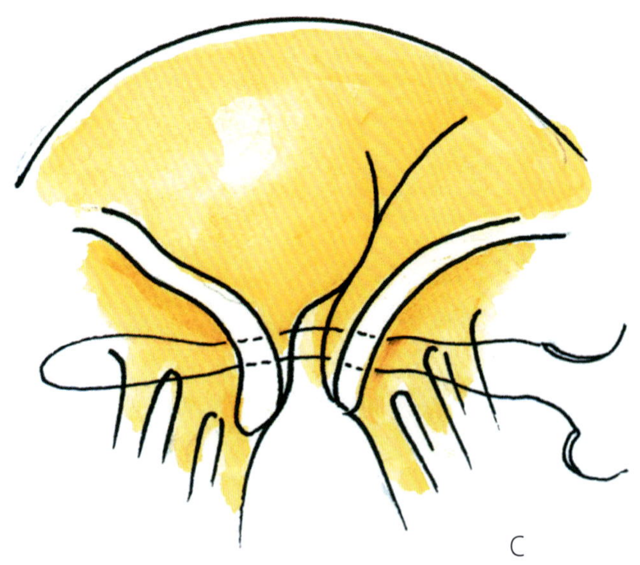

C. 缝合使两瓣叶的心房面对合。

C. During the suture, ensure the atrial surfaces of the anterior and septal leaflets are coapted.

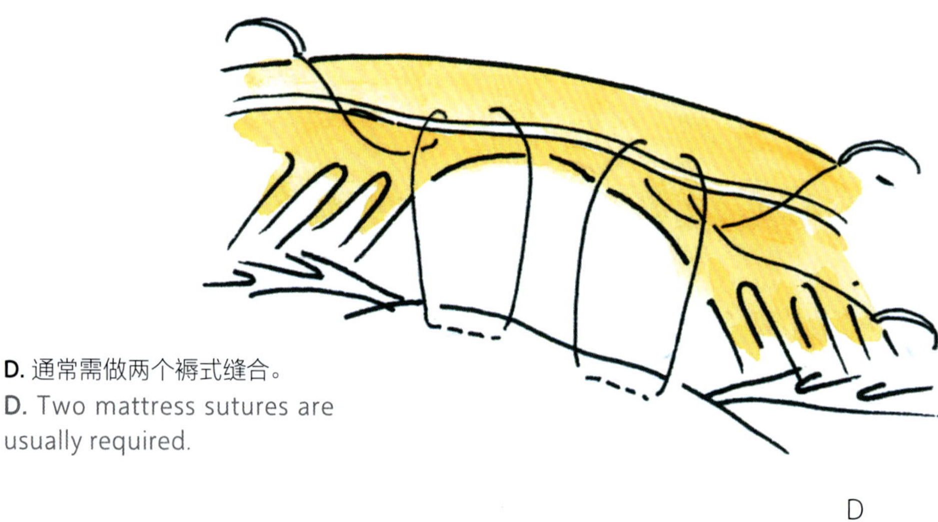

D. 通常需做两个褥式缝合。

D. Two mattress sutures are usually required.

E. 缝线安置完毕后分别结扎。

E. Sutures are placed and tied separately.

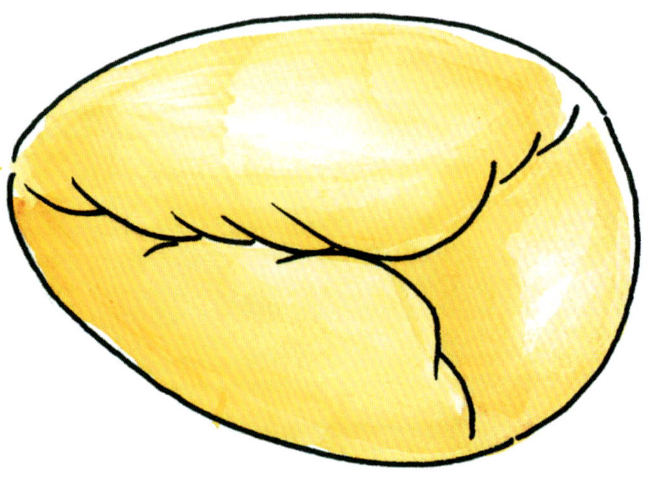

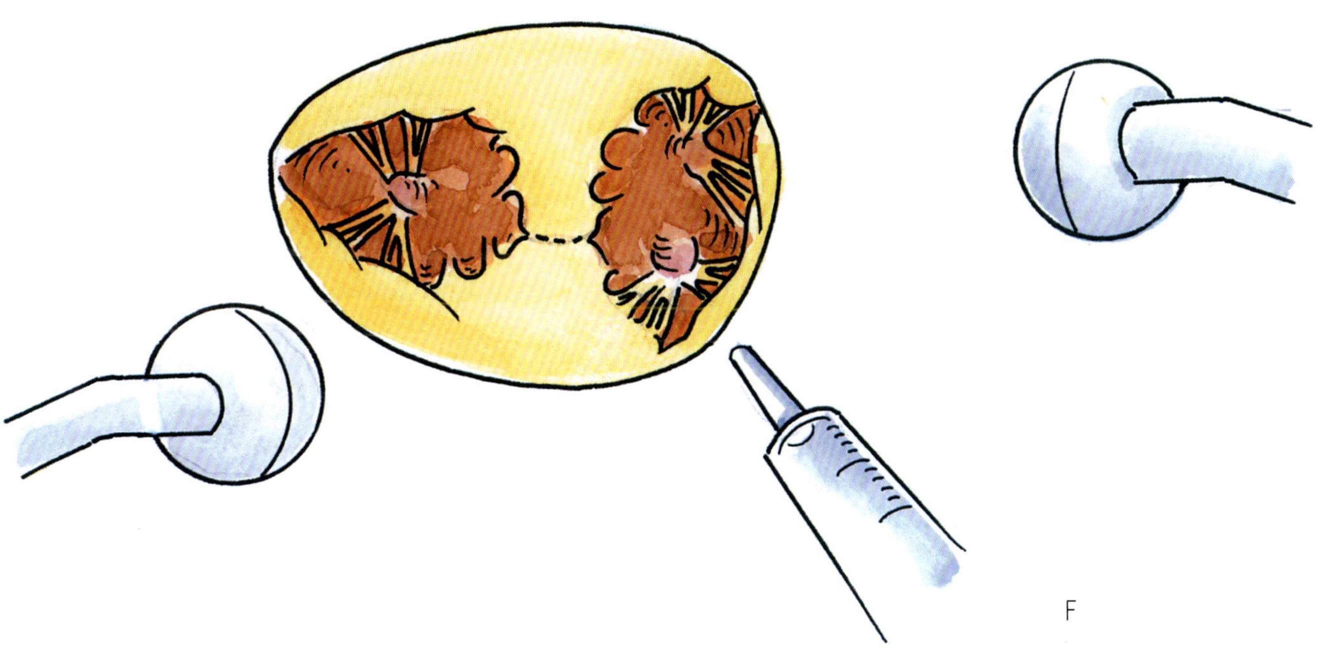

F. 三尖瓣形成两个开口，检查确认无关闭不全和狭窄。

F. With the formation of two tricuspid orifices, the absence of incomplete closure and stenosis is verified.

图 3-3-2　三尖瓣瓣环成形术（Hetzer-De Vega 法）

Figure 3-3-2　Tricuspid annuloplasty (Hetzer-De Vega procedure)

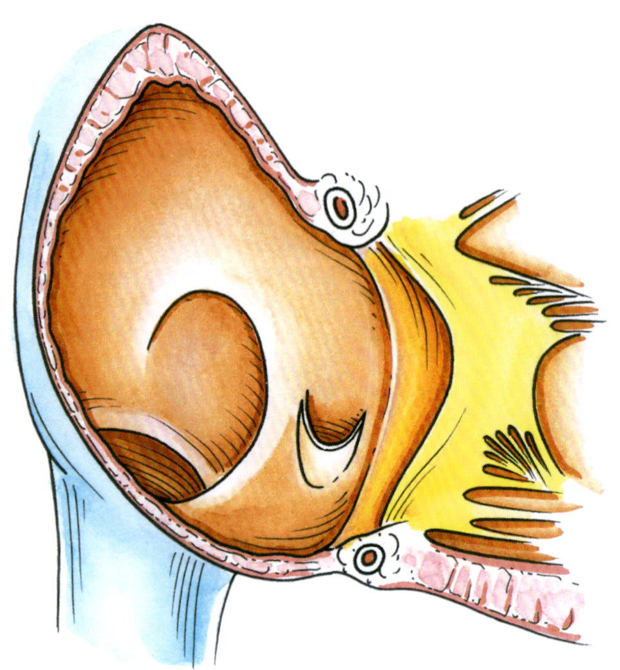

A. 三尖瓣位于右心房和右心室之间。三尖瓣隔瓣与冠状静脉窦口相邻。

A. The tricuspid valve is located between the right atrium and the right ventricle, and the tricuspid septal valve is next to the orifice of the coronary sinus.

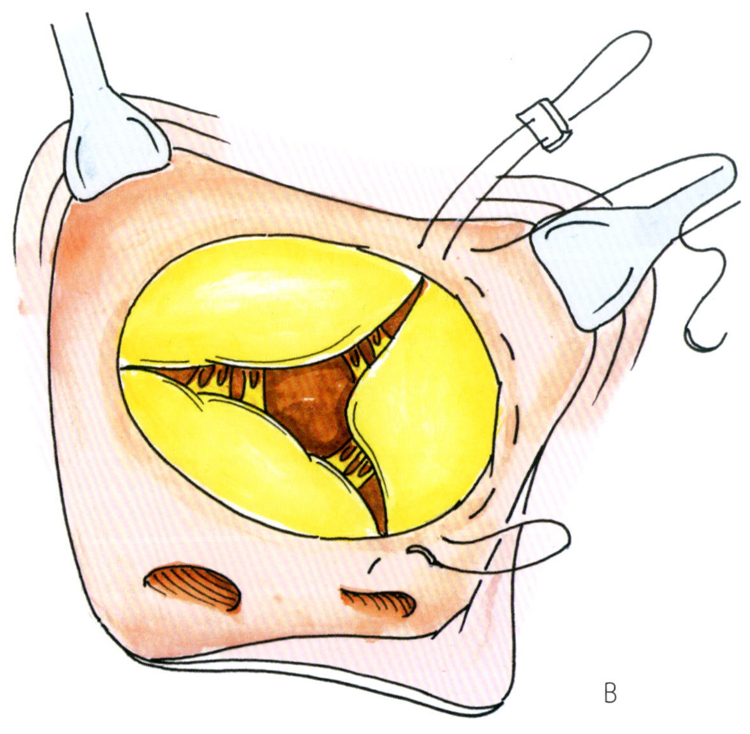

B. 三尖瓣环扩大，导致三尖瓣关闭不全。首先缩缝三尖瓣后瓣环。用带垫片双头缝针的一头沿三尖瓣后瓣环水平褥式缝合，两端超过瓣膜交界。

B. Tricuspid annular dilatation leads to tricuspid insufficiency. The suture is to be started at the posterior tricuspid annulus using the double-armed, horizontal mattress sutures with pledgets. One arm is sewn along the posterior tricuspid annulus with both ends beyond the valve commissure.

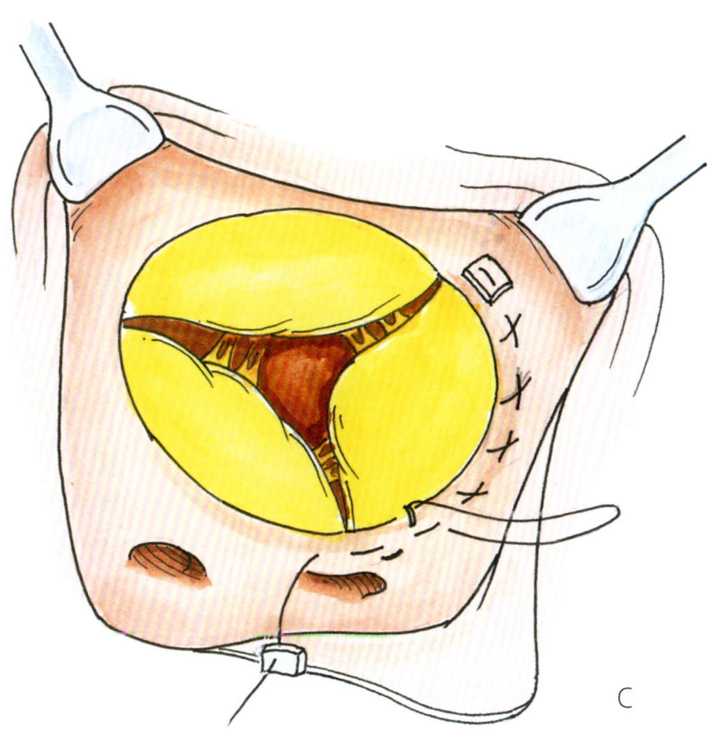

C. 再将双头缝针的另一头沿三尖瓣后瓣环与第一针的缝线交叉缝合。
C. The cross stitch is made by the other arm to the first suture line along the posterior tricuspid annulus.

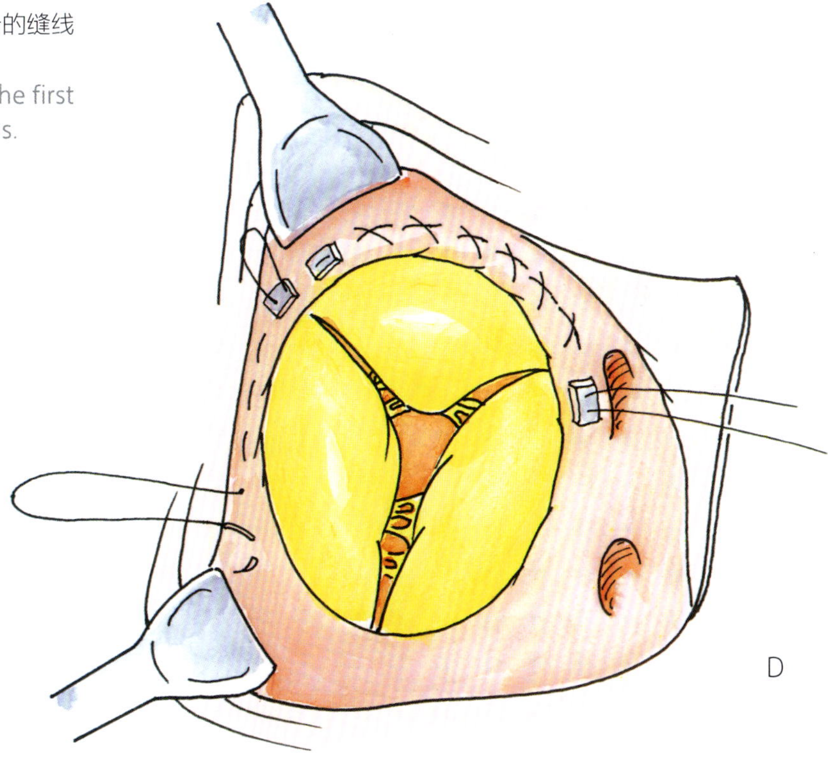

D. 另取一带垫片双头缝针沿三尖瓣前瓣环用同样方法缝合。
D. Another double-armed suture is used to suture the anterior tricuspid annulus in the same way.

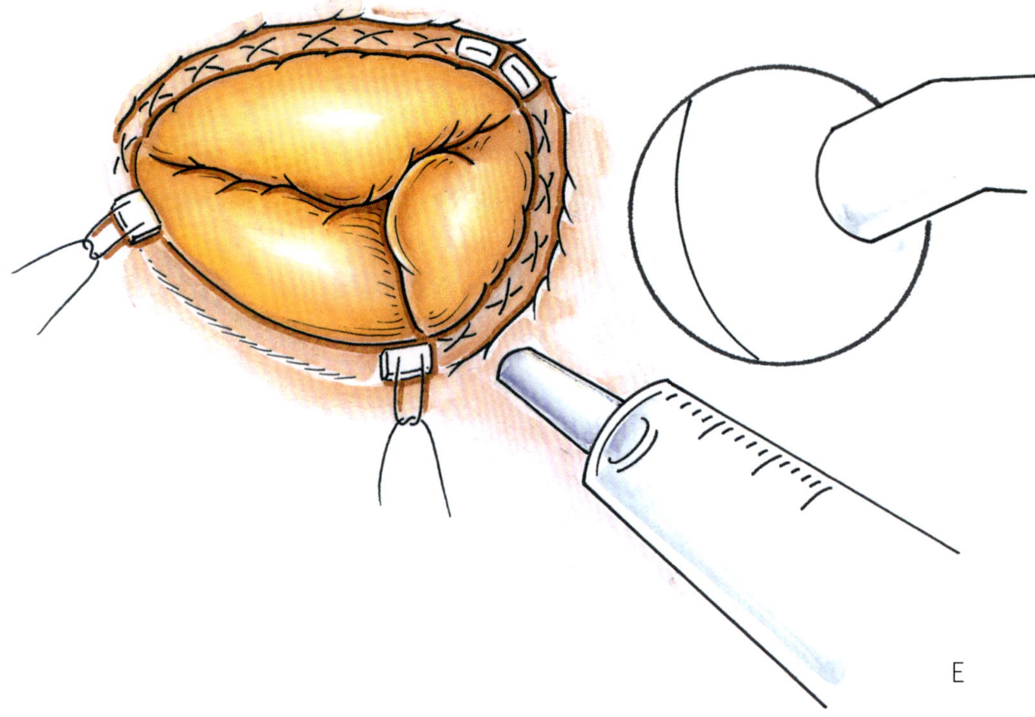

E. 逐渐分别收紧两缝线直至三尖瓣反流消失，予以结扎。检查三尖瓣确认无狭窄和关闭不全。

E. Tighten the sutures progressively until the disappearance of tricuspid regurgitation. Ligate the sutures. An examination is performed to verify there is no tricuspid valve stenosis or insufficiency.

图 3-3-3 三尖瓣后瓣环折叠缝合术（二瓣化）

Figure 3-3-3 Obliteration of posterior tricuspid annulus (bicuspidization)

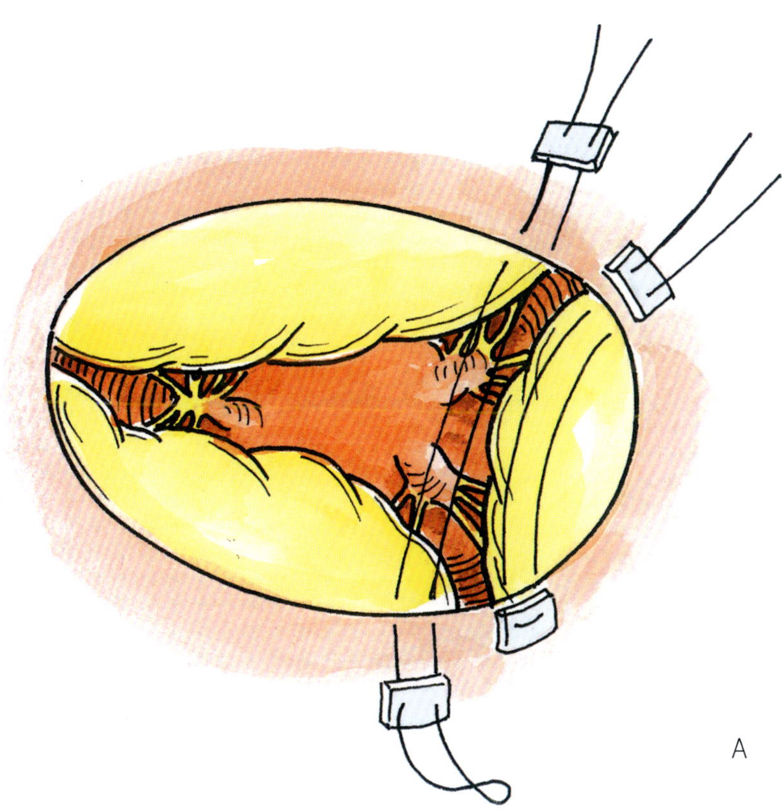

A. 首先在三尖瓣后瓣环两端瓣膜交界处做带垫片褥式缝合，首针要超过两交界，缝到三尖瓣前瓣环和隔瓣环。然后继续依次褥式缝合后瓣环。

A. A pledgeted mattress suture is first performed at the valve commissures at both ends of the posterior tricuspid annulus, with the first needle across the commissures and to the anterior annulus and septal annulus of the tricuspid valve. The posterior annulus is sutured in order.

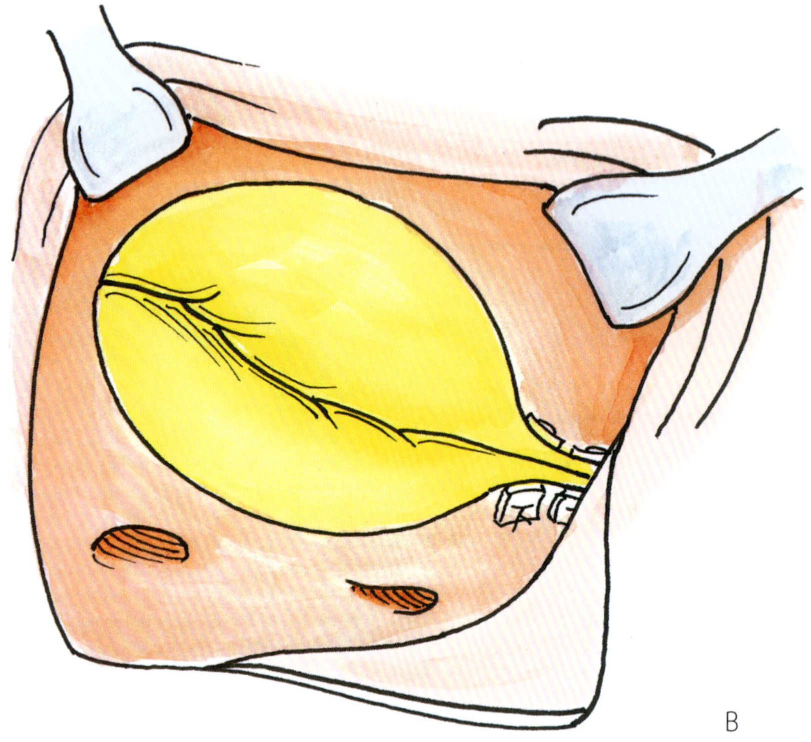

B. 将后瓣环全部缝上褥式缝合线，直至右心房亦缝置 1~2 针。结扎缝线，后瓣环折叠后三尖瓣呈二瓣状。

B. The posterior annulus is all sutured with mattress sutures, and the right atrium also needs 1-2 stitches. The suture is tied, and the posterior annulus is plicated to leave the tricuspid valve in a bicuspid shape.

图 3-3-4　直视三尖瓣狭窄交界分离术
Figure 3-3-4　Open commissurotomy for tricuspid stenosis

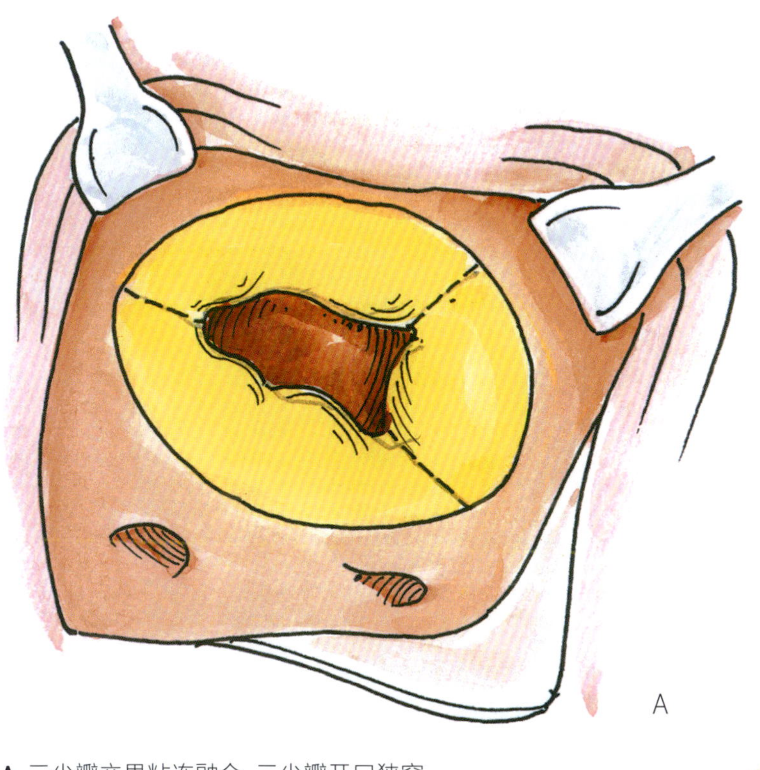

A. 三尖瓣交界粘连融合，三尖瓣开口狭窄。
A. Commissural fusion of tricuspid junction with tricuspid stenosis.

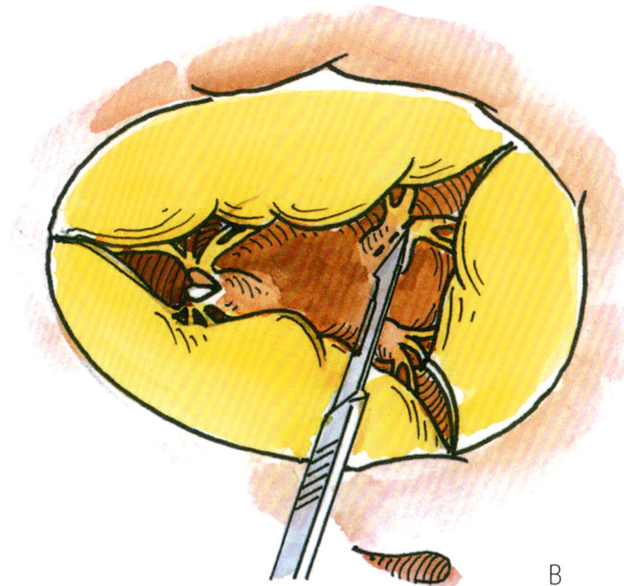

B. 循三个交界切开三尖瓣瓣叶的融合直至三尖瓣环，纵行劈开乳头肌松解三尖瓣腱索。
B. Dissect the commissural fusion along the tricuspid junction to the tricuspid annulus and longitudinally incise the papillary muscle to release the tricuspid chordae.

图 3-3-5　心内膜炎三尖瓣修补术
Figure 3-3-5　Tricuspid valve repair for endocarditis

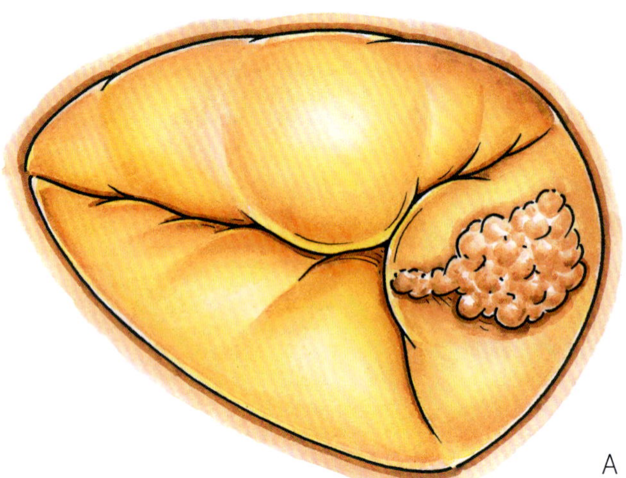

A. 心内膜炎三尖瓣后叶赘生物附着。

A. Vegetations attached to the posterior tricuspid leaflet in endocarditis.

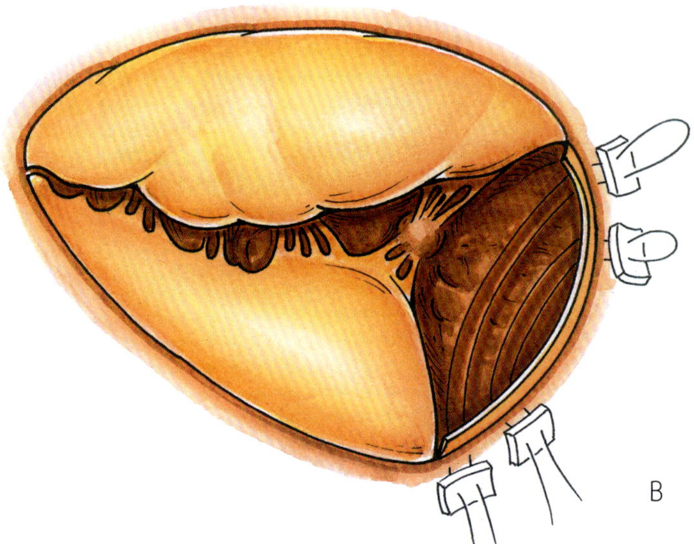

B. 完整切除三尖瓣后叶及其腱索，用带垫片褥式缝合将三尖瓣后瓣环予以折叠缝合，消除后瓣环。

B. The posterior leaflet of the tricuspid valve and its chordae tendineae are completely removed. The posterior tricuspid annulus is plicated and sutured with pledgeted mattress sutures, with the posterior annulus eliminated.

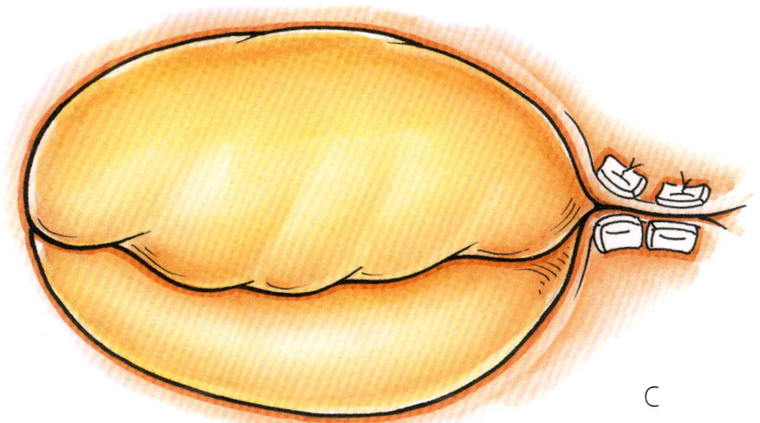

C. 结扎缝线，三尖瓣二瓣化。

C. Tie the sutures ，result in the bicuspidization of the tricuspid valve.

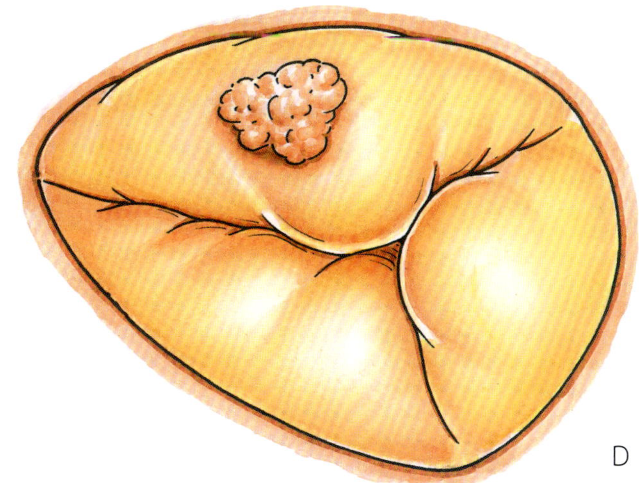

D. 心内膜炎三尖瓣前瓣叶赘生物附着。

D. Vegetations attached to the anterior leaflet of the tricuspid valve in endocarditis.

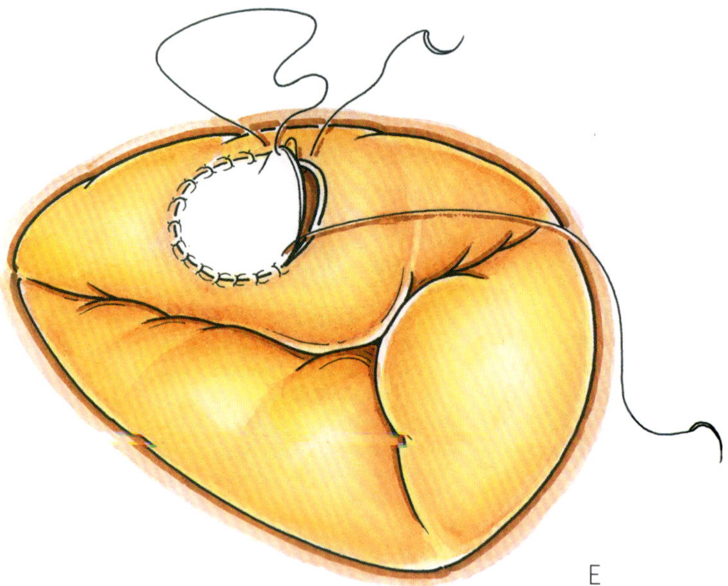

E. 切除三尖瓣前瓣叶赘生物附着处局部瓣叶，缺损用心包补片修补。

E. The anterior leaflet of the tricuspid valve is resected, and the defect is repaired with a pericardial patch.

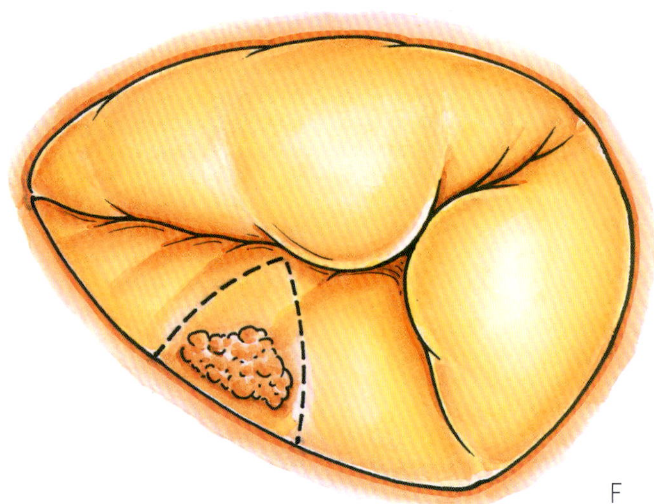

F. 心内膜炎三尖瓣隔瓣叶赘生物附着。

F. Vegetations attached to the septal leaflet of the tricuspid valve in endocarditis.

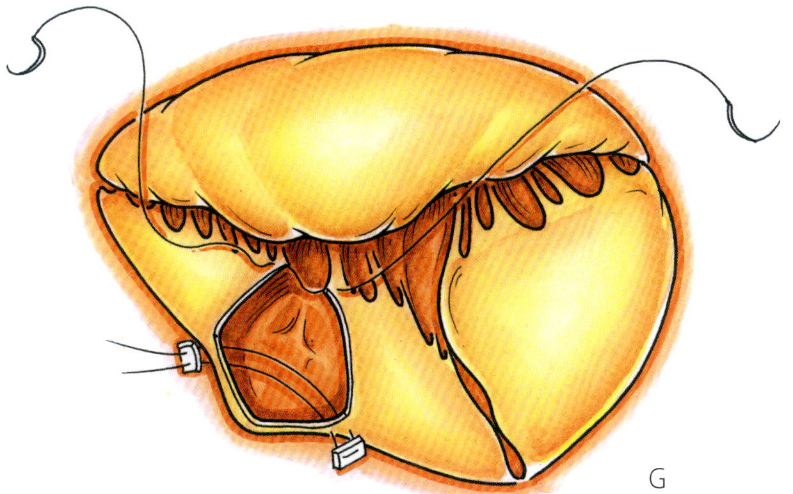

G. 楔形切除三尖瓣隔瓣叶赘生物附着处瓣叶，用带垫片褥式缝合将三尖瓣隔瓣环缺损处予以折叠缝合。

G. Wedge resection is performed to excise the septal leaflet of the tricuspid valve to which vegetations are attached, and the tricuspid septal annulus is plicated and sutured with pledgeted mattress sutures.

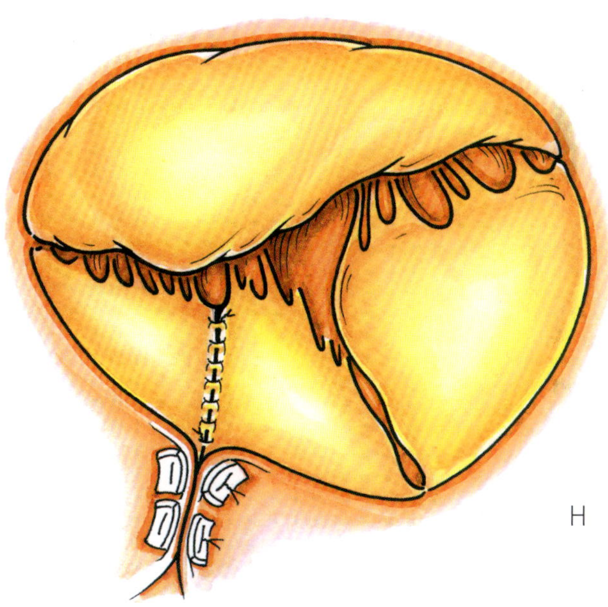

H. 间断缝合三尖瓣隔瓣叶。

H. Close the septal leaflet of the tricuspid valve with interrupted sutures.

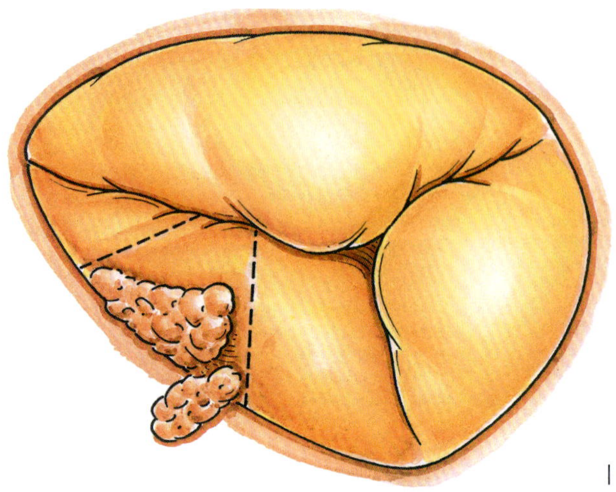

I. 心内膜炎三尖瓣隔瓣叶及其瓣环赘生物附着。

I. Vegetations attached to the septal leaflet of the tricuspid valve and its annulus in endocarditis.

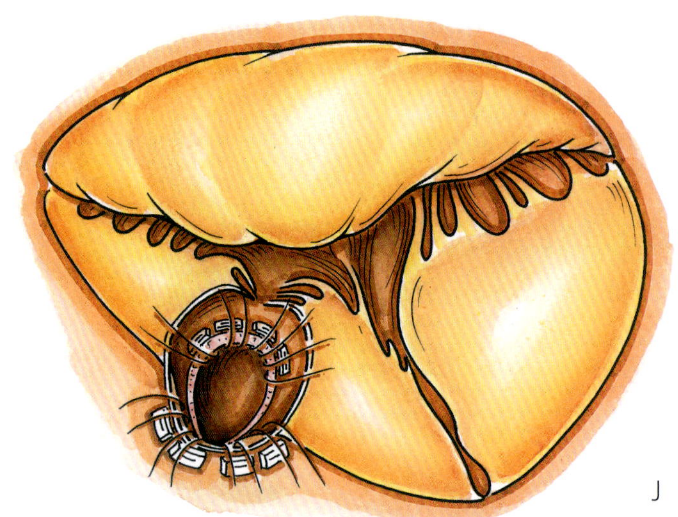

J. 切除三尖瓣隔瓣叶和及其瓣环赘生物，隔瓣下形成一室间隔缺损。沿室间隔缺损边缘用带垫片褥式缝合一周，隔瓣侧缝在隔瓣环上，其垫片留在右心房。

J. Vegetations on the septal leaflet of the tricuspid valve and its annulus are resected, and a ventricular septal defect is formed below the valve. The ventricular septal defect is sewn along its edge with pledgeted mattress sutures, and the side of the septal valve is sewn laterally to its annulus with the pledget left in the right atrium.

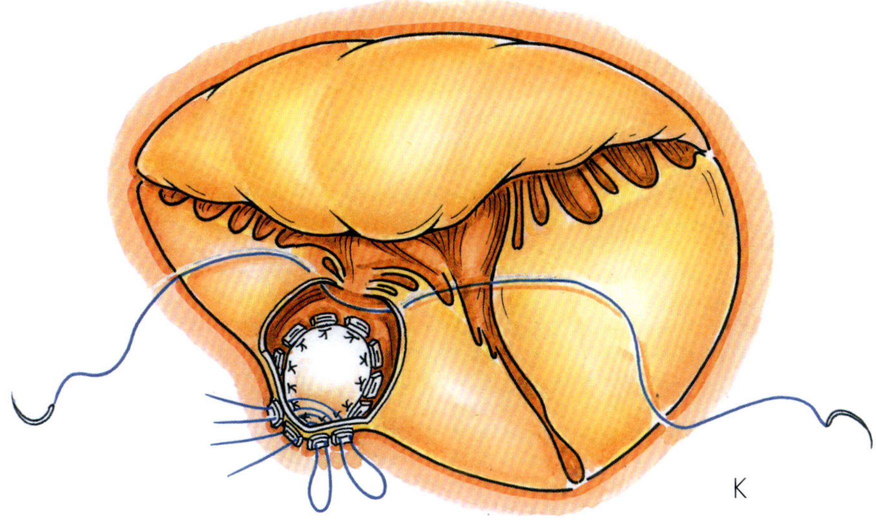

K. 修补室间隔缺损的补片推下后结扎。用带垫片褥式缝合将三尖瓣隔瓣环缺损处予以折叠缝合。间断缝合三尖瓣隔瓣叶。

K. A patch is pushed down to ventricular septal defects and ligated. The defect of the tricuspid septal annulus is plicated and sutured with a pledgeted mattress suture. Close the septal leaflet of the tricuspid valve with interrupted sutures.

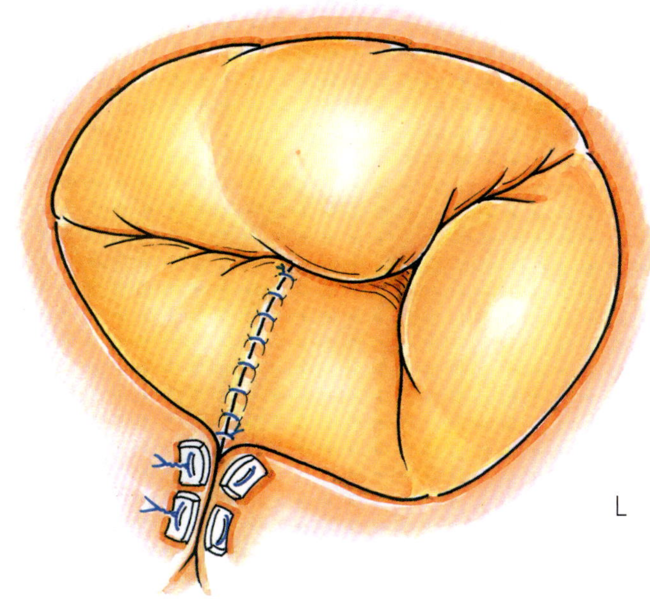

L. 三尖瓣修复完成。

L. Tricuspid valve repair is completed.

图 3-3-6　保留瓣下结构的三尖瓣置换术

Figure 3-3-6　Tricuspid valve replacement with subvalvular structure preserved

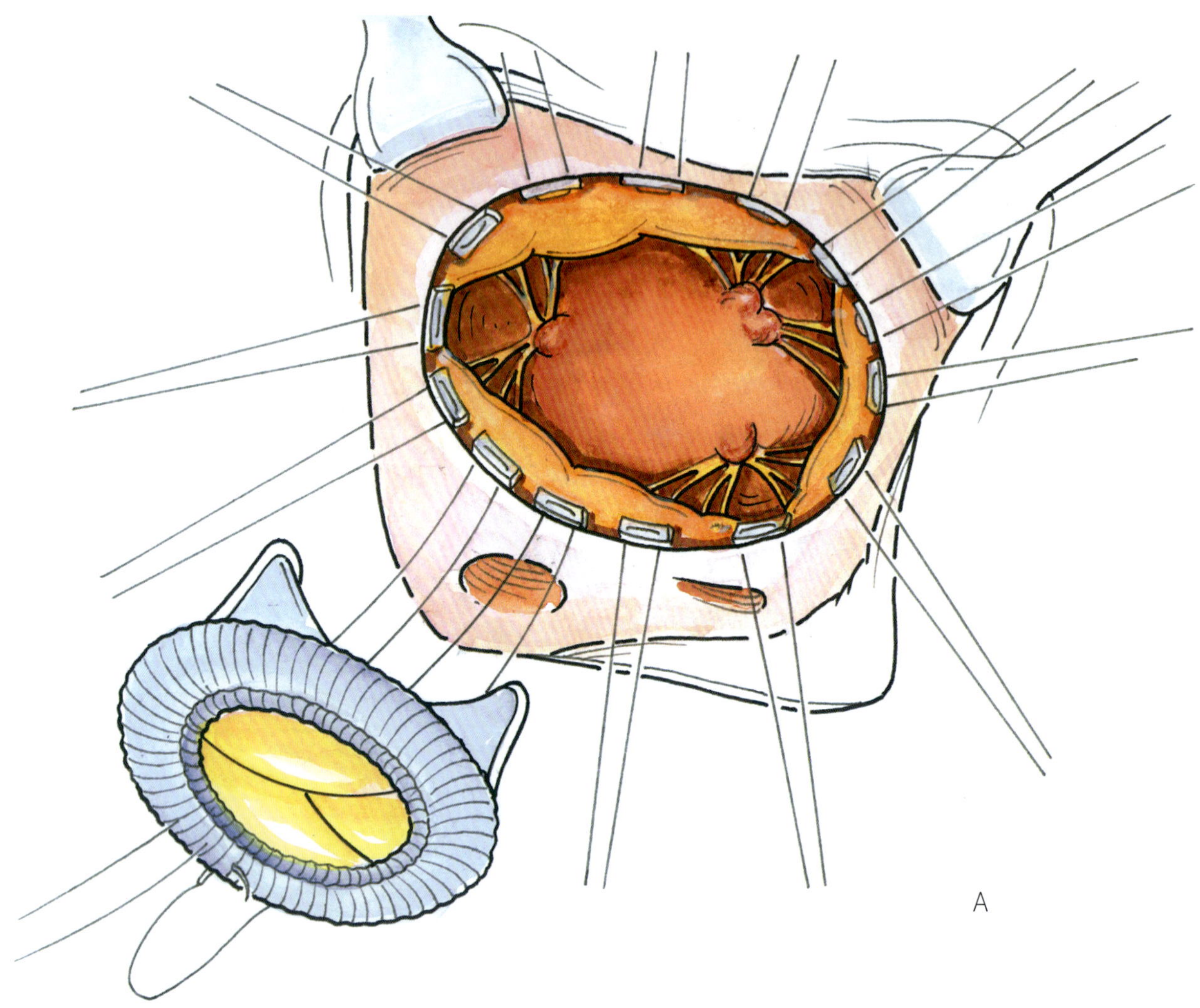

A. 三尖瓣瓣叶和瓣下结构不切除全部保留，带垫片双头瓣膜缝线由三尖瓣瓣叶进针，穿过三尖瓣环后由右心房出针，再缝到人工生物瓣缝合环。

A. The tricuspid valve leaflet and subvalvular structure are preserved, and the double-armed pledgeted suture is introduced into the tricuspid valve leaflet, passed through the tricuspid annulus to the right atrium, and sewed to the bioprosthetic valve suture ring.

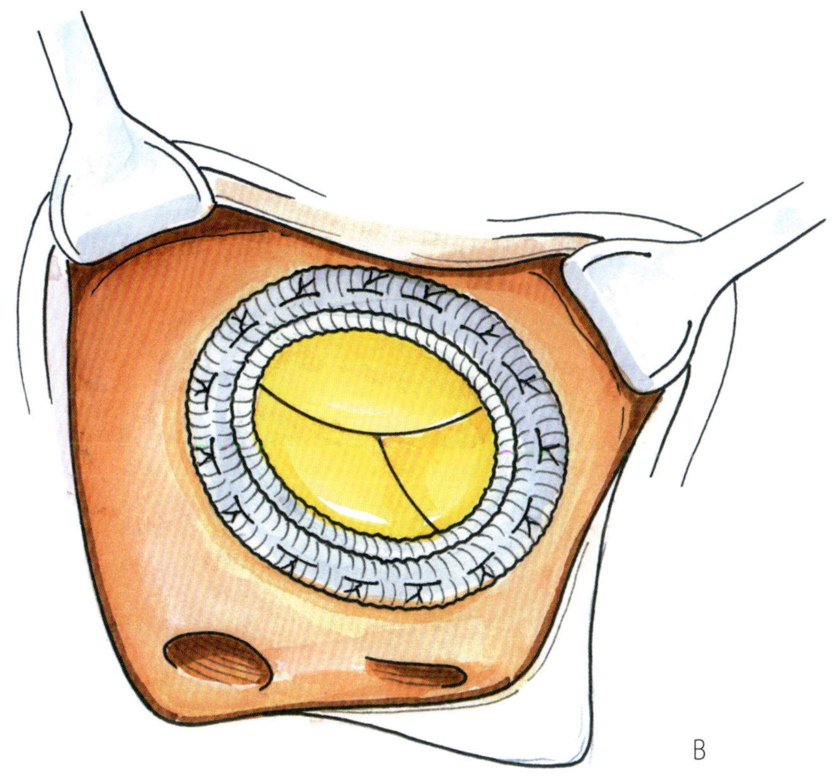

B. 人工生物瓣推下落位到三尖瓣口，逐一结扎缝线。

B. The bioprosthetic valve is pushed down to the tricuspid orifice, and the sutures are tied one by one.

第四章 主动脉疾病

Chapter 4 Aortic Disease

第一节　主动脉夹层
Section 1　Aortic Dissection

主动脉夹层是主动脉内膜破裂，在血流冲击下沿着主动脉中层剥脱，内膜与外膜分离把主动脉腔分隔成真腔和假腔而形成。

Aortic dissection is formed when there is a rupture in the tunica intima, the intima is stripped from the middle lamella under the impact of the blood flow, and the separation of the tunica intima and adventitia causes a false lumen and a true lumen.

主动脉夹层分离的范围不一，可以局限在某一段主动脉，也可能累及主动脉全长。Stanford 分型是最常用的主动脉夹层分型之一，根据夹层分离的范围将主动脉夹层分为 A、B 两型。

Classification of the aortic dissection varies. It can be confined to a segment of the aorta, or involve the full length of the aorta. The Stanford classification, one of the most used classifications, divides aortic dissections into types A and B according to the location of dissection separation.

图 4-1-1 主动脉夹层的分型

Figure 4-1-1 Classification of aortic dissection

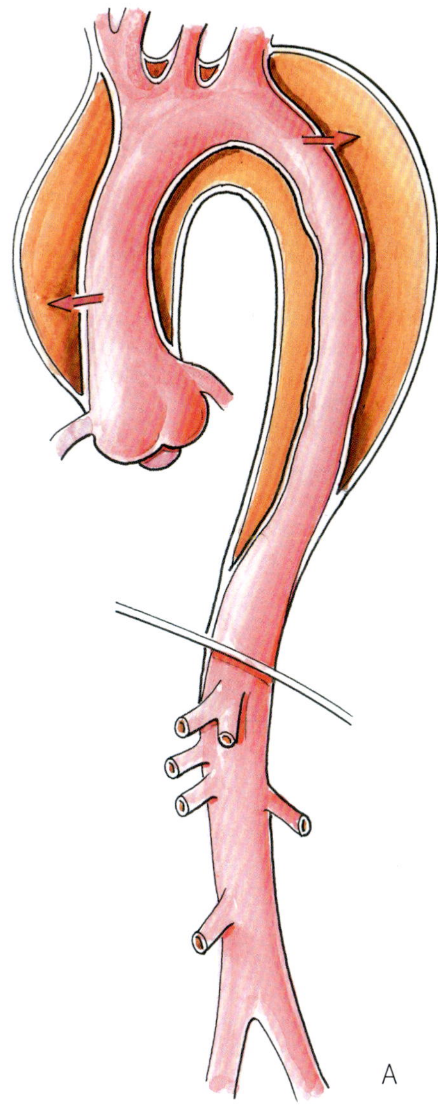

A. 凡夹层累及升主动脉，无论其远端到达哪里均为 A 型。

A. Type A: dissections involving the ascending aorta regardless of its distal end.

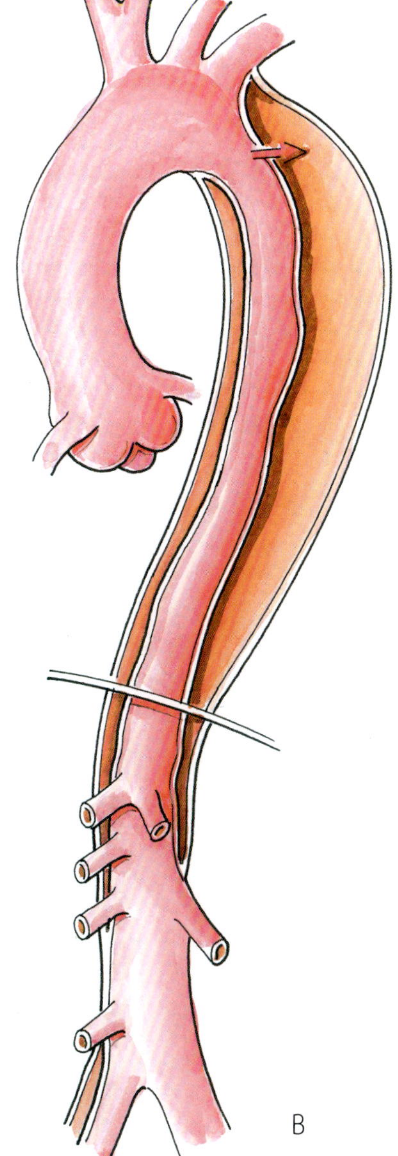

B. 夹层仅限于降主动脉为 B 型。

B. Type B: dissections confined to the descending aorta.

图 4-1-2 升主动脉人工血管置换和主动脉根部重建术
Figure 4-1-2 Ascending aorta graft replacement and aortic root reconstruction

A. 胸骨正中切口，切开心包。A 型夹层，内膜近、远端破口均位于升主动脉。右心耳插二级静脉引流管，股动脉插供血管，建立体外循环。

A. The pericardium is cut open through a median sternotomy. For the type A dissection with their proximal and distal intimal tear in the ascending aorta, a two-stage venous draining cannula is introduced in the right atrial appendage, and an arterial cannula is introduced into the femoral artery to establish extracorporeal circulation.

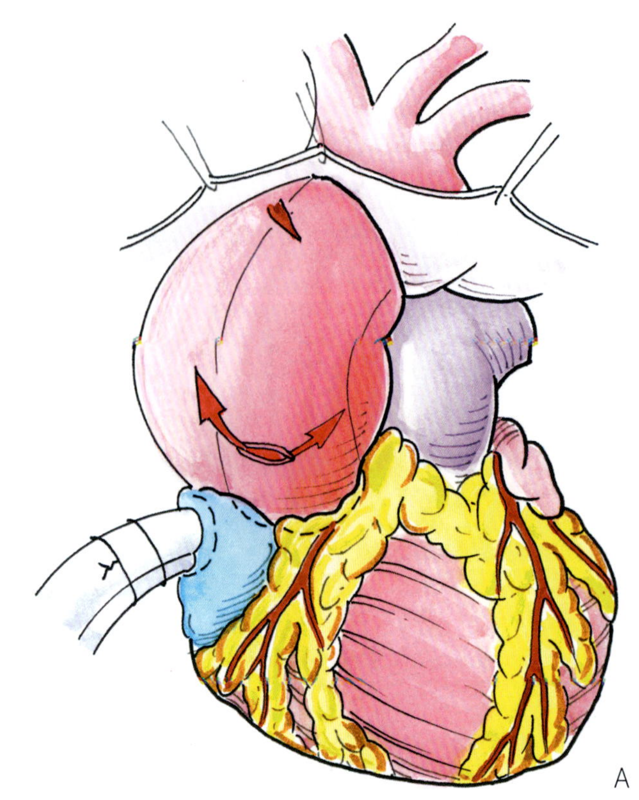

A

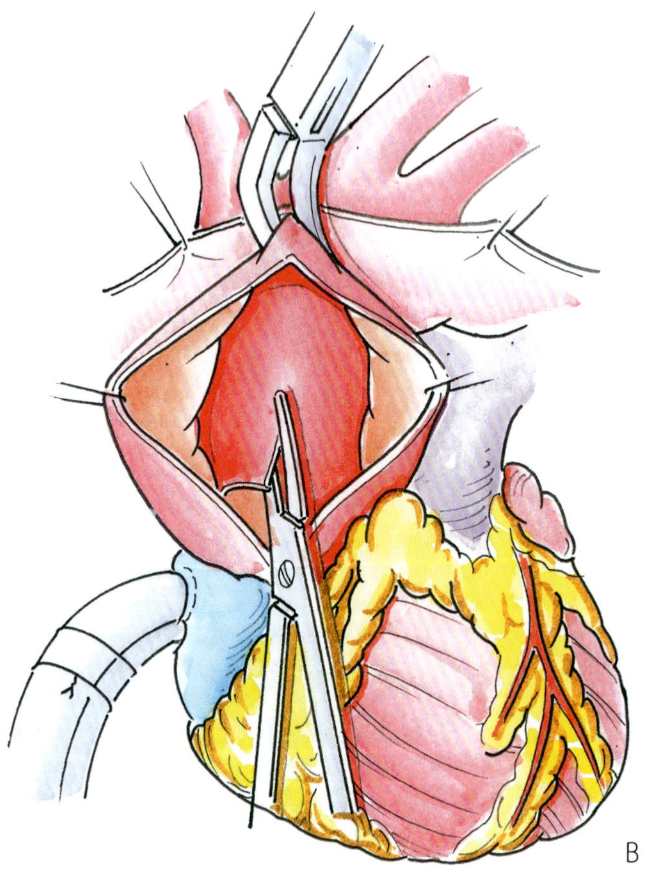

B

B. 升主动脉远端钳夹阻断主动脉，纵行切开升主动脉，清除夹层中的血栓，纵行剪开内膜。

B. With clamps placed on the distal end, the ascending aorta is incised longitudinally, the thrombus in the dissection removed, and the tunica intima cut longitudinally.

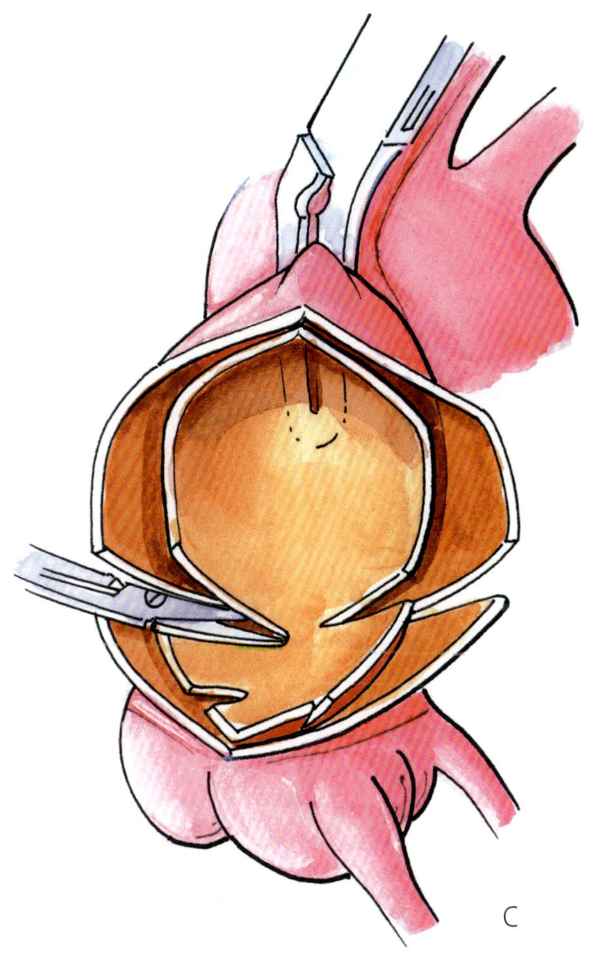

C. 于窦管交界处横行切断升主动脉。
C. The ascending aorta is transected at the sinotubular junction.

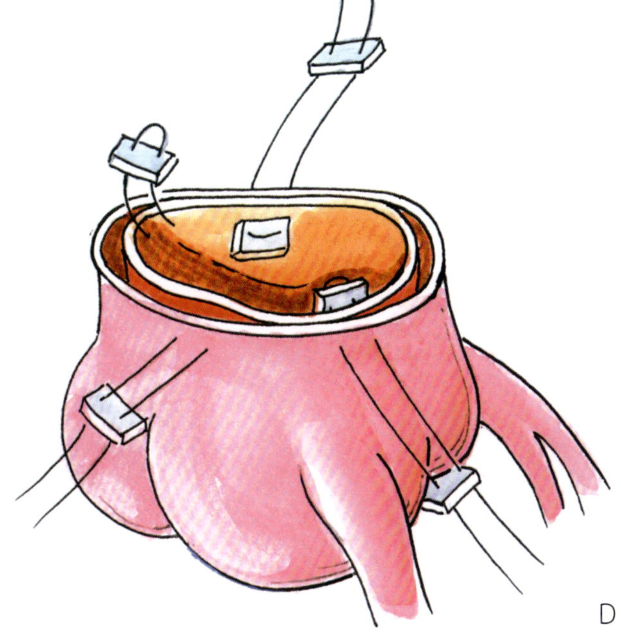

D. 主动脉窦夹层而未累及冠状动脉和主动脉瓣时，将主动脉瓣的三个交界用带垫片褥式缝合予以悬吊。
D. When the aortic sinus dissection does not involve the coronary artery and the aortic valve, the three commissures of the aortic valve are suspended with pledgeted mattress sutures.

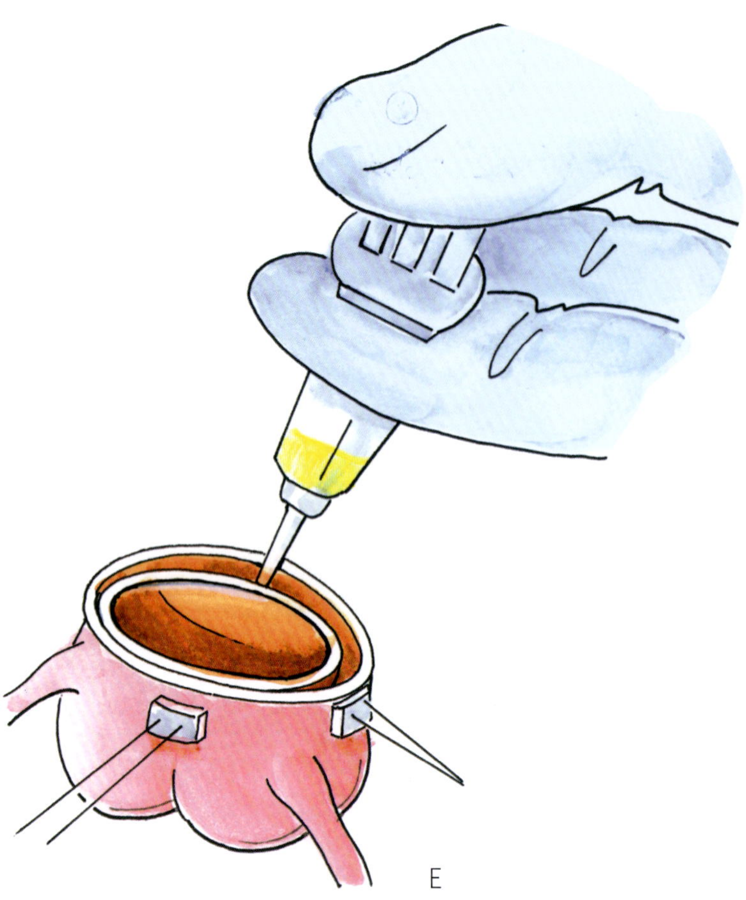

E. 继而在夹层中注入生物胶闭合夹层。

E. Then biological glue is injected into the dissection to close the rupture.

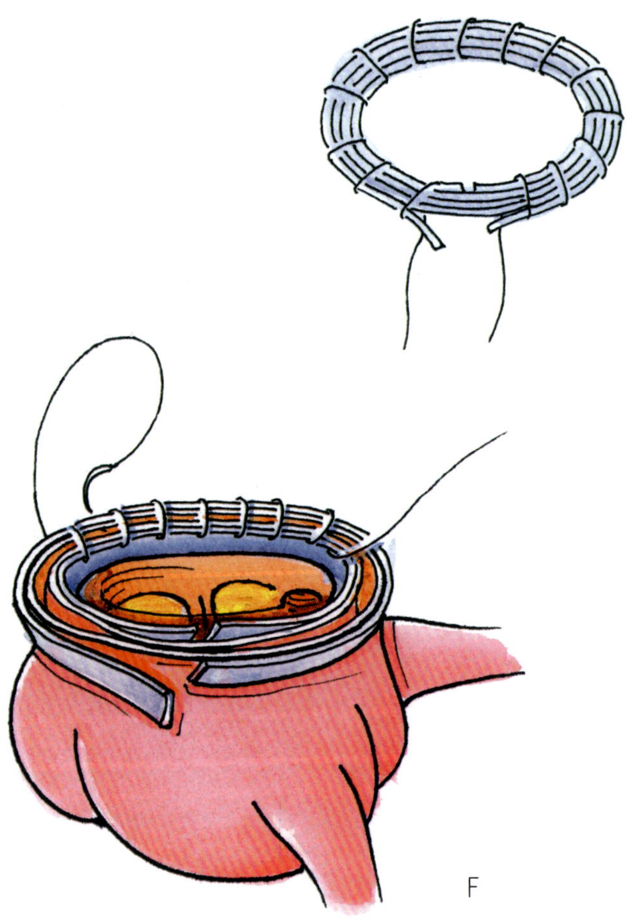

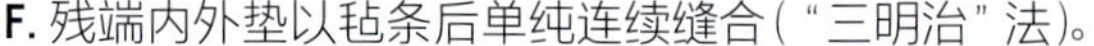

F. 残端内外垫以毡条后单纯连续缝合（“三明治”法）。

F. A felt strip is inserted into the internal and external layers of the stump and secured with simple continuous sutures (sandwich technique).

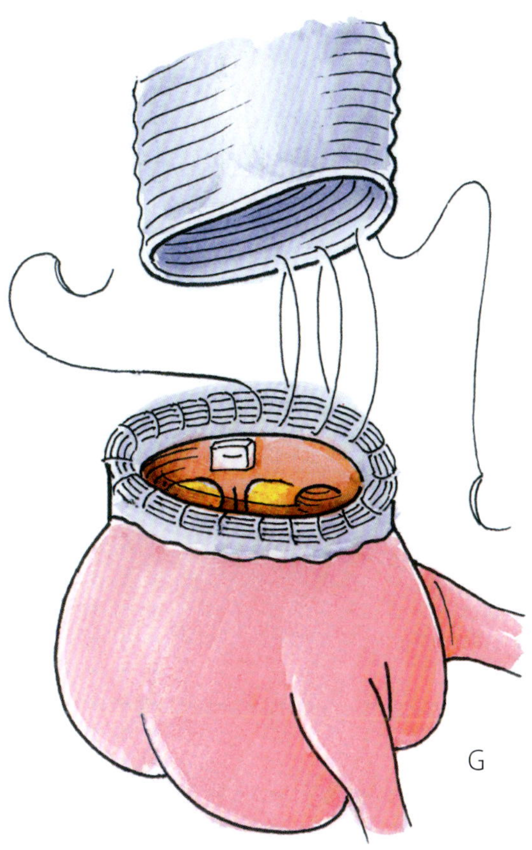

G. 用口径匹配的人工血管做近端吻合，4-0 Prolene 单纯连续缝合。

G. A proper-sized aortic graft is used. A proximal anastomosis is made with simple continuous sutures of 4-0 Prolene.

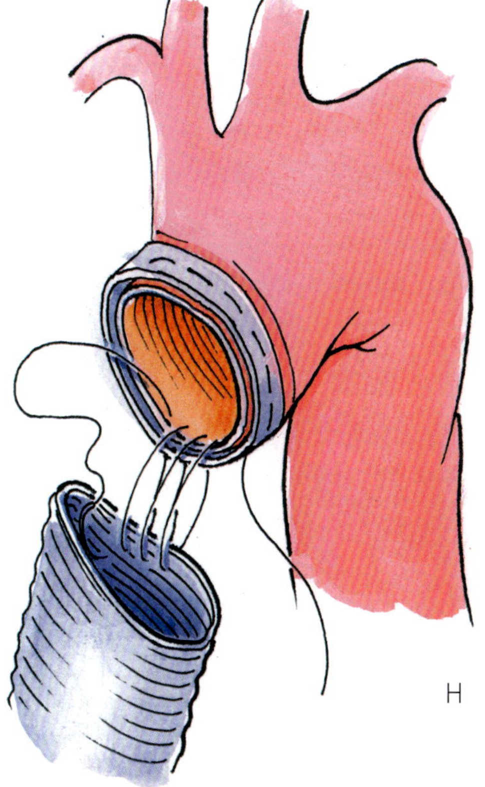

H. 横行切断升主动脉远端，断端用“三明治”法处理后与人工血管做端端吻合。

H. The distal end of the ascending aorta is transected, and the cut edge is treated with the sandwich technique and then anastomosed end-to-end to the aortic graft.

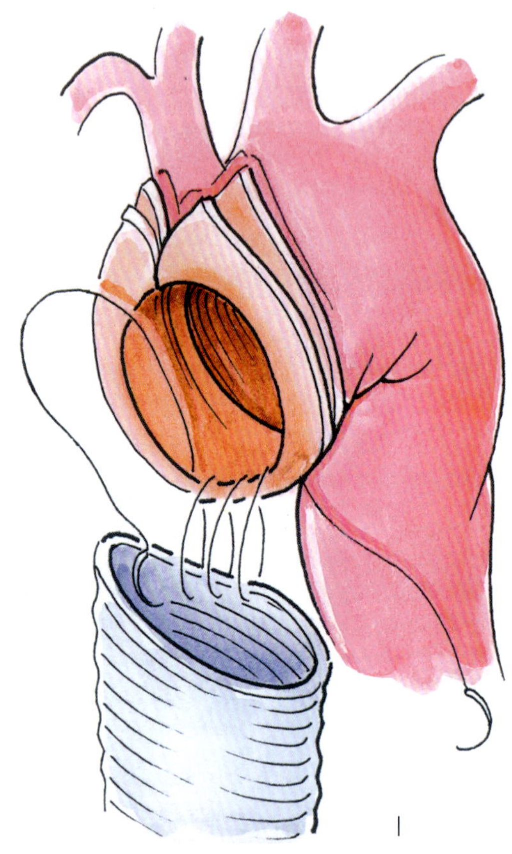

I. 若升主动脉远端仍有一定强度，亦可直接与人工血管端端吻合。

I. If the strength is feasible, the distal end of the ascending aorta can also be directly end-to-end anastomosed with the aortic graft.

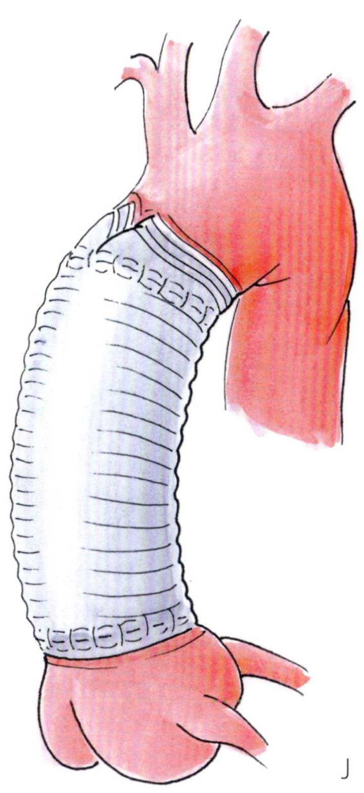

J. 升主动脉人工血管置换术完成。

J. The ascending aorta replacement with aortic graft is completed.

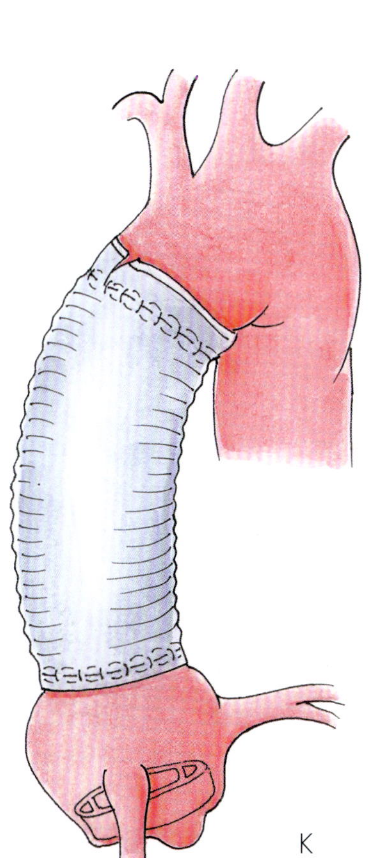

K. 累及主动脉窦的夹层可以造成主动脉瓣关闭不全，若主动脉三个交界悬吊后仍纠正不满意，须同时行主动脉瓣置换术。

K. Dissections involving the aortic sinus can cause aortic insufficiency, and if the suspension of the three aortic valve commissures still fails to reach satisfaction, aortic valve replacement must be performed at the same time.

图 4-1-3　带瓣外管道升主动脉置换术（Bentall 手术）

Figure 4-1-3　Ascending aortic graft replacement with a composite valved conduit (Bentall procedure)

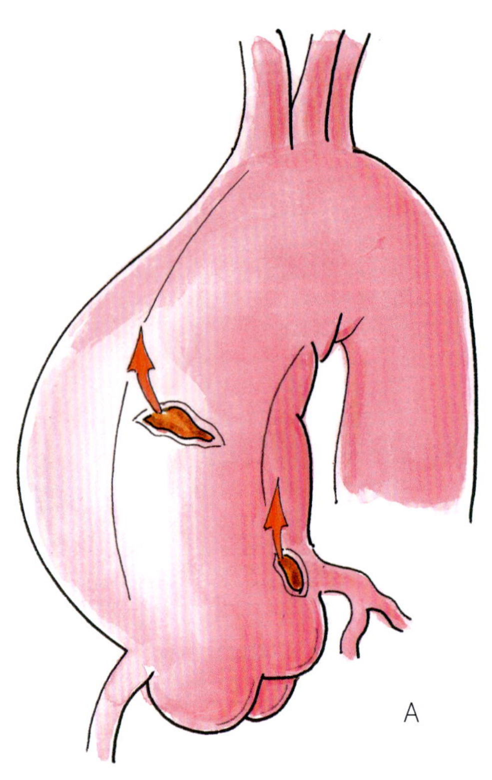

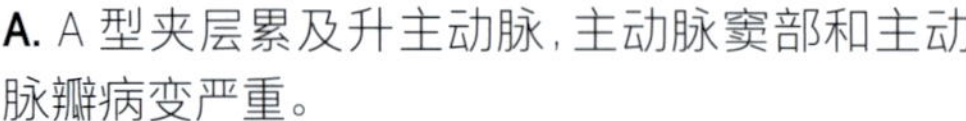

A. A 型夹层累及升主动脉，主动脉窦部和主动脉瓣病变严重。

A. Type A dissection involves the ascending aorta with severe lesions in the aortic sinus and aortic valve.

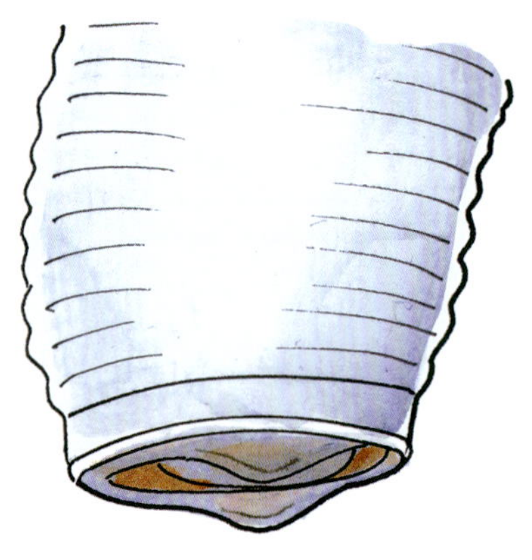

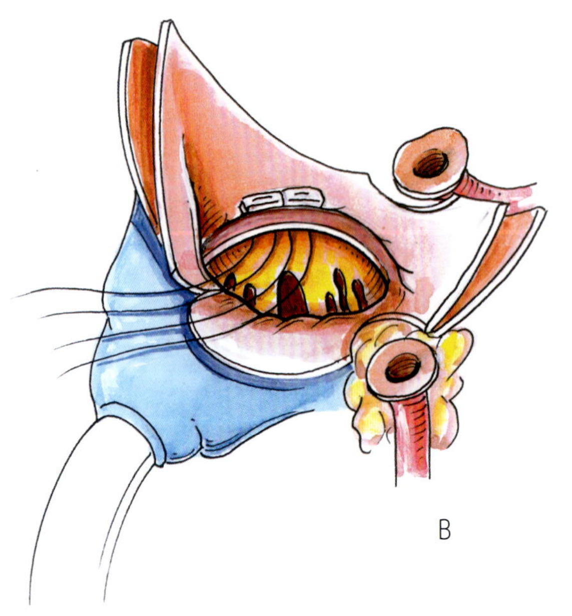

B. 建立体外循环，心脏停搏。纵行切开升主动脉，在主动脉窦内横断升主动脉。距冠状动脉开口约 5mm 将左、右冠状动脉开口连同主动脉壁做纽扣状分离。切除主动脉瓣叶。根据主动脉瓣环大小选择口径匹配的带瓣人工血管，用间断褥式缝合将其与主动脉瓣环缝合。

B. Extracorporeal circulation is established and the heart is stopped. The ascending aorta is incised longitudinally and transected within the aortic sinus. The left and right coronary artery ostia, together with the aortic wall, are cut off in a button shape at approximately 5 mm from the coronary artery ostia. The aortic leaflets are resected. Select a composite valved conduit which matches the size of the aortic annulus, and suture it to the aortic annulus with interrupted mattress sutures.

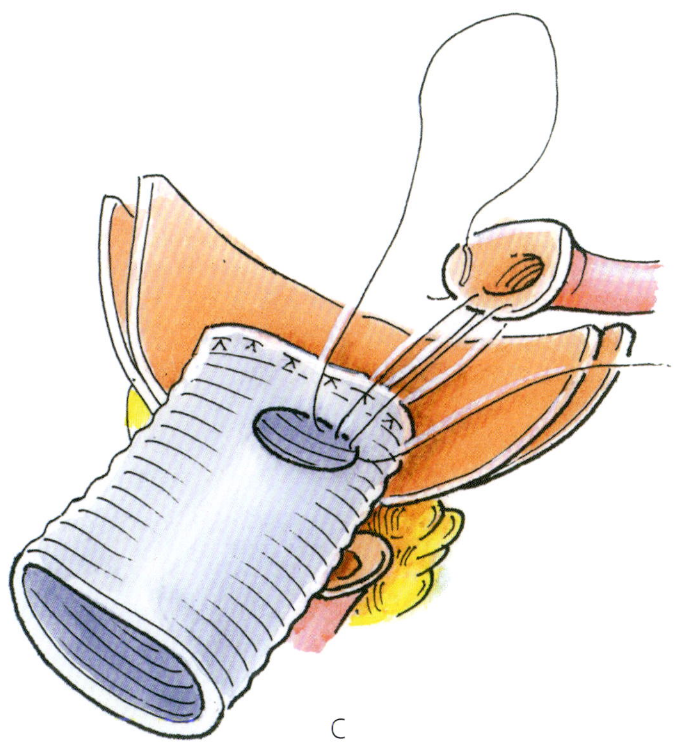

C. 带瓣人工血管缝入主动脉瓣环后，在对应左冠状动脉开口处开孔，将左冠状动脉与人工血管端侧吻合。

C. After sewing the composite valved conduit to the aortic annulus, openings are made in the corresponding to the left coronary ostia, and the left coronary artery is anastomosed end-to-side to the graft.

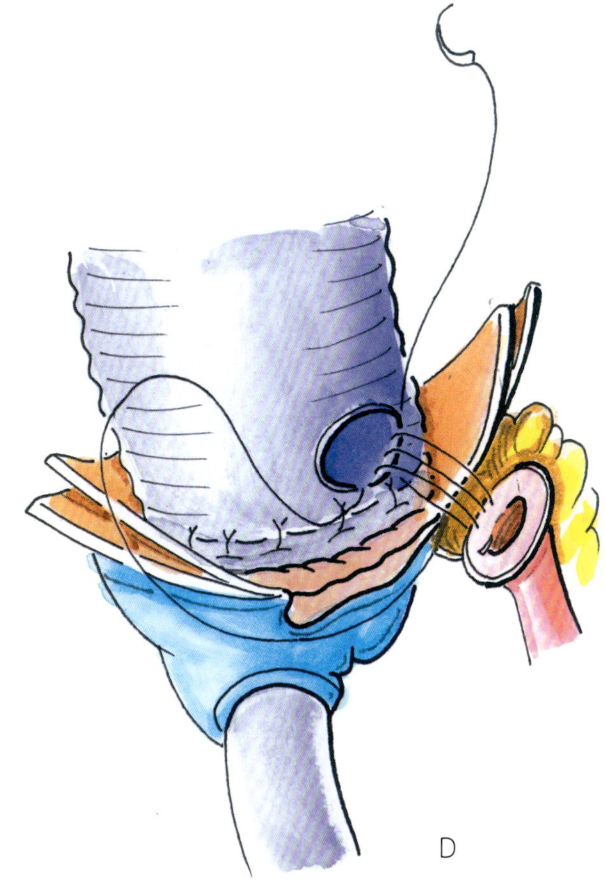

D. 带瓣人工血管对应右冠状动脉开口处开孔，将右冠状动脉与人工血管端侧吻合。

D. Openings are made in the composite valved conduit corresponding to the right coronary ostia, and the right coronary artery is anastomosed to the graft in an end-to-side fashion.

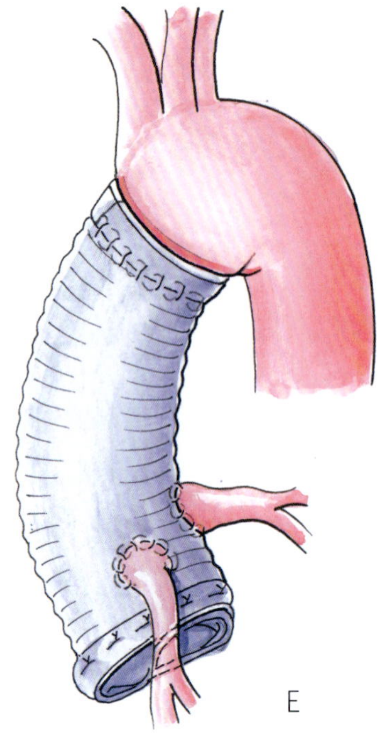

E. 升主动脉远端用“三明治”法处理后与人工血管端端吻合。

E. The distal end of the ascending aorta is treated with the sandwich technique and anastomosed end-to-end to the graft.

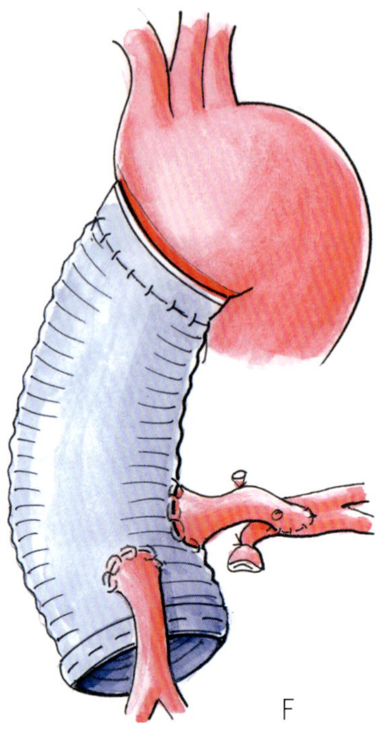

F. 若冠状动脉长度不足，为避免吻合口张力，可取一小段大隐静脉将冠状动脉与人工血管连接。

F. If the length of the coronary artery is insufficient, to avoid anastomotic tension, a small segment of the great saphenous vein is harvested to connect the coronary artery to the graft.

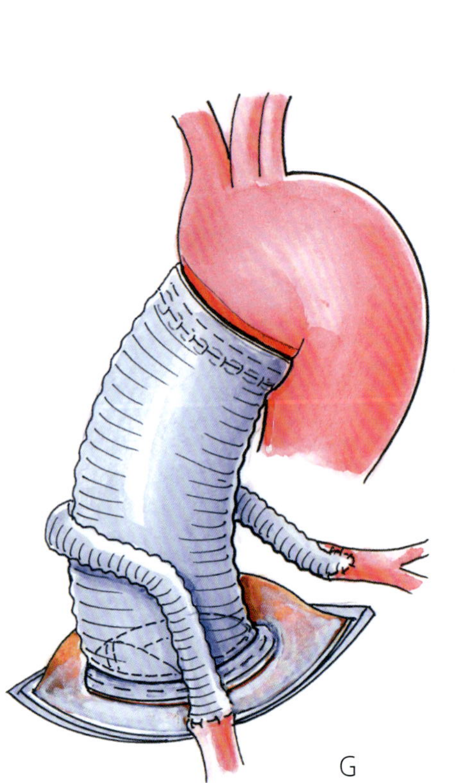

G. Cabrol 法：先将左、右冠状动脉开口分别与直径 0.8~1cm 的人工血管两端做端端吻合，然后再将该人工血管与带瓣人工血管做侧侧吻合。

G. Cabrol technique: The ostia of the left and right coronary arteries are sutured to both ends of a artificial vessel of a diameter of 0.8-1 cm in an end-to-end fashion, respectively, and then the graft is anastomosed side-to-side with the composite valved conduit.

图 4-1-4 主动脉弓顶岛状修复术
Figure 4-1-4 Repair of transverse aortic arch

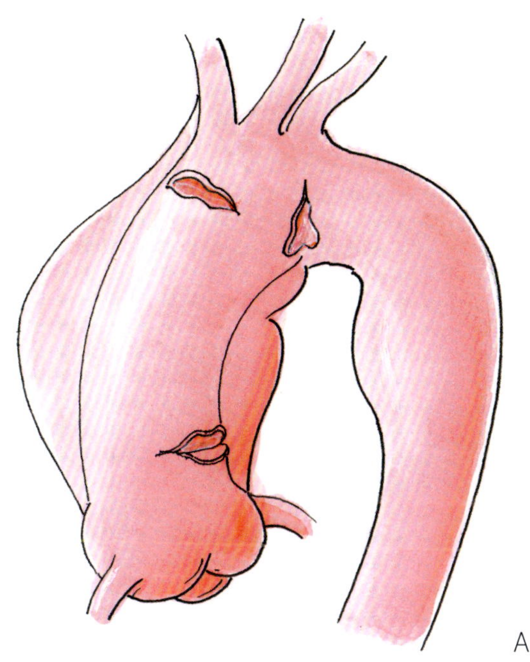

A. A 型夹层，内膜近端破口在升主动脉，远端破口在主动脉弓部。

A. Type A dissection with a proximal intimal rupture in the ascending aorta and a distal rupture in the aortic arch.

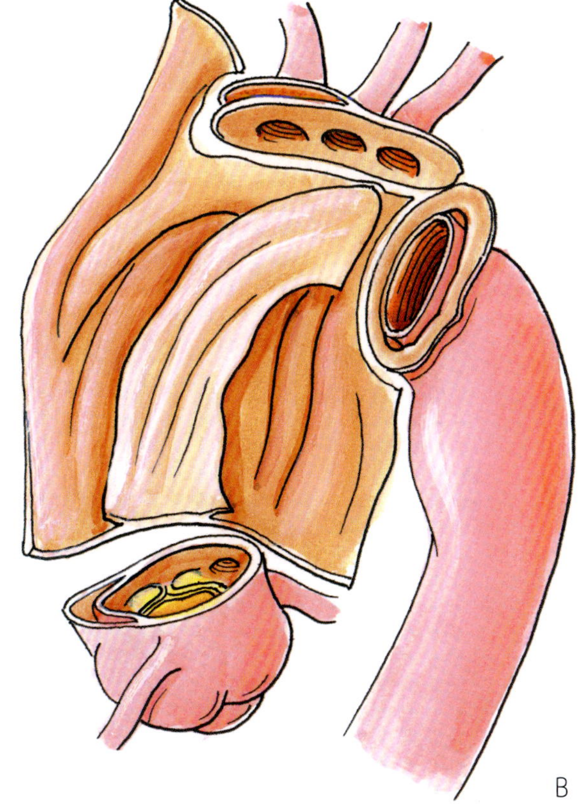

B. 深低温停循环。切开升主动脉和主动脉弓前壁。分别在窦管交界处和弓降部横断主动脉。主动脉弓顶部连同其三大分支岛状游离。

B. With deep hypothermia circulatory arrest, the anterior wall of ascending aorta and aortic arch are incised. The aorta is transected at the sinotubular junction and the descending part of aortic arch, respectively. The aortic arch roof, together with its three branches, is dissociated in an island shape.

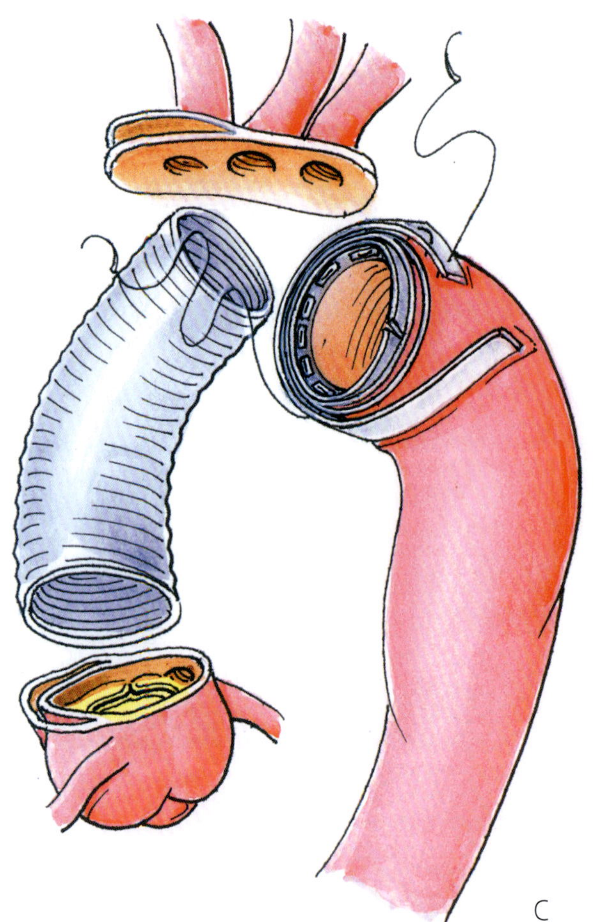

C. 主动脉弓降部断端经"三明治"法处理后，与合适口径的人工血管做端端吻合。

C. After treatment with the sandwich technique, the stump of descending aortic arch is anastomosed end-to-end to an appropriate artificial vessel.

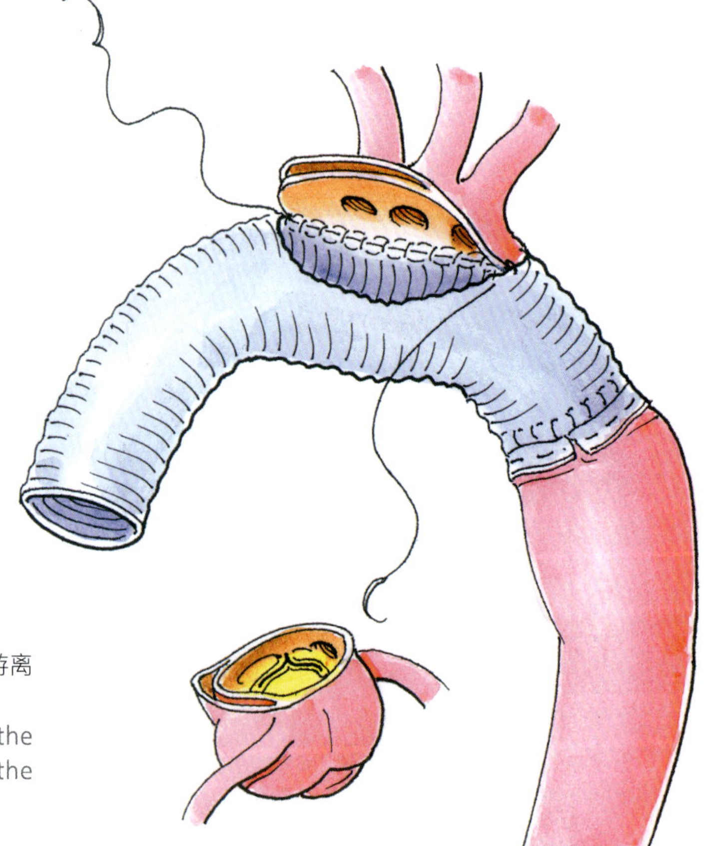

D. 人工血管上壁剪一椭圆形开口，将主动脉顶部岛状游离片与其吻合。

D. An oval opening is made on the upper wall of the artificial aortic graft, and the freed island flap of the aorta arch roof is anastomosed to the graft.

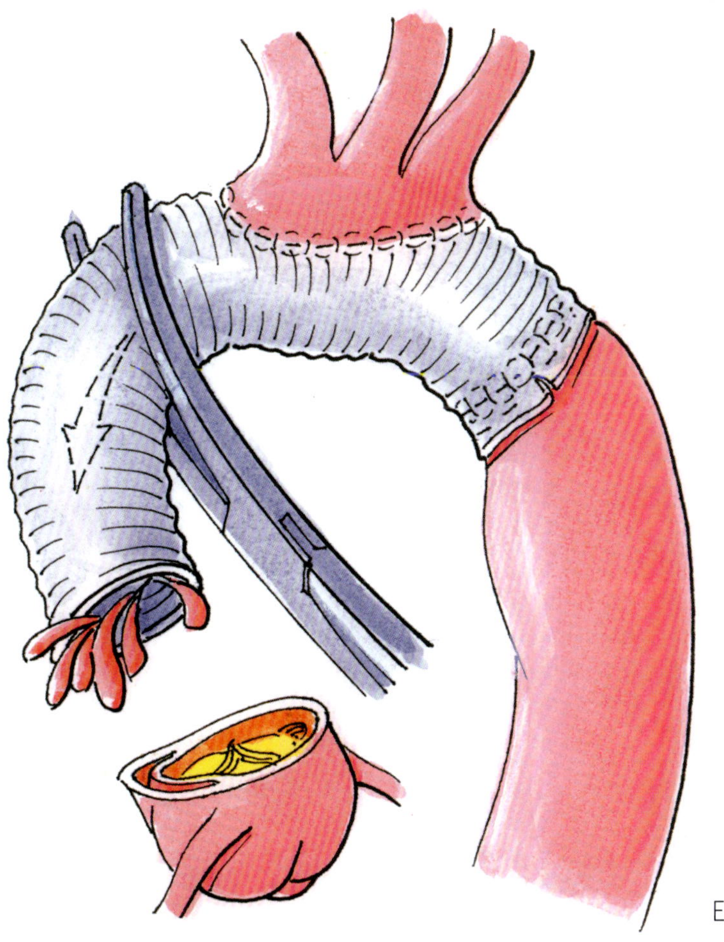

E. 恢复体外循环，人工血管排气后钳夹阻断。

E. Extracorporeal circulation is restored, and clamps are placed on the artificial aortic graft after de-airing.

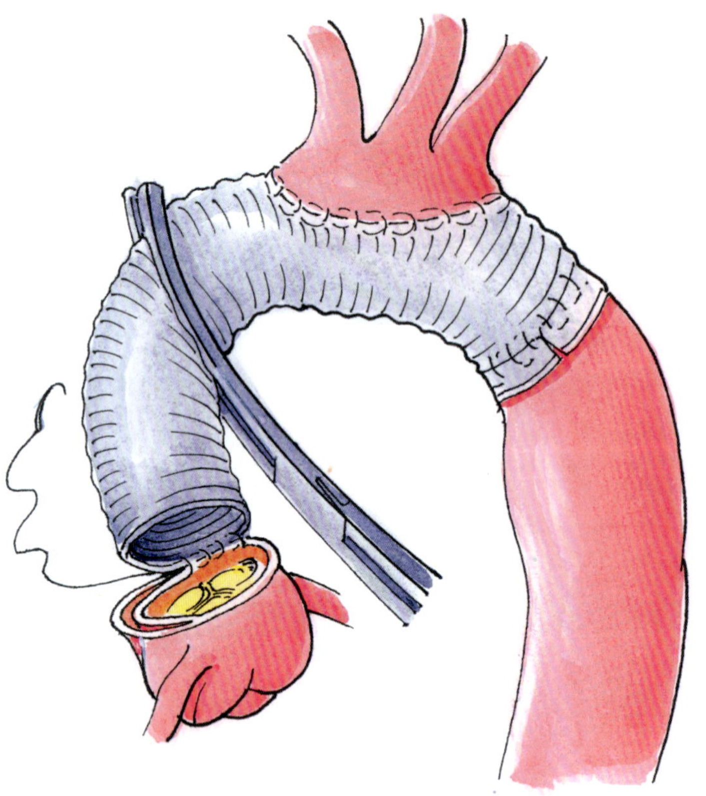

F. 人工血管与升主动脉窦管交界处断端行端端吻合。

F. End-to-end anastomosis is performed at the graft and the stump of the ascending aortic at the sinotubular junction.

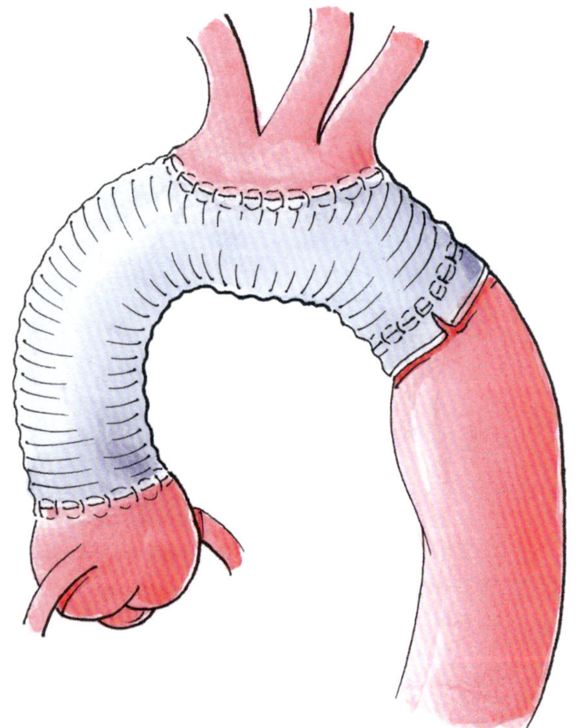

G. 吻合完成。

G. Anastomosis is completed.

图 4-1-5 胸降主动脉人工血管置换术
Figure 4-1-5 Descending thoracic aorta graft replacement

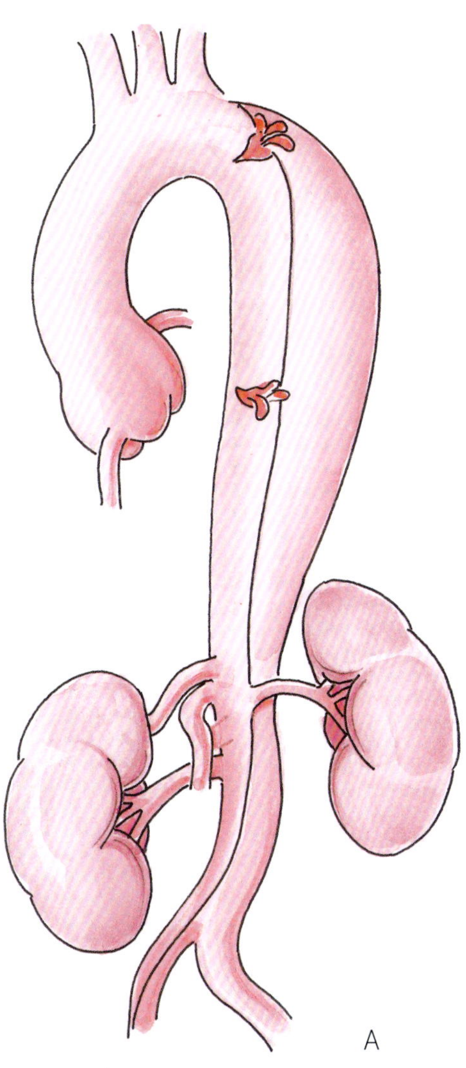

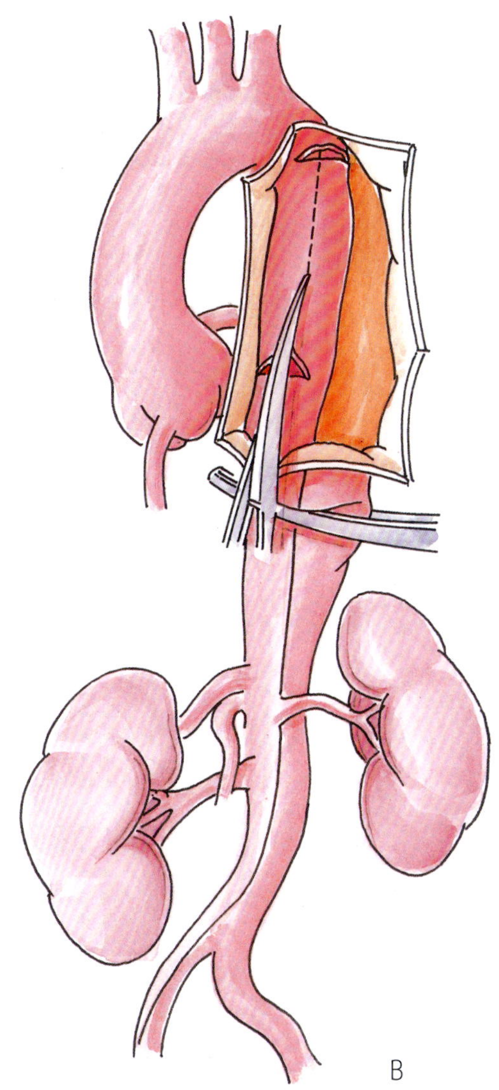

A. 急性 B 型夹层累及降主动脉全长，内膜近、远端破口均位于胸降主动脉。

A. Acute Type B dissection involves the entire length of the descending aorta, with proximal and distal intimal ruptures in the descending thoracic aorta.

B. 左心转流下，主动脉弓左颈总动脉和左锁骨下动脉之间钳夹做近端阻断。胸降主动脉远端钳夹阻断。切开胸降主动脉前壁。

B. Under left cardiac bypass, proximal occlusion is performed by placing clamps between the left common carotid artery and the left subclavian artery of the aortic arch. Block the distal end of the descending thoracic aorta, and cut open the anterior wall of the descending thoracic aorta.

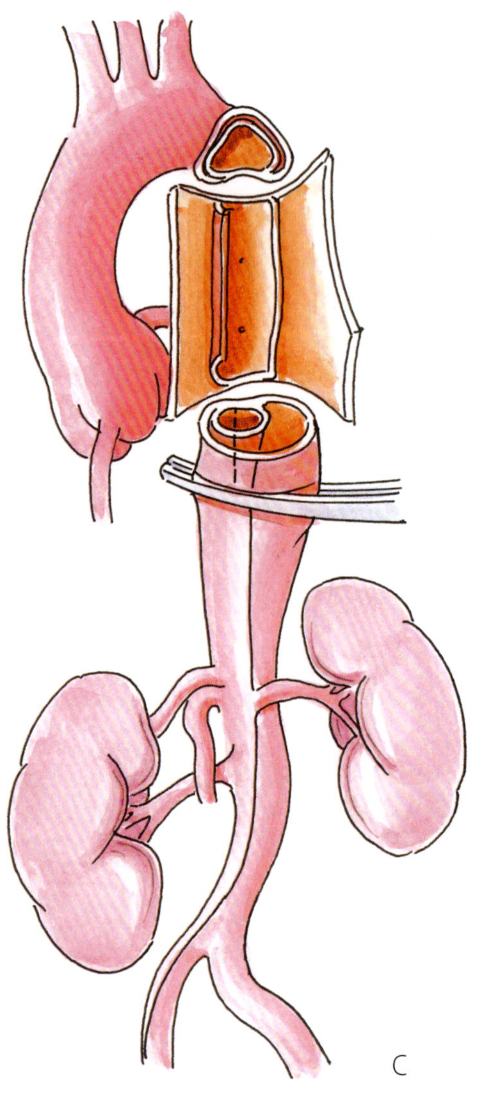

C. 胸降主动脉两端横断。

C. Both ends of the descending thoracic aorta are transected.

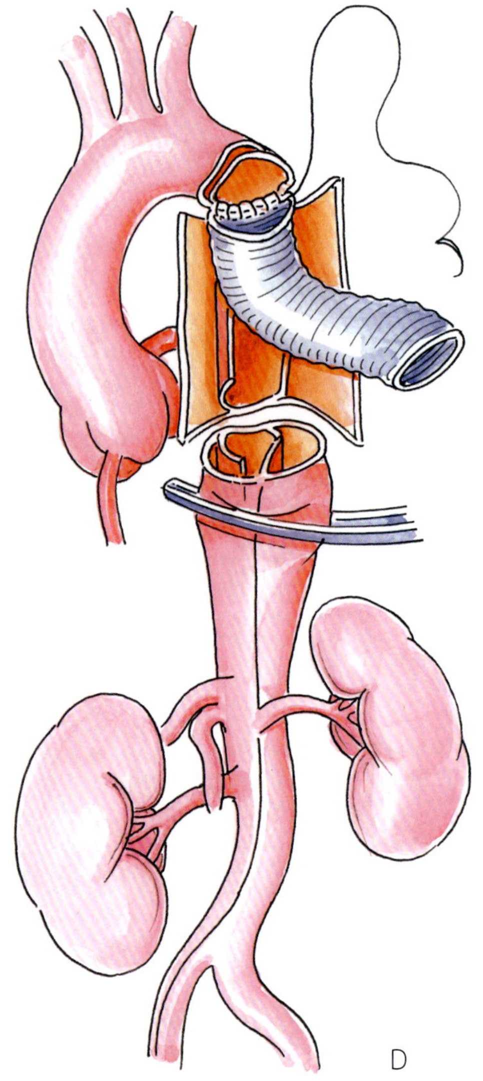

D. 选择合适口径的人工血管，与弓降部断端做端端吻合。

D. A properly sized artificial aortic graft is sutured to the stump of the descending aortic arch in an end-to-end fashion.

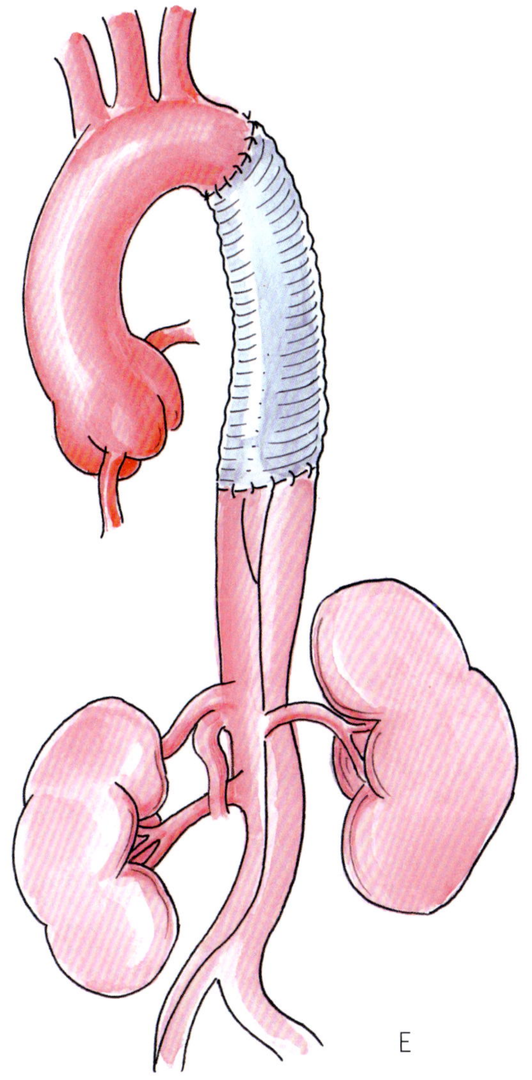

E. 慢性 B 型夹层真腔通常较小，有些分支已与真腔分离，而由假腔供血，此时若封闭假腔，会引起这些分支供应的器官缺血坏死。处理方法是将真假腔之间的内膜斜行剪开一个缺口，使真腔与假腔贯通。人工血管与胸降主动脉远侧断端行端端吻合，部分吻合仅缝在真腔壁。

E. In chronic type B dissection, the true lumen is usually small, with some branches separated from the true lumen and supplied by a false lumen. In such cases, the blocking of the false lumen causes ischemic necrosis of the organs supplied by these branches. The treatment is to make an oblique incision between the true and false lumens to connect both lumens. End-to-end anastomosis is performed between the artificial vessel and the distal stump of the descending thoracic aorta, partially sutured to the true lumen wall only.

图 4-1-6　急性 B 型夹层降主动脉人工血管置换术
Figure 4-1-6　Descending aorta graft replacement for acute type B dissection

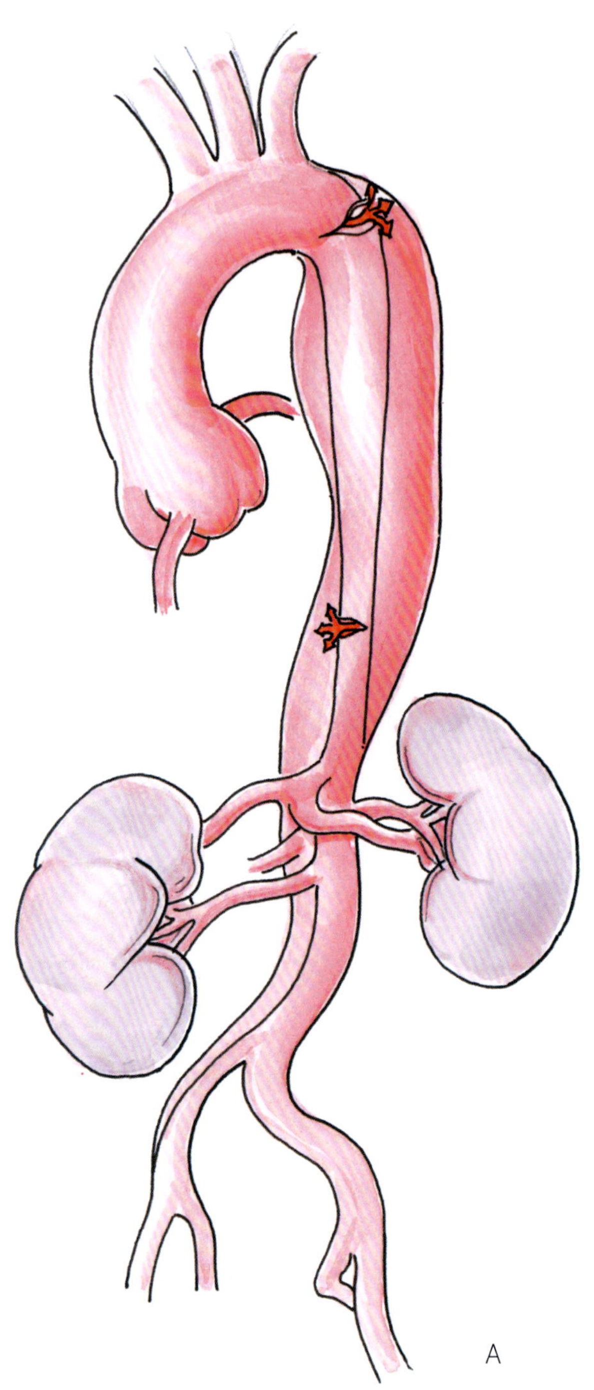

A. 急性 B 型夹层累及降主动脉全长。内膜近端破口位于弓降部，远端破口在膈肌水平。

A. Acute type B dissection involves the entire length of the descending aorta with proximal intimal ruptures in the descending arch and distal ruptures at the diaphragm level.

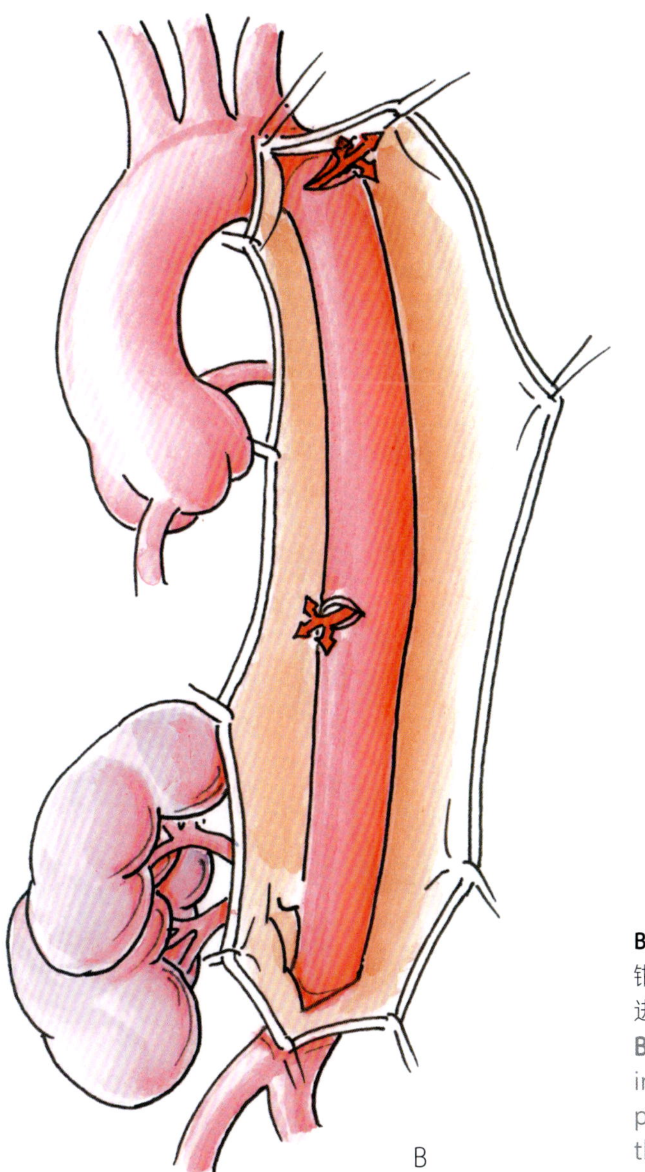

B. 胸腹联合切口。降主动脉近、远端钳夹阻断。切开降主动脉前壁外膜，进入假腔，清除血栓。

B. Make a thoracoabdominal incision and place clamps on the proximal and distal descending thoracic aorta respectively. Open the anterior wall adventitia of the descending aorta, enter the false lumen, and clear the thrombus.

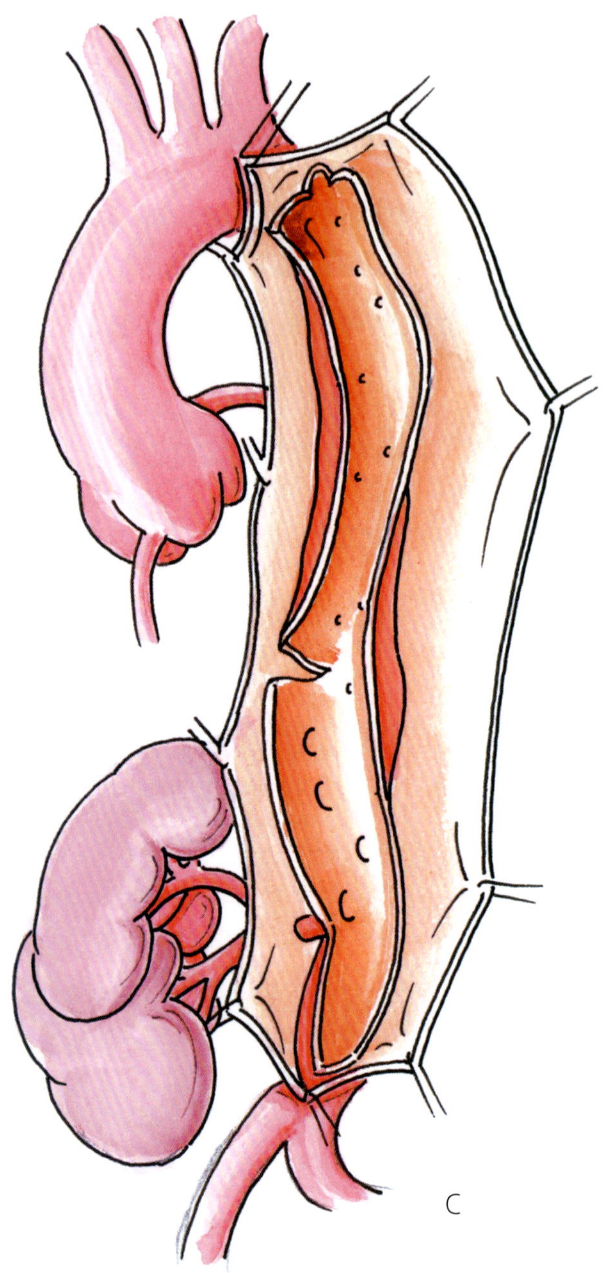

C. 切开降主动脉内膜，进入真腔，辨认其主要分支开口。
C. Incise the tunica intima of the descending aorta, access the true lumen, and identify the ostium of its major branches.

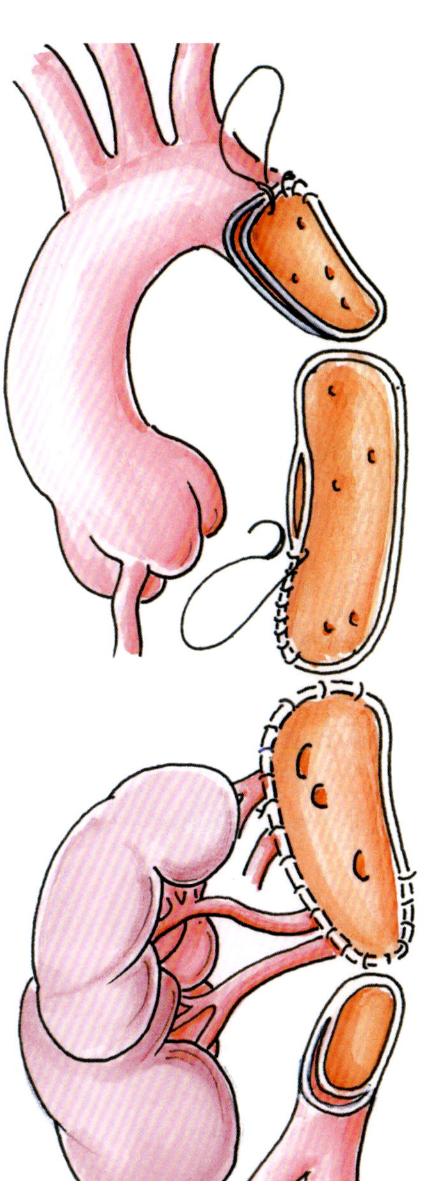

D. 弓降部斜行切断主动脉，保留有肋间动脉开口的主动脉后壁。胸降主动脉后壁做长段岛状保留，其中含肋间动脉开口。腹降主动脉在腹腔干和左右肾动脉开口处做岛状保留。降主动脉远端亦斜行切断，保留其后壁的分支血供。

D. An oblique transection of the aorta is made at the descending arch, preserving the posterior wall of the aorta with ostia of intercostal arteries. The posterior wall of descending thoracic aorta is preserved with the ostia of the intercostal arteries in the shape of a long island. The abdominal descending aorta is preserved in an island shape at the celiac trunk and the ostia of the left and right renal arteries. The distal end of descending aorta is also obliquely transected while preserving its posterior wall branches supplying the blood.

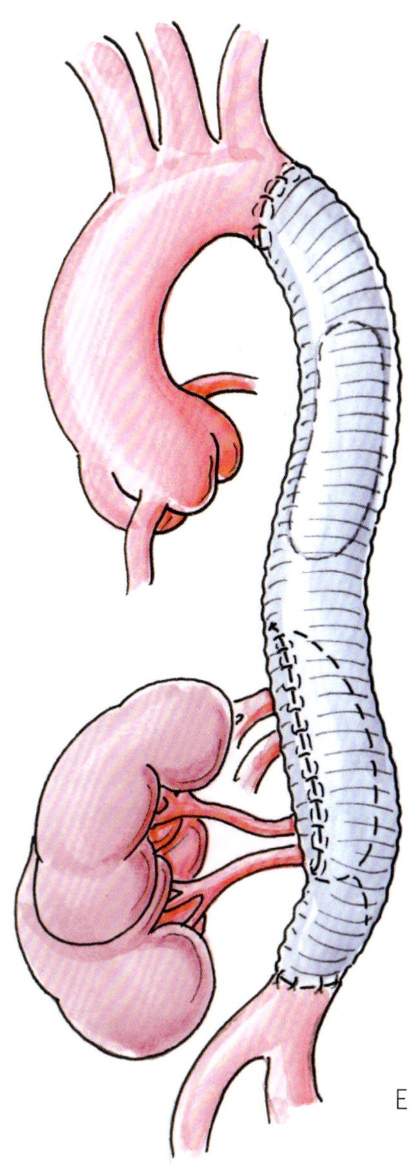

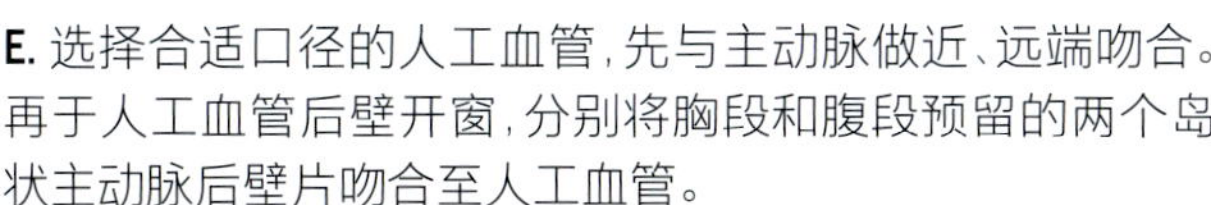
E. 选择合适口径的人工血管，先与主动脉做近、远端吻合。再于人工血管后壁开窗，分别将胸段和腹段预留的两个岛状主动脉后壁片吻合至人工血管。

E. An appropriately sized artificial vessel is anastomosed with the aorta proximally and distally. Two fenestrations are made in the posterior wall of the graft, and the island posterior aortic walls of the thoracic and abdominal segments are anastomosed to the graft respectively.

图 4-1-7 慢性 B 型夹层降主动脉人工血管置换术
Figure 4-1-7 Descending aorta graft replacement for chronic type B dissection

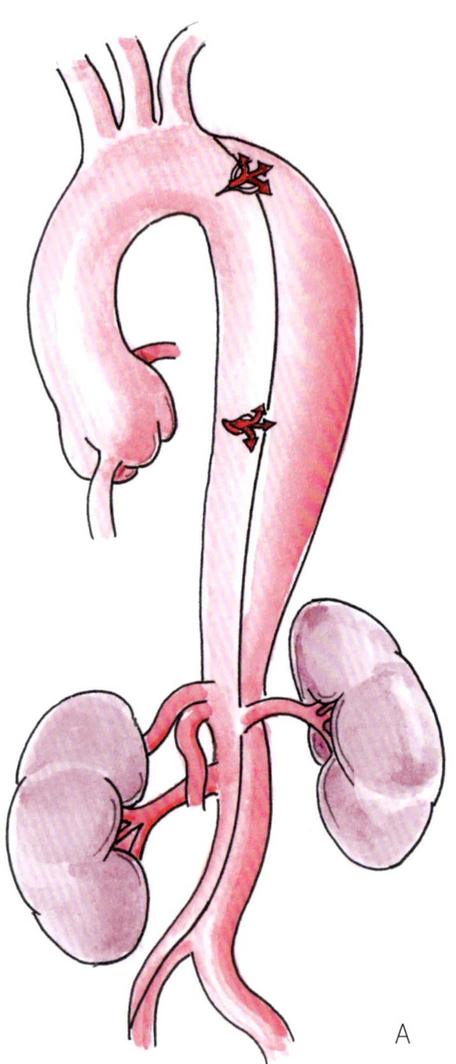

A. 慢性 B 型夹层累及降主动脉全长，内膜近、远端破口均位于胸降主动脉。

A. Chronic type B dissection involves the entire length of the descending aorta, with its proximal and distal intimal tears located in the descending thoracic aorta.

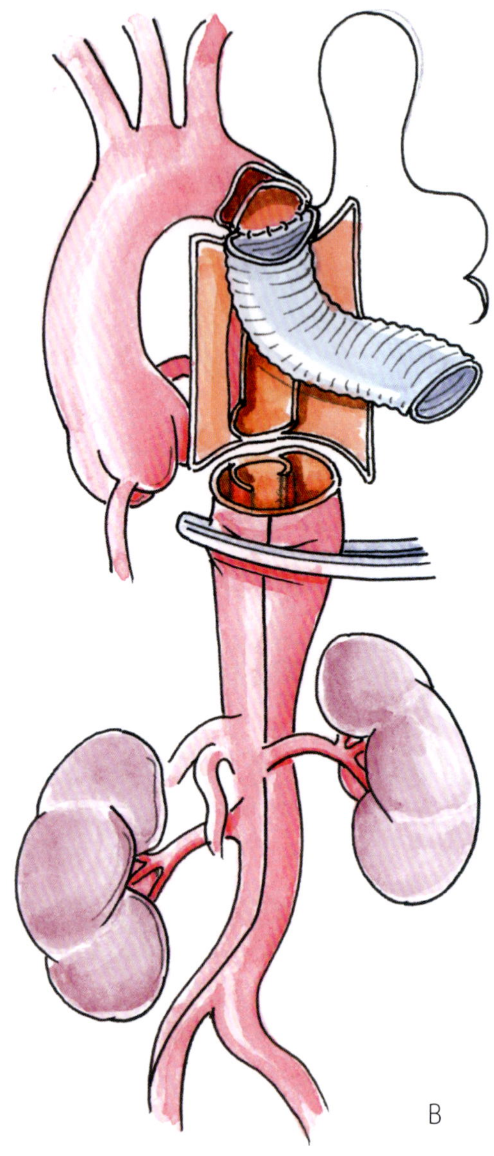

B. 切开胸降主动脉前壁，两端横断。选择合适口径的人工血管与降主动脉近侧断端行端端吻合。将真假腔之间的内膜斜行剪开一个缺口，使真腔与假腔贯通。

B. The anterior wall of the descending thoracic aorta is cut and transected at both ends. An appropriately sized artificial vessel is anastomosed end to end to the proximal stump of the descending aorta. An oblique incision is placed on the intima between the true and false lumens to connect them.

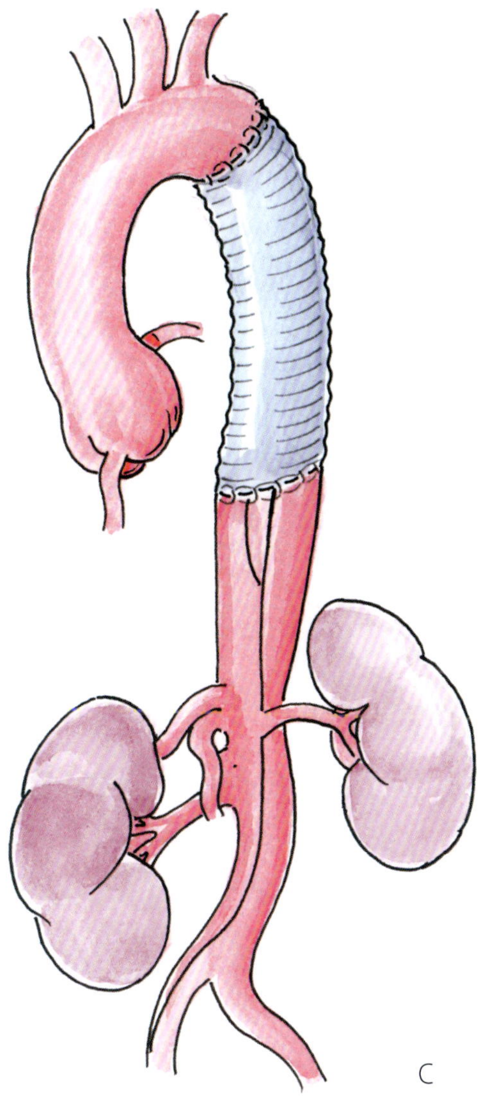

C. 人工血管与降主动脉远侧断端行端端吻合。
C. End-to-end anastomosis is performed between the graft and the distal stump of the descending aorta.

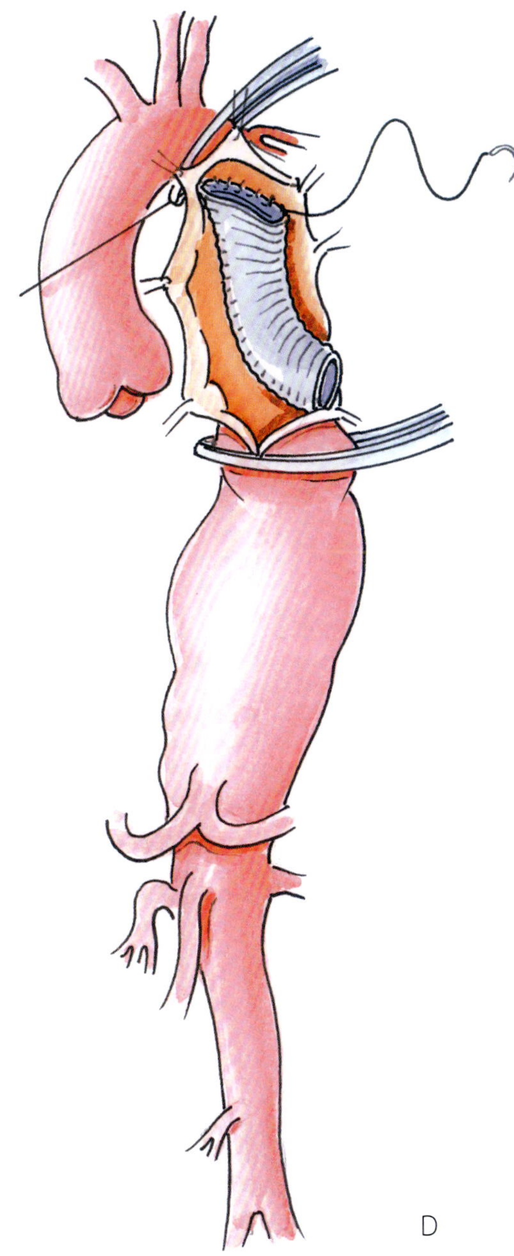

D. 主动脉两端亦可不离断，切开主动脉前壁后先做近端的端端吻合。
D. The two ends of the aorta may not be dissected, and the proximal end-to-end anastomosis is performed after an incision is made on the anterior wall of the aorta.

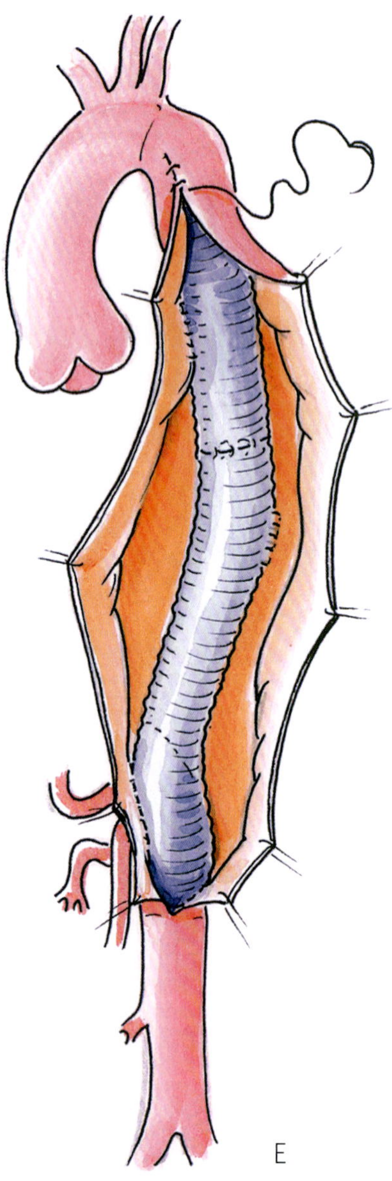

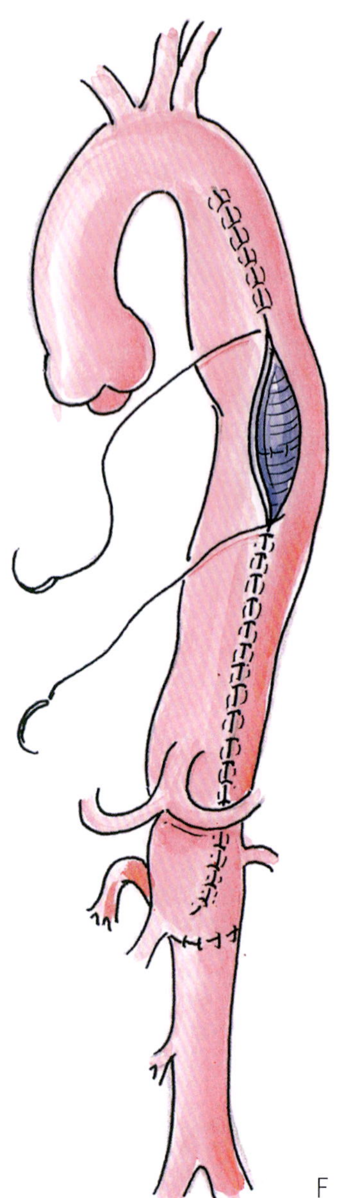

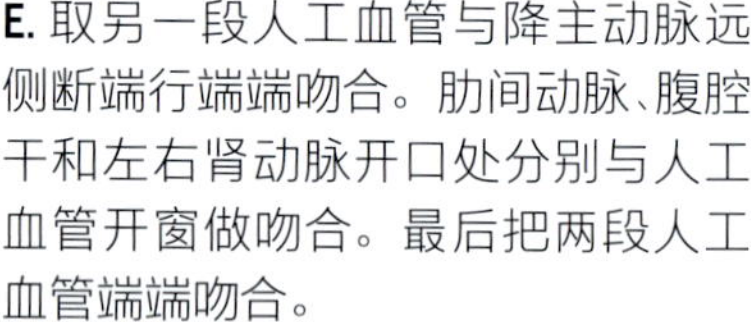
E. 取另一段人工血管与降主动脉远侧断端行端端吻合。肋间动脉、腹腔干和左右肾动脉开口处分别与人工血管开窗做吻合。最后把两段人工血管端端吻合。

E. Another segment of the graft is anastomosed end-to-end to the distal cut edge of the descending aorta. The fenestration is placed in the ostia of the intercostal artery, celiac trunk, and left and right renal arteries for anastomosis with the grafts, respectively. Finally, end-to-end anastomosis of the two grafts is performed.

F. 缝合切开的降主动脉，包埋人工血管。

F. Close the incision on the descending aorta and embed the grafts.

图 4-1-8 A 型夹层一期杂交修复术
Figure 4-1-8 One-stage hybrid repair for type A dissection

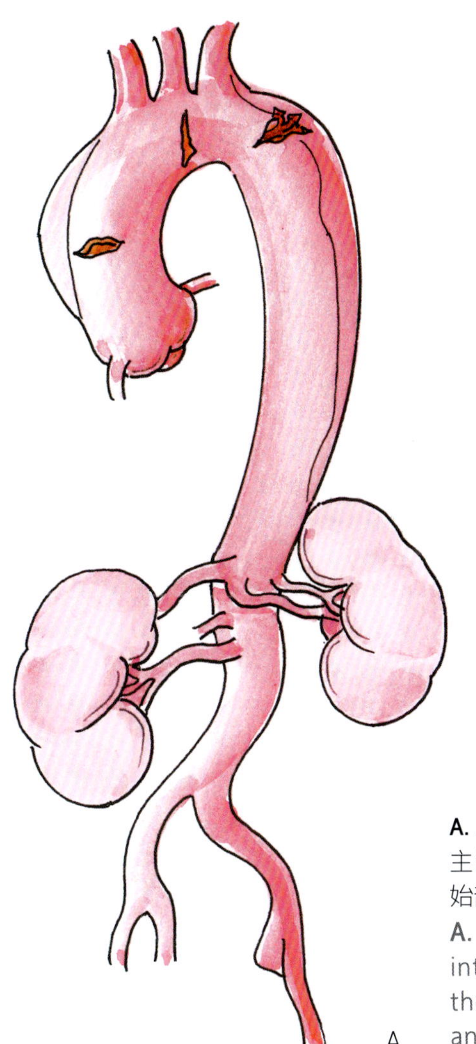

A

A. A 型夹层，主动脉内膜破口位于升主动脉、主动脉弓部和降主动脉起始部。

A. Type A dissection with aortic intimal ruptures in the origin of the ascending aorta, aortic arch, and descending aorta.

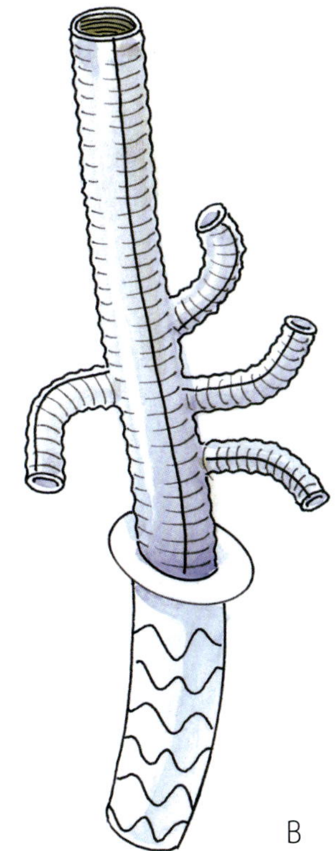

B

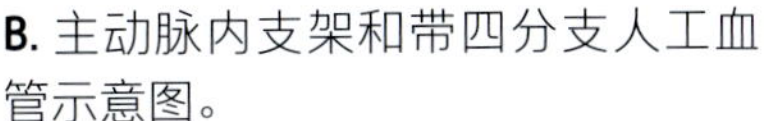

B. 主动脉内支架和带四分支人工血管示意图。

B. Diagram of the intra-aortic stent graft and a four-branched artificial vessel.

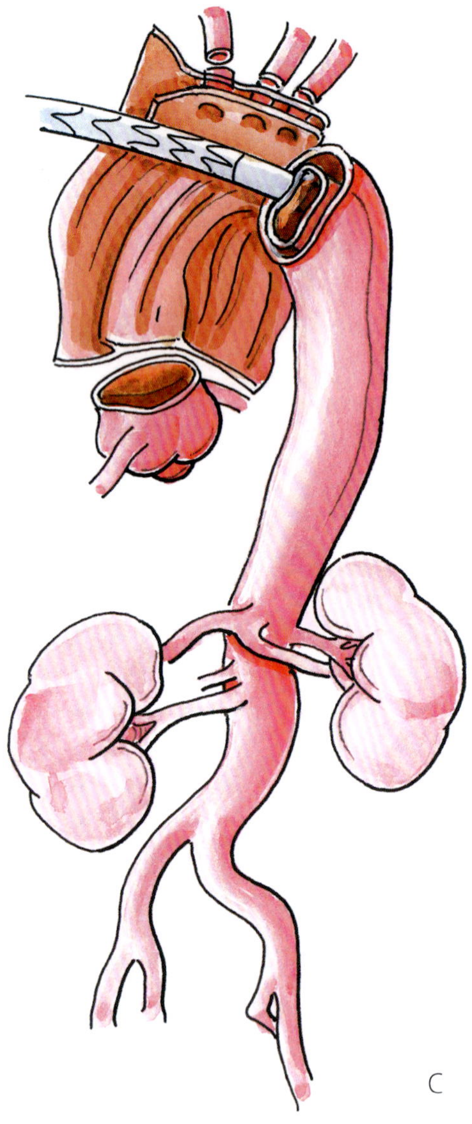

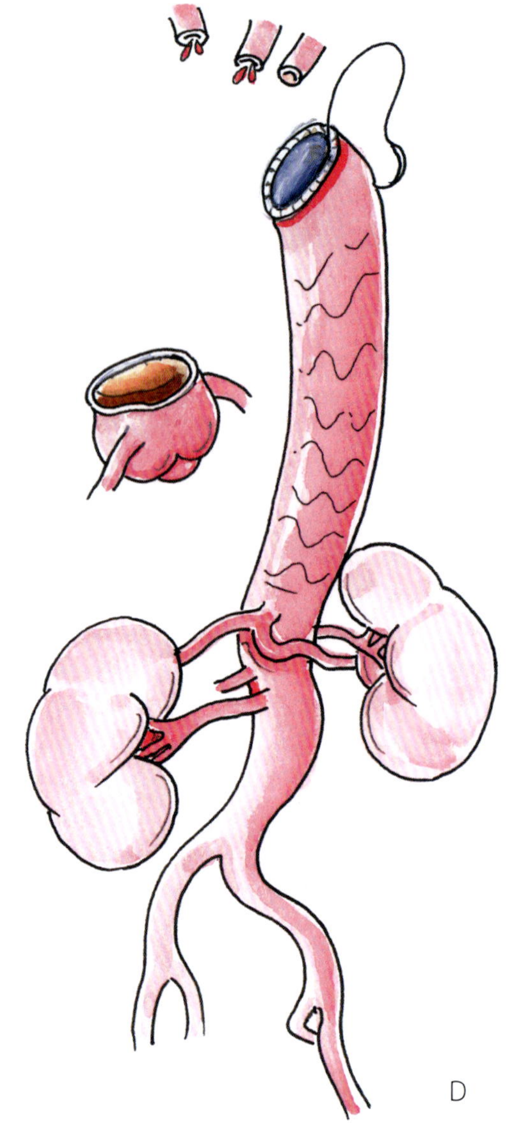

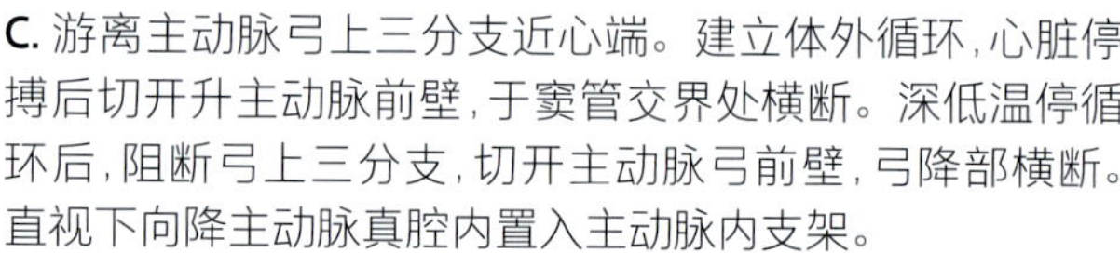

C. 游离主动脉弓上三分支近心端。建立体外循环，心脏停搏后切开升主动脉前壁，于窦管交界处横断。深低温停循环后，阻断弓上三分支，切开主动脉弓前壁，弓降部横断。直视下向降主动脉真腔内置入主动脉内支架。

C. Free the proximal ends of three supra-aortic arch branches. Under extracorporeal circulation and cardiac arrest, the anterior wall of the ascending aorta is incised and transected at the sinotubular junction. After deep hypothermic circulatory arrest, the three supra-aortic arch branches are blocked, the anterior wall of the aortic arch cut, and the descending arch transected. An intra-aortic stent is placed into the true lumen of the descending aorta under direct vision.

D. 主动脉内膜支架到位后释放，其缝合环与降主动脉做单纯连续缝合。

D. After the aortic intimal stent is placed, the suture ring is sutured to the descending aorta with simple continuous sutures.

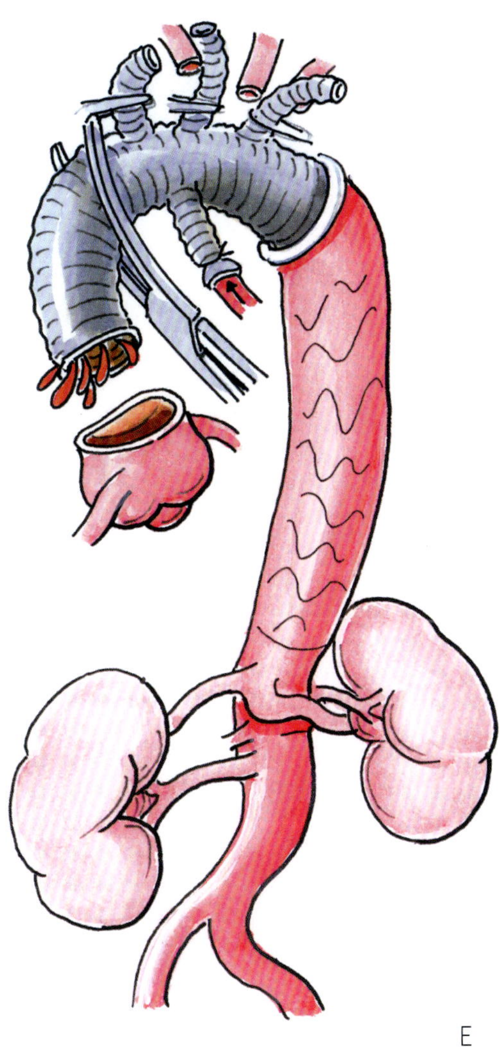

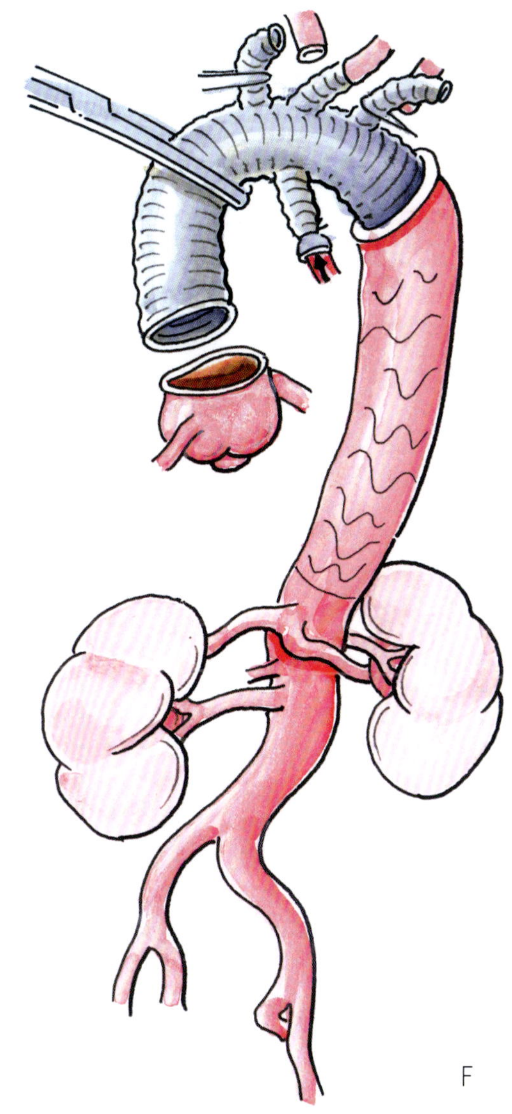

E. 带四分支人工血管远端与降主动脉和主动脉内支架缝合环连续缝合。恢复体外循环，人工血管排气后钳夹阻断人工血管，体外循环改换至经人工血管分支供血。

E. The distal end of the four-branched artificial vessel is attached to a descending aortic and intra-aortic stent with a continuous suture loop. Extracorporeal circulation is resumed, and the graft is vented and clamped. Extracorporeal circulation is switched to blood supply by the graft branch.

F. 人工血管分支与左颈总动脉吻合，恢复脑部供血。

F. The branch of the artificial vessel is sutured to the left common carotid artery to restore cerebral blood supply.

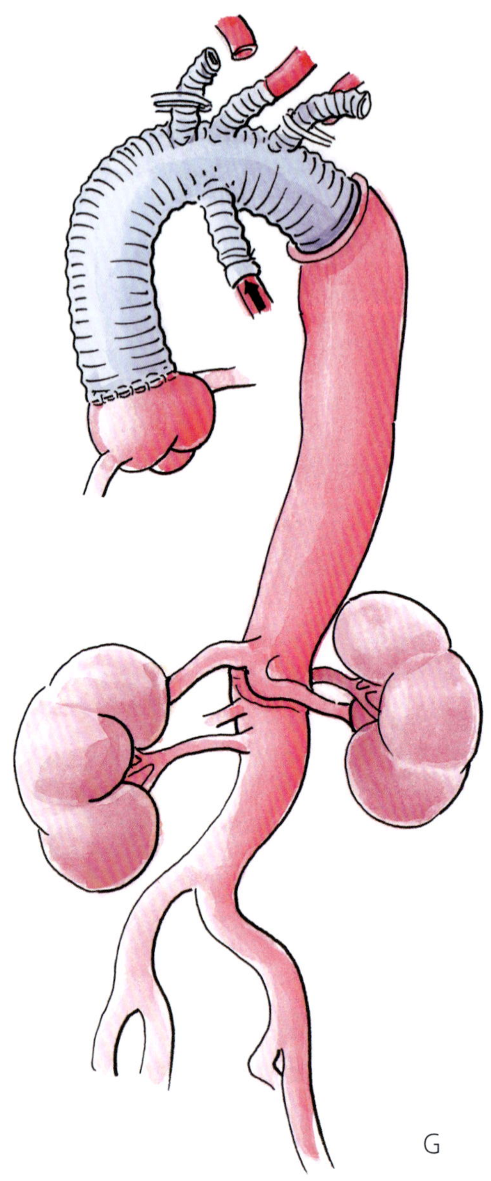

G. 人工血管与升主动脉做近端吻合。开放人工血管阻断钳，恢复冠状动脉供血。

G. The graft is anastomosed proximally to the ascending aorta. Release the vascular blocking forceps and restore coronary artery supply.

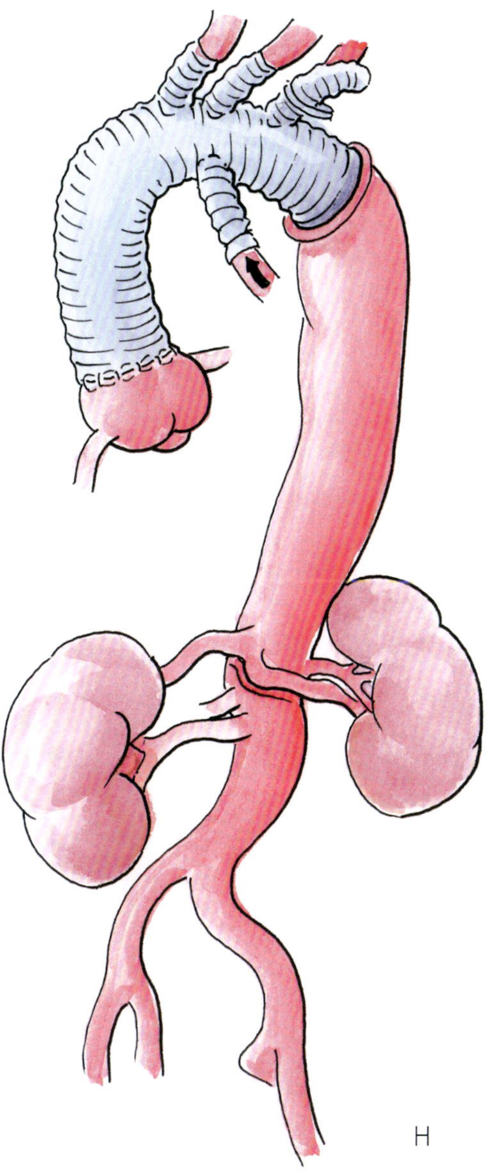

H. 人工血管分支与头臂干吻合。

H. The graft branch is anastomosed to the brachiocephalic trunk.

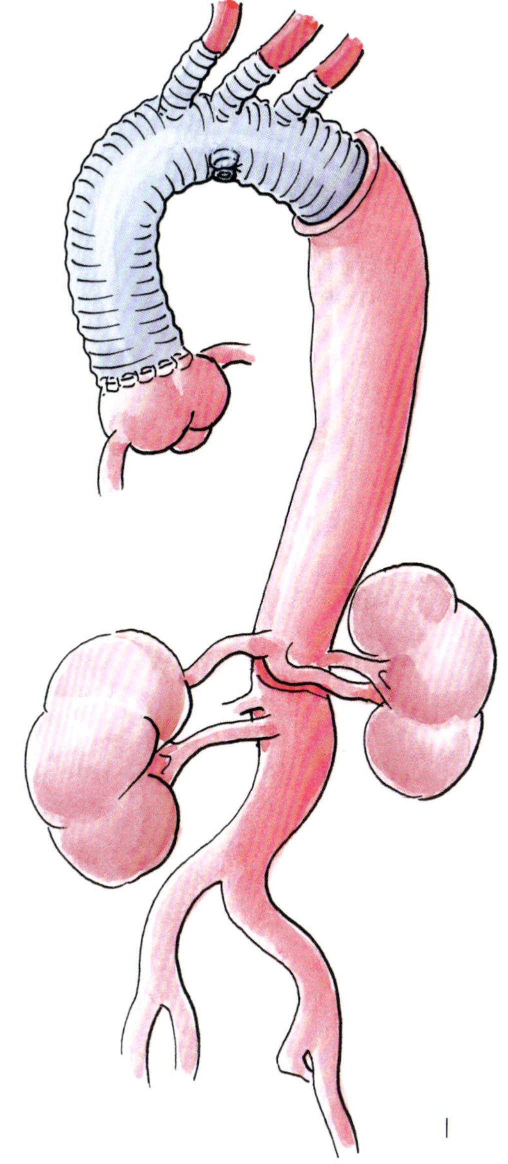

I. 最后将人工血管分支与左锁骨下动脉吻合。 撤除体外循环后将供血分支人工血管缝闭。

I. Finally, the graft is anastomosed to the left subclavian artery. After removing extracorporeal circulation, close the graft branch supplying blood.

第 二 节　升主动脉瘤和主动脉根部手术
Section 2　Ascending Aortic Aneurysm and Aortic Root Surgery

图 4-2-1　升主动脉人工血管置换术
Figure 4-2-1　Ascending aorta graft replacement

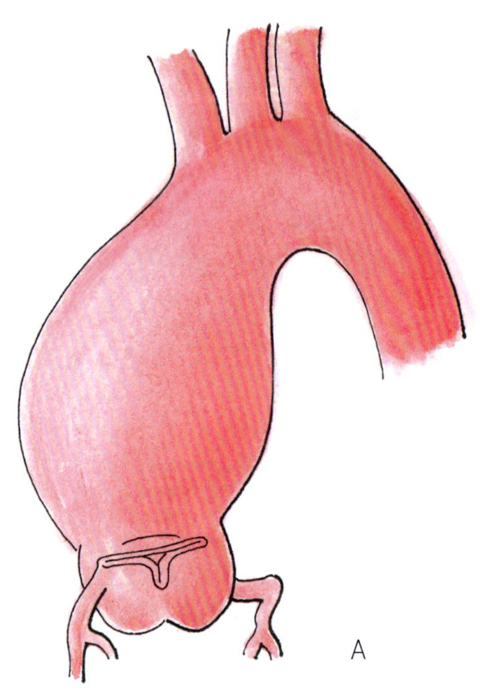

A. 升主动脉瘤，主动脉根部正常。

A. Ascending aortic aneurysm with normal aortic root.

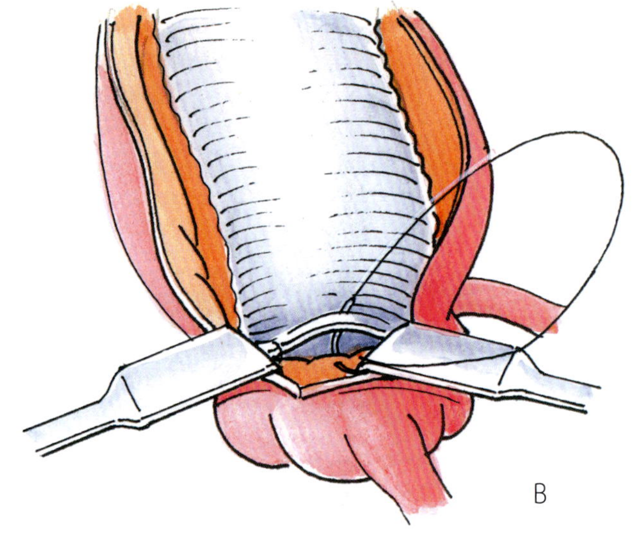

B. 建立体外循环，心脏停搏后纵行切开升主动脉瘤。选择合适口径的人工血管，在动脉瘤腔内将人工血管与升主动脉做近端吻合。

B. Extracorporeal circulation is established, and the ascending aortic aneurysm is incised longitudinally after cardiac arrest. An appropriately sized artificial vessel is anastomosed proximally to the ascending aorta in the aneurysm cavity.

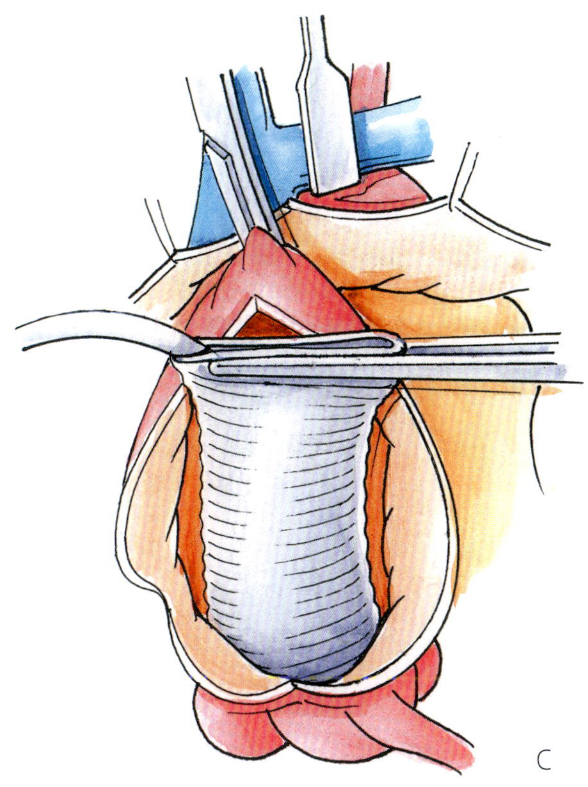

C. 加压注液检查近端吻合口，若有漏液予以修补。

C. Pressure injections are performed to assess the proximal anastomosis quality, and an anastomotic leak is to be repaired if present.

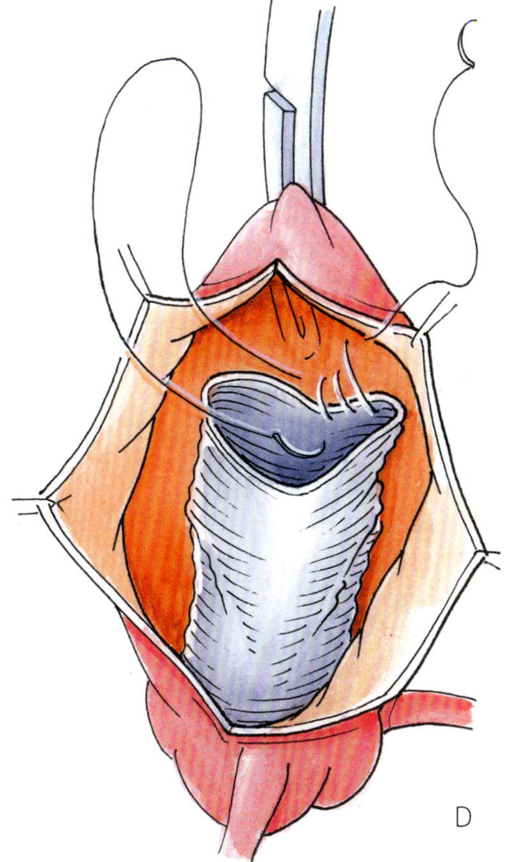

D. 人工血管另一端与升主动脉的远端做端端吻合。

D. The other end of the graft is anastomosed end-to-end to the distal end of the ascending aorta.

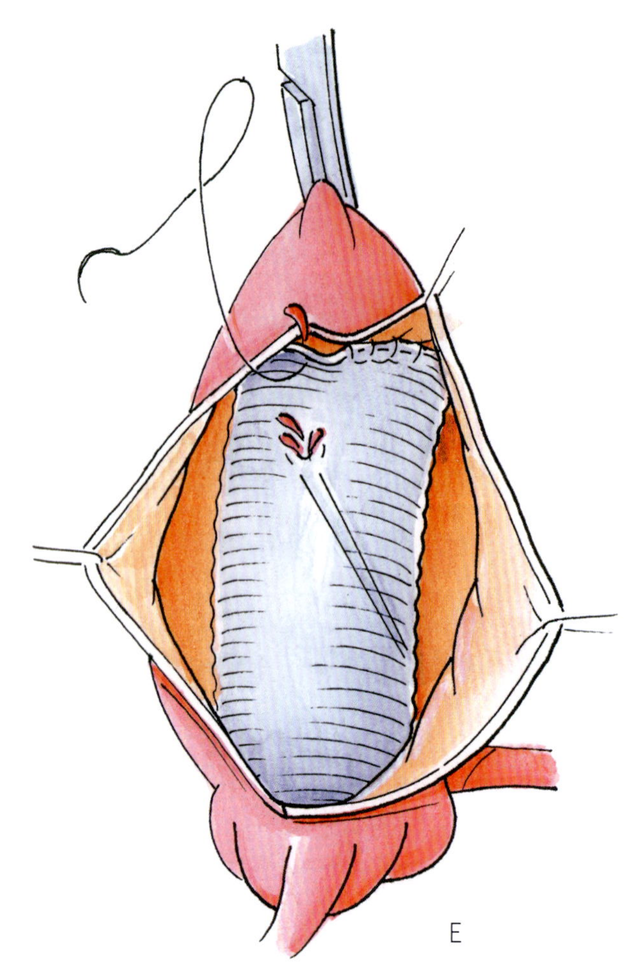

E. 远端吻合口结扎前放松一下主动脉阻断钳，排出人工血管中的空气。人工血管前壁戳排气孔排出残余空气，留荷包缝合备用。

E. Release the aortic cross-clamping forceps before ligation and distal anastomosis, and expel air from the graft. The anterior wall of the graft is punctured to vent the residual air, reserving the purse-string suture as a backup.

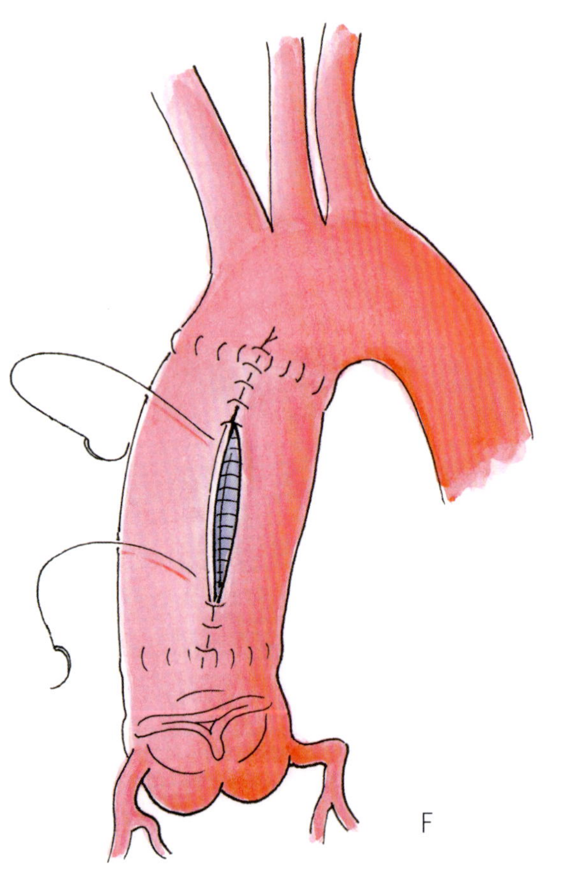

F. 开放主动脉阻断钳。心脏复跳，排气、撤除体外循环、中和肝素后，检查吻合口无漏血。剪去多余的动脉瘤壁，将其缝合包埋人工血管。

F. Unclamp the aortic blocking forceps. Heartbeat is resumed, and ventilation, extracorporeal circulation withdrawal, and heparin neutralization are finished. Anastomotic testing is performed to assure the absence of the anastomotic leakage. The redundant aneurysm wall is cut off, and the graft is embedded and sutured.

图 4-2-2　升主动脉人工血管置换加半弓重建术

Figure 4-2-2　Ascending aorta graft replacement with hemi-arch reconstruction

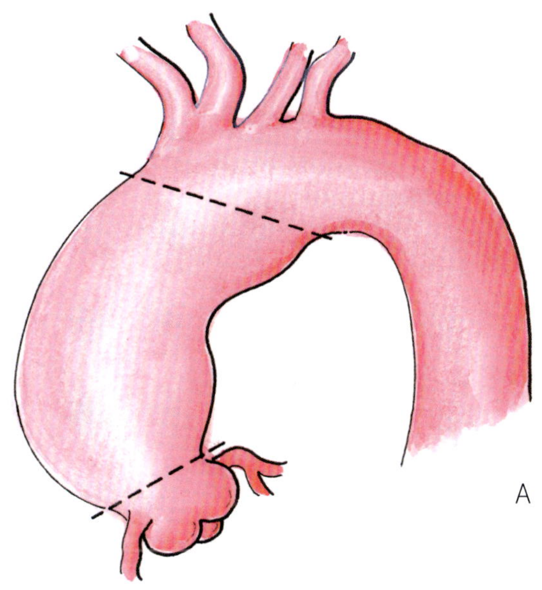

A. 升主动脉瘤，其病变延伸到主动脉弓下缘。虚线示拟行吻合的位置，即吻合口要做在超过动脉瘤的正常血管壁。

A. Ascending aortic aneurysm extends to the inferior margin of the aortic arch. The dotted line indicates the anastomotic site, i.e., the anastomosis to be placed at the normal vessel wall beyond the aneurysm.

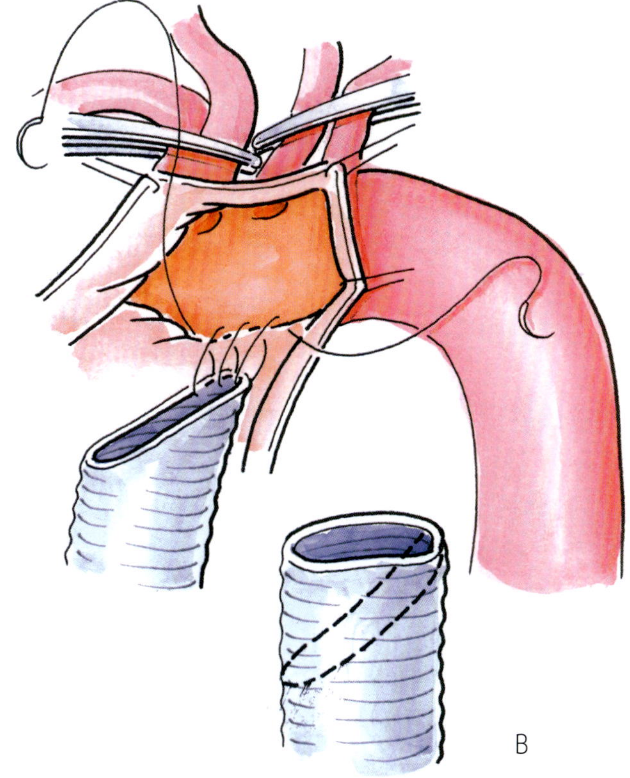

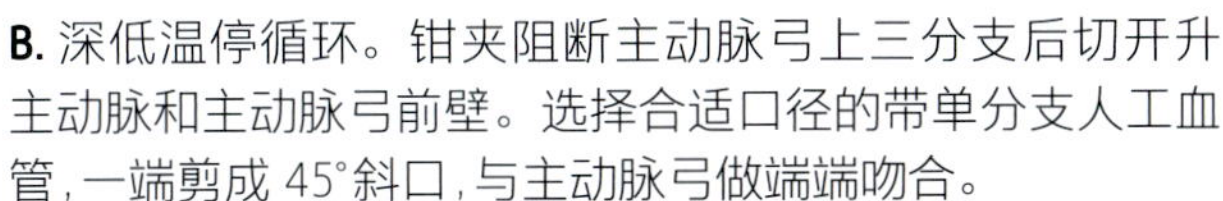
B. 深低温停循环。钳夹阻断主动脉弓上三分支后切开升主动脉和主动脉弓前壁。选择合适口径的带单分支人工血管，一端剪成 45°斜口，与主动脉弓做端端吻合。

B. With the deep hypothermic circulatory arrest, the ascending aorta and the anterior wall of the aortic arch are incised after the block of three supra-aortic arch branches. An appropriate single-branched graft is obliquely cut at a 45-degree angle at one end and sutured to the aortic arch with end-to-end anastomosis.

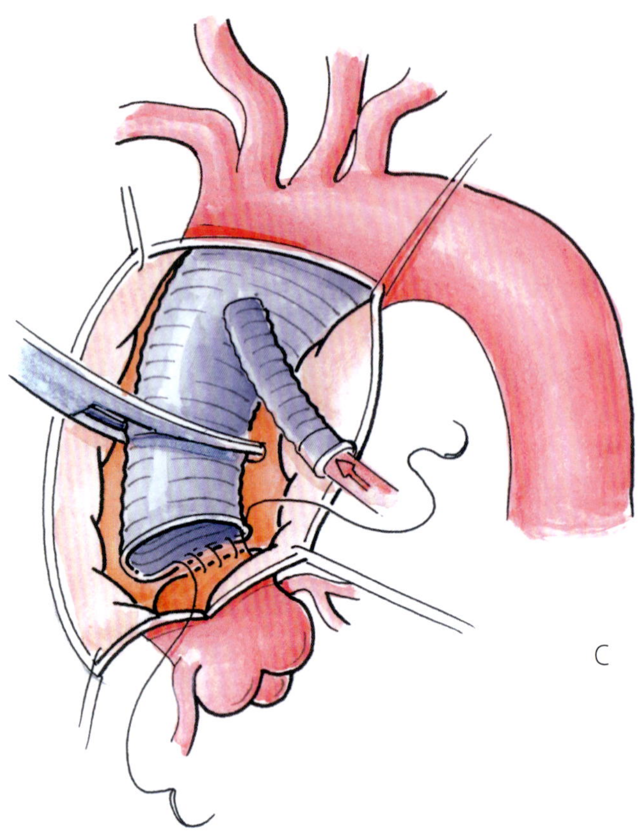

C. 恢复体外循环，人工血管排气后体外循环改换为经人工血管分支供血。人工血管与升主动脉近端做端端吻合。

C. Extracorporeal circulation is resumed and then changed to blood supply by the graft branch after its de-airing. An end-to-end anastomosis is performed between the graft and the proximal end of the ascending aorta.

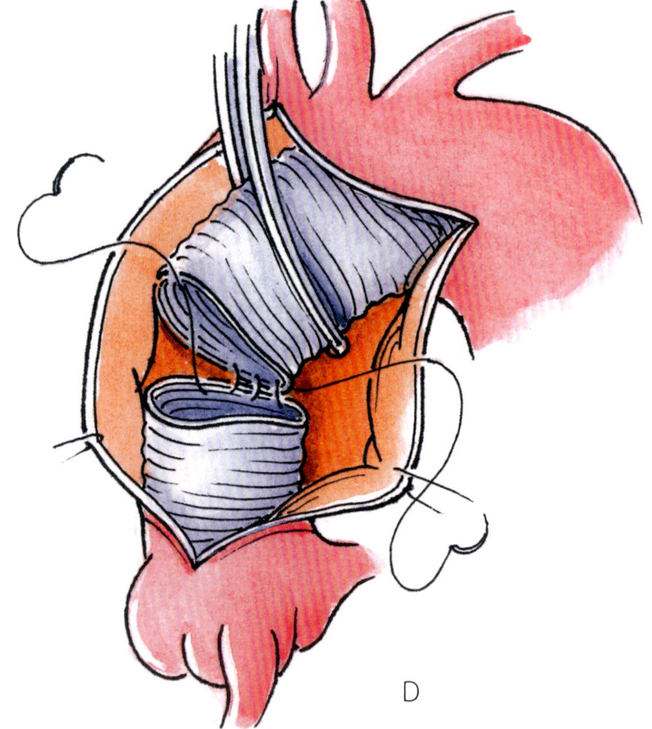

D. 也可用两段人工血管分别做近、远端吻合，再将两段人工血管端端吻合。

D. Alternatively, perform proximal and distal anastomosis with two segments of graft and then connect them with end-to-end anastomosis.

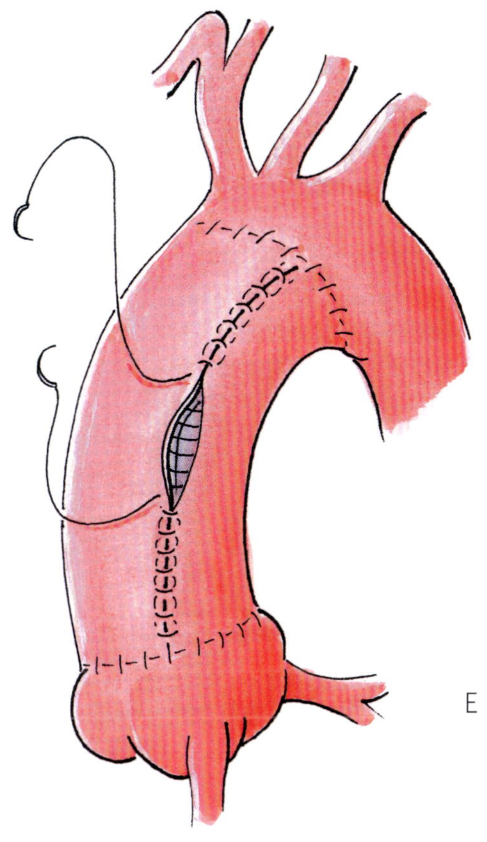

E. 撤除体外循环后结扎人工血管分支。止血后缝合动脉瘤壁将人工血管包埋，若有多余的动脉瘤壁先行剪除。

E. Ligate the branch vessel of the graft after extracorporeal circulation is weaned. After hemostasis, the aneurysm wall is sutured, and the graft is embedded. The redundant aneurysm wall is excised first if present.

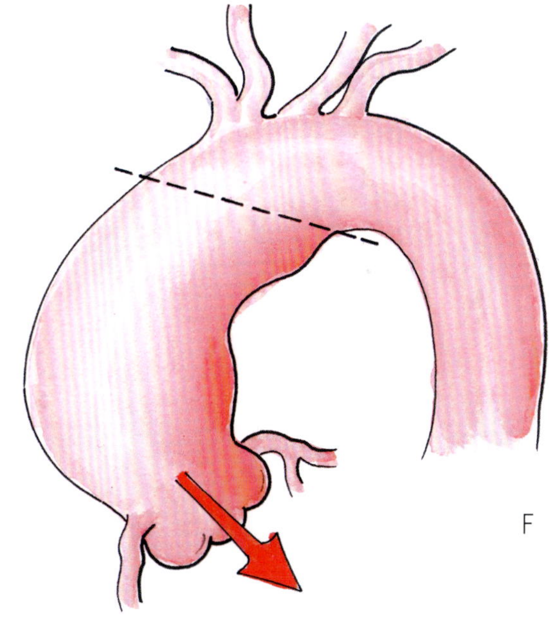

F. 升主动脉瘤，其病变近端累及主动脉窦，造成主动脉瓣关闭不全；病变远端延伸到主动脉弓下缘。

F. The proximal end of the ascending aortic aneurysm may involve the aortic sinus, which may result in aortic insufficiency. The lesion's distal end extends to the inferior margin of the aortic arch.

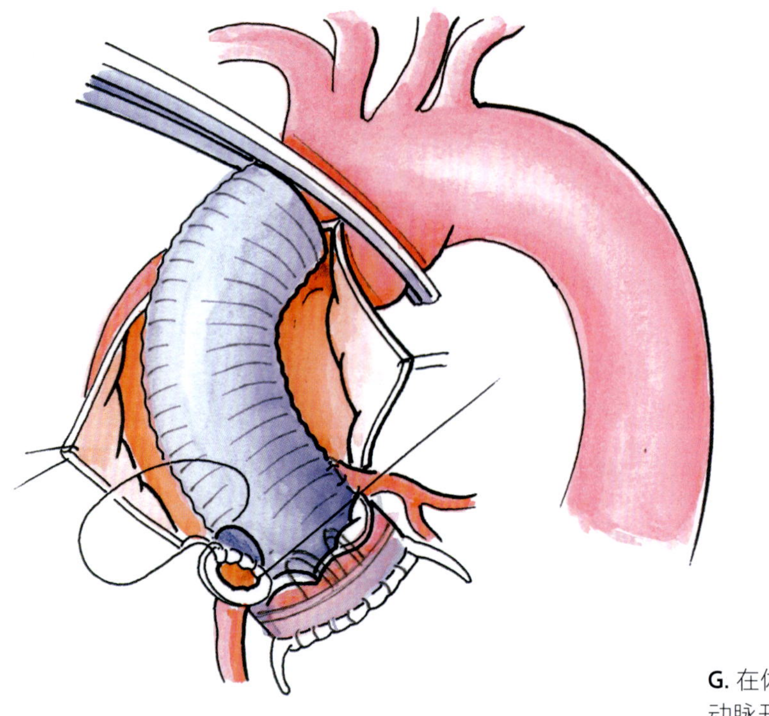

G. 在体外循环心脏停搏下切开升主动脉。游离左、右冠状动脉开口。剪去主动脉瓣叶，带垫片间断褥式缝合植入合适口径的带瓣外导管。左、右冠状动脉分别与带瓣外导管开口端侧吻合。

G. The ascending aorta is incised under extracorporeal circulation and cardiac arrest. Free the left and right coronary arteries ostia. The aortic valve leaflets are excised and an appropriately sized composite valved conduit is introduced by using interrupted pledgeted mattress sutures with its open end laterally anastomosed to the left and right coronary arteries.

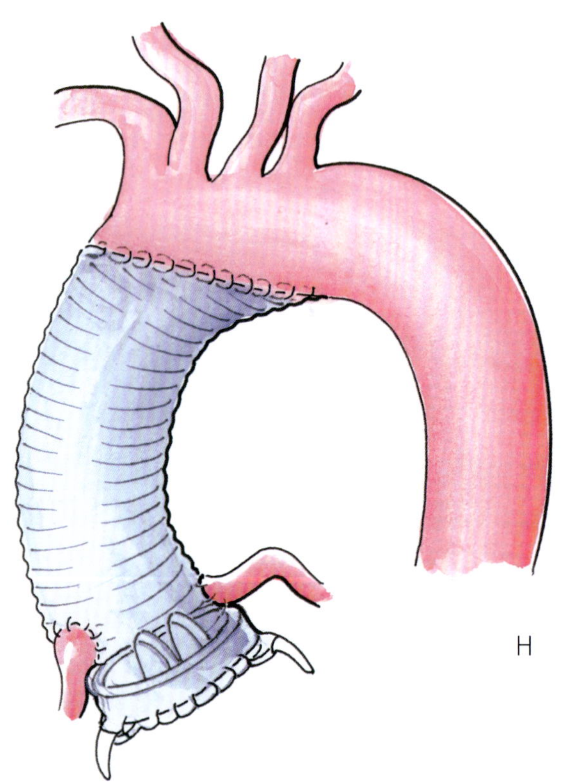

H. 深低温停循环，开放主动脉阻断钳。切除动脉瘤壁，斜行修剪主动脉弓，带瓣外导管远端亦剪成相应的斜口与主动脉弓端端吻合。

H. With the deep hypothermic circulatory arrest, the aortic clamping forceps are released, the aneurysm wall resected, and the aortic arch clipped obliquely. The distal end of the valved conduit is also trimmed correspondingly and sutured to the aortic arch with end-to-end anastomosis.

图 4-2-3　主动脉根部扩张保留瓣膜的修复术（Hetzer 法）
Figure 4-2-3　Valve-sparing operation in aortic root ectasia (Hetzer procedure)

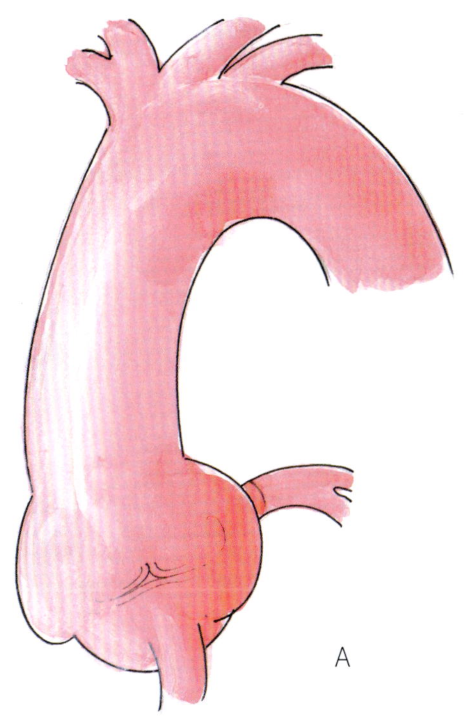

A. 主动脉窦严重扩张而主动脉环无明显扩张，主动脉瓣关闭良好。

A. Severe dilation of the aortic sinus without significant dilation of the aortic ring but with good aortic valve closure.

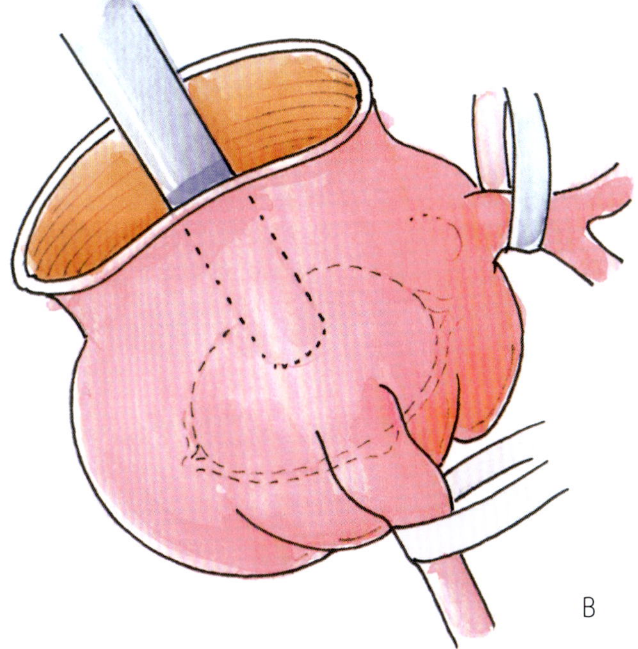

B. 游离主动脉根部至主动脉瓣环水平，左、右冠状动脉起始段也一并游离。窦管交界处横断升主动脉，测量主动脉瓣环内径。

B. Free the aortic root to the level of the aortic annulus, as well as the initial segments of the left and right coronary arteries. The ascending aorta is transected at the sinotubular junction, and the inner diameter of the aortic annulus is sized.

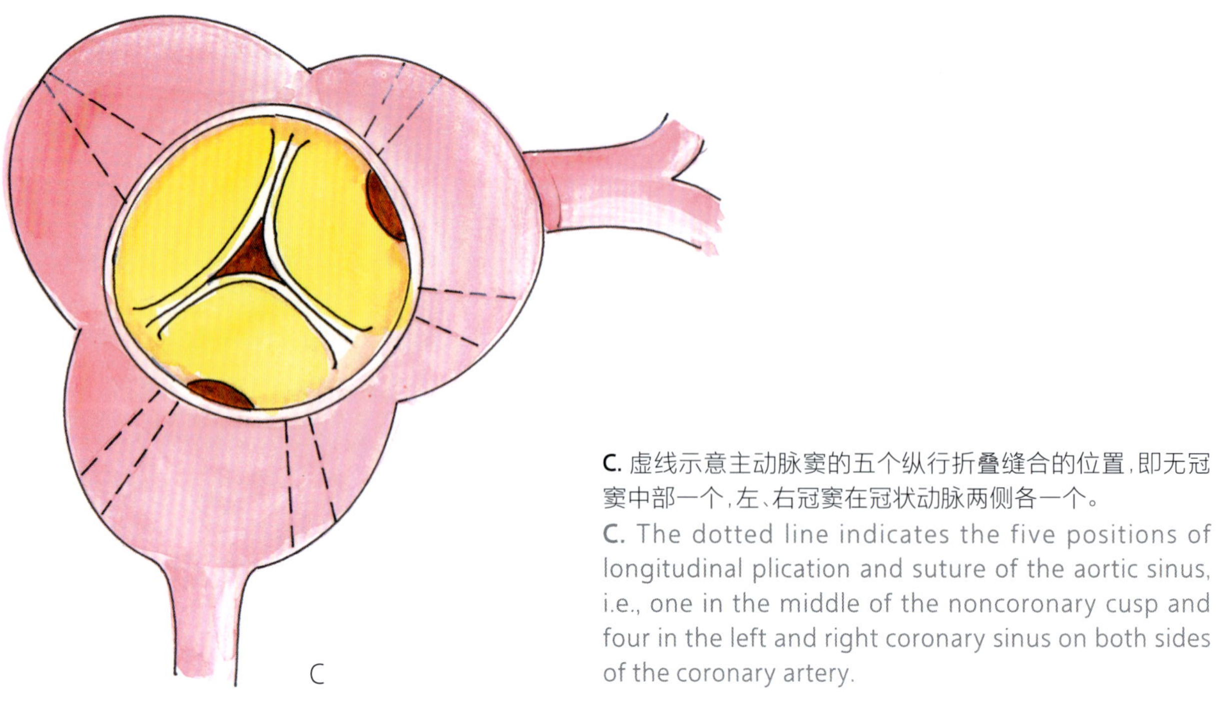

C. 虚线示意主动脉窦的五个纵行折叠缝合的位置，即无冠窦中部一个，左、右冠窦在冠状动脉两侧各一个。

C. The dotted line indicates the five positions of longitudinal plication and suture of the aortic sinus, i.e., one in the middle of the noncoronary cusp and four in the left and right coronary sinus on both sides of the coronary artery.

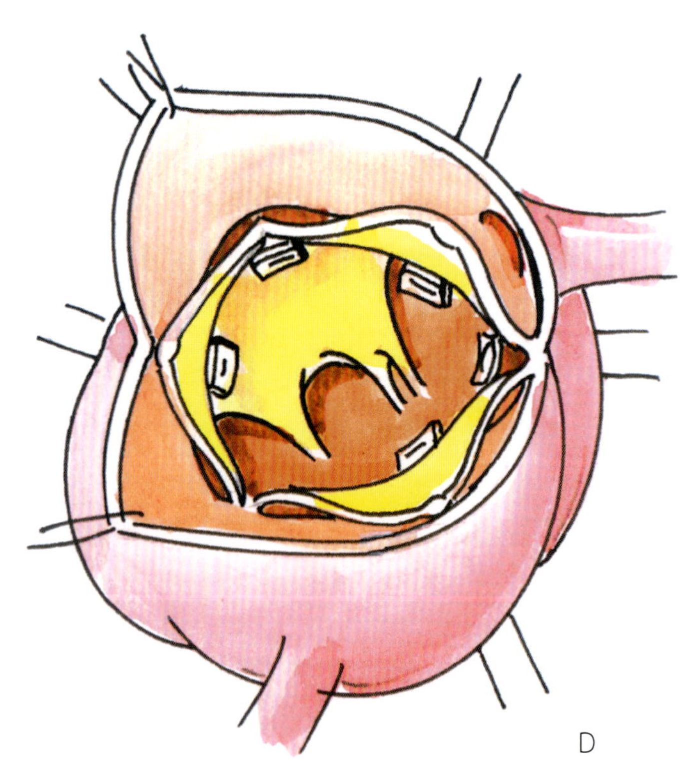

D. 经主动脉瓣环预置瓣环缝线，由内向外水平褥式缝合。

D. Annular suture is preset through the aortic valve annulus with an inside-out horizontal mattress suture.

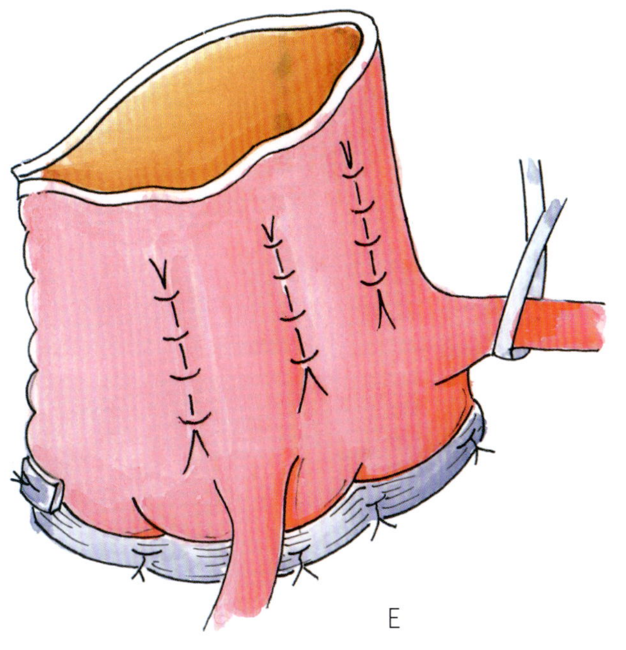

E. 在主动脉窦扩张部位做五条纵行折叠缝合，将主动脉窦的直径缩小到接近正常大小。用一毡条在左、右冠状动脉下穿过，在主动脉根部形成一个缝合环，预置的褥式缝线再由该缝合环穿出，逐一结扎。

E. Five longitudinal plications and sutures are performed at the dilated aortic sinus to narrow the diameter of the sinus. A felt strip is passed through the left and right coronary arteries, forming a suture ring at the aortic root, and the preset mattress suture is passed through the ring and ligated one by one.

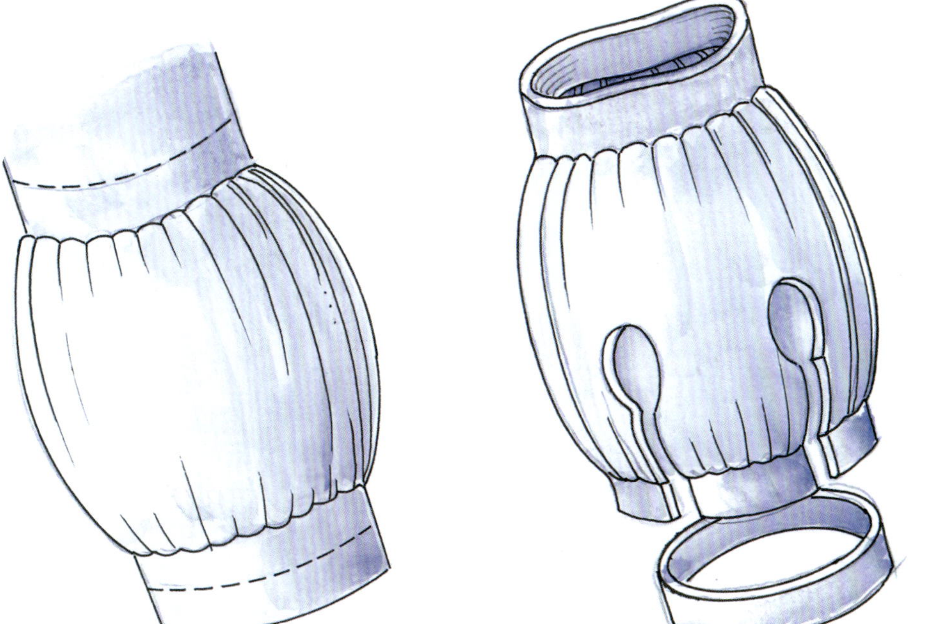

F. 选择一适当口径的球笼状人工血管，比照左、右冠状动脉的相应位置剪开。

F. Select a spherical cage-shaped artificial vessel with an appropriate diameter, and cut it according to the corresponding positions of the left and right coronary arteries.

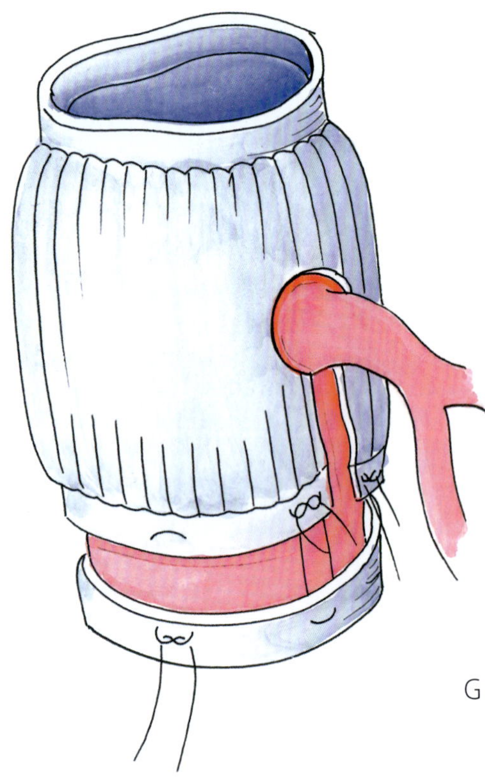

G. 剪开的球笼状人工血管循左、右冠状动脉向下插入，下端与根部缝合环做数针间断褥式缝合以固定人工血管。注意勿造成左、右冠状动脉的压迫和扭曲。

G. The incised spherical cage-shaped artificial vessel is inserted downward along the left and right coronary arteries, and its lower end is anastomosed to the root suture ring with interrupted mattress sutures to fix the position of the grafts. Care is taken to avoid compression and distortion of the left and right coronary arteries.

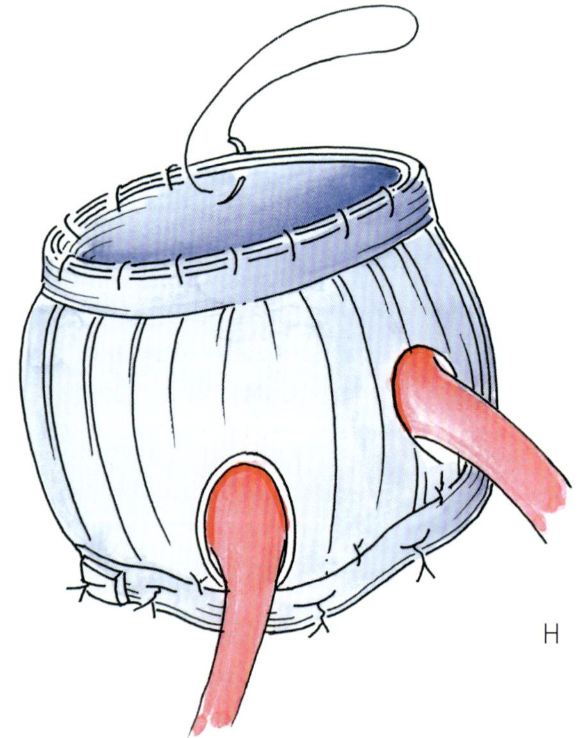

H. 人工血管远端与升主动脉近侧断端做一圈单纯连续缝合。

H. The distal end of the artificial vessel is anastomosed to the proximal stump of the ascending aorta with a simple continuous suture.

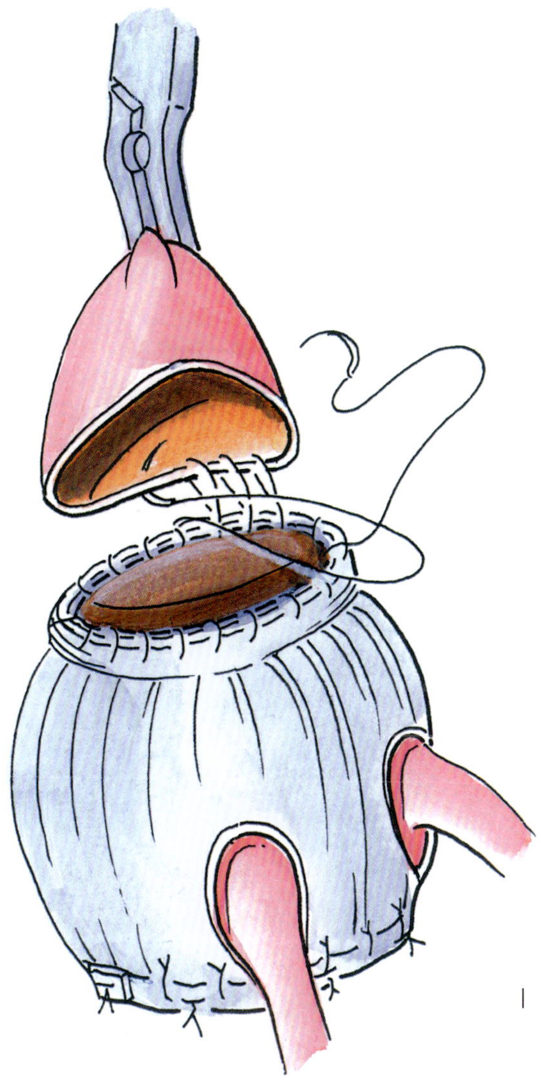

I. 再与升主动脉远侧断端行端端吻合。

I. An end-to-end anastomosis is performed between the artificial vessel and the distal stump of the ascending aorta.

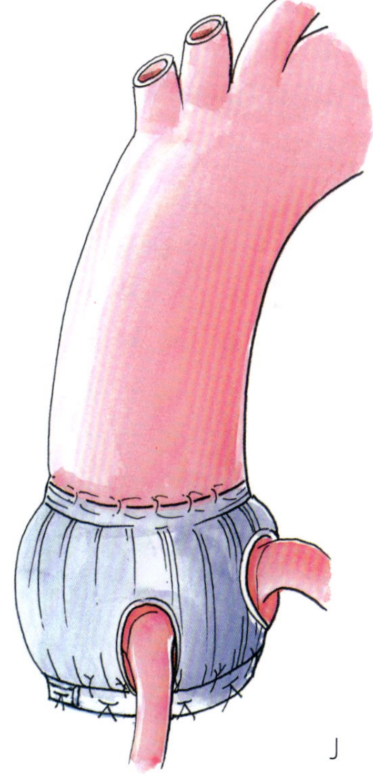

J. 吻合完成。

J. Anastomosis is completed.

图 4-2-4　保留瓣膜的升主动脉人工血管置换术

Figure 4-2-4　Ascending aorta graft replacement with valve-sparing technique

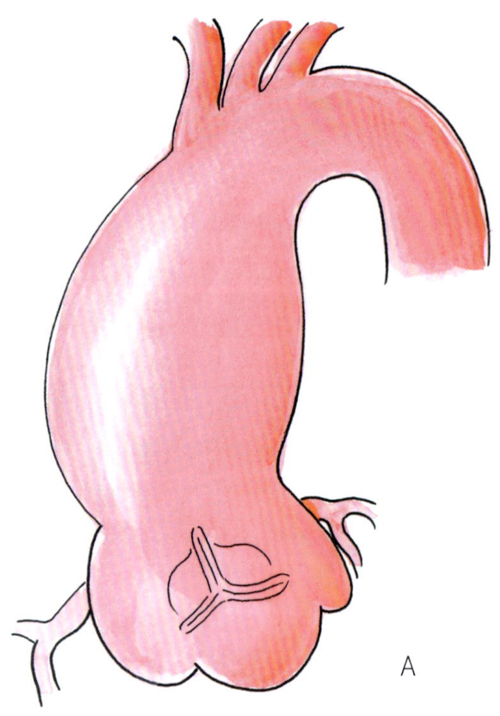

A. 升主动脉和主动脉窦同时扩张而主动脉环无明显扩张，主动脉瓣正常。

A. The ascending aorta and aortic sinus are dilated simultaneously without significant aortic ring dilation but with a normal aortic valve.

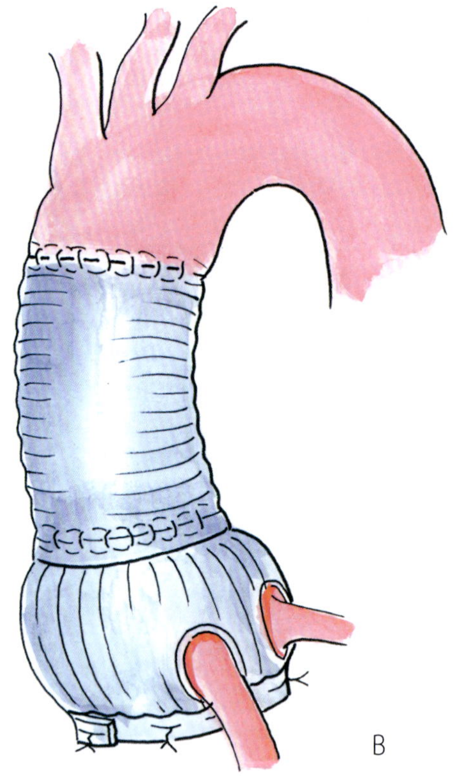

B. 在 Hetzer 法修复主动脉根部的基础上，切除升主动脉，植入另一段直筒型的人工血管。

B. Based on Hetzer repair of the aortic root, the ascending aorta is excised, and another straight artificial vessel is implanted.

图 4-2-5　升主动脉置换和主动脉瓣置换术
Figure 4-2-5　Separate replacement of ascending aorta and aortic valve

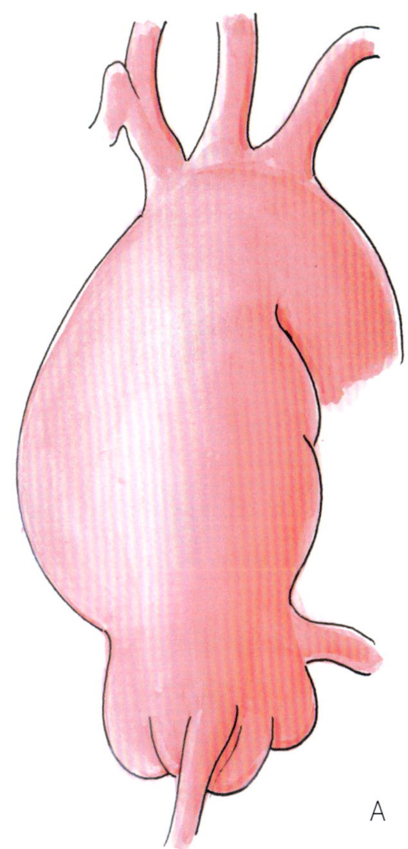

A. 主动脉瓣病变合并升主动脉瘤样扩张。
A. Aortic valve disease with ascending aortic aneurysm.

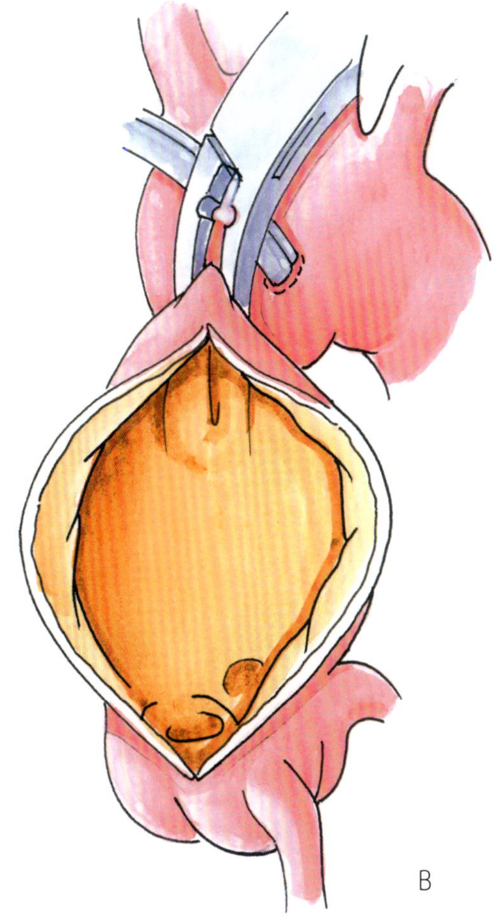

B. 体外循环下纵行切开升主动脉。
B. A longitudinal incision is made on the ascending aorta under extracorporeal circulation.

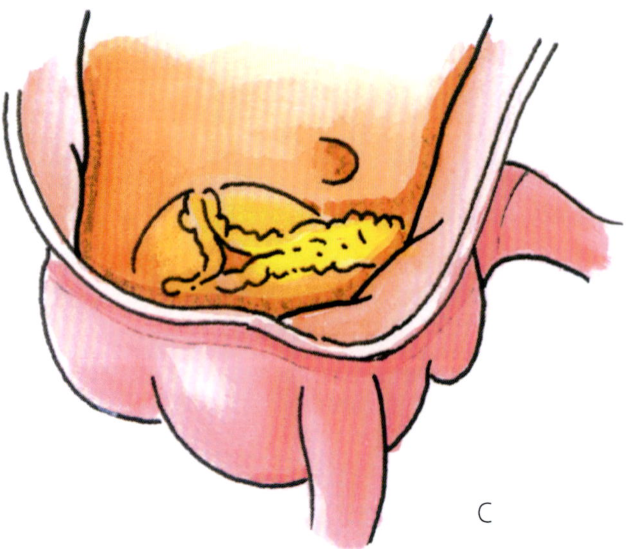

C. 检视并切除主动脉瓣叶。

C. Inspect and excise the aortic leaflets.

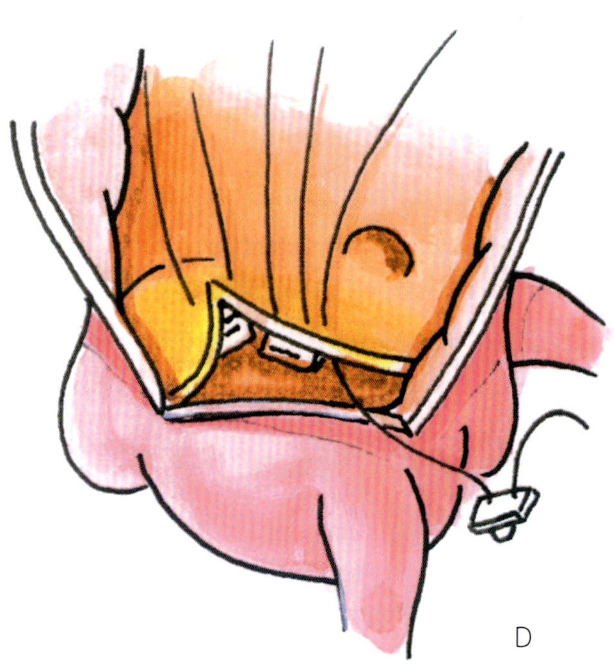

D. 带垫片间断褥式缝合植入匹配的人工瓣膜。

D. Implant a matched prosthetic valve and sew it with interrupted pledgeted mattress sutures.

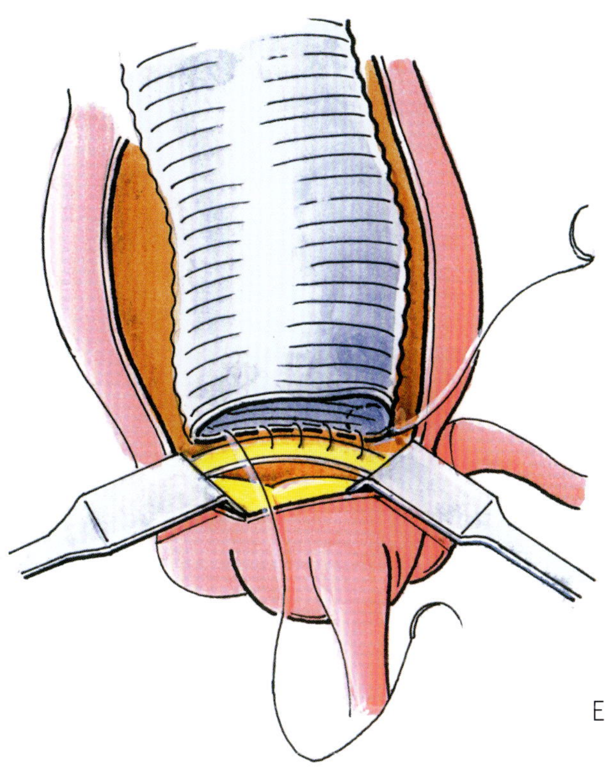

E. 选择一合适口径的人工血管，在窦管交界处与主动脉端端吻合。

E. An appropriate artificial vessel is anastomosed end to end to the aorta at the sinotubular junction.

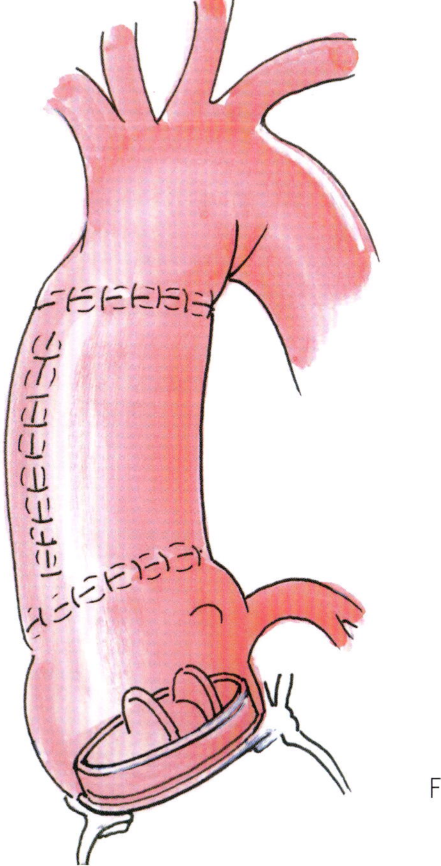

F. 人工血管另一端与升主动脉远端做端端吻合。修剪多余的主动脉壁，缝合包埋人工血管。

F. The other end of the graft is anastomosed end-to-end to the distal end of the ascending aorta. The redundant aortic wall is trimmed, and the graft is embedded and sutured.

图 4-2-6　带瓣外管道主动脉根部置换术(Bentall 手术)
Figure 4-2-6　Aortic root replacement with a composite valved conduit (Bentall procedure)

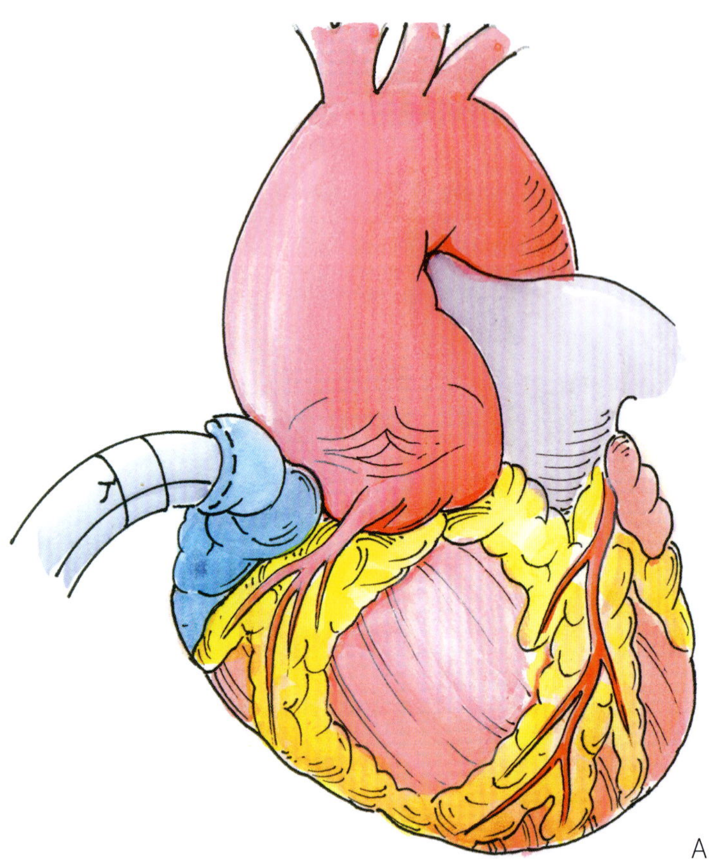

A. 主动脉根部病变伴升主动脉扩张。右心耳插二级静脉引流管,股动脉插供血管,建立体外循环。

A. Aortic root disease with dilated ascending aorta. A two-stage venous drainage cannula is inserted into the right atrial appendage, and the femoral artery is cannulated to establish extracorporeal circulation.

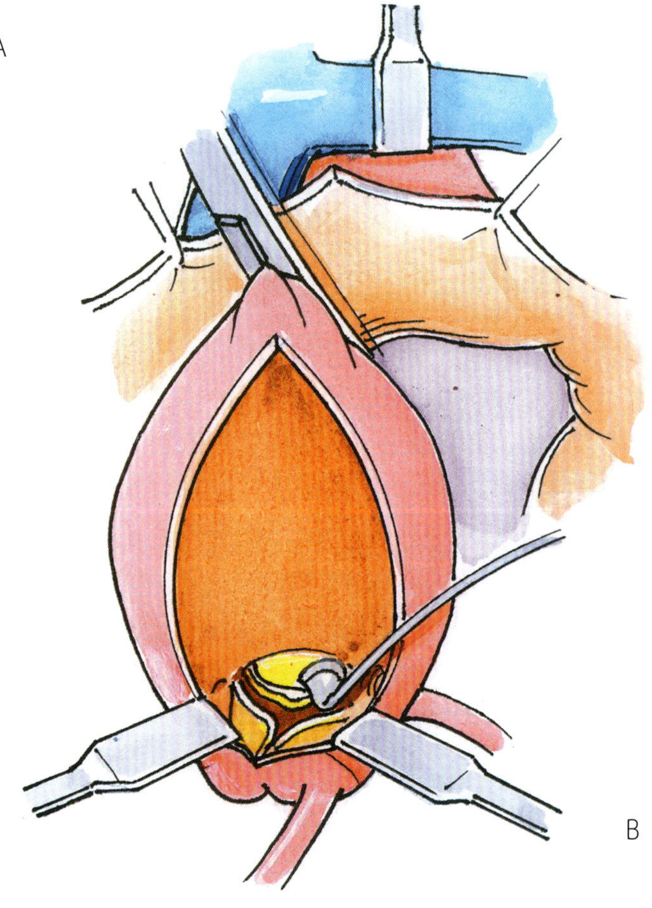

B. 升主动脉远端钳夹阻断,纵行切开升主动脉,经左、右冠状动脉开口灌注心肌保护液,心脏停搏。

B. The distal end of the ascending aorta is clamped and the ascending aorta is incised longitudinally. The cardioplegic solution is perfused through the ostia of the left and right coronary arteries, and the heart arrests.

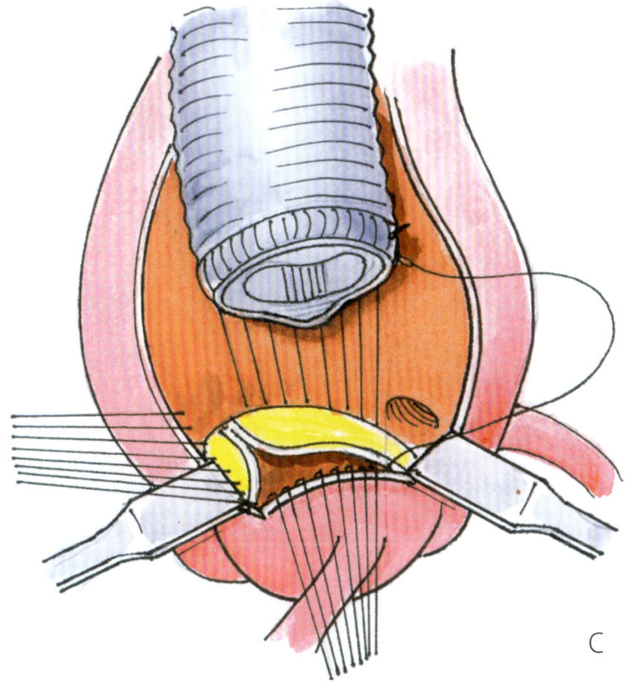

C. 切除主动脉瓣叶。根据主动脉瓣环大小选择合适口径的带瓣人工血管，用间断褥式缝合将其与主动脉瓣环缝合。

C. Resect the aortic leaflet. With interrupted mattress sutures, the aortic annulus is anastomosed to a valved artificial vessel appropriately sized by the aortic annulus.

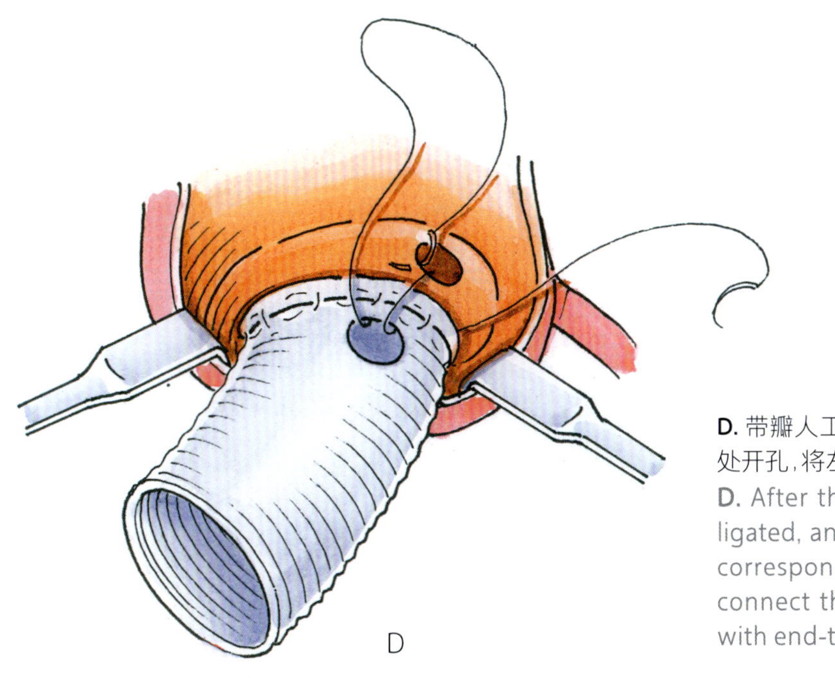

D. 带瓣人工血管推下结扎缝线后，在对应左冠状动脉开口处开孔，将左冠状动脉与人工血管端侧吻合。

D. After the valved artificial vessel is pushed down, ligated, and sutured, and a hole is made on the graft corresponding to the left coronary artery ostium to connect the left coronary artery and the prosthesis with end-to-side anastomosis.

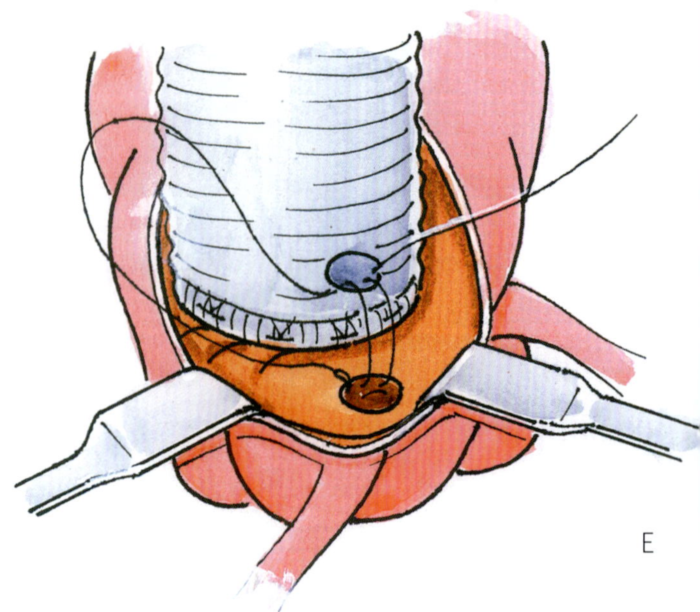

E. 人工血管对应右冠状动脉开口处开孔，将右冠状动脉与人工血管端侧吻合。

E. Another hole is made on the artificial vessel corresponding to the right coronary artery ostium. An end-to-side anastomosis of the right coronary artery to the artificial vessel is performed.

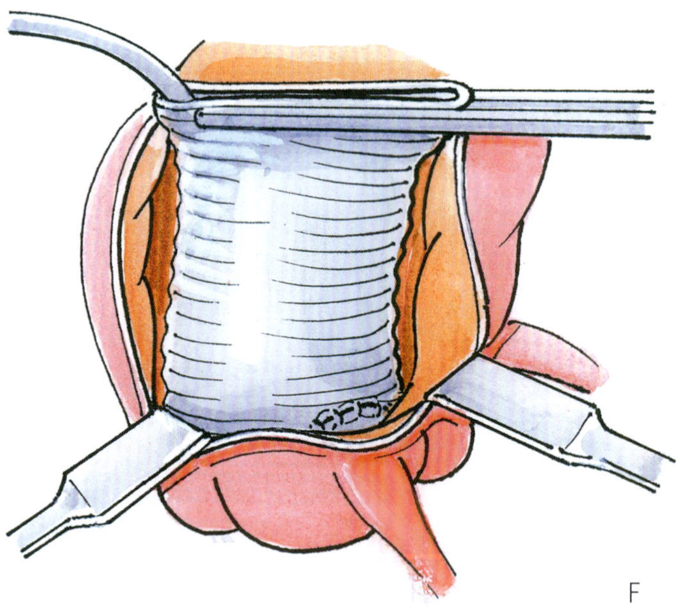

F. 加压注液检查吻合口无漏液。

F. Pressure injection is performed to assess the proximal anastomosis quality to avoid leakage.

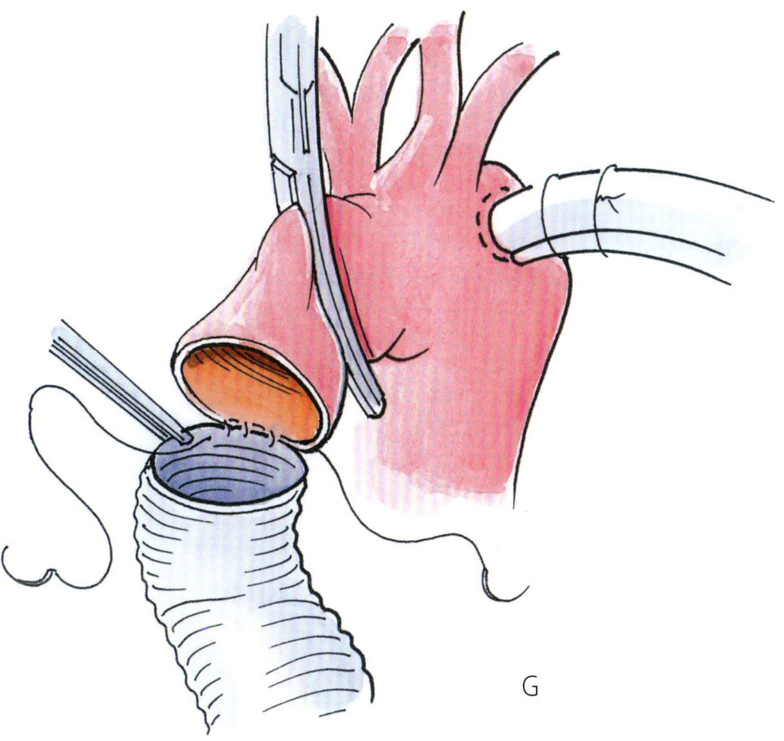

G. 升主动脉远端横断，与人工血管端端吻合。
G. The ascending aorta is transected distally and anastomosed end-to-end to the artificial vessel.

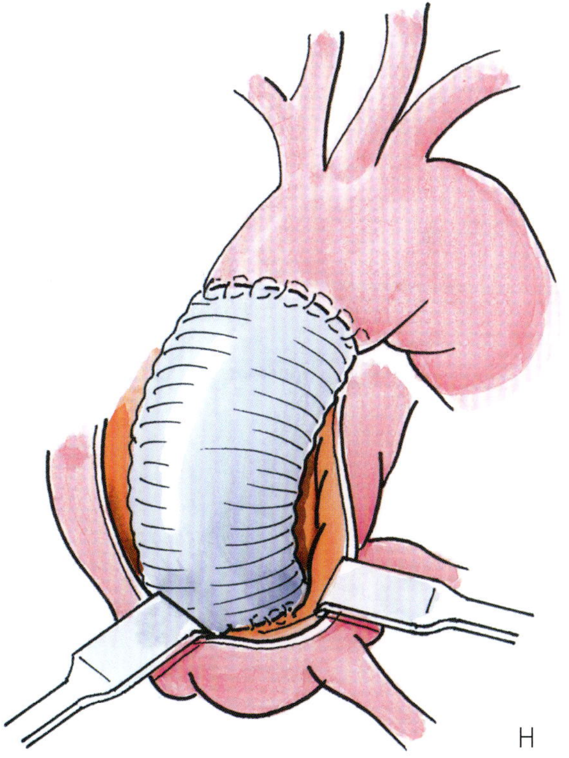

H. 吻合完毕。
H. Anastomosis is completed.

图 4-2-7 Cabrol 技术重建冠状动脉血流
Figure 4-2-7 Cabrol technique for reestablishment of coronary flow

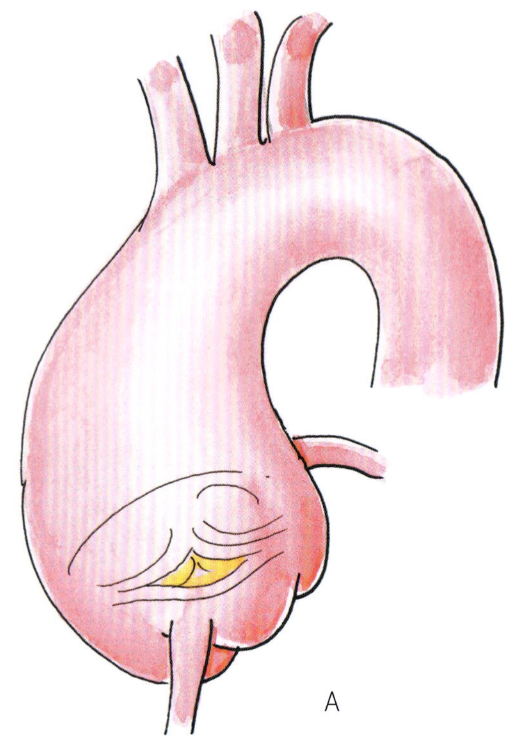

A. 主动脉根部病变累及主动脉瓣。
A. Aortic root disease involves the aortic valve.

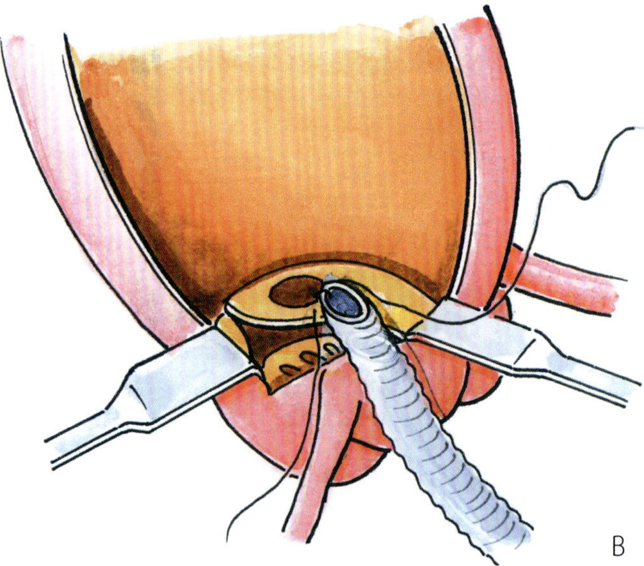

B. 切除主动脉瓣叶。为避免冠状动脉吻合口张力，将左、右冠状动脉开口分别与直径 0.8~1cm 的人工血管两端做端端吻合。先做左冠状动脉与人工血管的吻合。
B. Remove the aortic leaflet. In order to avoid the tension of the coronary artery anastomotic site, end-to-end anastomosis is performed between the left and right coronary artery ostia and both ends of 0.8-1 cm-diameter artificial vessels. The left coronary artery is first anastomosed to the artificial vessel.

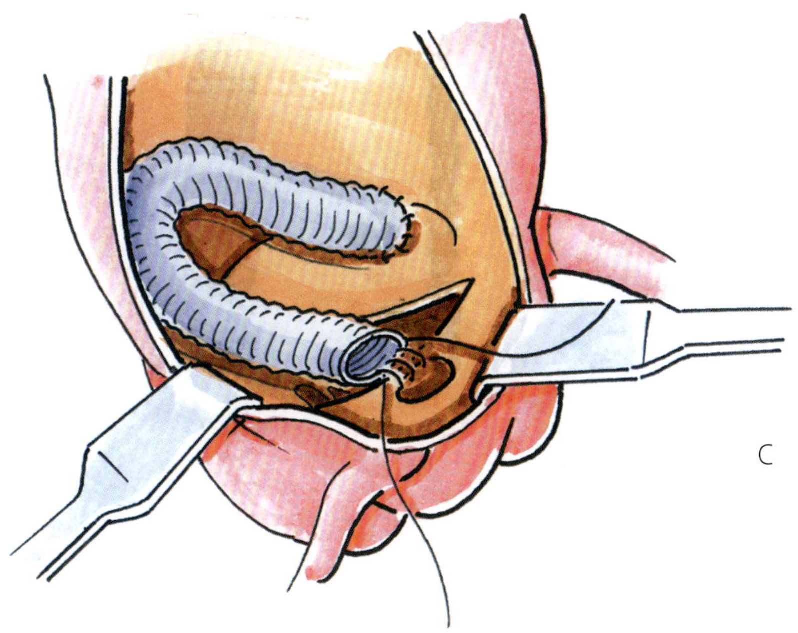

C. 再做右冠状动脉与人工血管的端端吻合。
C. The right coronary artery is sutured to the graft by using an end-to-end anastomosis.

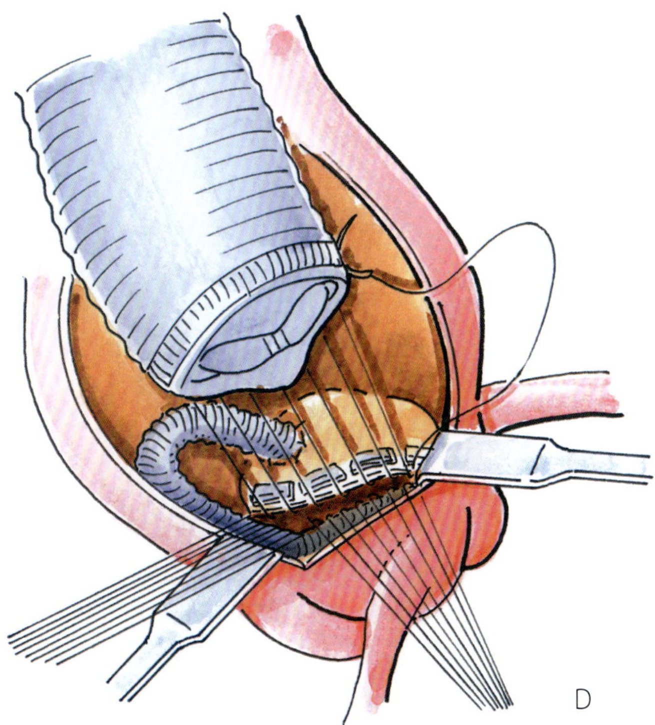

D. 带垫片间断褥式缝合将带瓣人工血管缝至主动脉瓣环。
D. The valved artificial vessel is attached to the aortic annulus with pledgeted interrupted mattress sutures.

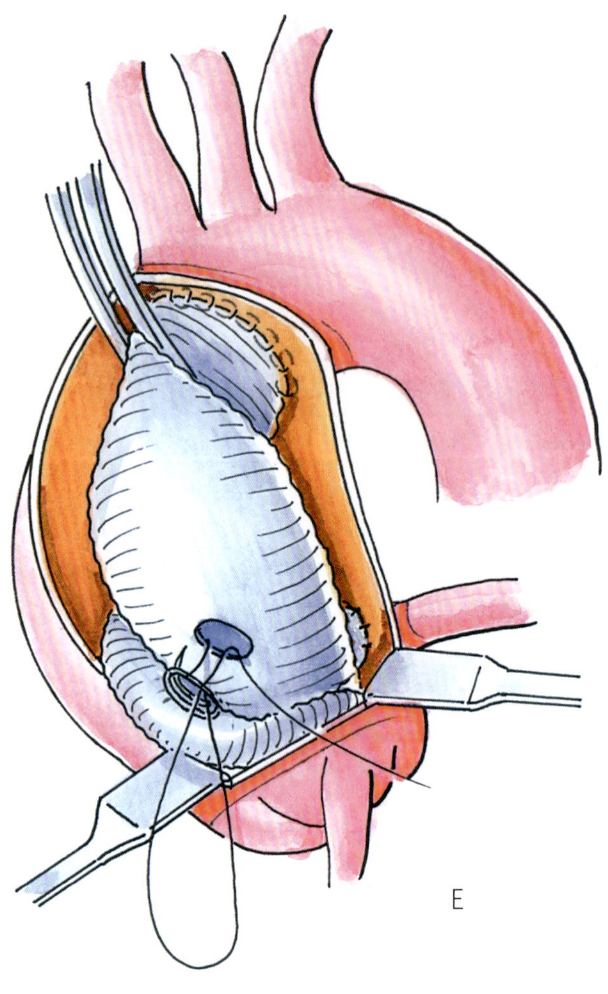

E. 人工血管另一端与远端升主动脉端端吻合。将连接冠状动脉的人工血管与带瓣人工血管分别开口做侧侧吻合。

E. The other end of the valved artificial vessel is anastomosed end-to-end to the distal ascending aorta. An opening is made in the two grafts respectively, connecting them with side-to-side anastomosis.

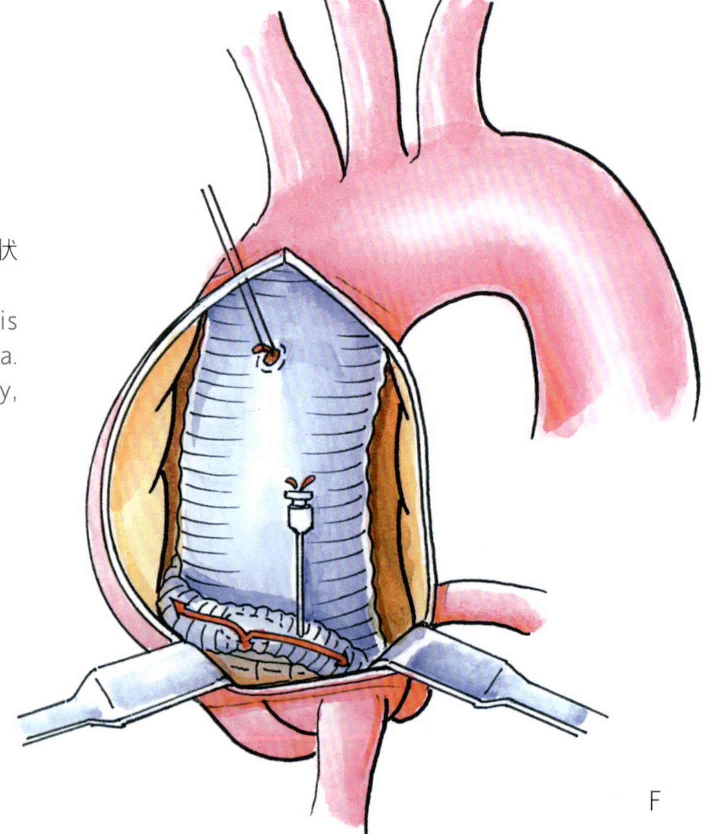

F. 两人工血管分别戳孔，开放主动脉阻断钳，排气后缝闭人工血管戳孔。

F. Poke a hole in the two grafts respectively, release the aortic blocking forceps, and repair the hole after venting.

图 4-2-8 主动脉窦部分切除成形术
Figure 4-2-8 Partial resection and angioplasty of aortic sinus

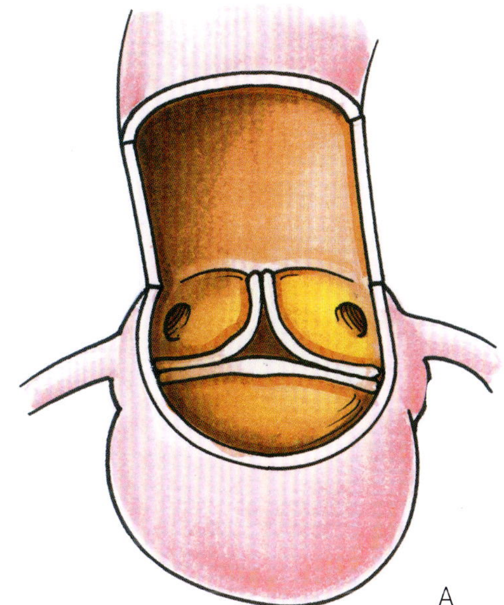

A. 主动脉无冠窦扩大。
A. Enlargement of noncoronary aortic cusp.

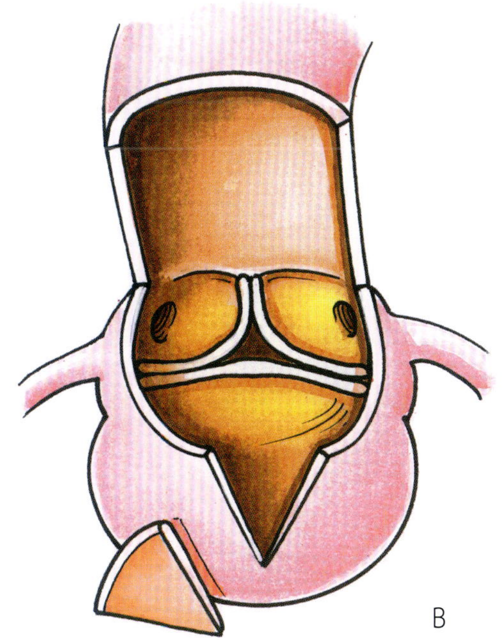

B. 无冠窦壁做一三角形切除。
B. A triangular resection of the noncoronary aortic cusp wall is performed.

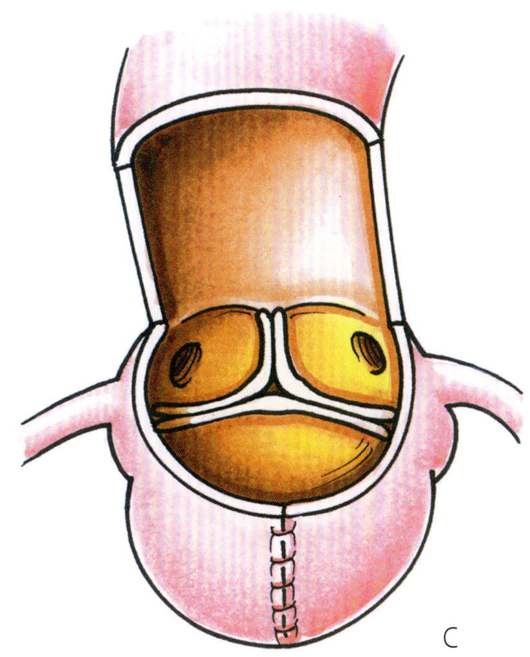

C. 连续缝合无冠窦切口。
C. Close noncoronary sinus incision with running sutures.

图 4-2-9　保留瓣膜的主动脉瓣根部置换术(David 手术)
Figure 4-2-9　Valve-sparing aortic root replacement (David procedure)

保留瓣膜的主动脉瓣根部置换术(valve-sparing aortic root replacement, VSRR)用于治疗瓣膜质地良好的主动脉根部病变,David 手术是 VSRR 的主要术式之一,亦称主动脉根部再植入术。

Valve-sparing aortic root replacement (VSRR) is used for the treatment of aortic root diseases with good valve quality. The David procedure is one of the main surgical approaches for VSRR, also known as aortic root reimplantation.

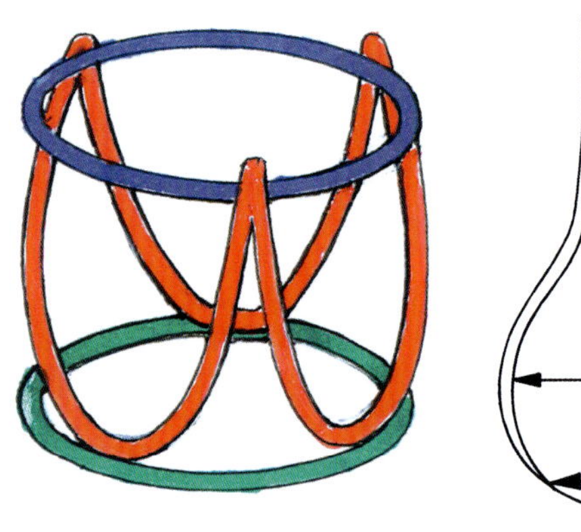

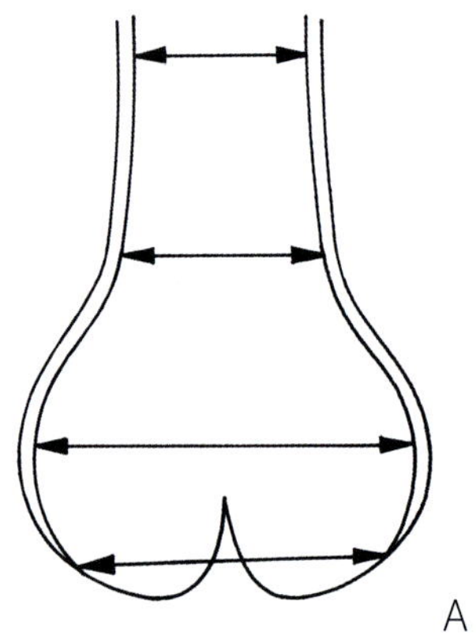

A

A. 主动脉根部包括左心室主动脉连接、主动脉窦、主动脉瓣环、主动脉瓣叶和窦管交界(sinotubular junction, STJ)五部分。

A. Aortic root consists of five parts: left ventricular-aortic junction, Valsalva sinus, aortic annulus, aortic valve leaflet, and sinotubular junction (STJ).

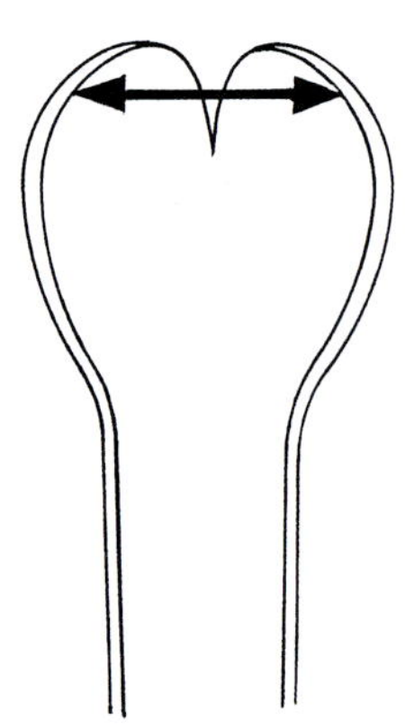

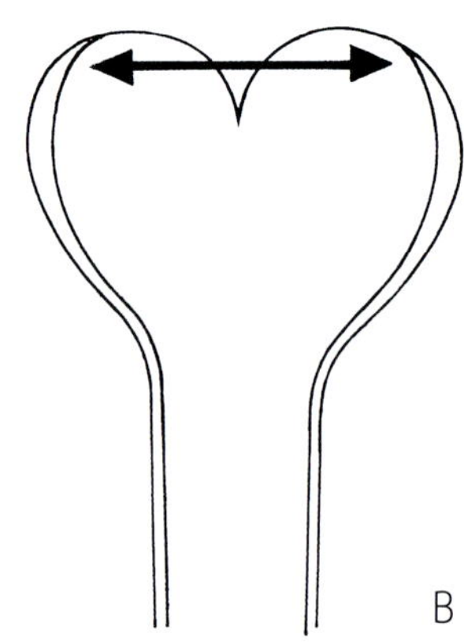

B

B. David 手术适用于伴有左心室主动脉连接扩张的主动脉根部病变,主动脉瓣叶本身无明显病变。

B. The David procedure is indicated for aortic root lesions with dilation of left ventricular aortic connections, with no significant lesions in the aortic leaflets.

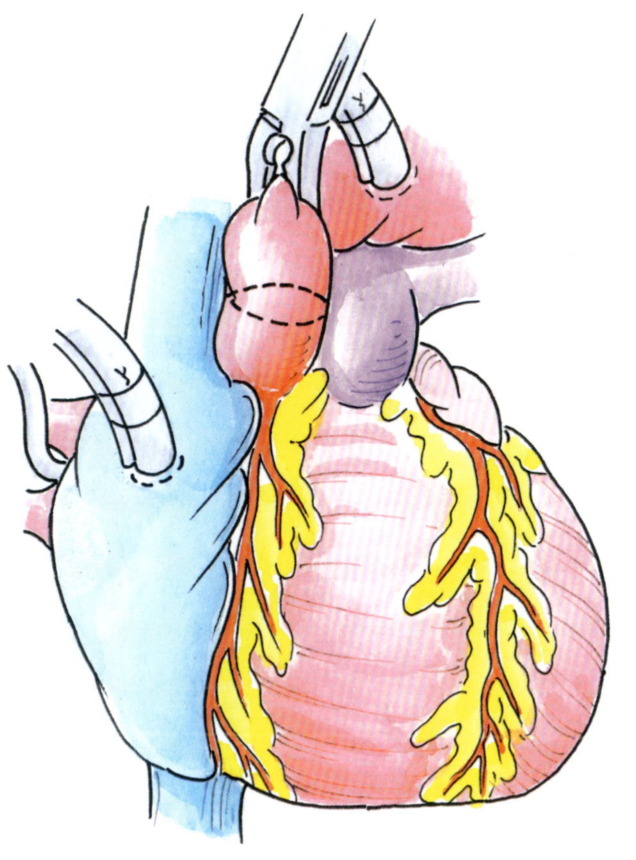

C. 建立体外循环，心脏停搏后在窦管交界上方 1cm 横断升主动脉。

C. With extracorporeal circulation established, the ascending aorta is transected 1 cm above the STJ after cardiac arrest.

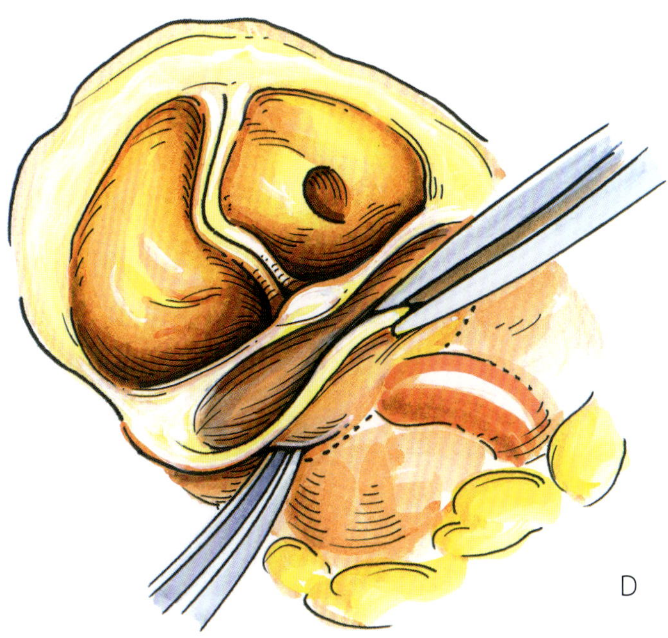

D. 游离主动脉根部至主动脉瓣环水平。

D. Free aortic root to the level of the aortic annulus.

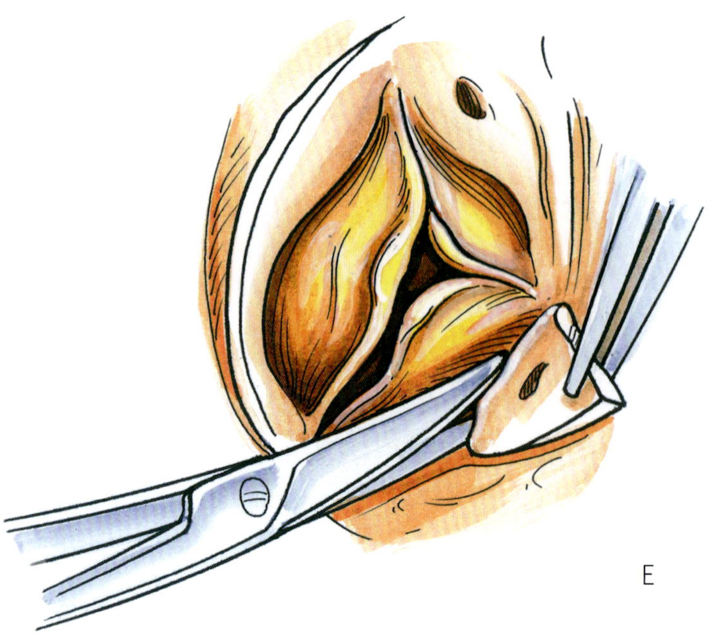

E. 左、右冠状动脉开口纽扣状分离。
E. Button-like separation of left and right coronary ostia.

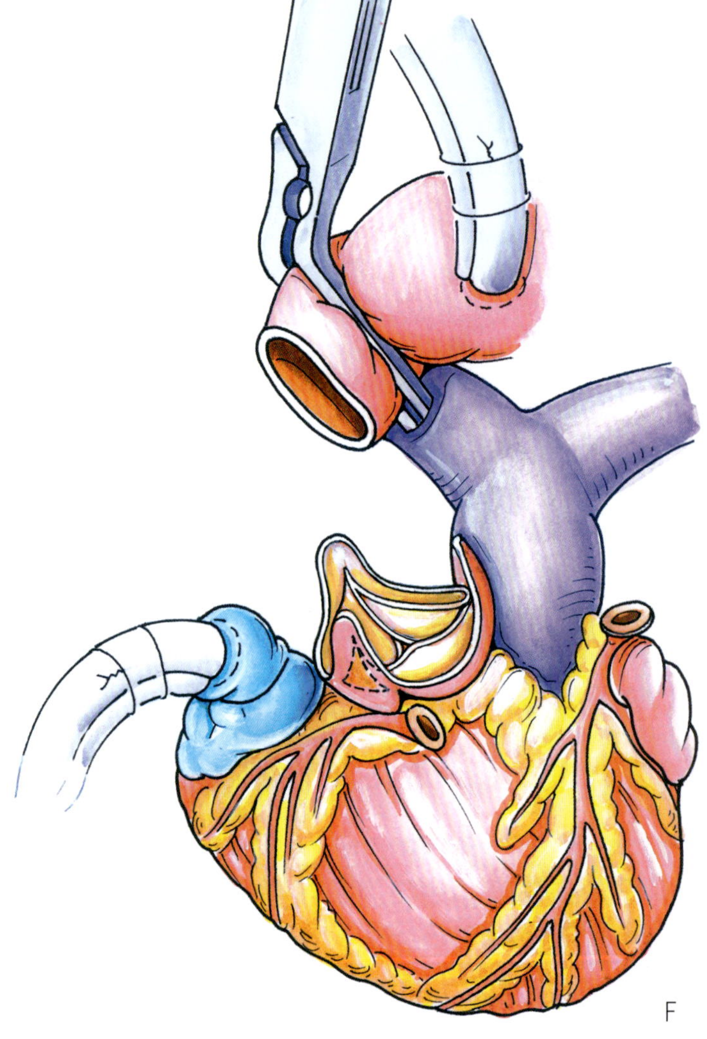

F. 距主动脉瓣环约 5mm 切除主动脉窦壁。
F. The aortic sinus wall is resected about 5 mm to the aortic annulus.

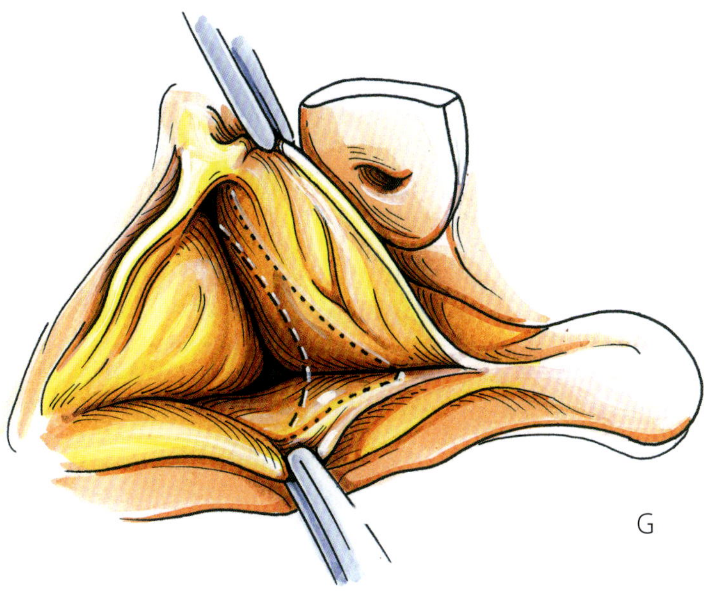

G. 牵开主动脉瓣叶，显露左心室主动脉连接，插入测瓣器测量左心室主动脉连接内径。选用大于测量值 3~5mm 直径的人工血管。

G. Retract the aortic valve leaflet, expose the left ventricular aortic connection, and insert a sizer to measure the inner diameter of the left ventricular aortic connection. Select a artificial vessel with a diameter 3-5 mm larger than the measured value.

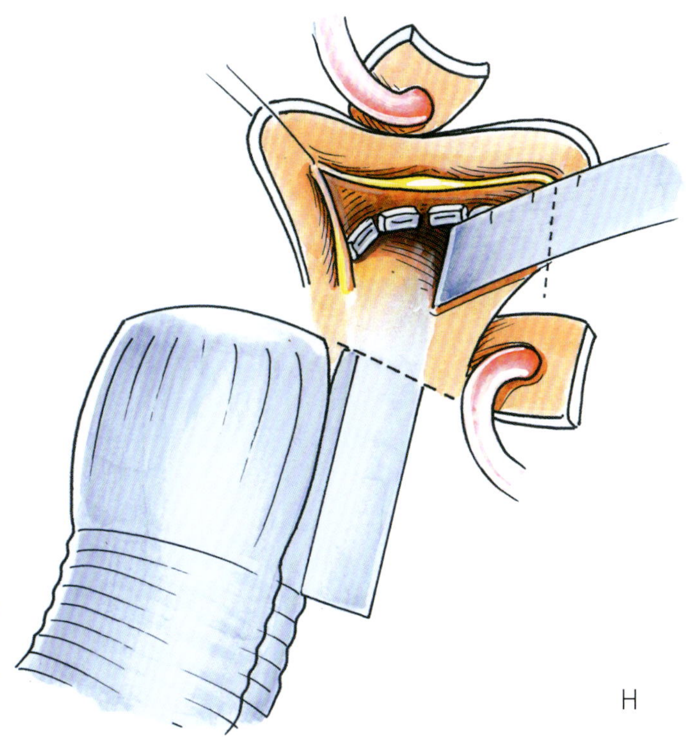

H. 测量左心室主动脉连接到主动脉瓣交界的距离，以此确定人工血管膨出部分的长度。

H. The length of the graft bulge is determined by the distance between the left ventricular aortic connection and the aortic valve junction.

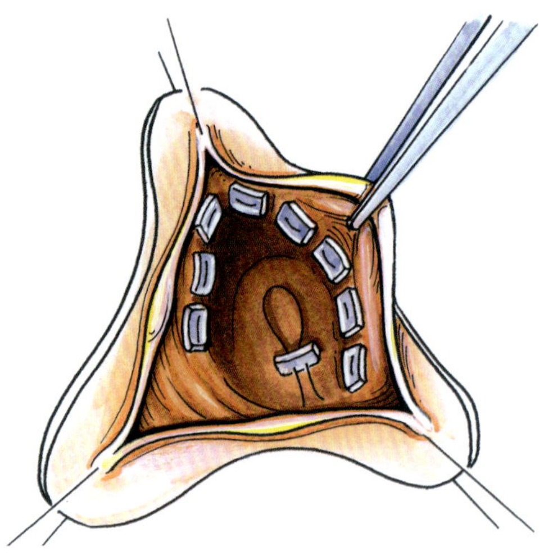

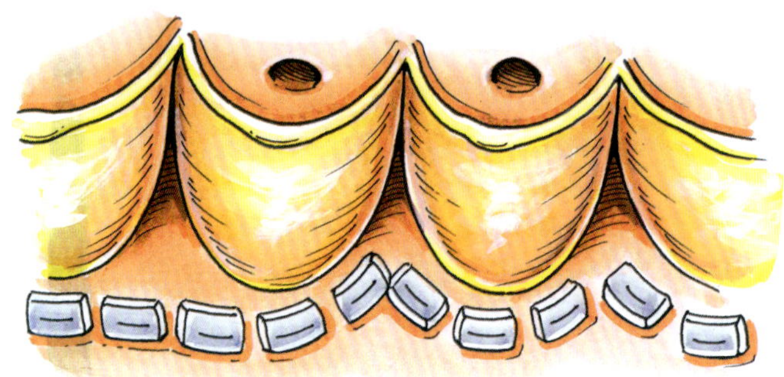

I. 沿左心室主动脉连接由心内向心外置入一圈带垫片褥式缝线。

I. A loop of pledgeted mattress sutures is placed in the heart from inside to outside along the left ventricular aortic connection.

I

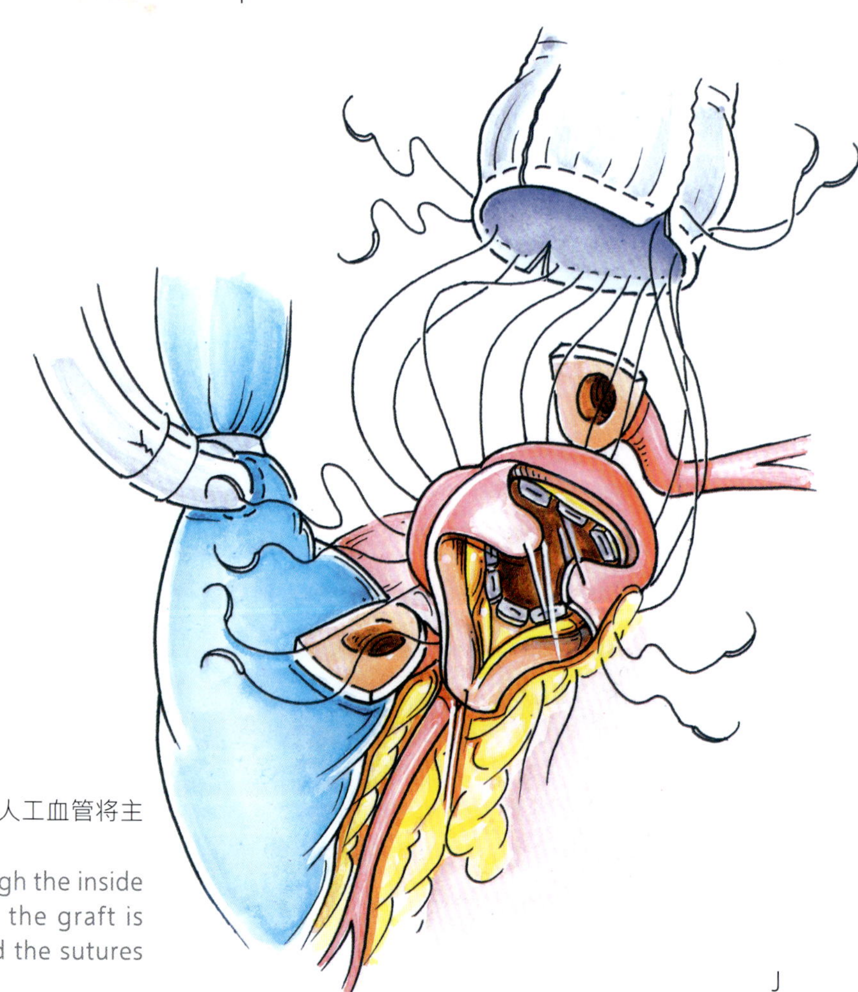

J

J. 褥式缝线从人工血管由内向外缝出，推下人工血管将主动脉残端套入，逐一结扎缝线。

J. The mattress sutures are passed through the inside of the artificial vessel to the outside, the graft is pushed down into the aortic stump and the sutures are ligated one by one.

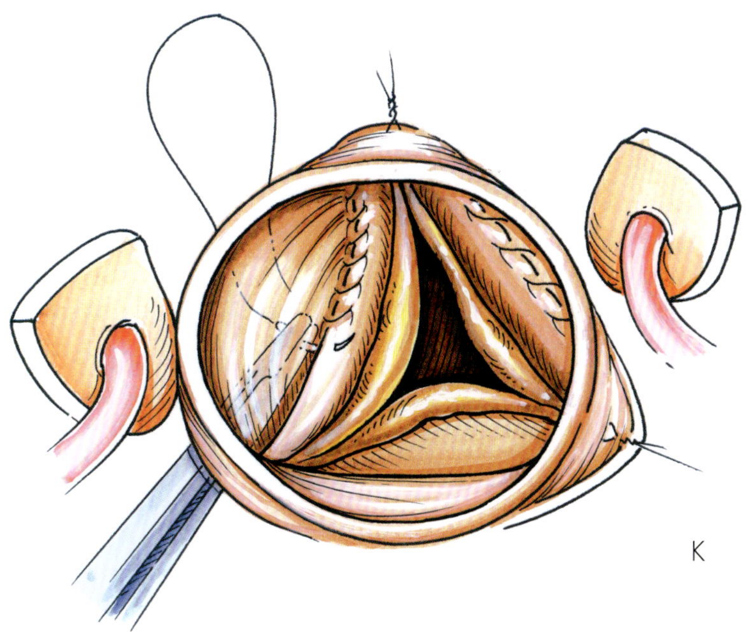

K. 先将主动脉瓣交界缝到人工血管对应位置，勿使血管扭曲，确保主动脉瓣对合良好。然后将主动脉窦壁残端缝到人工血管上。

K. Sew the aortic valve commissures to the corresponding position of the graft first, and do not distort the graft to ensure that the aortic valve is well aligned. The stump of the aortic sinus wall is then sutured to the graft.

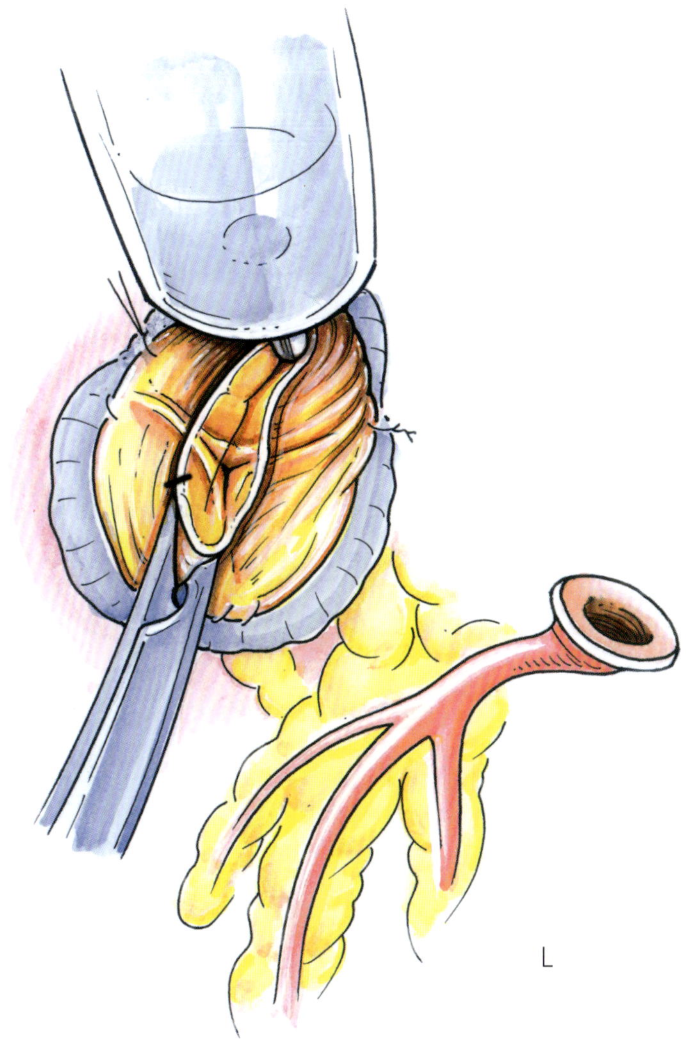

L. 加压注水检查主动脉瓣闭合情况和吻合口有无漏血。

L. Pressure injection is performed to check for aortic valve closure and anastomotic leakage.

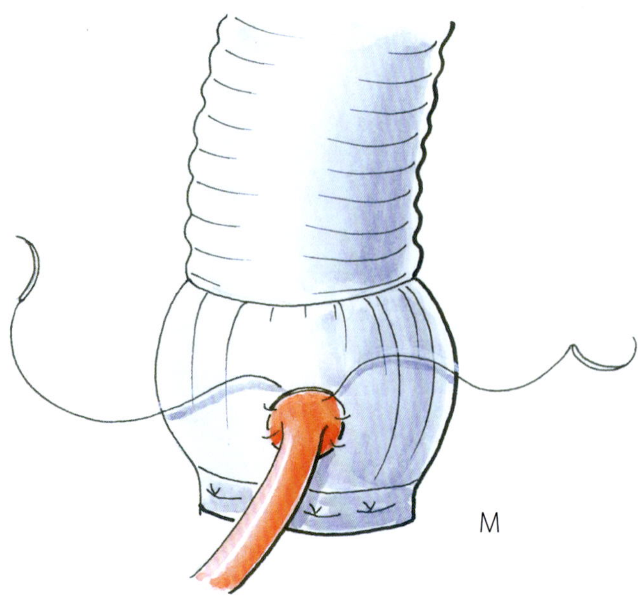

M. 人工血管开孔完成与左、右冠状动脉的吻合。

M. After making holes, the graft is anastomosed to the left and right coronary arteries.

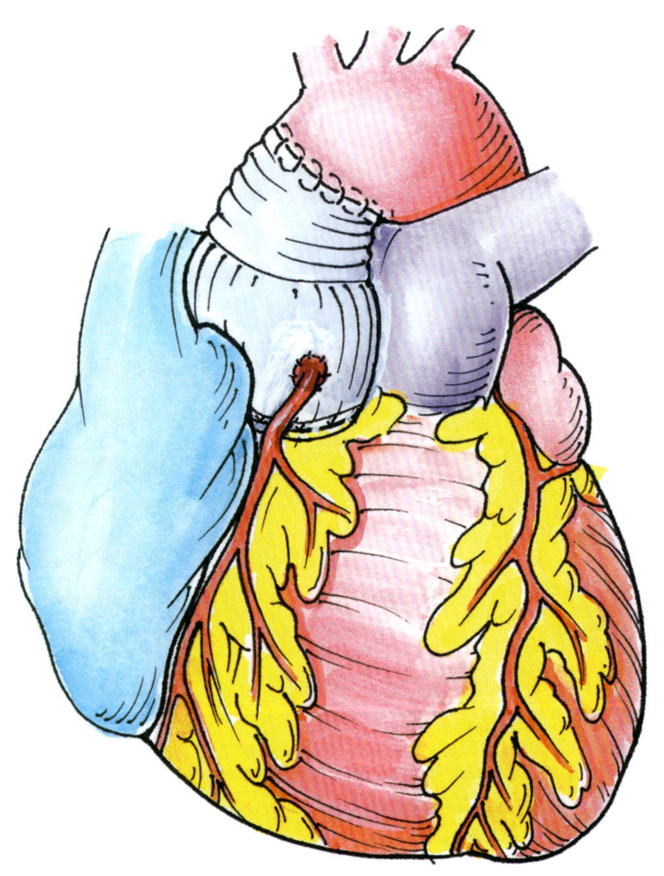

N. 人工血管与升主动脉端端吻合。

N. The graft is anastomosed end-to-end to the ascending aorta.

图 4-2-10 保留瓣膜的主动脉瓣根部置换术（Yacoub 手术）
Figure 4-2-10 Valve-sparing aortic root replacement (Yacoub technique)

Yacoub 手术是 VSRR 的另一主要术式，亦称主动脉根部重塑术。该手术操作相对 David 手术较为简单，但由于不对主动脉瓣环加以限制，远期瓣环进行性扩大导致瓣膜关闭不全复发的风险较大。

The Yacoub procedure is another major procedure for VSRR, also known as aortic root remodeling. The Yacoub procedure is simpler than David's, but it usually has a greater risk of recurrent valve insufficiency due to the progressive enlargement of the long-term annulus without restrictions on the aortic annulus.

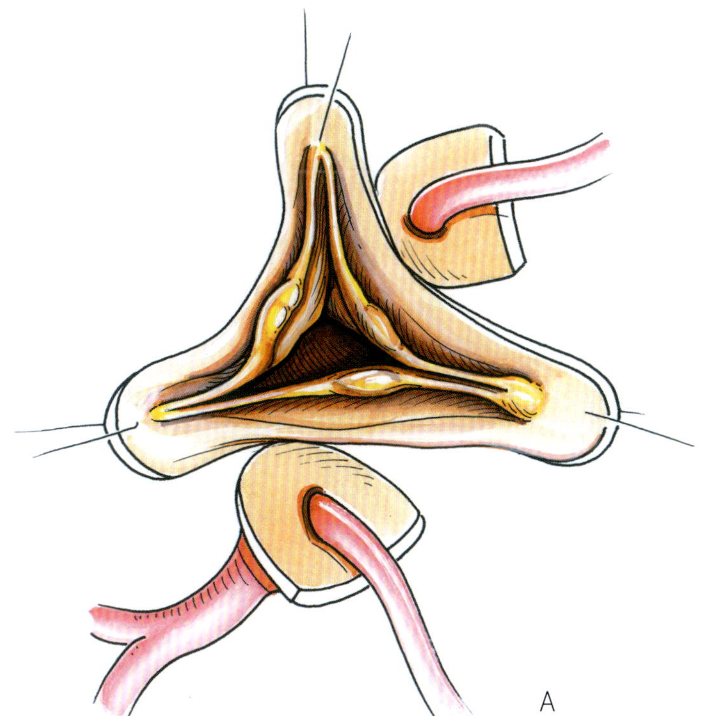

A. 彻底切除主动脉根部病变组织，仅保留距主动脉瓣环 5mm 左右主动脉窦壁，左、右冠状动脉开口纽扣状分离。

A. Radical resection of the diseased tissue at the aortic root is performed, only about 5 mm of the aortic sinus wall away from the aortic annulus is preserved, and button-like separation is made on the left and right coronary artery ostia.

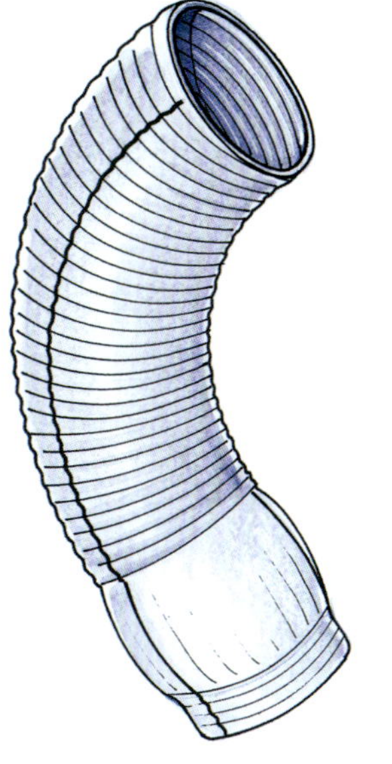

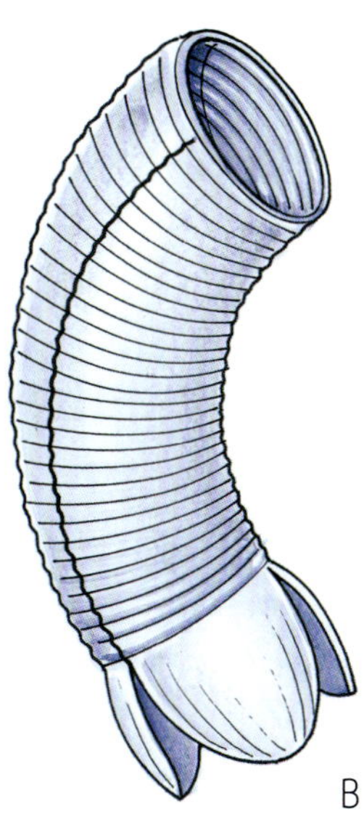

B. 如果没有主动脉瓣环扩张和主动脉瓣关闭不全，就按照窦管交界的直径选用人工血管，人工血管下端裁剪成新的主动脉窦壁。

B. With the absence of aortic annular dilatation and aortic valve insufficiency, an artificial vessel is chosen depending on the STJ diameter, and its lower end is clipped into a new aortic sinus wall.

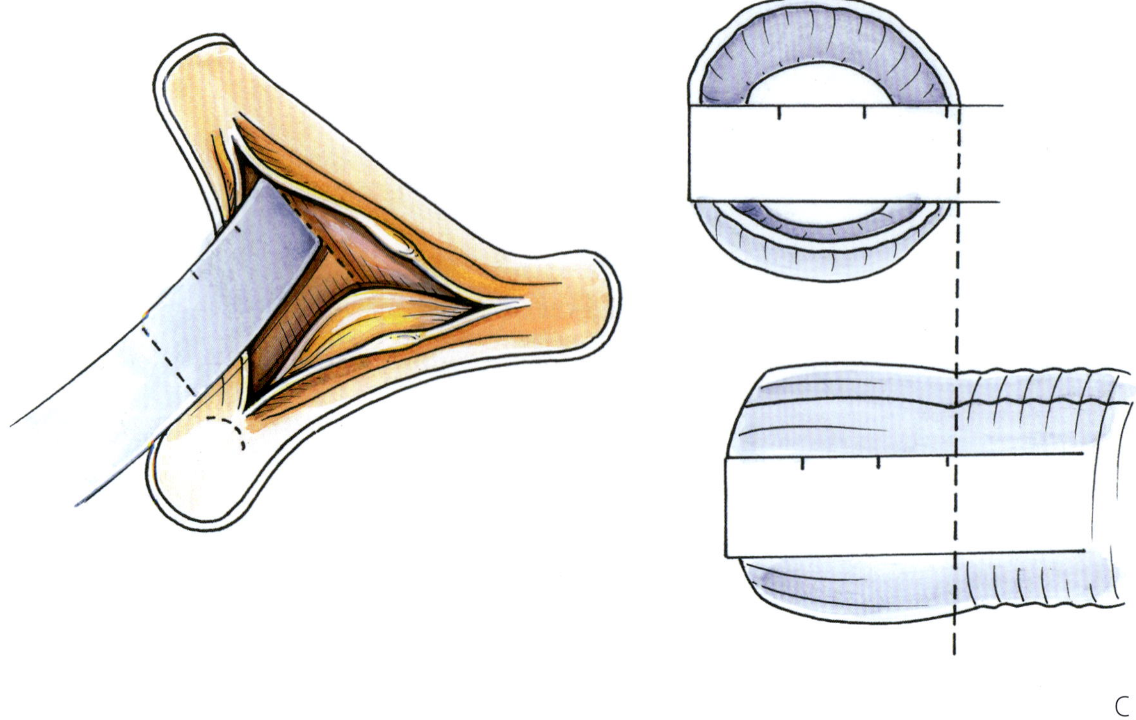

C. 新主动脉窦壁的高度约等于人工血管的直径。

C. The height of the new aortic sinus wall is approximately equal to the diameter of the graft.

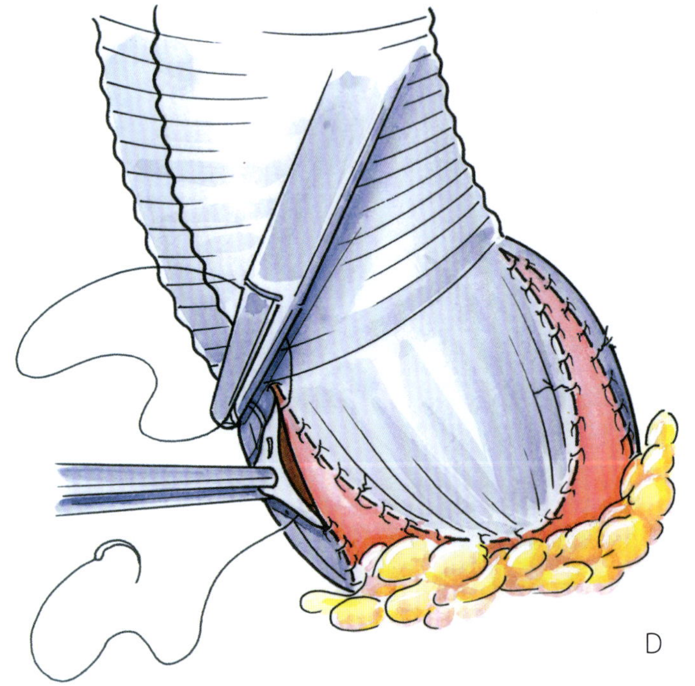

D. 先将三个交界缝到人工血管上，然后将人工血管与残留的主动脉窦壁连续缝合。

D. Three commissures are sutured to the graft and the graft is attached to the residual aortic sinus wall with continuous sutures.

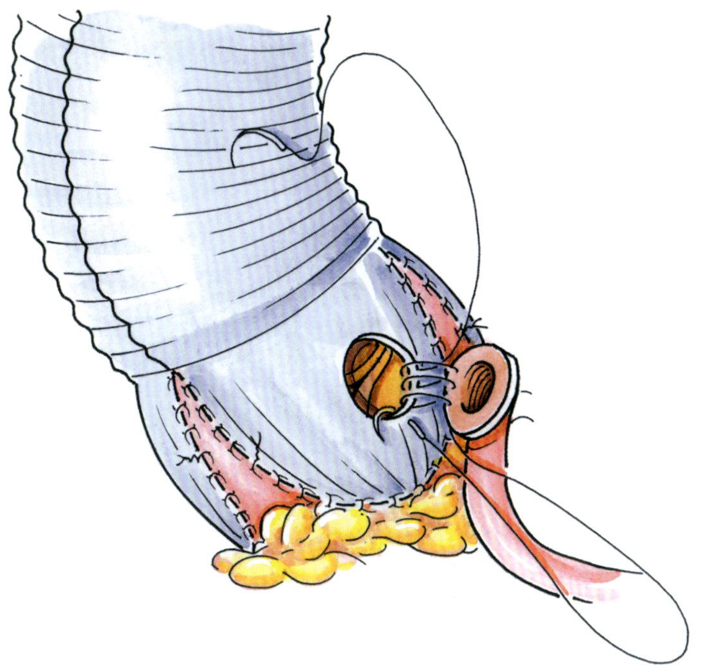

E. 人工血管开孔，与左、右冠状动脉纽扣片端侧吻合。

E. When holes in the graft are made, end-to-side anastomoses of the graft and the left and right coronary artery with buttons are performed.

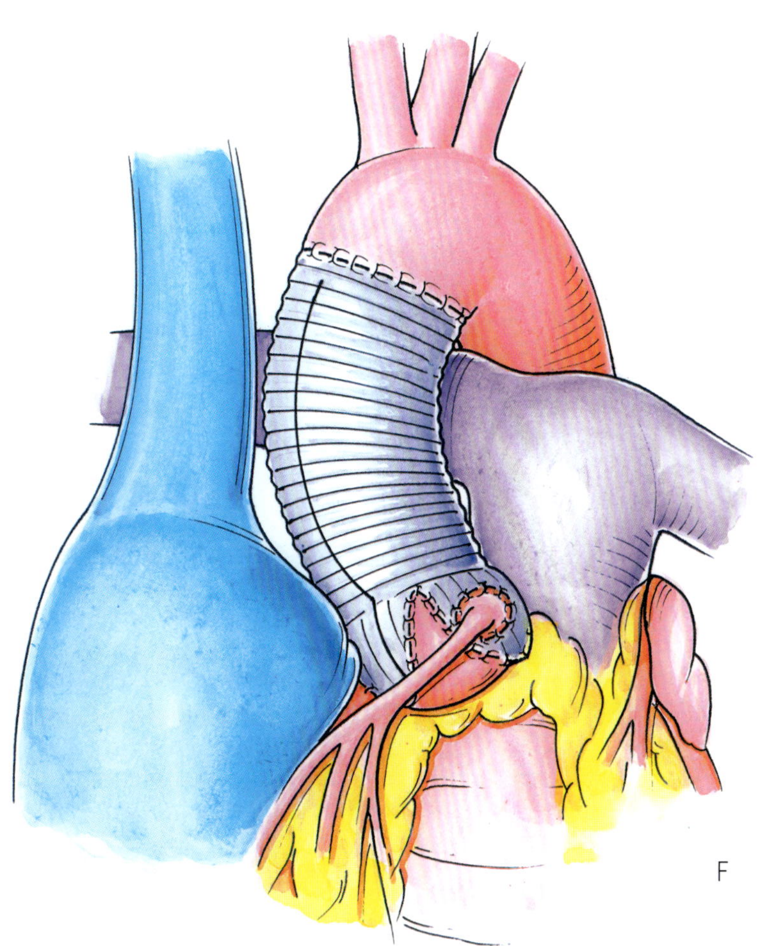

F. 人工血管与升主动脉端端吻合。

F. The graft is anastomosed end-to-end to the ascending aorta.

第 三 节　主动脉弓动脉瘤
Section 3　Aortic Arch Aneurysm

图 4-3-1　主动脉弓人工血管置换术
Figure 4-3-1　Aortic arch graft replacement

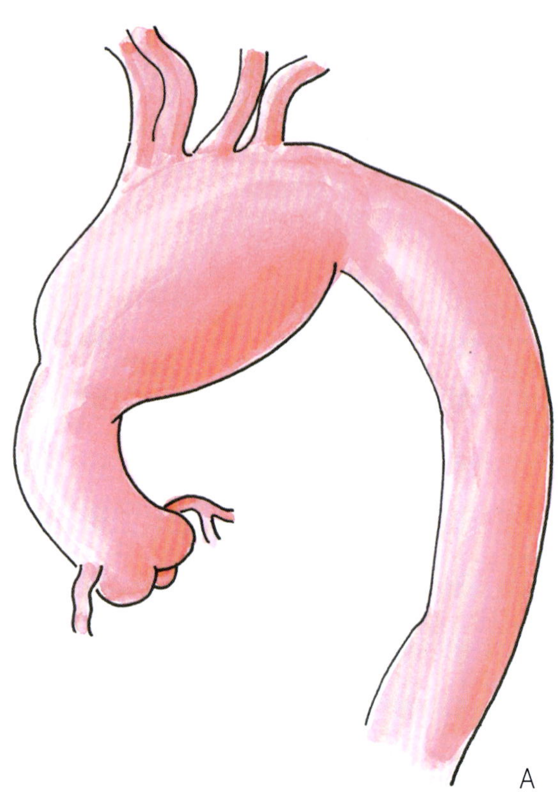

A. 主动脉弓梭形动脉瘤。
A. Fusiform aortic aneurysm.

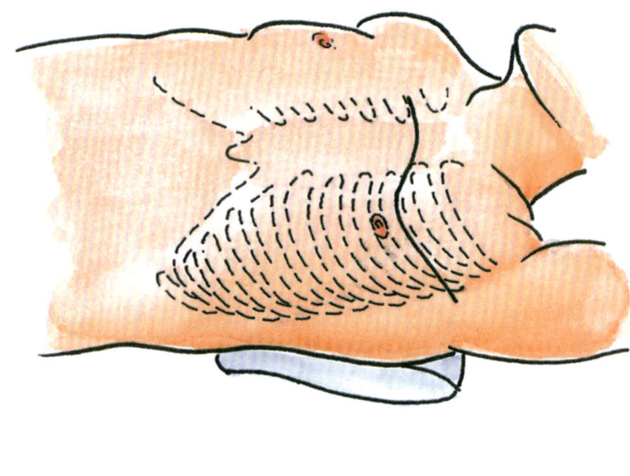

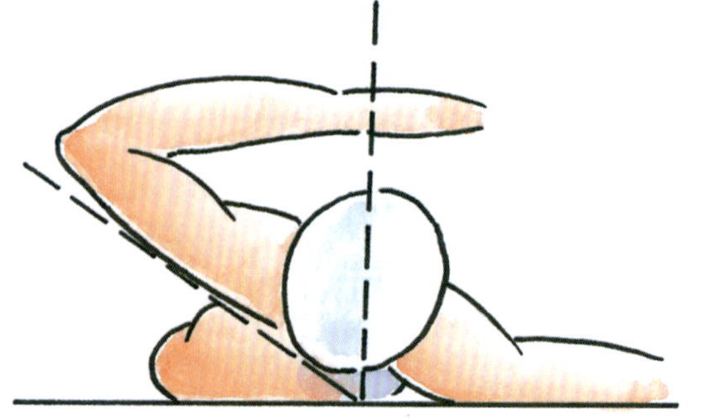

B. 仰卧位，左胸垫高。左前胸第 3 肋间切口，向右横断胸骨至右胸第 2 肋间。
B. In the supine position, the patient's left chest is elevated. An incision is placed at the third intercostal space of the left anterior chest and extended to the right and across the sternum to the second intercostal space of the right chest.

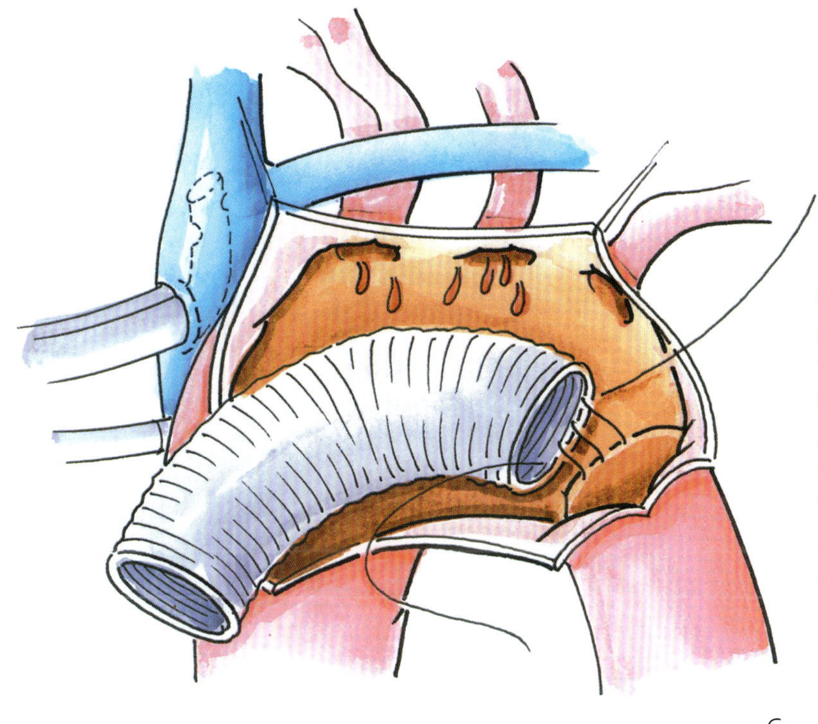

C. 深低温停循环，切开远段升主动脉，切口向主动脉弓延长至弓降部。选择合适口径的人工血管与降主动脉端端吻合。

C. Under deep hypothermic circulatory arrest, an incision is placed at the distal segment of the ascending aorta and extended toward the aortic arch to the descending arch. An appropriate aortic graft is used for end-to-end anastomosis with the descending aorta.

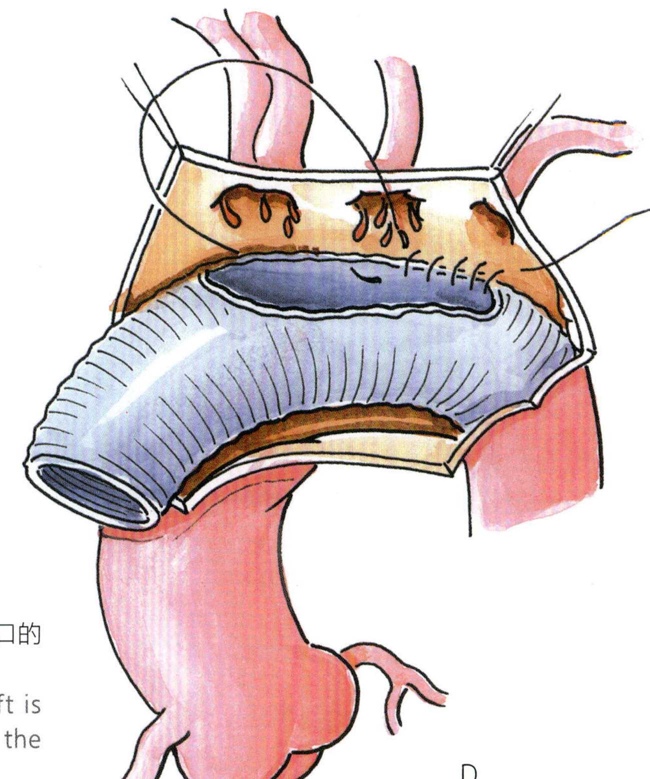

D. 人工血管顶部椭圆形开窗，与包含三个头臂动脉开口的主动脉弓顶部吻合。

D. With oval fenestration on the roof, the graft is anastomosed with the roof of the arch containing the ostia of the three brachiocephalic arteries.

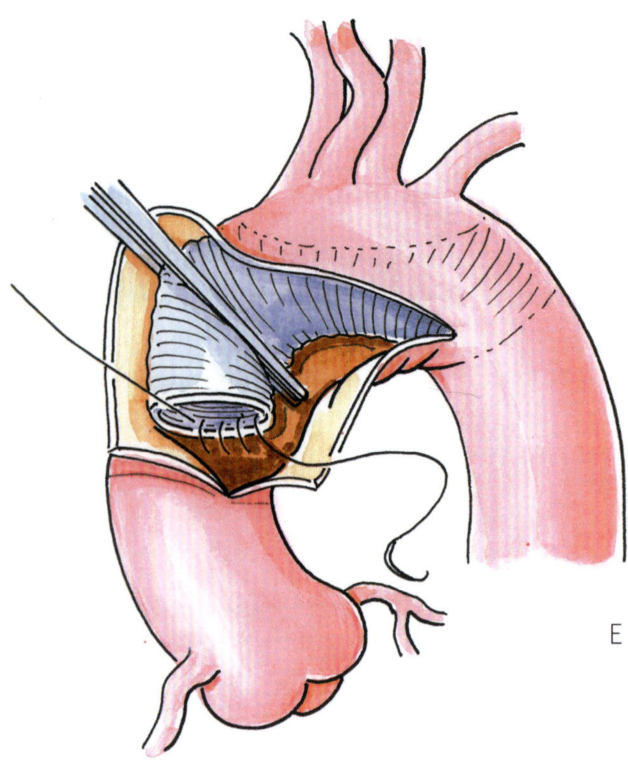

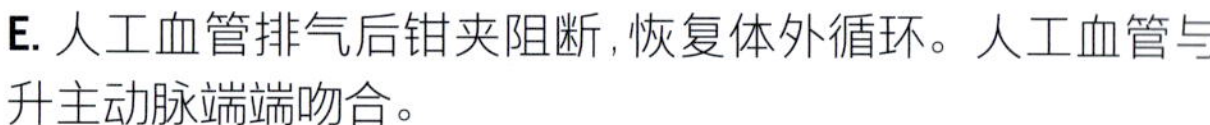
E. 人工血管排气后钳夹阻断，恢复体外循环。人工血管与升主动脉端端吻合。

E. The graft is occluded with clamps after ventilation, and extracorporeal circulation is resumed. The end-to-end anastomosis of the graft to the ascending aorta is made.

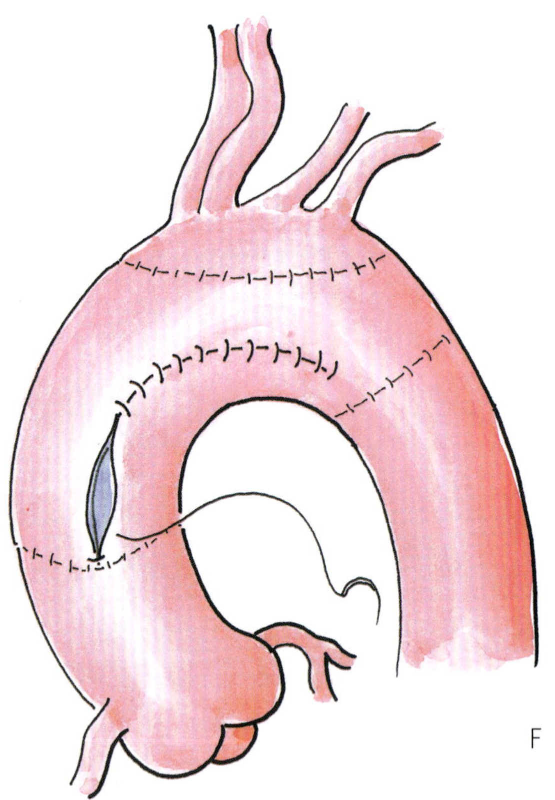

F. 剪除多余的动脉瘤壁，缝合包埋人工血管。

F. The excess aneurysm walls are cut off, and the artificial blood vessel is sutured and embedded.

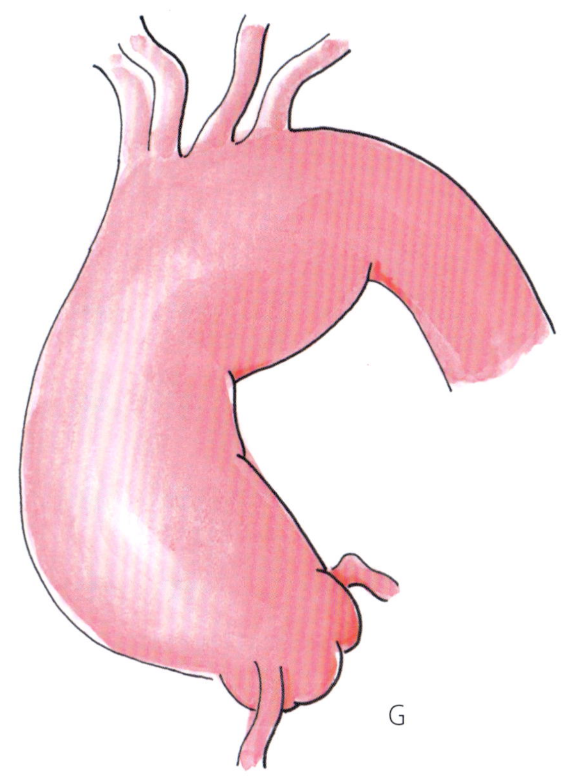

G. 梭形动脉瘤累及主动脉弓和升主动脉。

G. The fusiform aneurysm involves the aortic arch and the ascending aorta.

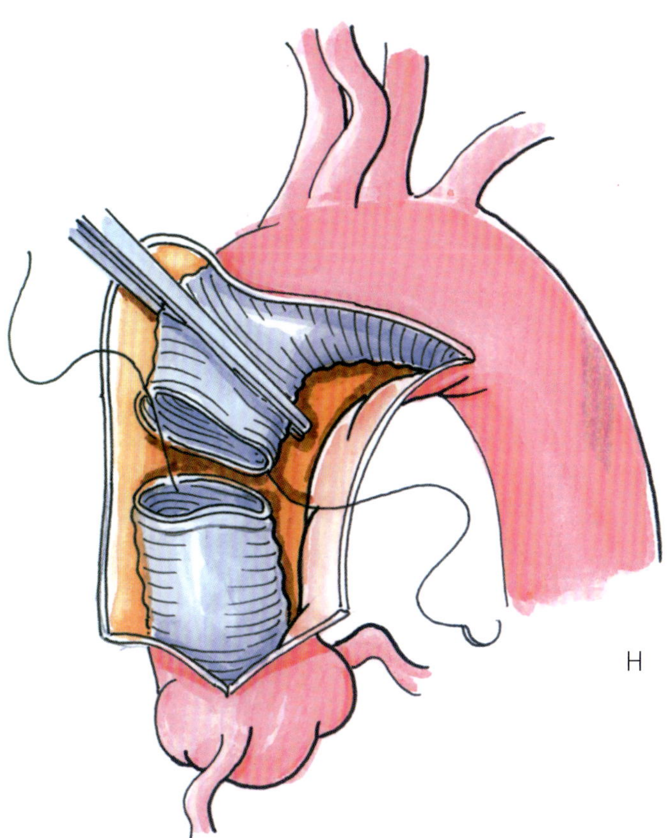

H. 在深低温停循环下完成远端和弓顶的吻合后，在体外循环下用另外一段人工血管做升主动脉替换，先在近端与升主动脉起始部端端吻合，然后两人工血管端端吻合。

H. After completing anastomosis between the distal end and archtop under deep hypothermic circulatory arrest, the ascending aorta is replaced with another artificial vessel under extracorporeal circulation. The proximal end is sutured to the origin of the ascending aorta with end-to-end anastomosis, and then the two grafts are connected in an end-to-end fashion.

图 4-3-2　主动脉弓人工血管置换加象鼻术
Figure 4-3-2　Aortic arch graft replacement with elephant trunk reconstruction

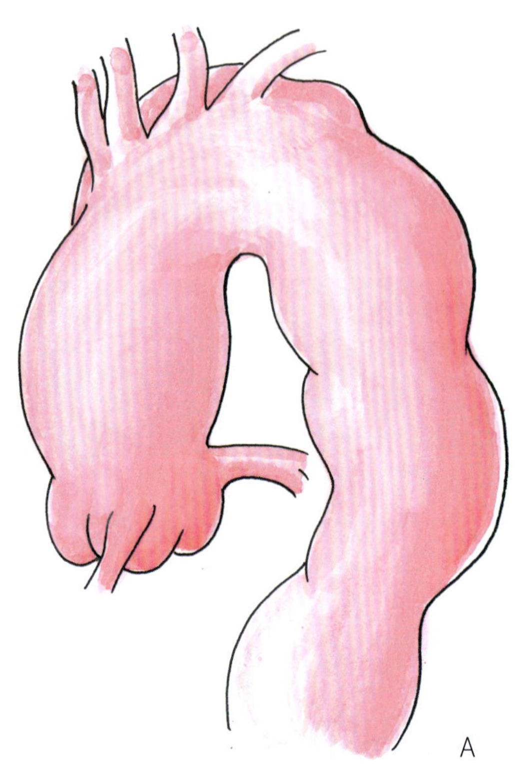

A. 长段主动脉瘤，累及升主动脉、主动脉弓和降主动脉。

A. A long-segmental aortic aneurysm involves the ascending aorta, aortic arch, and descending aorta.

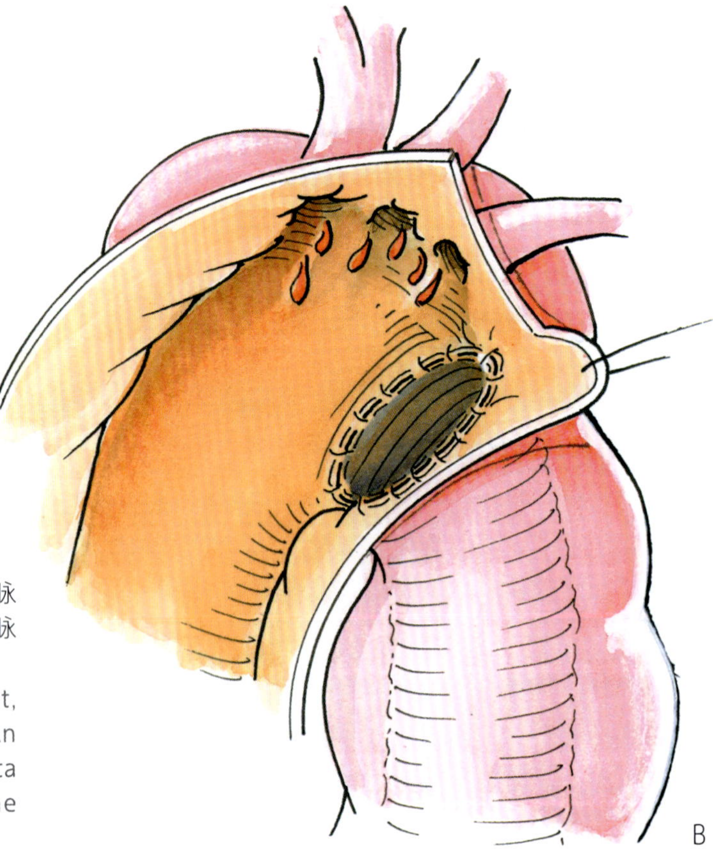

B. 深低温停循环后切开升主动脉和主动脉弓。向降主动脉内置入人工血管，在主动脉弓降部将人工血管与降主动脉缝合。

B. With the deep hypothermic circulatory arrest, the ascending aorta and aortic arch are incised. An artificial vessel is placed into the descending aorta and anastomosed to the descending aorta at the descending aortic arch.

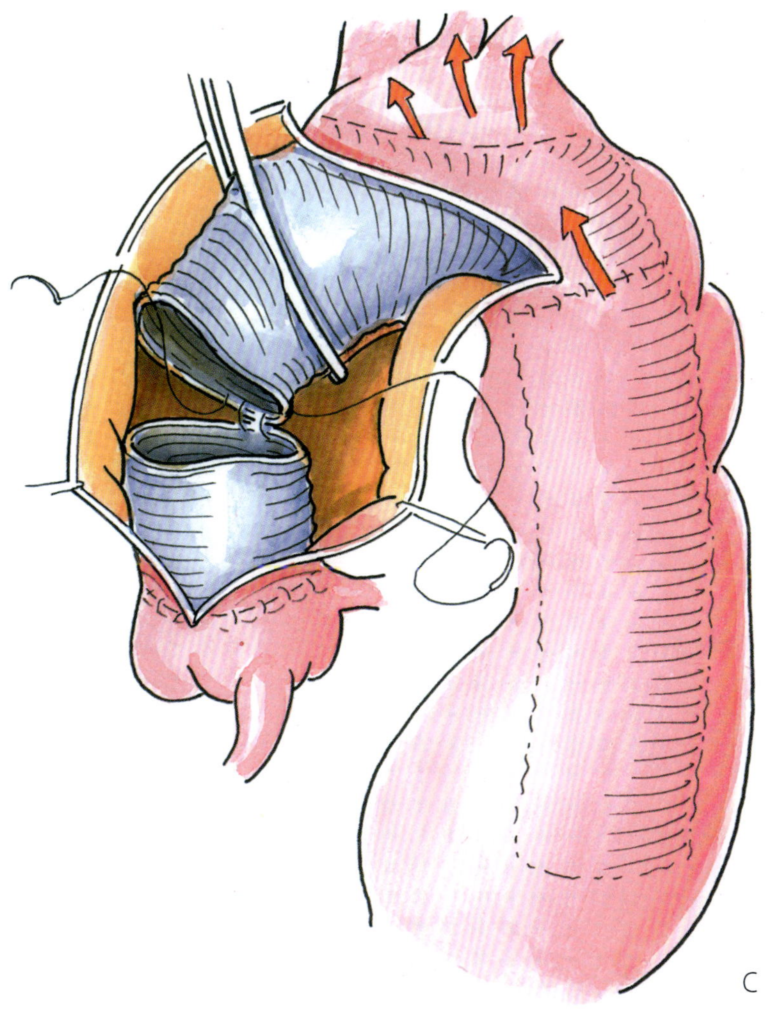

C. 选择合适口径的人工血管在弓降部和降主动脉吻合。人工血管顶部开窗，与包含三个头臂动脉开口的主动脉弓顶部吻合。人工血管排气后钳夹阻断，恢复体外循环。人工血管与升主动脉移植的人工血管端端吻合。

C. An appropriately sized graft is anastomosed to the descending aorta at the descending arch. With fenestration on the roof, the graft is anastomosed to the roof of the aortic arch containing three brachiocephalic arteries ostia. The artificial vessel is occluded with clamps after ventilation, and extracorporeal circulation is resumed. The artificial vessel is anastomosed end-to-end to the artificial vessel of the ascending aorta.

图 4-3-3 主动脉弓上分支重建加主动脉弓内支架术

Figure 4-3-3 Translocation of the supra-aortic vessels and stent grafting of the aortic arch

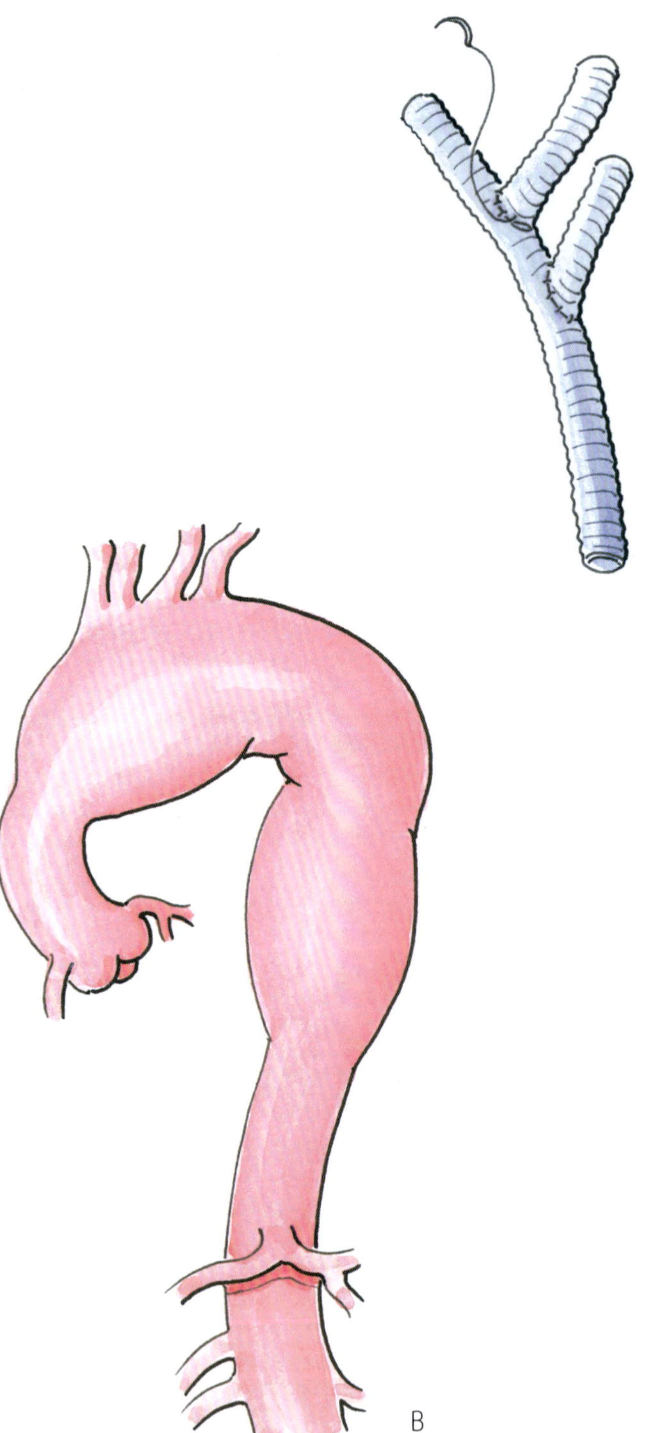

A. 准备带三分叉的人工血管，若无成品亦可自行手工缝制。

A. Prepare trifurcated artificial vessel or hand-make some.

A

B. 主动脉梭形动脉瘤，病变广泛，起自升主动脉远段止于胸降主动脉末端。

B. Aortic fusiform aneurysm with extensive lesions originates from the distal segment of the ascending aorta to the distal end of the descending thoracic aorta.

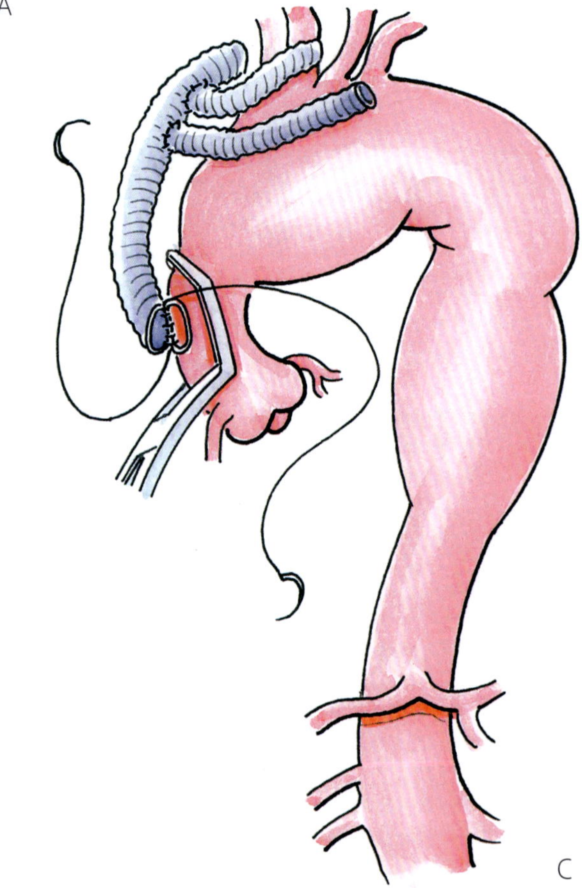

C. 常温下升主动脉上侧壁钳，切除一小块椭圆形的主动脉壁，在此与人工血管做端侧吻合。

C. At room temperature, a side-biting vascular clamp is placed on the ascending aorta, a small oval of the aortic wall is removed, and an end-to-side anastomosis is performed there between the artery and an artificial vessel.

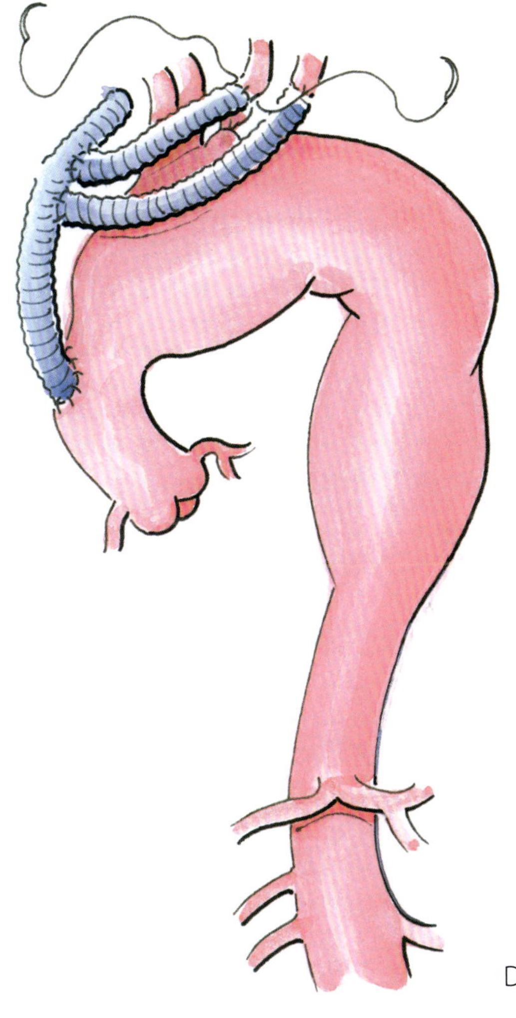

D. 起始部横断左锁骨下动脉，近端缝扎，远端与人工血管分支端端吻合。然后依法切断左颈总动脉并与人工血管分支端端吻合。

D. After the origin of the left subclavian artery is transected, its proximal end is closed, and its distal end anastomosed end-to-end with one branch of the artificial vessel. The left common carotid artery is then cut off and sutured to the other branch of the graft in end-to-end anastomosis.

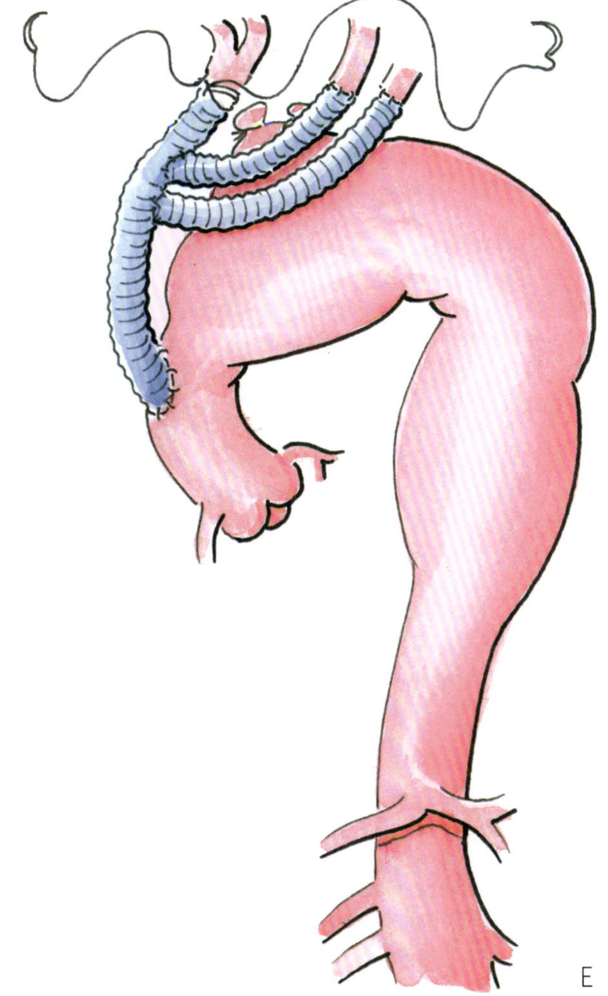

E. 最后切断头臂干并与人工血管端端吻合。

E. The brachiocephalic trunk is finally cut off and anastomosed end to end to the graft.

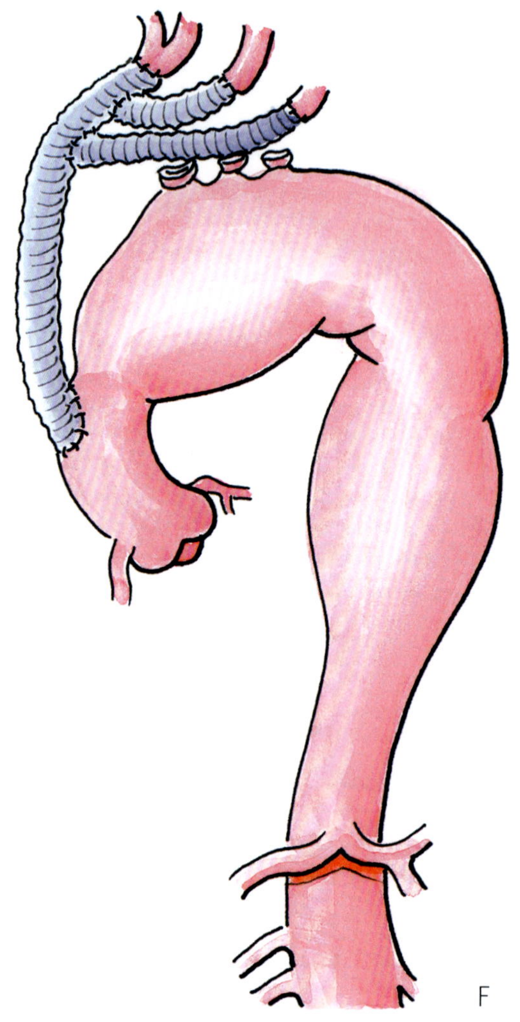

F. 主动脉弓去分支及弓上分支重建完成，主动脉弓上分支由人工血管供血。

F. The aortic arch is debranched, and the supra-aortic vessels are reconstructed, which are supplied by the artificial vessels.

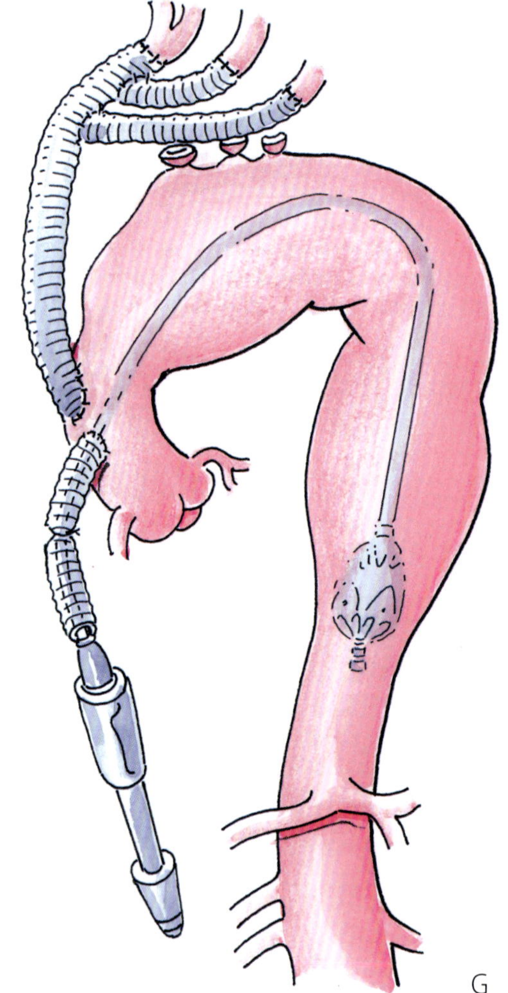

G. 经升主动脉插入支架导管。

G. Insert a stent catheter via the ascending aorta.

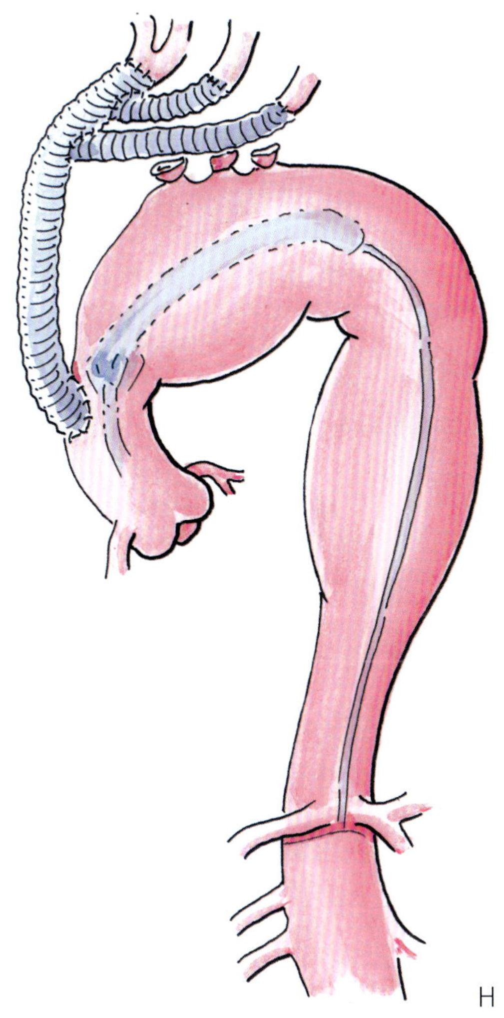

H. 支架导管亦可经股动脉插入。

H. The stent catheter can also be inserted through the femoral artery.

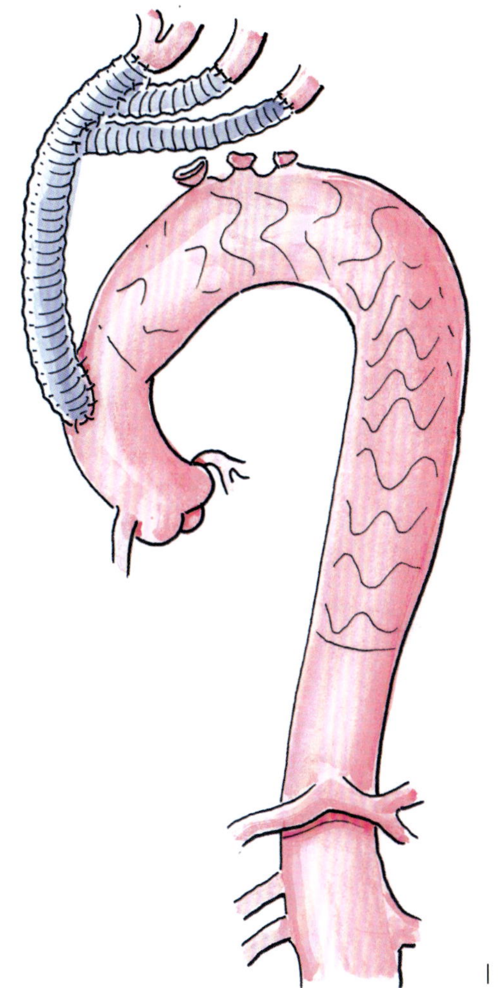

I. 主动脉内支架定位后释放，在主动脉腔内覆盖动脉瘤全长。

I. The intra-aortic stent is released after positioning, and it covers the entire length of the aneurysm in the aortic lumen.

图 4-3-4　**升主动脉置换、主动脉弓上分支重建加主动脉弓内支架术**

Figure 4-3-4　**Ascending aortic graft replacement, translocation of the supra-aortic vessels, and stent grafting of the aortic arch**

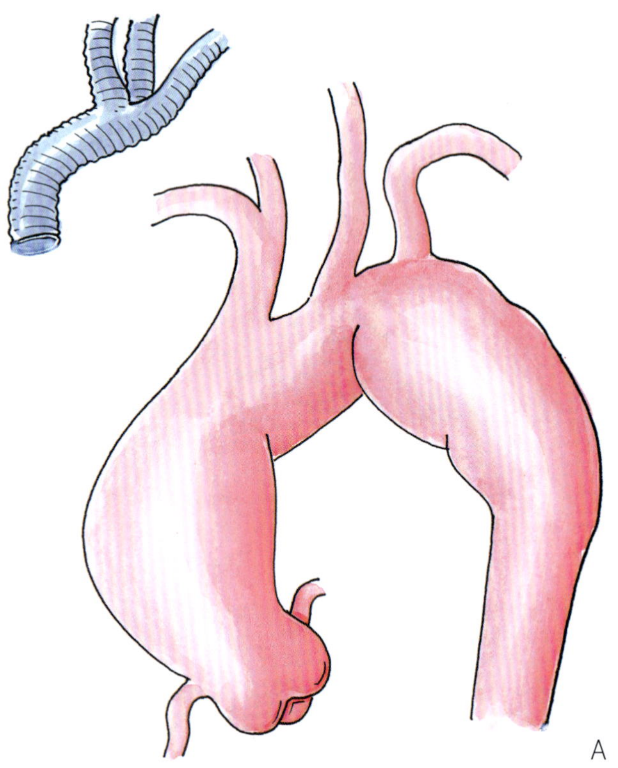

A. 主动脉梭形动脉瘤，病变广泛，起自升主动脉近端止于胸降主动脉末端。备三分叉人工血管。

A. Aortic fusiform aneurysm has extensive lesions from the proximal end of the ascending aorta to the distal end of the descending thoracic aorta. A trifurcated artificial vessel is prepared.

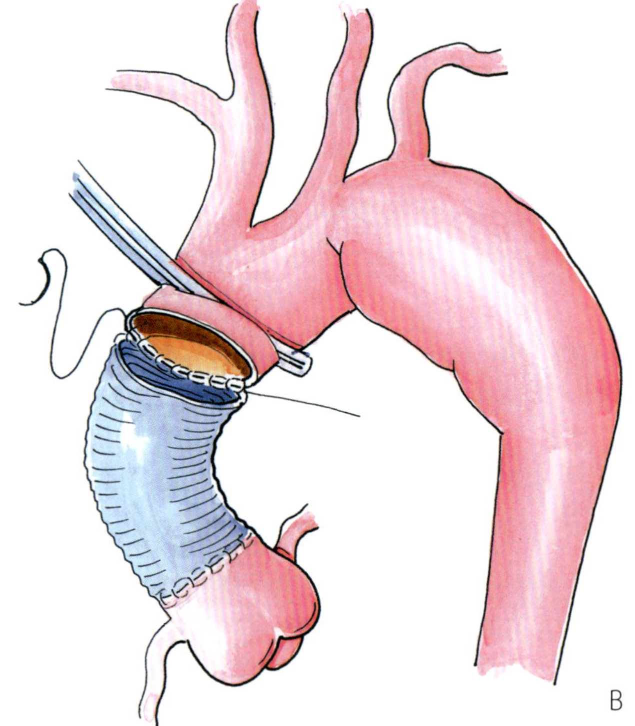

B. 体外循环心脏停搏下用人工血管置换升主动脉。

B. The ascending aorta is replaced with the graft under extracorporeal circulation and cardiac arrest.

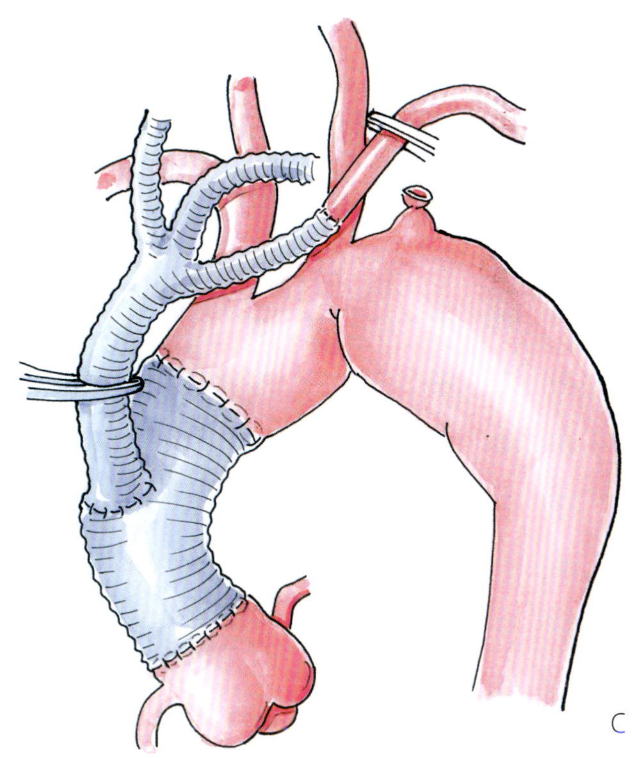

C. 三分叉人工血管与升主动脉人工血管端侧吻合。于起始部横断左锁骨下动脉，近端缝扎，远端与人工血管端端吻合。

C. The trifurcation graft is sutured to the ascending aorta graft with end-to-side anastomosis. The left subclavian artery is transected at the original portion, with its proximal end sutured, and the distal end sutured to a branch of the graft using end-to-end anastomosis.

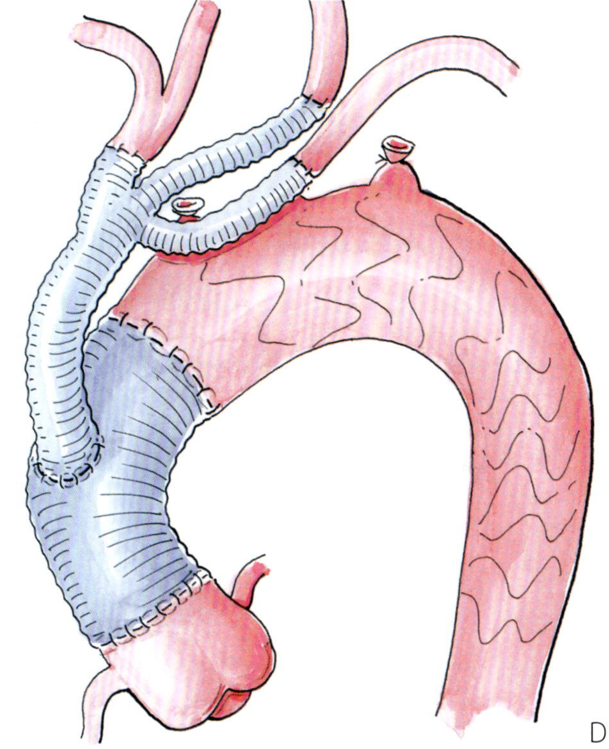

D. 切断左颈总动脉并与人工血管端端吻合，切断头臂干也与人工血管端端吻合。经股动脉插入支架导管，主动脉内支架覆盖主动脉弓和降主动脉。

D. The left common carotid artery is cut and sutured to another branch of the artificial vessel with end-to-end anastomosis. The brachiocephalic trunk is incised and is anastomosed to the third graft branch in an end-to-end fashion. Stent catheters are inserted via the femoral artery, and the intra-aortic stent is covers the aortic arch and the descending aorta.

图 4-3-5　主动脉弓囊状动脉瘤切除修补术
Figure 4-3-5　Aortic arch saccular aneurysm resection and repair

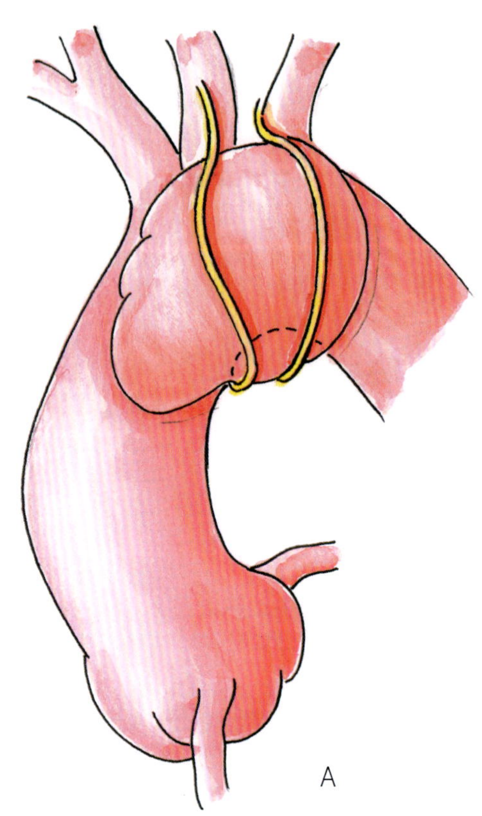

A. 主动脉弓动脉瘤囊袋样突出，其基底有一缩小的颈部与主动脉弓相通。

A. An aortic arch aneurysm has a saccular bulge with a narrowed neck at its base connecting to the aortic arch.

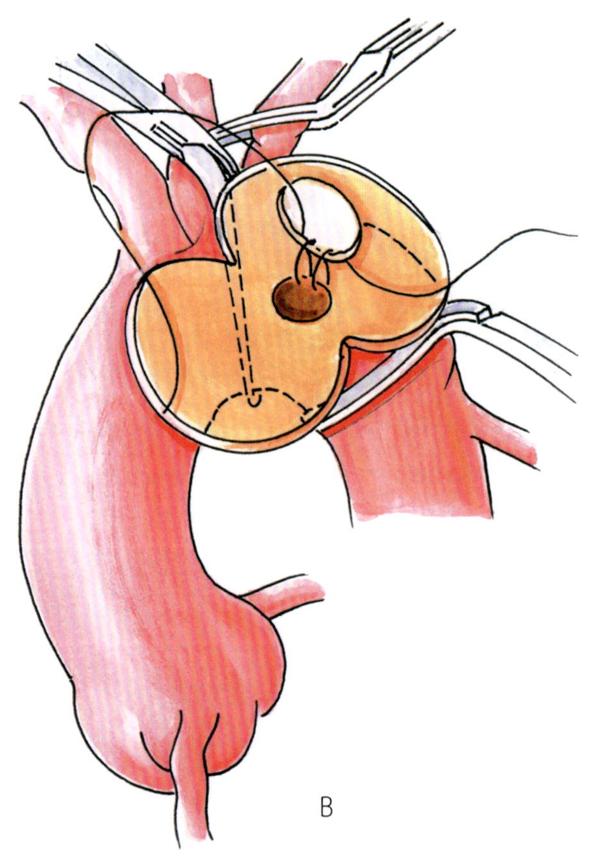

B. 体外循环心脏停搏，在动脉瘤两端阻断主动脉弓，阻断相关的主动脉弓分支左锁骨下动脉。切开动脉瘤，补片修补基底部与主动脉弓相通的缺损，单纯连续缝合。

B. Under extracorporeal circulation and cardiac arrest, occlude the aortic arch at both ends of the aneurysm and the left subclavian artery, a branch of the aortic arch. The aneurysm is incised, and the defect whose basilar part communicates with the aortic arch is repaired with patches using simple continuous sutures.

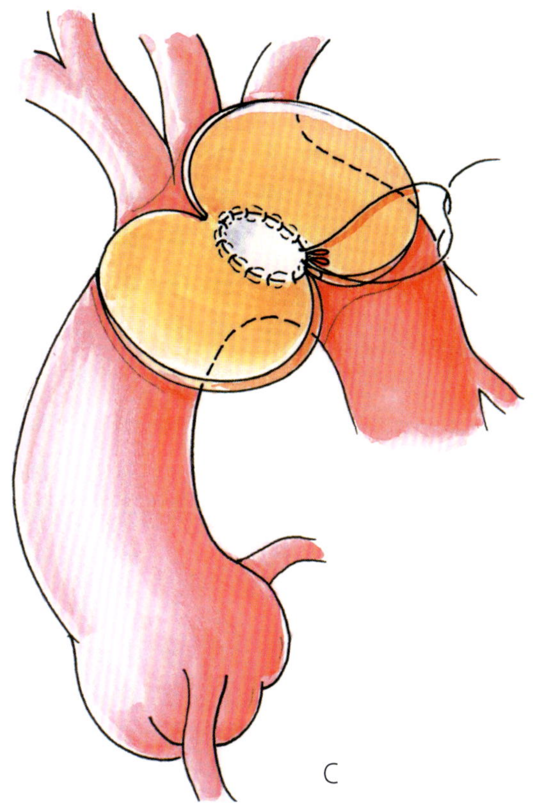

C. 开放主动脉阻断钳和左锁骨下动脉阻断钳，排气后结扎。

C. Release the aortic clamp and left subclavian artery clamp. Ligate after venting.

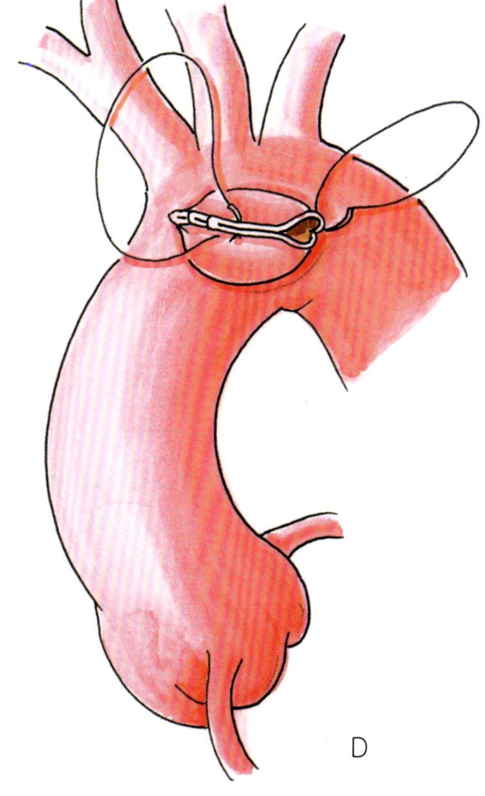

D. 切除部分动脉瘤壁，剩余部分缝合覆盖补片。

D. Portion of the aneurysm wall is removed, and the remaining portion is overlaid by a patch.

第四节 降主动脉瘤
Section 4 Descending Aortic Aneurysm

图 4-4-1 降主动脉人工血管置换加半弓重建术
Figure 4-4-1 Descending aortic graft replacement and hemi-arch reconstruction

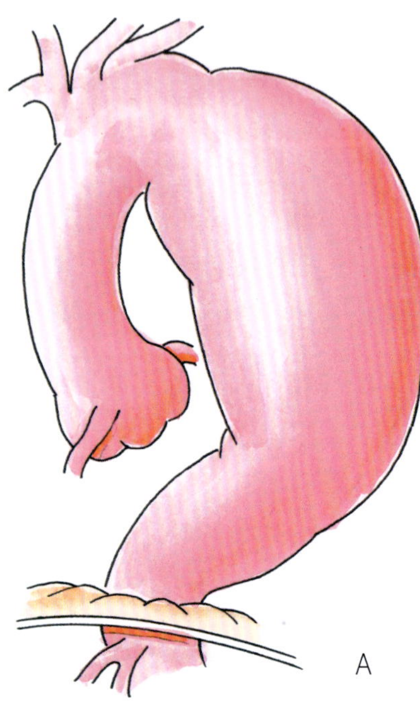

A. 胸降主动脉巨大梭形动脉瘤。

A. Giant fusiform aneurysm of the descending thoracic aorta.

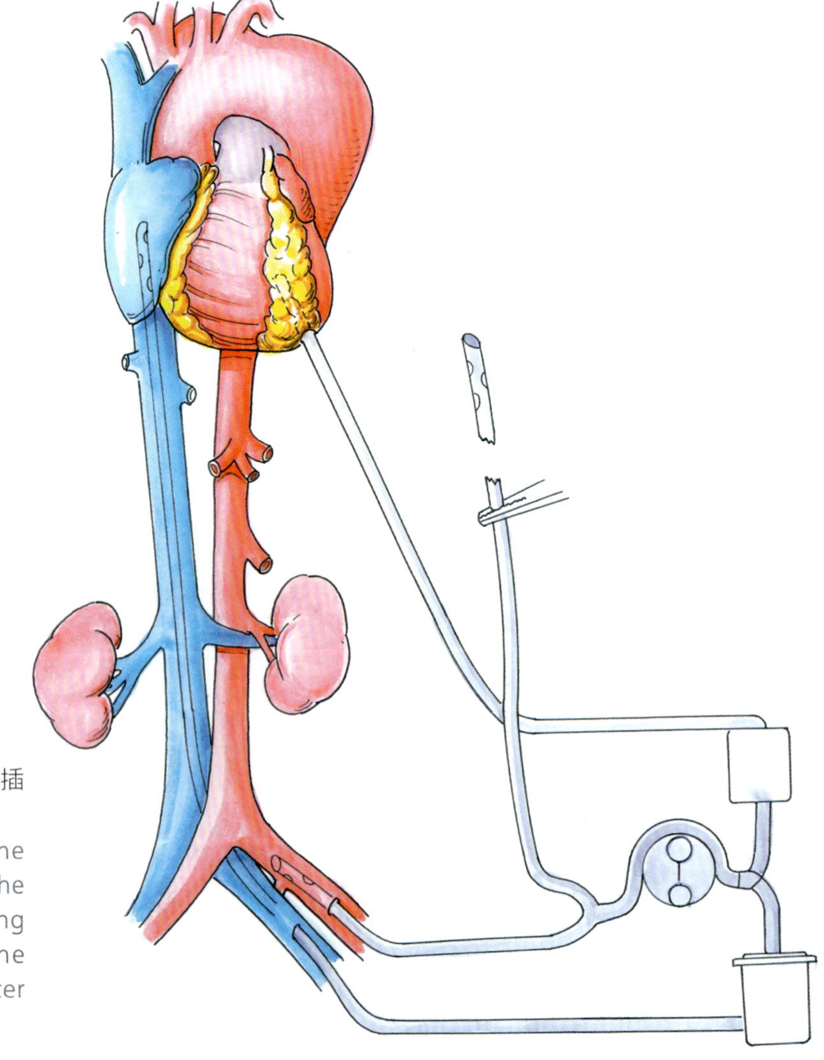

B. 股动脉插供血管，股静脉插引流管，心尖插左心减压管。供血管留一头备用。

B. Arterial cannulation is placed in the femoral artery, a drainage cannula in the femoral vein, and a left cardiac venting catheter in the apex. One arm of the arterial cannulation is reserved for later use.

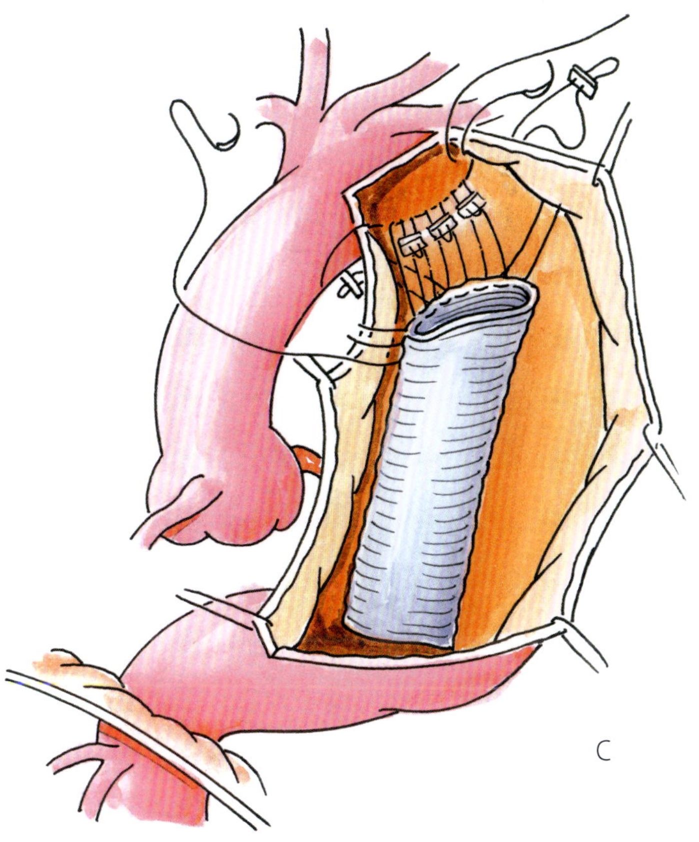

C. 深低温停循环下纵行切开动脉瘤全长。带垫片间断褥式缝合将人工血管与主动脉弓末端做端端吻合。先缝后壁，缝针的垫片放在主动脉腔内，即主动脉腔内进针、腔内出针。

C. A longitudinal incision is made over the entire length of the aneurysm under deep hypothermic circulatory arrest. The artificial vessel is end-to-end anastomosed to the aortic arch with interrupted pledgeted mattress sutures. Suturing the back part first, the pledget of the suture is placed in the aortic lumen, that is, the needle is introduced into the aortic lumen and out of the lumen.

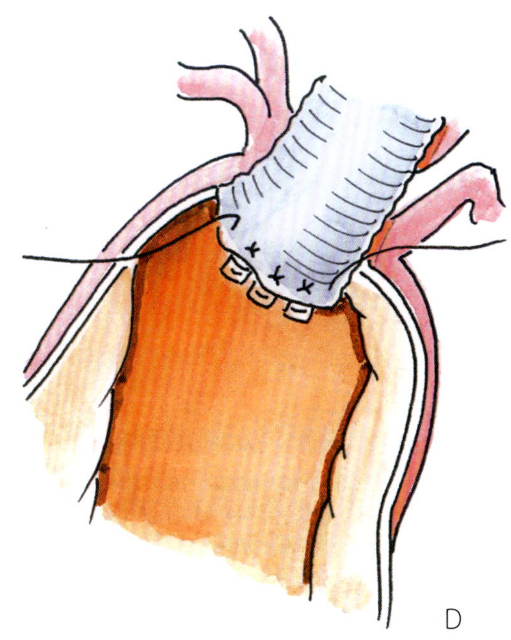

D. 人工血管推下后继续缝合。

D. Suture proceeds after the artificial vessel is pushed down.

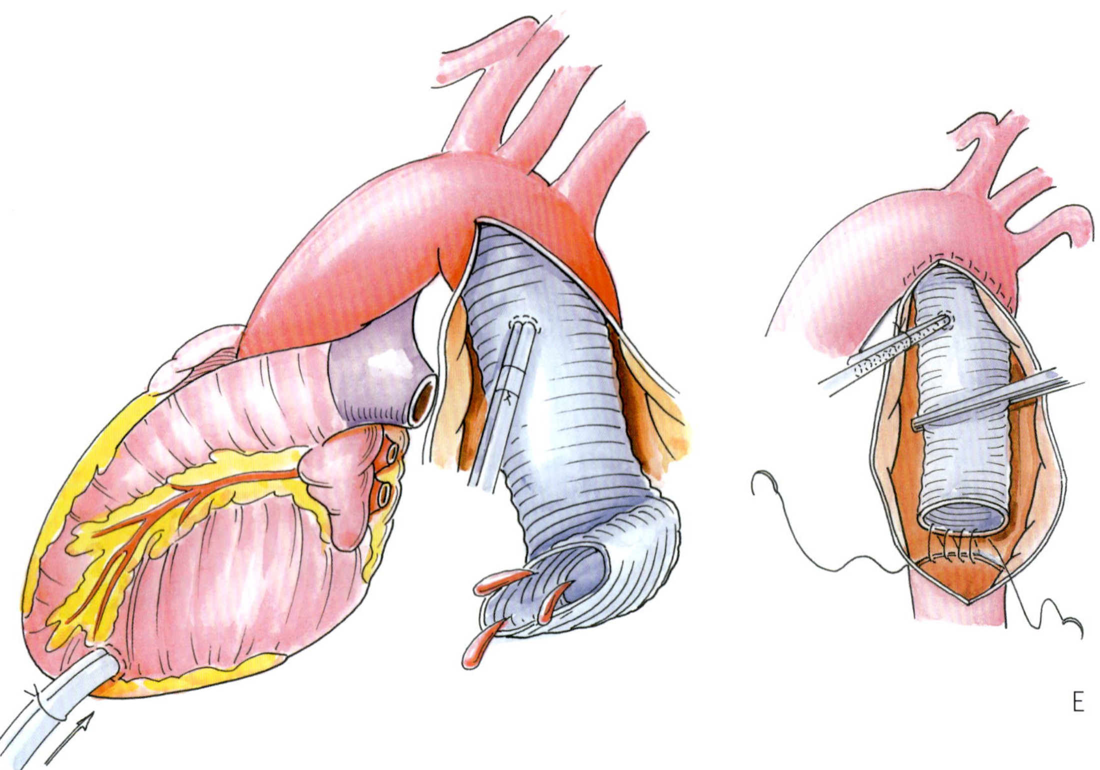

E. 近端吻合完成后，将供血管的备用头插入人工血管，排气后启动体外循环，复温。人工血管与胸降主动脉远端做端端吻合，单纯连续缝合。

E. After completing the proximal anastomosis, insert the spare head of the arterial cannulation into the graft, initiate extracorporeal circulation after de-airing, and restore body temperature. The graft is end-to-end anastomosed with the distal end of the descending thoracic aorta with simple continuous sutures.

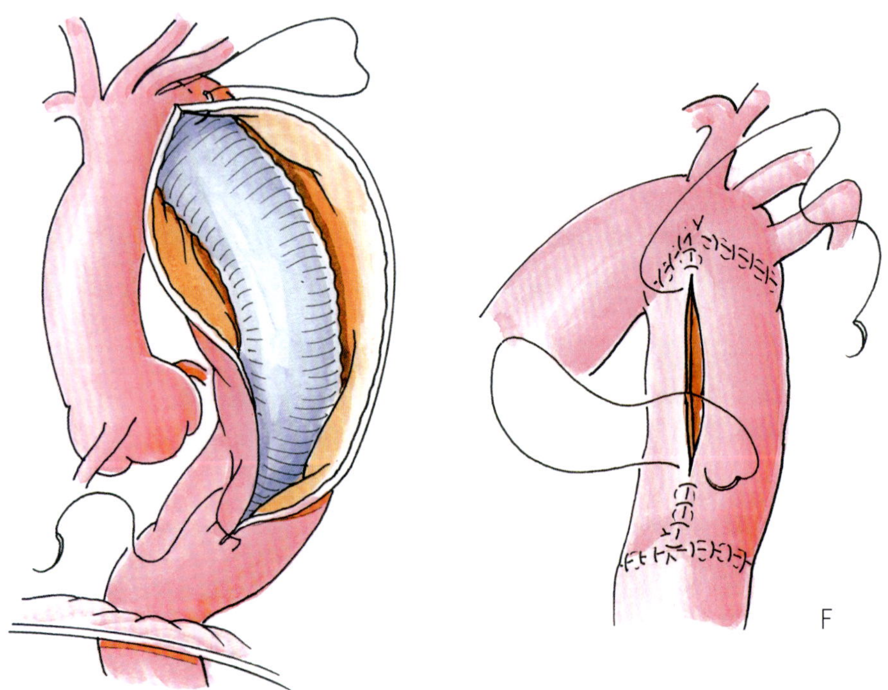

F. 体外循环撤离后，剪去部分动脉瘤壁后缝合包埋人工血管。

F. After removing extracorporeal circulation, part of the aneurysm wall is cut, and the artificial vessel is then embedded and sutured.

图 4-4-2 单纯阻断技术降主动脉人工血管置换术

Figure 4-4-2 Descending aorta graft replacement with simple clamping technique

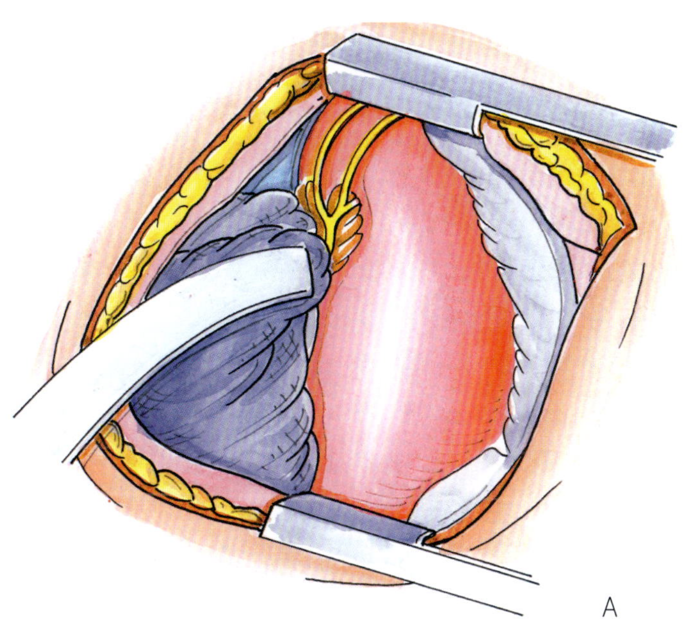

A. 左胸后外侧切口第 6 肋间进胸，显露降主动脉瘤。

A. On the left side of the chest, make a posterolateral incision at the sixth intercostal space, exposing the descending aortic aneurysm.

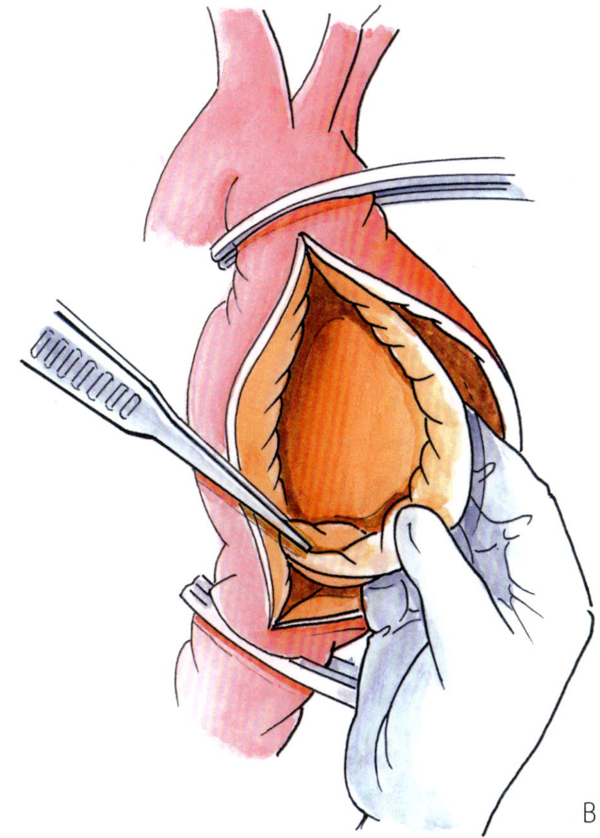

B. 体外循环或左心转流下，在动脉瘤两端正常降主动脉处钳夹阻断。

B. Under extracorporeal circulation or left cardiac bypass, clamps are placed on the normal descending aorta at both ends of the aneurysm.

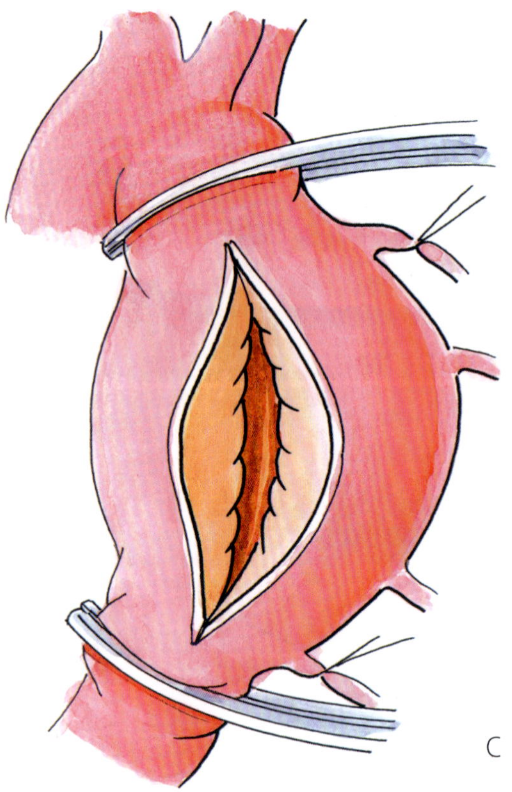

C. 纵行切开动脉瘤，剥离清除增厚的内膜。

C. The aneurysm is incised longitudinally, and the thickened intima is dissected.

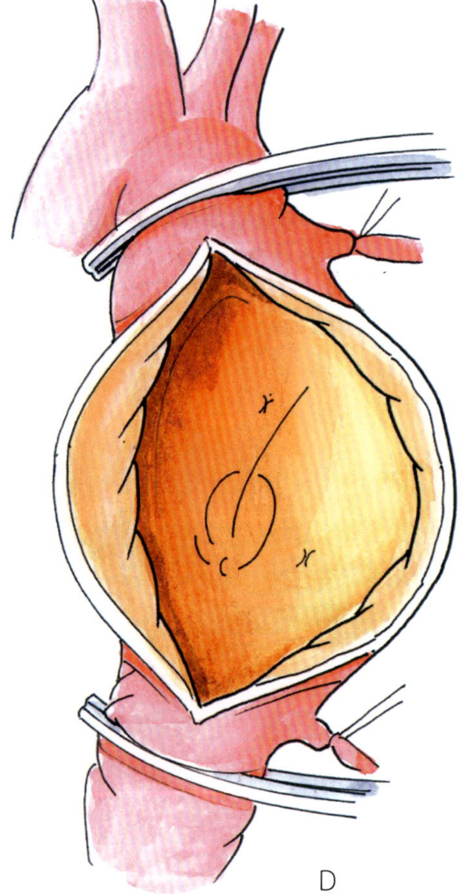

D. 肋间动脉开口予以缝扎。

D. The ostia of the intercostal arteries are sutured.

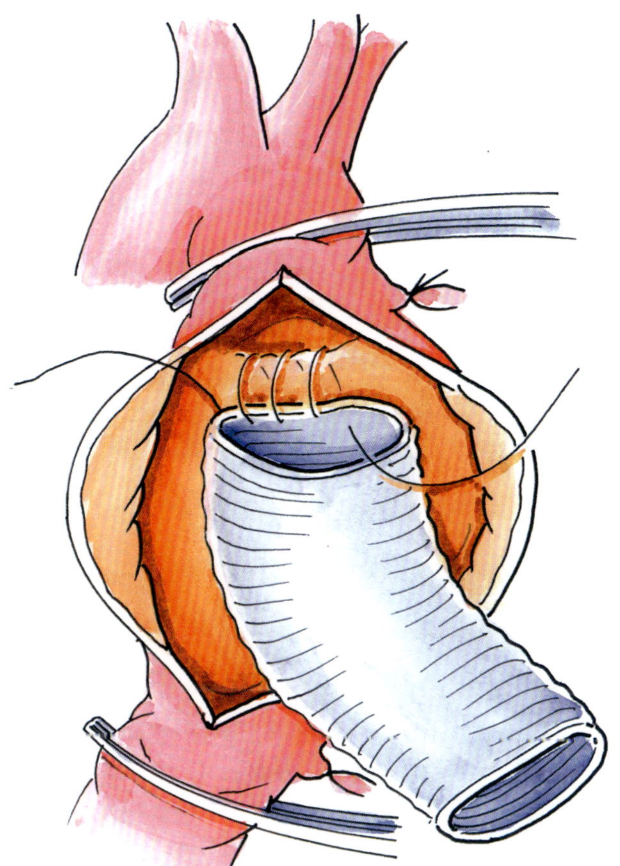

E. 人工血管与降主动脉近端做端端吻合，单纯连续缝合。

E. An end-to-end anastomosis is performed between the graft and the proximal end of the descending aorta with simple continuous sutures.

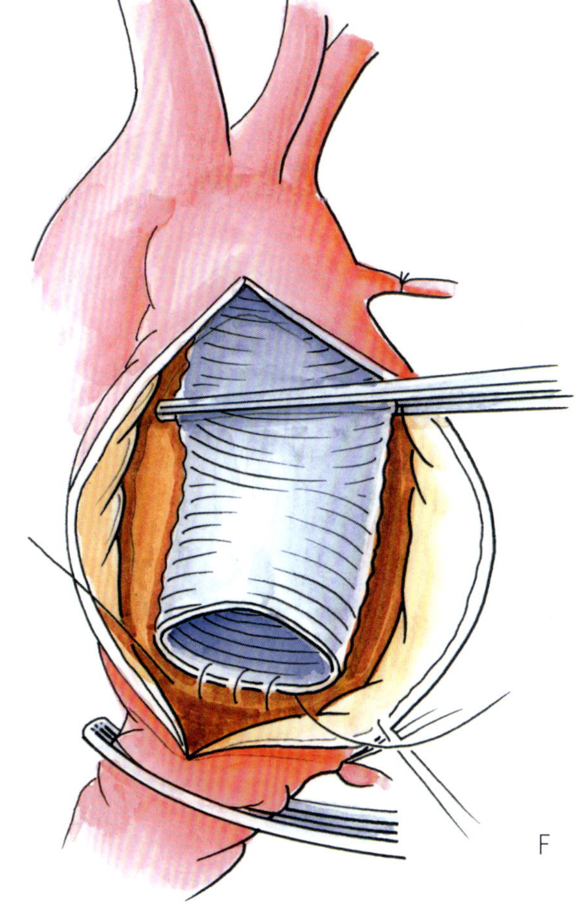

F. 近端阻断钳换到人工血管上，单纯连续缝合吻合人工血管与胸降主动脉远端。

F. With the proximal clamps switched on the graft, the graft is anastomosed to the distal end of the descending thoracic aorta with simple continuous sutures.

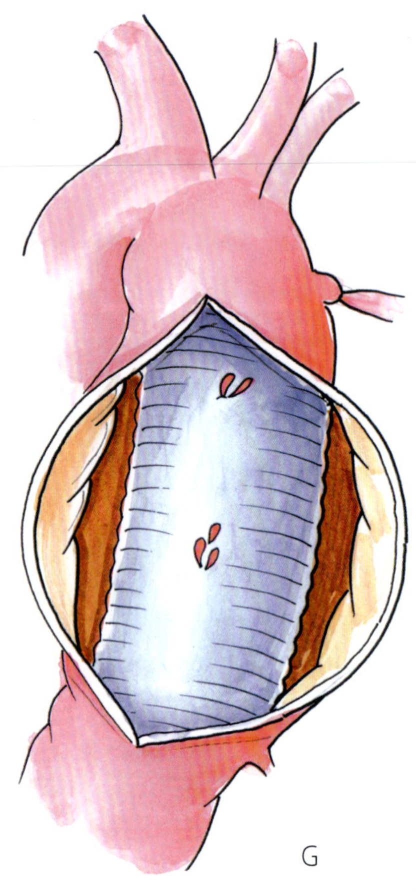

G. 去除二阻断钳，人工血管戳孔排气。

G. Release the two blocking forceps, poke a hole at the graft, and de-air.

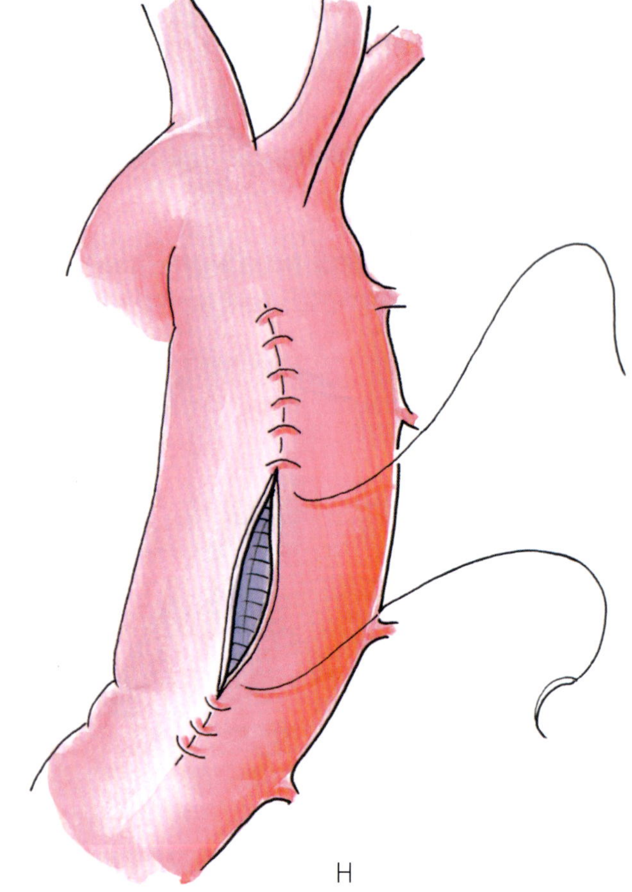

H. 剪去部分动脉瘤壁后缝合包埋人工血管。

H. Part of the aneurysm wall is removed, and the artificial vessel is embedded and sutured.

图 4-4-3 分段阻断技术降主动脉人工血管置换术

Figure 4-4-3 Descending aorta graft replacement with subsection simple clamping technique

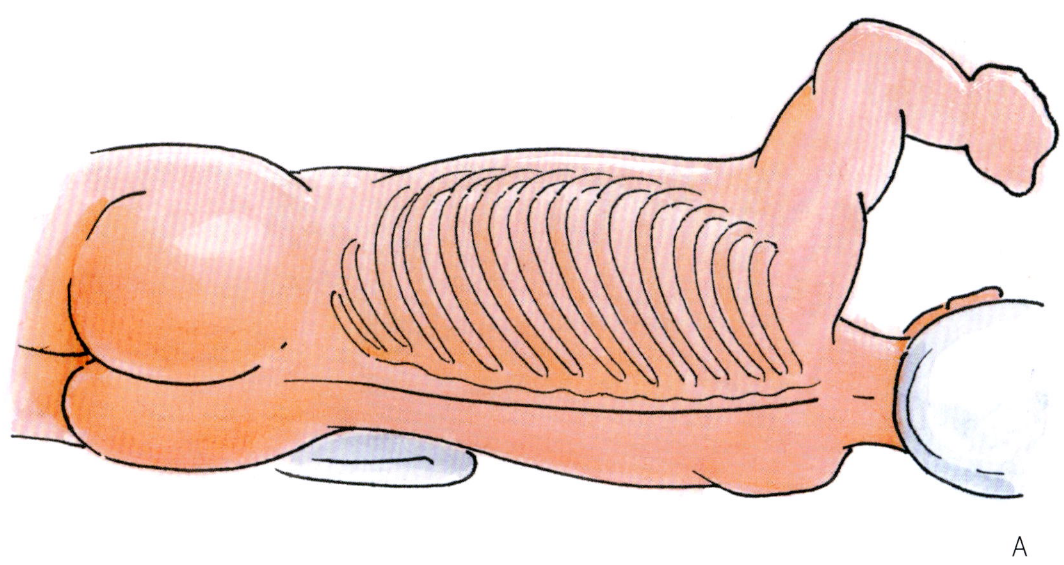

A. 右侧卧位，腰下垫软枕。

A. With the patient lying in the right lateral recumbent position, a soft pillow is to be placed under the waist.

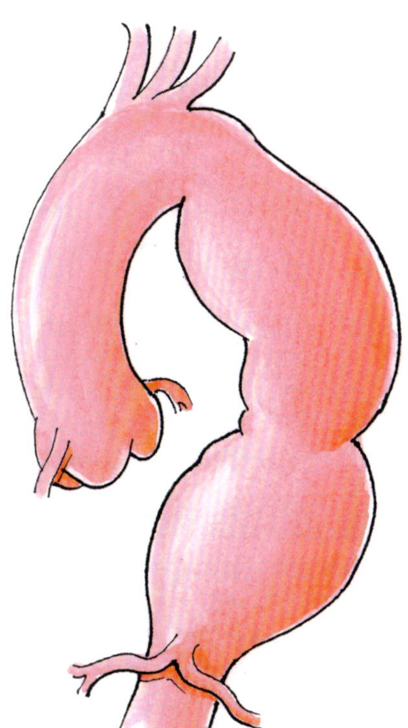

B. 降主动脉瘤，起自弓降部延伸到腹腔干上水平。

B. A descending aortic aneurysm starts from the descending arch and extends to the level above the abdominal trunk.

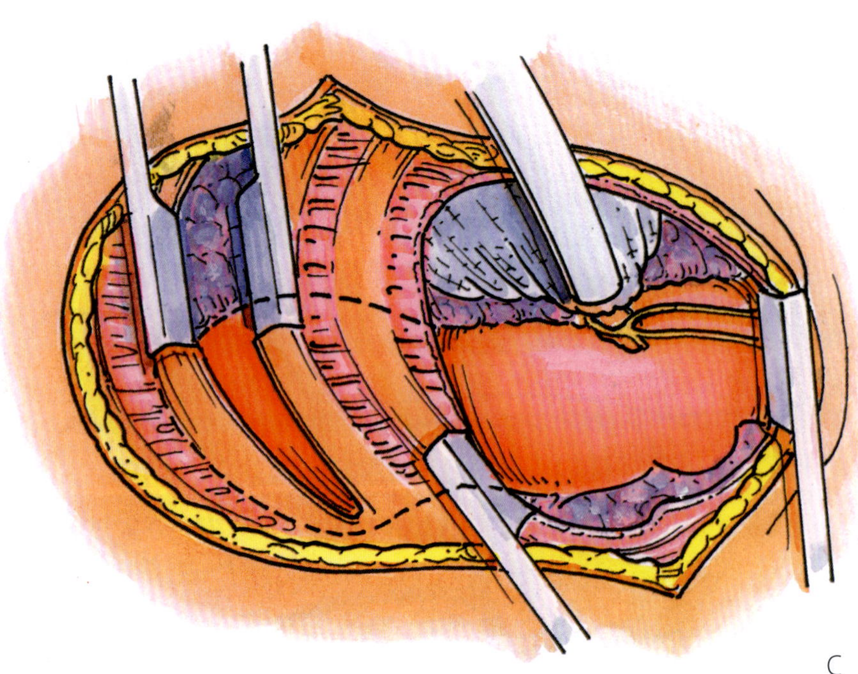

C. 左胸后外侧切口，第 4 肋间进胸显露并处理动脉瘤近端，第 7 肋间切开处理动脉瘤远端。

C. On the left side of the chest, a posterolateral incision is made at the fourth intercostal space to enter the chest, exposing and treating the proximal end of the aneurysm. Another incision is made at the seventh intercostal space to treat the distal end.

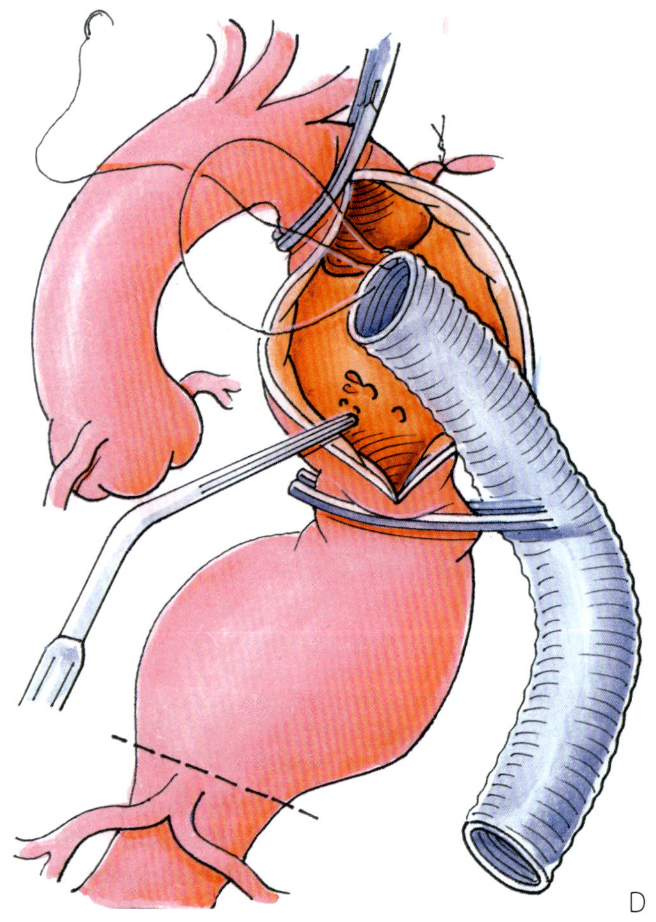

D. 建立体外循环或左心转流。先在弓降部和胸降主动脉中部分别上阻断钳阻断降主动脉血流。单纯连续缝合做人工血管与降主动脉的近端吻合。

D. Establish extracorporeal circulation or left cardiac bypass. The blood flow of the descending aorta is blocked by placing clamping forceps on the descending arch and the middle part of the descending thoracic aorta, respectively. A simple continuous suture is performed to anastomose a graft with the proximal end of the descending aorta.

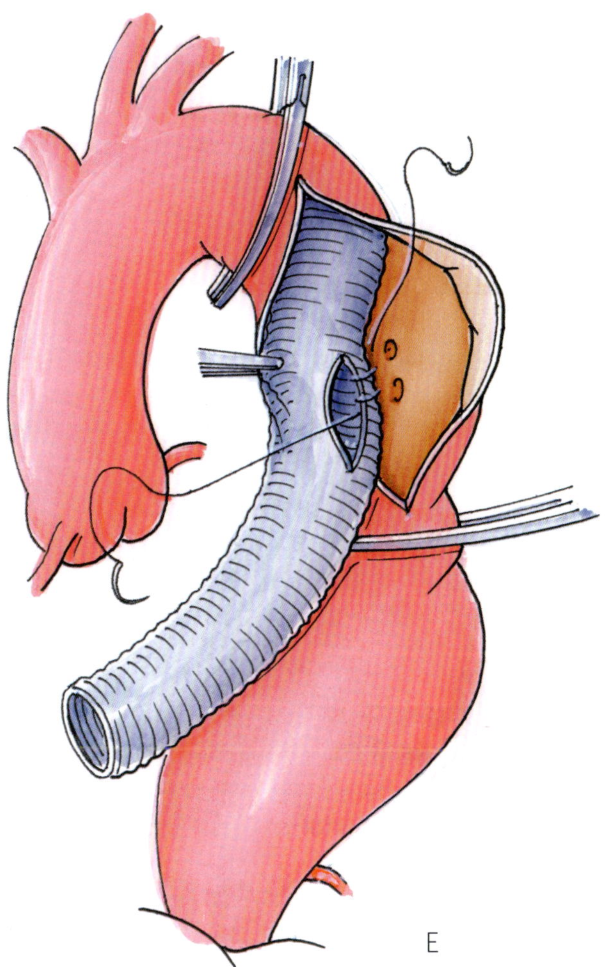

E. 将人工血管上段后壁开窗，与肋间动脉开口吻合。

E. The upper posterior wall of the graft is fenestrated and anastomosed with the ostia of the intercostal artery.

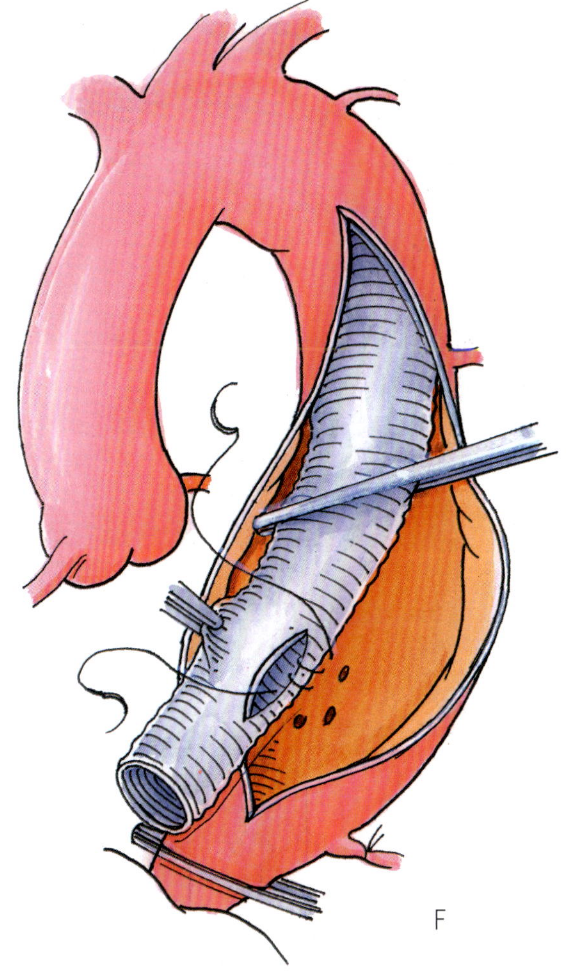

F. 近端主动脉阻断钳下移到人工血管，远端主动脉阻断钳下移到动脉瘤远侧的正常降主动脉上。

将人工血管下段后壁开窗，与肋间动脉开口吻合。最后，人工血管与降主动脉做远侧端端吻合。

F. Proximal aortic clamping forceps are moved down to the graft, and distal aortic clamping forceps are moved down to the normal descending aorta distal to the aneurysm.

The inferior posterior wall of the graft is fenestrated and anastomosed to the ostia of the intercostal artery. A final end-to-end anastomosis of the graft to the distal end of the descending aorta is made.

第五节 胸-腹主动脉瘤
Section 5 Thoraco-Abdominal Aortic Aneurysm

图 4-5-1 带分支人工血管移植和肋间动脉重建术
Figure 4-5-1 Branched graft implantation and intercostal arteries reconstruction

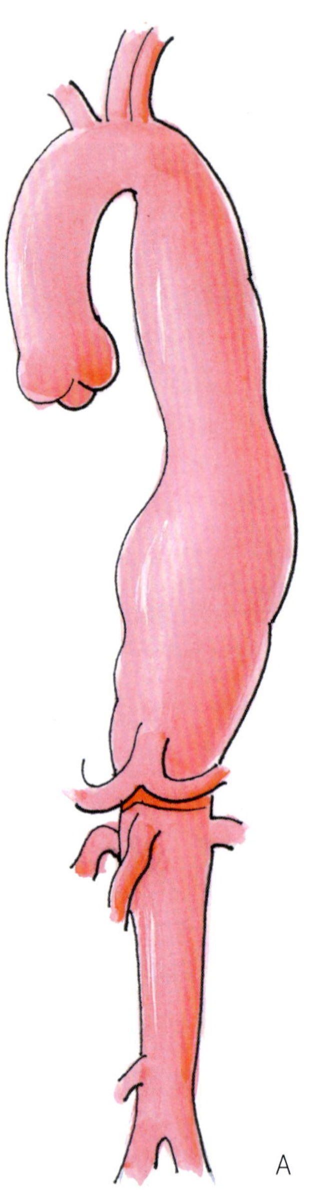

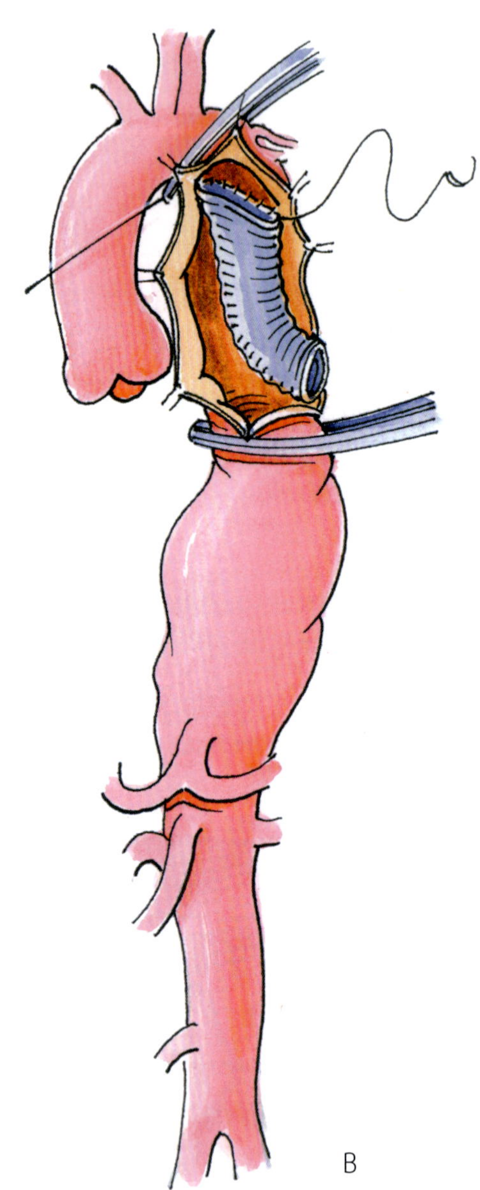

A. 胸 - 腹主动脉瘤，起自降主动脉起始段，向下延伸到肠系膜上动脉开口远端。

A. Thoraco-abdominal aortic aneurysm originates from the origin of the descending aorta and advances downwards to the distal end of the superior mesenteric artery ostium.

B. 体外循环下，在胸降主动脉两端钳夹阻断主动脉。人工血管与降主动脉近端做端端吻合。

B. Under extracorporeal circulation, an aortic cross-clamp is applied to both ends of the descending thoracic aorta. End-to-end anastomosis is performed between a artificial vessel and the proximal end of the descending aorta.

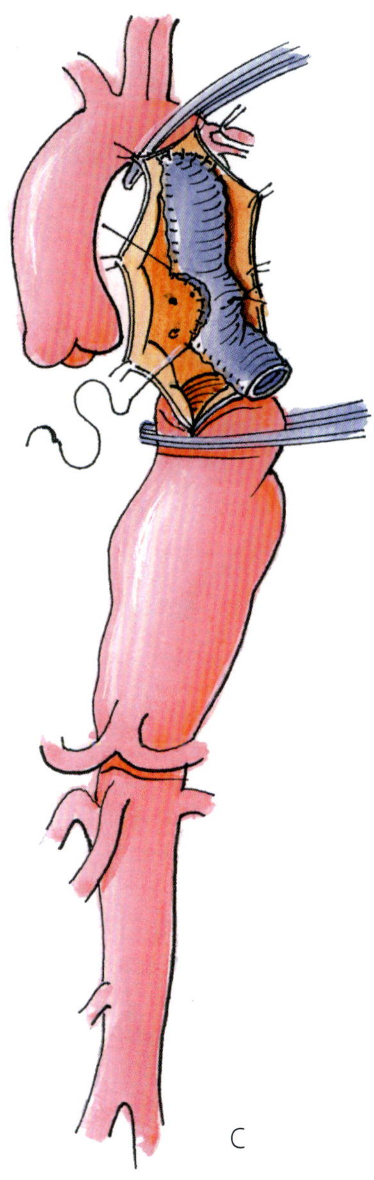

C. 将人工血管后壁开窗，与肋间动脉开口吻合。

C. The posterior wall of the graft is fenestrated and anastomosed to the intercostal artery ostia.

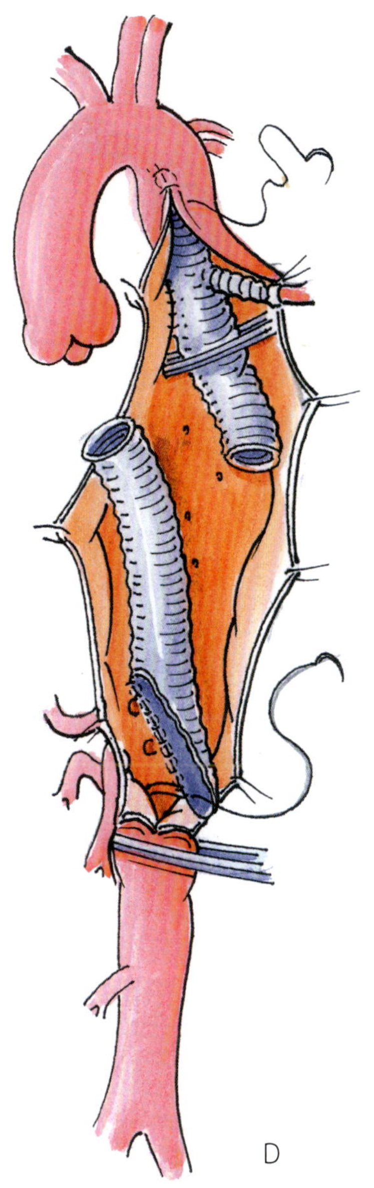

D. 近端主动脉阻断钳下移到人工血管。经人工血管的分支供血。远端主动脉阻断钳下移到动脉瘤远侧的正常降主动脉上。取另外一段人工血管，一端剪成斜口包绕腹腔干、肠系膜上动脉和肾动脉与降主动脉做远端吻合。

D. The aortic cross-clamp at the proximal end is moved down to the graft. Blood is supplied via a branch of the graft. The aortic clamp at the distal end is lowered onto the normal descending aorta distal to the aneurysm. Another artificial vessel is needed with one end trimmed obliquely, and used to encircle the celiac trunk, superior mesenteric artery, and renal artery with distal anastomosis with the descending aorta.

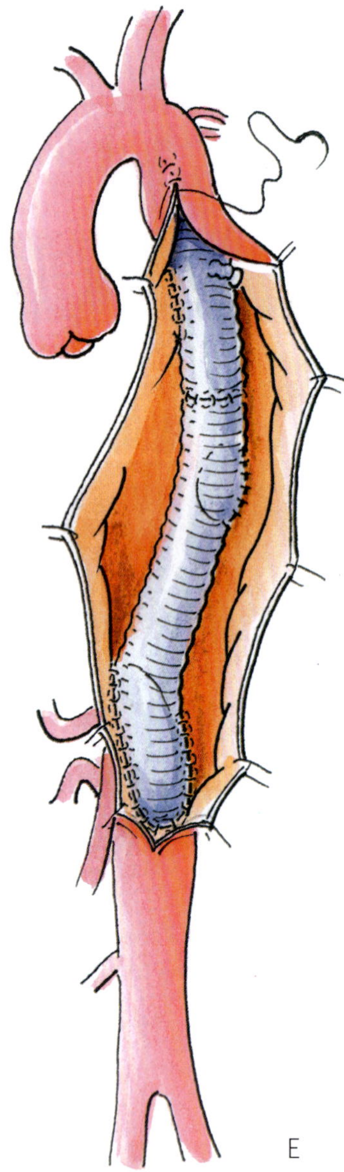

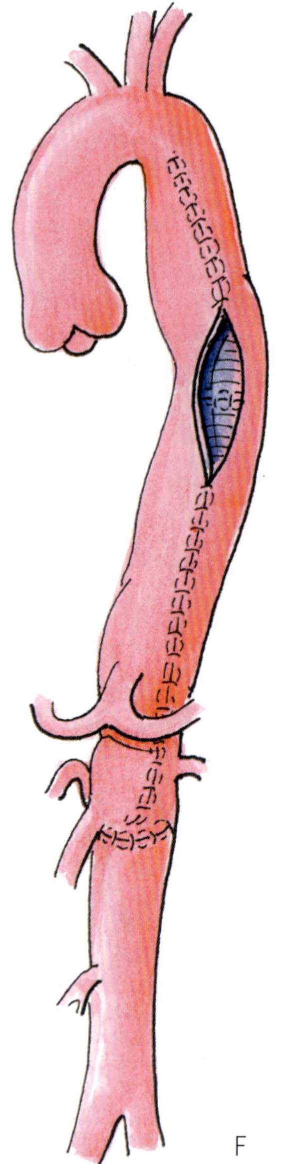

E. 腹腔侧人工血管上段开窗与肋间动脉开口吻合，然后将两人工血管端端吻合。人工血管内排气，撤除主动脉阻断钳和人工血管分支供血。

E. The upper segment of the fenestrated abdominal artificial vessel is anastomosed with the ostia of the intercostal arteries, and then the two artificial vessels are connected. The artificial vessel is vented, the aortic clamp is removed, and the artificial vessel branch is used to supply blood.

F. 剪去部分动脉瘤壁后缝合、包埋人工血管。

F. Part of the aneurysm wall is removed, and the grafts are sutured and embedded.

图 4-5-2 胸 - 腹主动脉瘤直视修复术

Figure 4-5-2 Open thoraco-abdominal aortic aneurysm repair

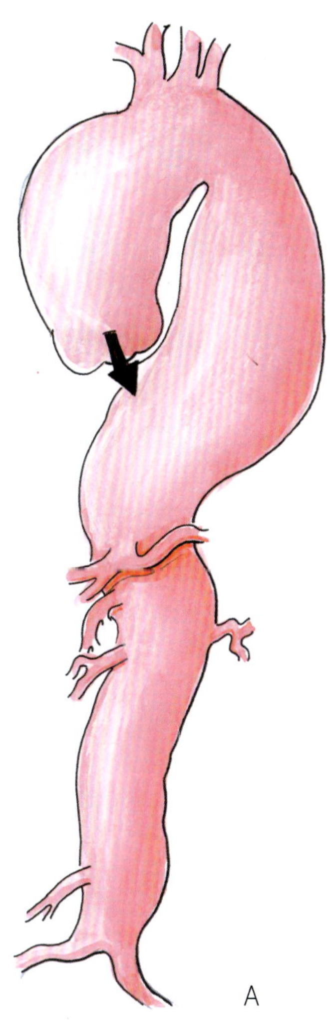

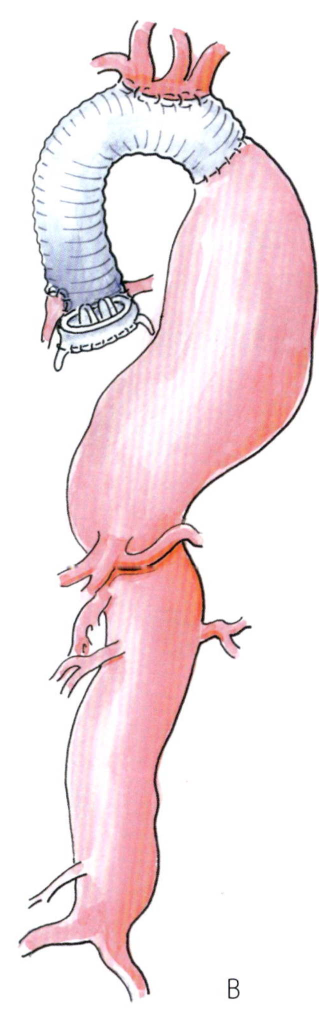

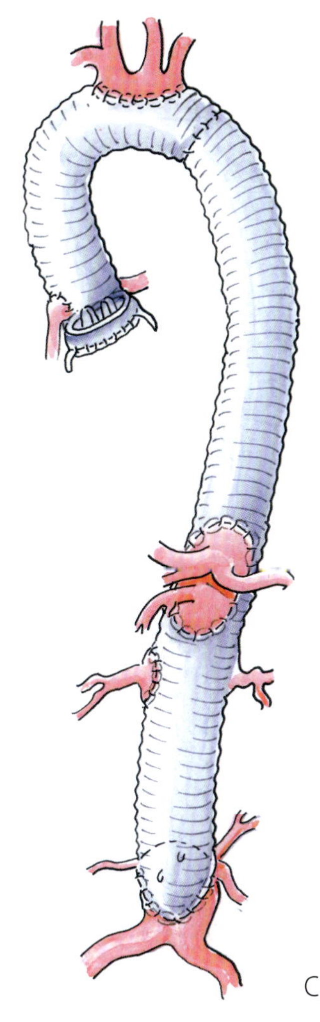

A. 主动脉瘤由升主动脉一直延伸到腹主动脉，同时合并主动脉瓣关闭不全。

A. Aortic aneurysm extends from the ascending aorta to the abdominal aorta with concomitant aortic insufficiency.

B. 升主动脉和主动脉弓置换，主动脉根部采用 Bentall 手术方法，主动脉弓顶部连同主动脉弓上三大分支一并分离后与人工血管吻合。降主动脉的病变留置。

B. The ascending aorta and aortic arch is replaced, and the part of aortic root is replaced by using the Bentall procedure. Three major supra-aortic arch branches together with the roof of aortic arch are dissected and anastomosed with the artificial vessel, retaining the lesions of the descending aorta.

C. 彻底的术式是全主动脉置换。即在上述手术的基础上再用人工血管置换降主动脉，降主动脉的主要分支肋间动脉、腹腔干和肠系膜上动脉、左右肾动脉，分别与人工血管开窗吻合。

C. Total aortic replacement is radical surgery. Based on the above-mentioned operation, the descending aorta is replaced by a graft. Its main branches-intercostal arteries, celiac trunk, superior mesenteric artery and left and right renal arteries, are anastomosed with the graft fenestration respectively.

图 4-5-3　带多分支人工血管主动脉直视修复术

Figure 4-5-3　Open aortic repair with multibranched graft

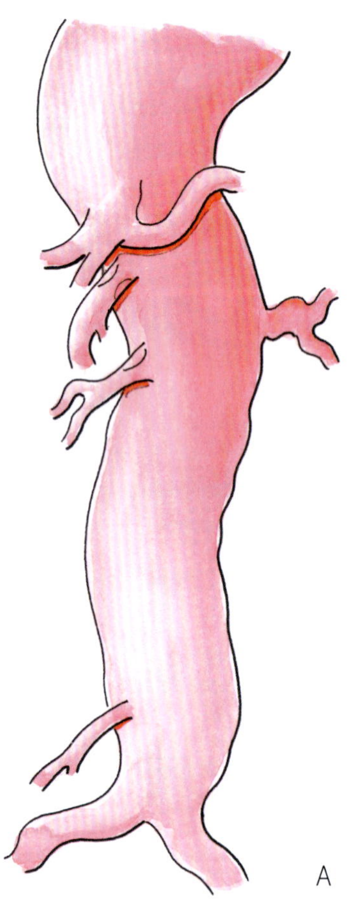

A. 降主动脉动脉瘤累及降主动脉全长。

A. A descending aortic aneurysm involves the full length of the descending aorta.

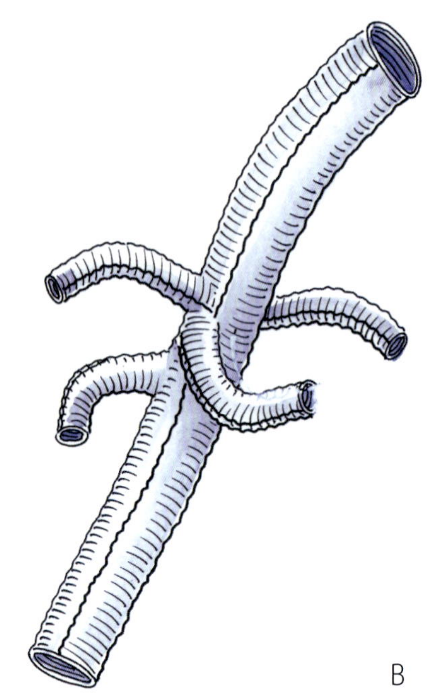

B. 带四分支人工血管。

B. A four-branched artificial vessel.

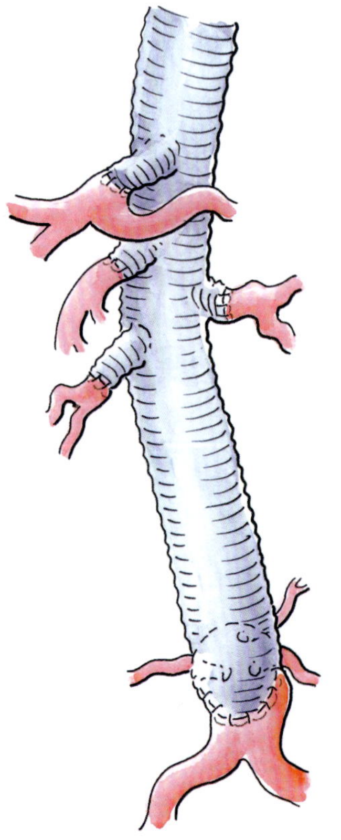

C. 人工血管上端与降主动脉近端做端端吻合。人工血管下端剪成斜口与降主动脉远端做端端吻合，远端分支动脉予以保留。腹腔干、肠系膜上动脉、左右肾动脉分别与人工血管分支吻合。

C. The upper end of the graft is anastomosed end-to-end to the proximal end of the descending aorta, and the lower end trimmed into oblique orifice is anastomosed end-to-end to the distal end of the descending aorta, with the distal branch artery preserved. The celiac trunk, superior mesenteric artery, and left and right renal arteries are anastomosed with the branches of the graft.

第六节 腹主动脉瘤
Section 6 Abdominal Aortic Aneurysm

图 4-6-1 肾动脉下腹主动脉瘤人工血管置换术
Figure 4-6-1 Aortic graft repair for infrarenal abdominal aortic aneurysm

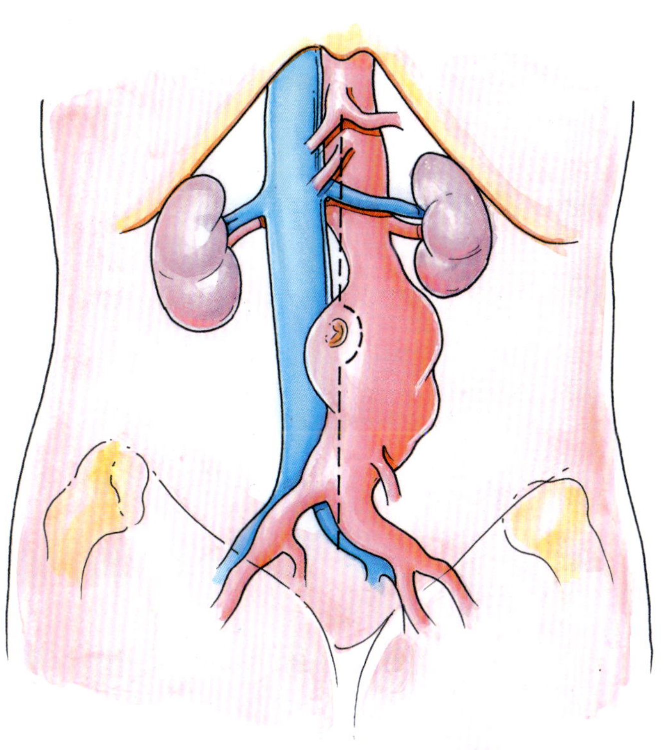

A. 腹主动脉瘤位于肾动脉开口下方。腹白线切口进入腹腔。

A. The abdominal aortic aneurysm is located below the opening of the renal artery. Make an incision through the linea alba (abdomen) to gain access to the peritoneal cavity.

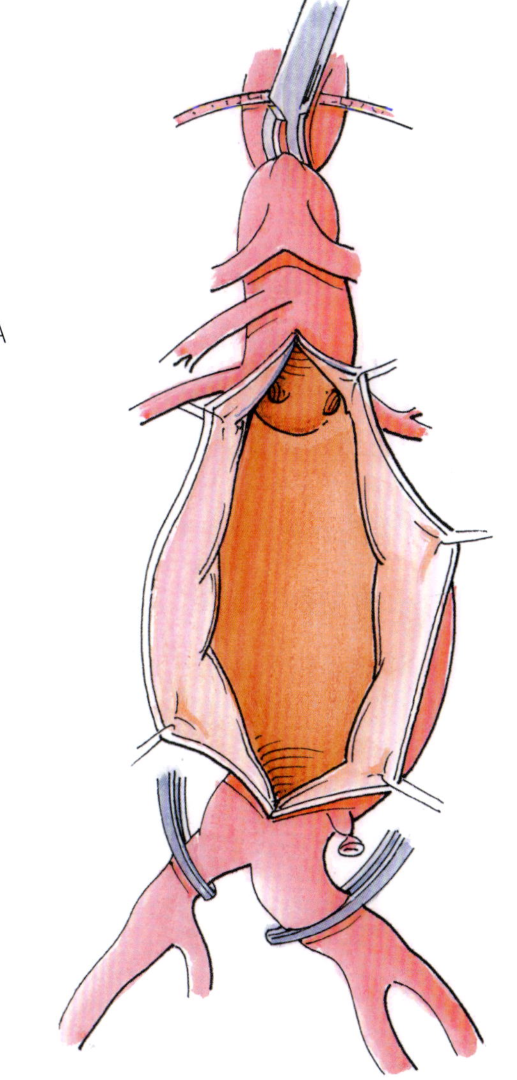

B. 分别阻断腹主动脉近端和左、右髂动脉。切开动脉瘤。

B. Cross-clamp the proximal end of the abdominal aorta and the left and right iliac arteries and incise the aneurysm.

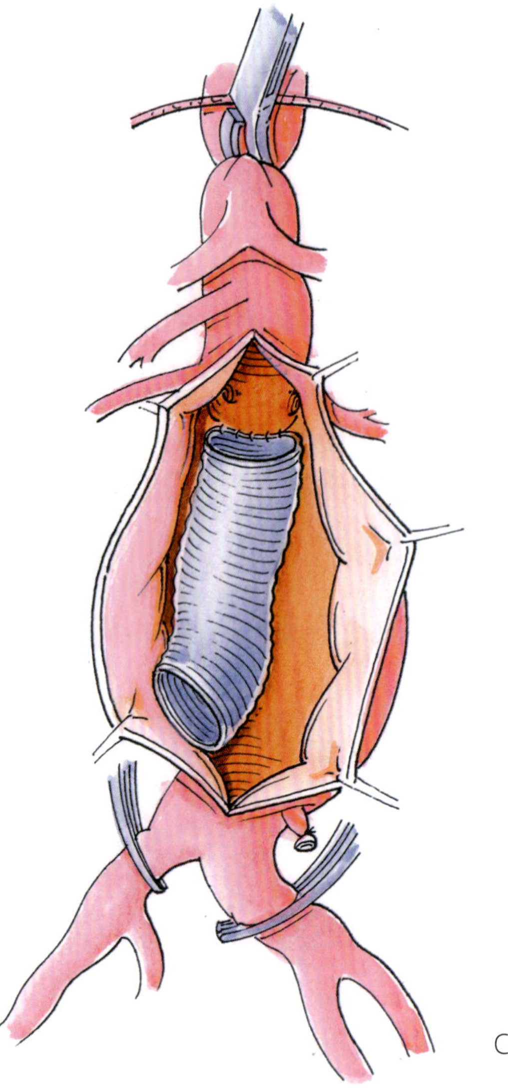

C. 取一段口径匹配的人工血管，在肾动脉水平下与腹主动脉做近端吻合。然后做人工血管腹主动脉远端吻合。

C. A proper artificial vessel is anastomosed proximally to the abdominal aorta under the renal artery level. A distal anastomosis between the graft and the abdominal aorta is then performed.

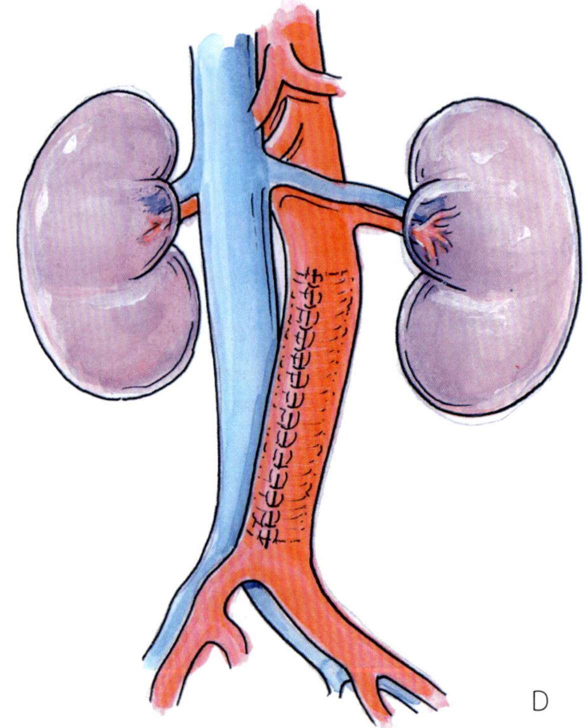

D. 用腹主动脉血管壁将人工血管包埋。

D. The artificial vessel is embedded in the abdominal aortic wall.

图 4-6-2　肾动脉下腹主动脉瘤 Y 形人工血管置换术
Figure 4-6-2　Y-shaped graft repair for infrarenal abdominal aortic aneurysm

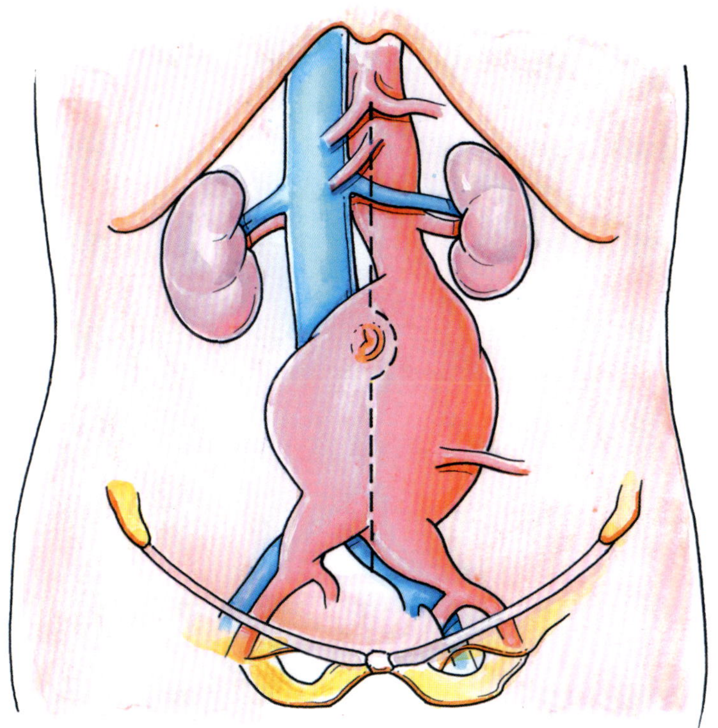

A. 腹主动脉瘤位于肾动脉开口下方，远端至双侧髂动脉。腹白线切口进入腹腔。

A. The abdominal aortic aneurysm is located below the opening of the renal artery, and its distal end reaches the bilateral iliac artery. An incision through the linea alba is performed to access the abdominal cavity.

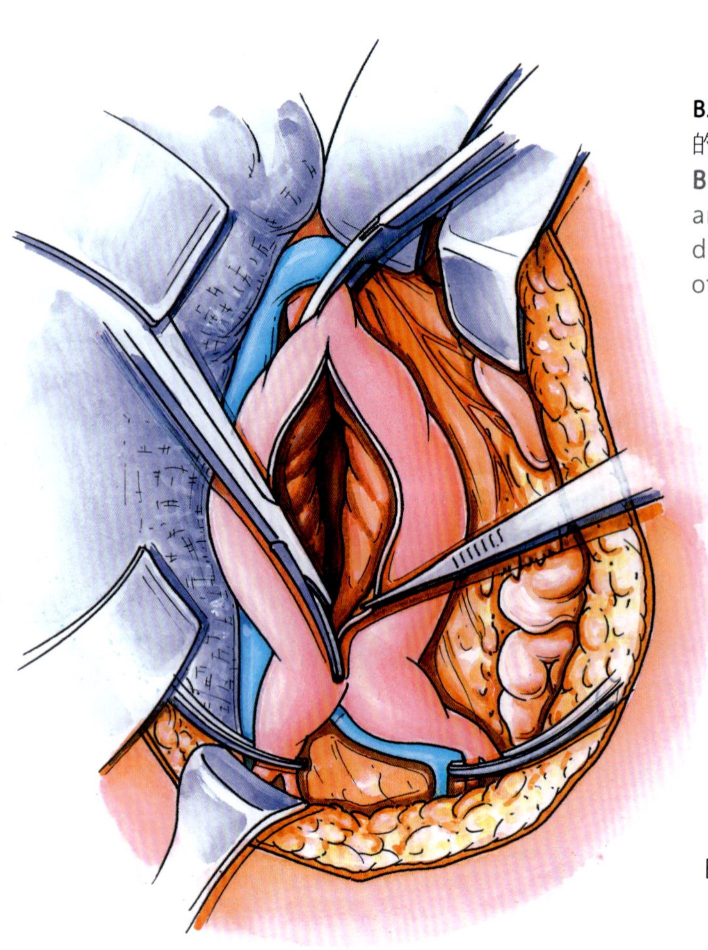

B. 切开后腹膜显露动脉瘤。钳夹阻断近端腹主动脉和远端的两支髂动脉，纵行切开动脉瘤全长。

B. The retroperitoneum is incised to expose the aneurysm. The proximal abdominal aorta and two distal iliac arteries are clamped, and the entire length of the aneurysm is longitudinally incised.

B

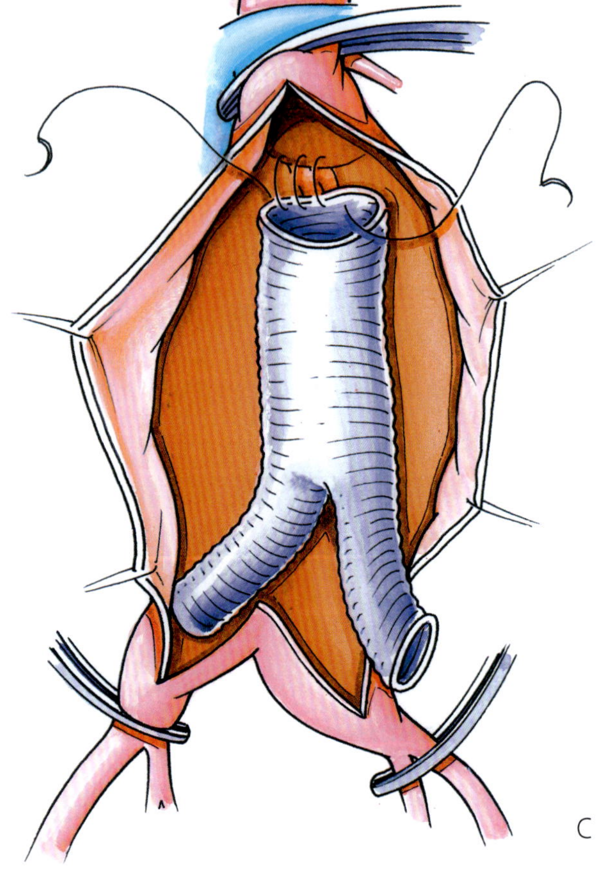

C

C. 选择一口径合适的带二分叉人工血管，将人工血管与腹主动脉近端做端端吻合。

C. A proper Y-shaped bifurcated artificial vessel is utilized and sutured to the proximal end of the abdominal aorta in an end-to-end fashion.

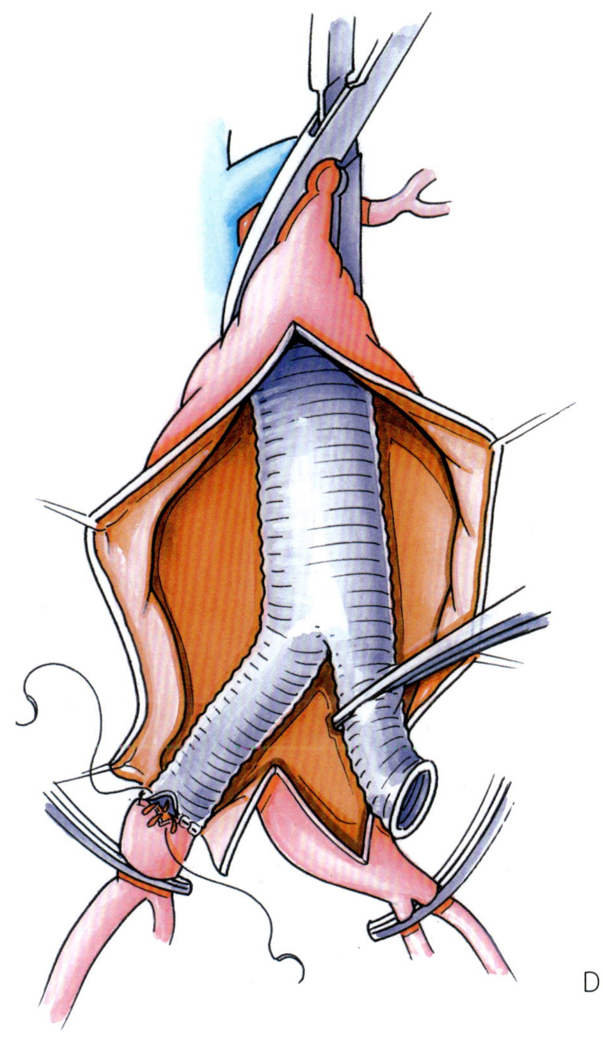

D. 再将人工血管的两个分叉分别与右、左髂动脉做远端吻合。

D. The two limbs of the bifurcated graft are anastomosed distally to the right and left iliac arteries.

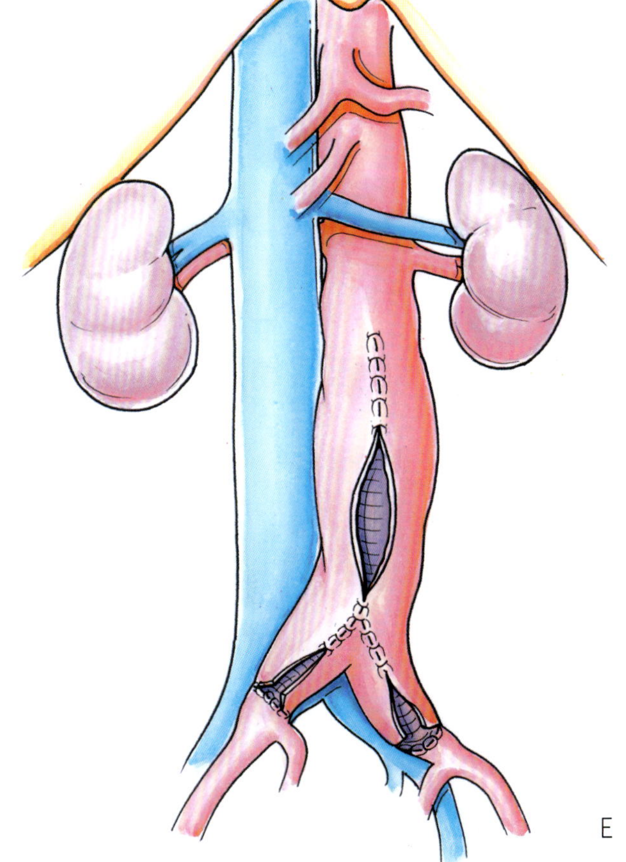

E. 缝合动脉瘤壁包埋人工血管。

E. Suture the aneurysm wall and embed the grafts.

图 4-6-3 肾动脉下腹主动脉瘤伴髂动脉狭窄 Y 形人工血管置换术

Figure 4-6-3 Y-shaped graft repair for infrarenal abdominal aortic aneurysm with iliac artery stenosis

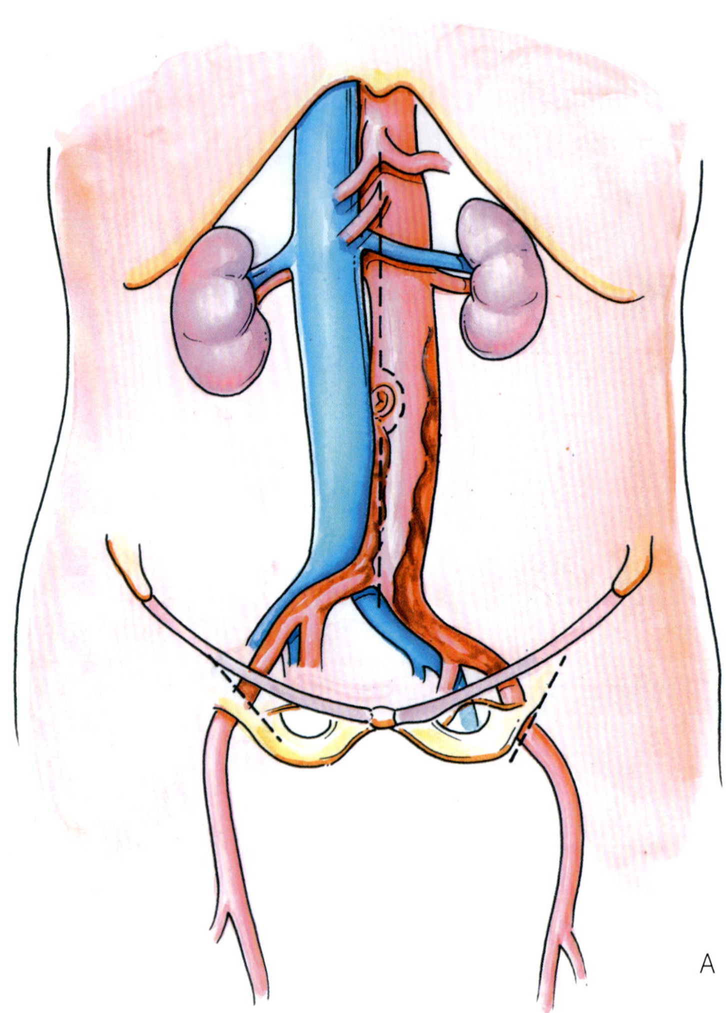

A. 腹主动脉瘤位于肾动脉开口下方，双侧髂动脉狭窄并累及髂外动脉。腹白线切口进入腹腔。

A. An abdominal aortic aneurysm is located below the opening of the renal artery, with bilateral iliac stenosis and involvement of the external iliac artery. Enter the abdominal cavity through an incision into the linea alba.

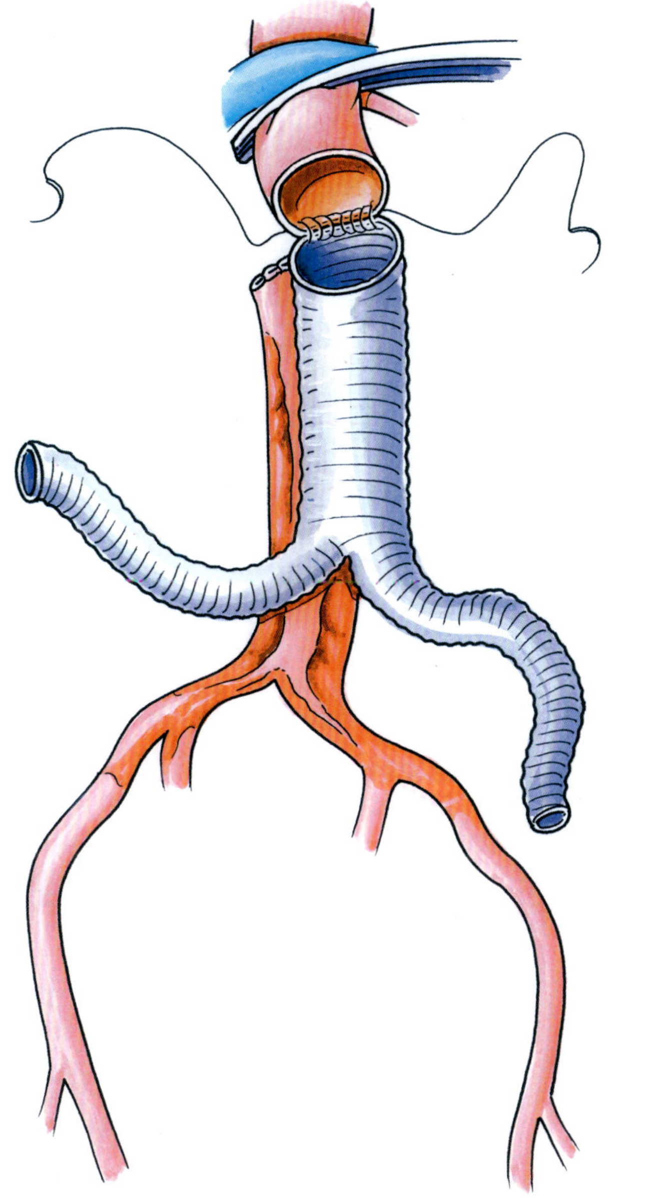

B. 切开后腹膜显露动脉瘤。钳夹阻断近、远端腹主动脉，近端正常腹主动脉处横断，与合适口径的二分叉人工血管端端吻合。腹主动脉远侧断端缝闭。

B. The retroperitoneum is opened to expose the aneurysm. With the proximal and distal abdominal aorta clamped, the proximal normal abdominal aorta is transected and anastomosed to a properly sized bifurcated graft. The distal stump of the abdominal aorta is closed.

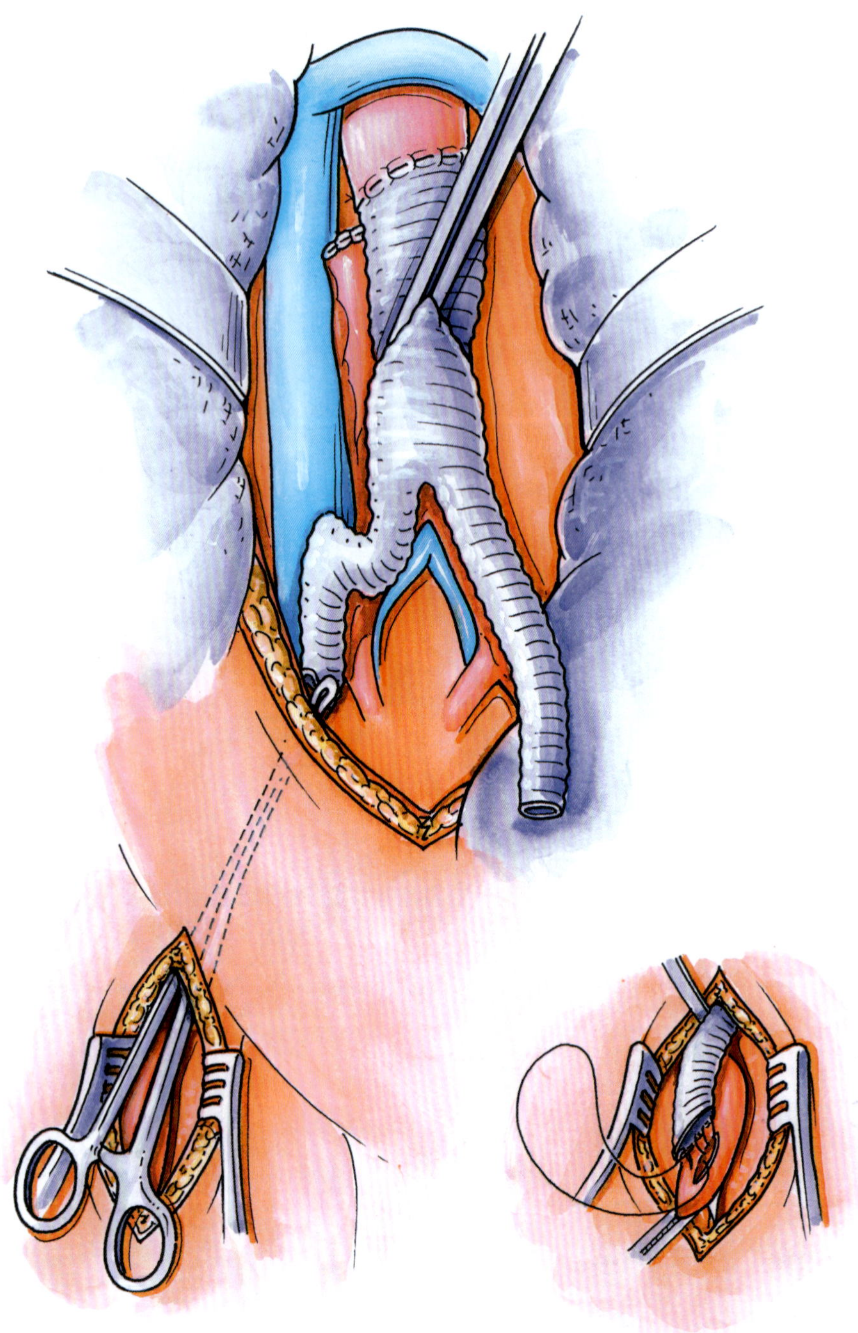

C. 近端主动脉阻断钳下移到人工血管，检查近端吻合口，若有漏血予以补充缝合。双侧腹股沟下循股动脉表面分别做纵行切口。显露股动脉。经皮下隧道将人工血管的分支从腹腔拉到腹股沟切口内。股动脉钳夹阻断后切开，与人工血管端侧吻合。

C. The proximal aortic blocking clamp is moved down to the artificial vessels. The proximal anastomosis is examined, and the anastomotic leakage, if present, is to be repaired with sutures. Longitudinal incisions are performed along the surface of the femoral arteries underneath the bilateral groins to expose the femoral artery. The branch of the graft is brought from the abdominal cavity into the inguinal incision through a subcutaneous tunnel. The femoral artery is clamped and cut open and anastomosed with the graft in an end-to-side fashion.

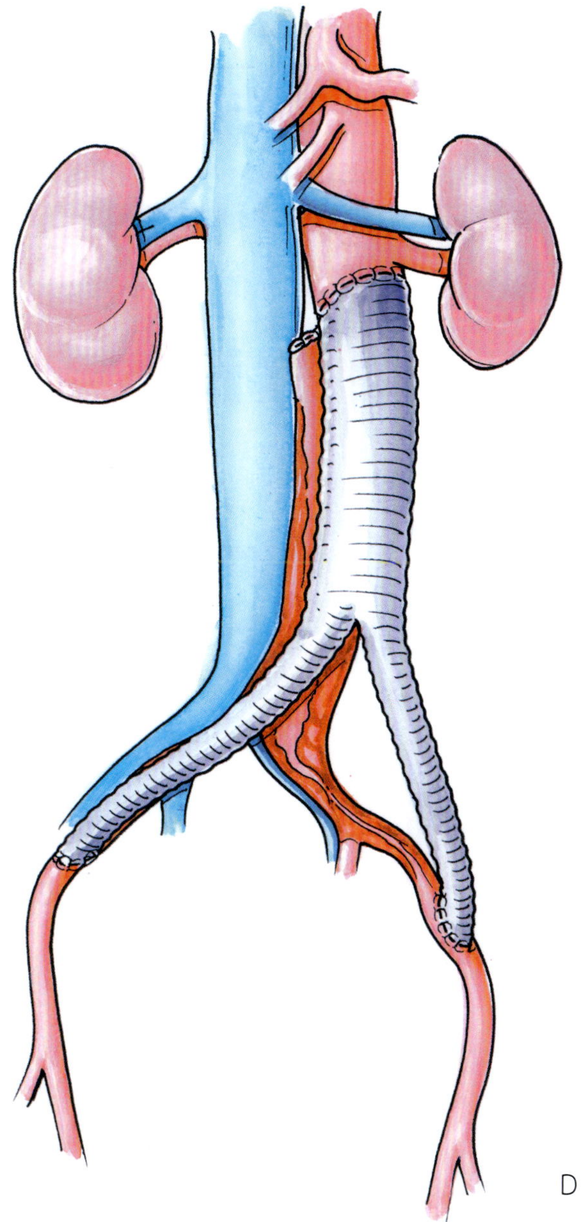

D. 吻合完成。

D. Anastomosis is completed.

图 4-6-4 肾动脉上腹主动脉瘤人工血管置换术（胸 - 腹联合切口）

Figure 4-6-4 Aortic graft repair vascular for suprarenal abdominal aortic aneurysm (thoraco-abdominal incision)

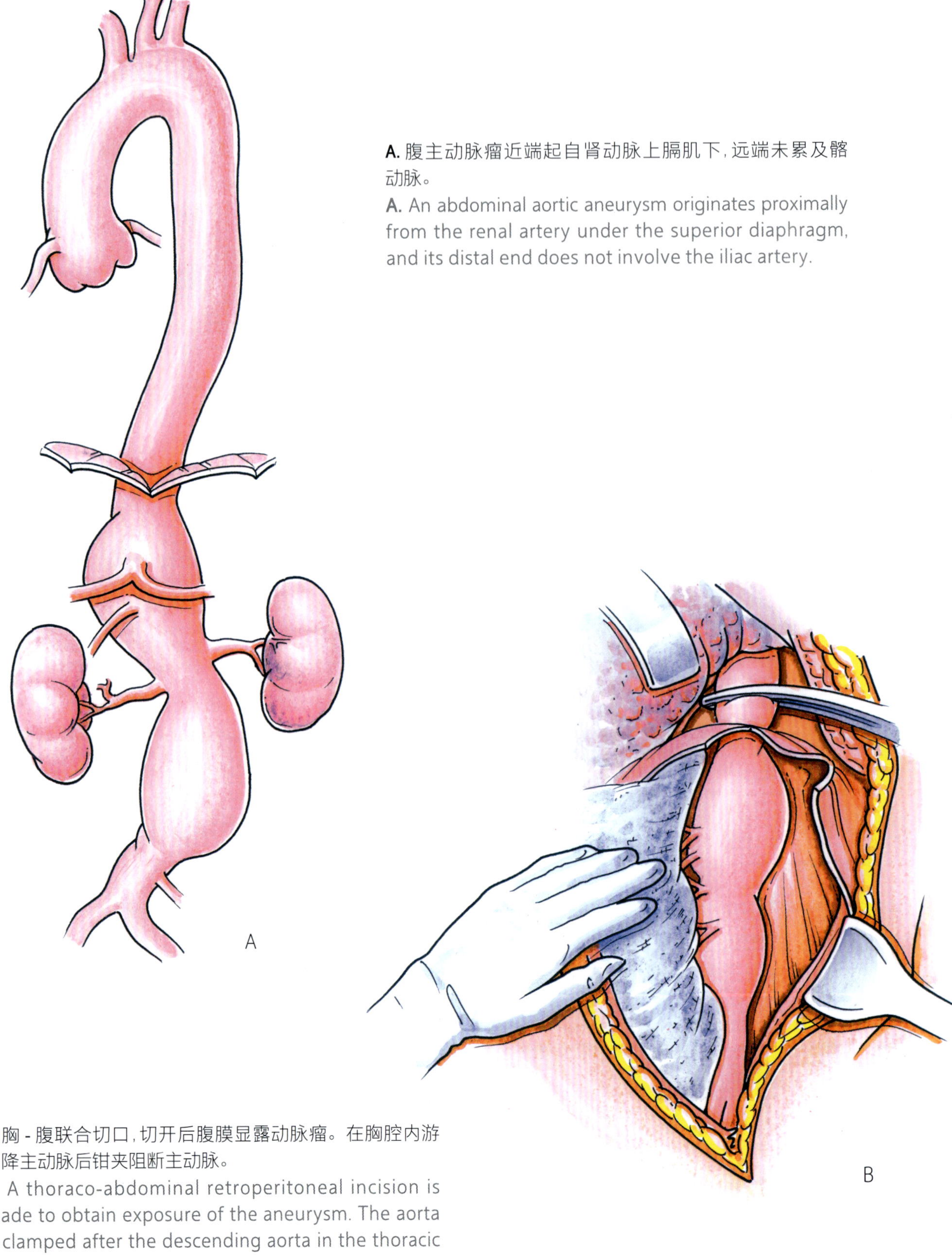

A. 腹主动脉瘤近端起自肾动脉上膈肌下，远端未累及髂动脉。

A. An abdominal aortic aneurysm originates proximally from the renal artery under the superior diaphragm, and its distal end does not involve the iliac artery.

B. 胸 - 腹联合切口，切开后腹膜显露动脉瘤。在胸腔内游离降主动脉后钳夹阻断主动脉。

B. A thoraco-abdominal retroperitoneal incision is made to obtain exposure of the aneurysm. The aorta is clamped after the descending aorta in the thoracic cavity is freed.

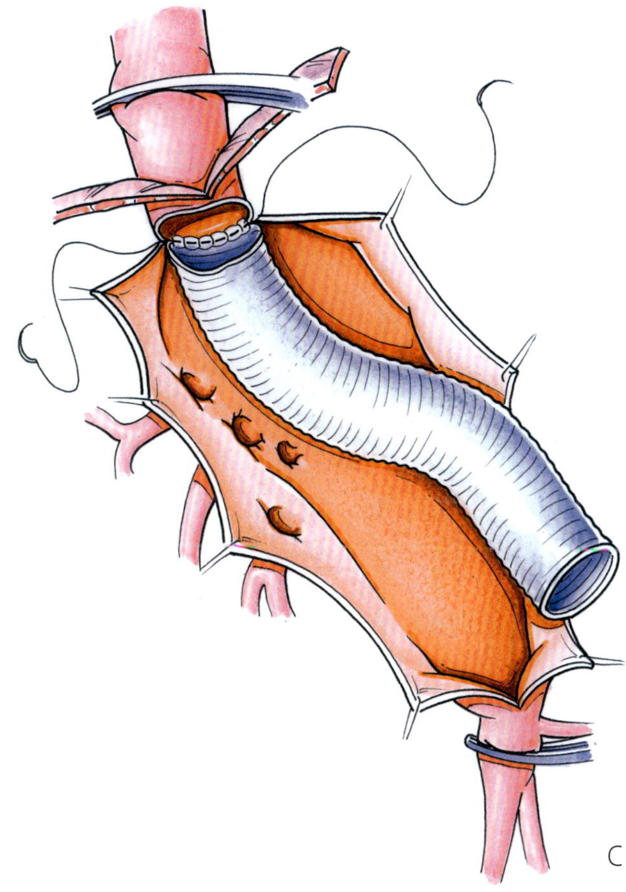

C. 降主动脉远端上钳阻断，纵行切开动脉瘤全长，选择合适口径的人工血管与降主动脉做近端吻合。

C. The distal end of the descending aorta is clamped with forceps, and the entire length of the aneurysm is incised longitudinally. A proper graft is selected for proximal anastomosis with the descending aorta.

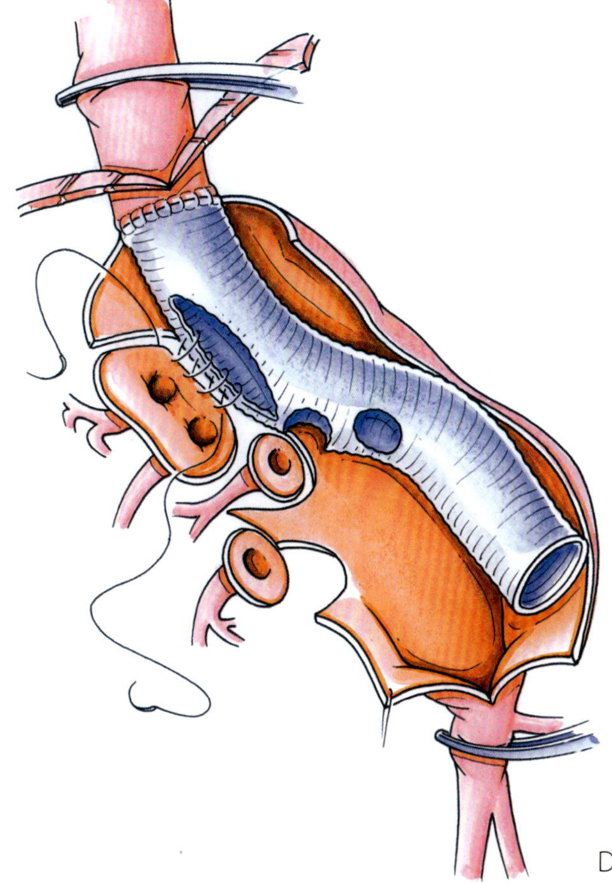

D. 腹主动脉的主要分支腹腔干和肠系膜上动脉、左右肾动脉、肠系膜下动脉分别与人工血管开口吻合。

D. The main branches of the abdominal aorta- celiac artery, superior mesenteric artery, left and right renal arteries, and inferior mesenteric artery are anastomosed with the opening of artificial vessel, respectively.

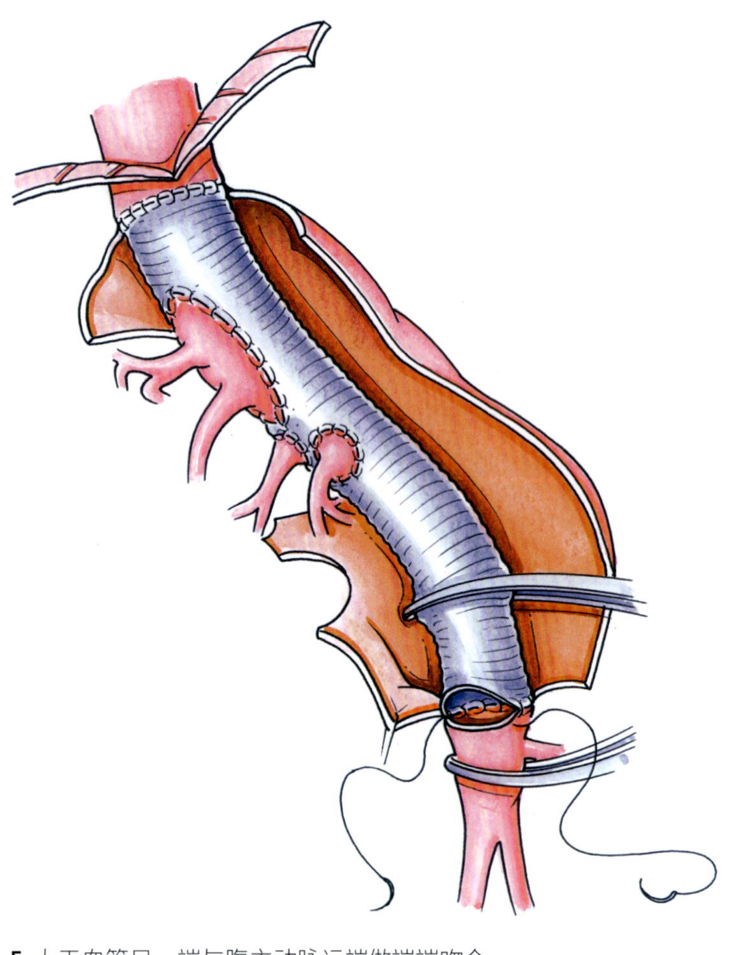

E. 人工血管另一端与腹主动脉远端做端端吻合。

E. An end-to-end anastomosis is performed between the other end of the graft and the distal end of the abdominal aorta.

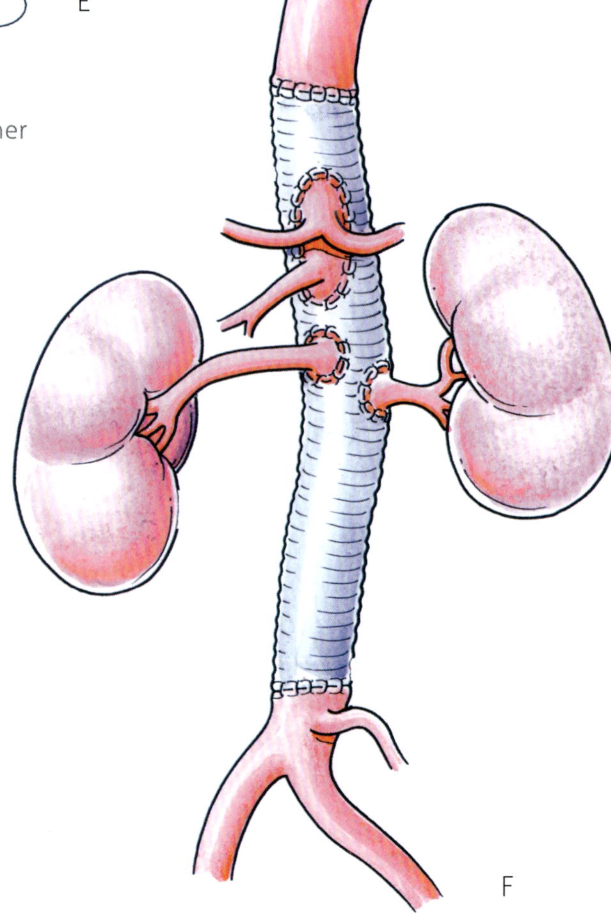

F. 吻合完成。

F. Anastomosis is completed.

图 4-6-5 肾动脉上腹主动脉瘤人工血管置换术（腹部切口）

Figure 4-6-5 Aortic graft repair for suprarenal abdominal aortic aneurysm (abdominal incision)

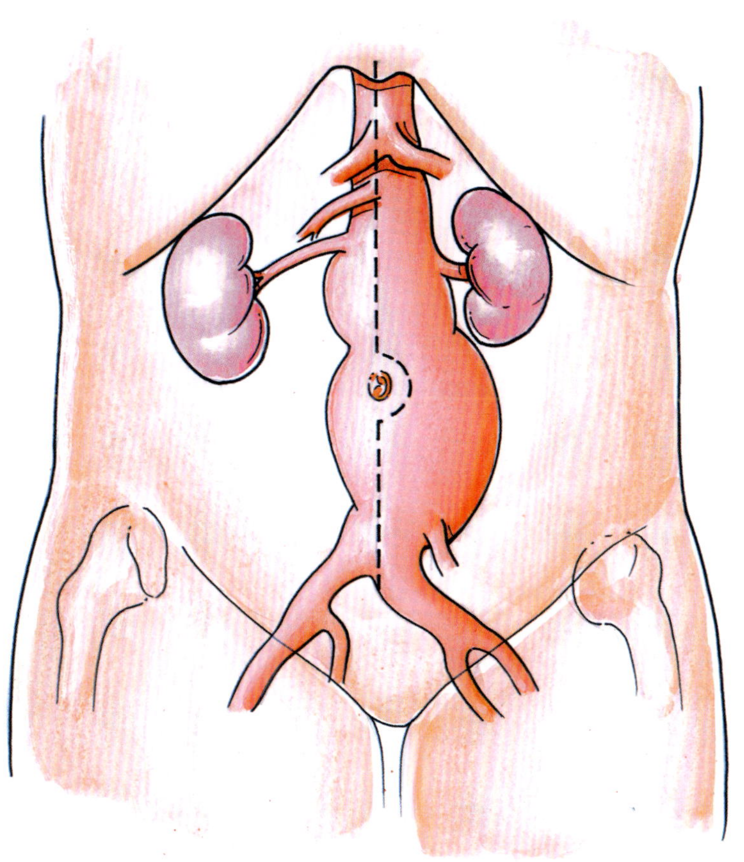

A. 腹主动脉瘤上端达肾动脉开口水平，远端至腹主动脉末段。腹白线切口进入腹腔。

A. The upper end of the abdominal aortic aneurysm reaches the level of the renal artery ostium, and its distal end reaches the end of the abdominal aorta. Make an incision through the linea alba to gain access to the peritoneal cavity.

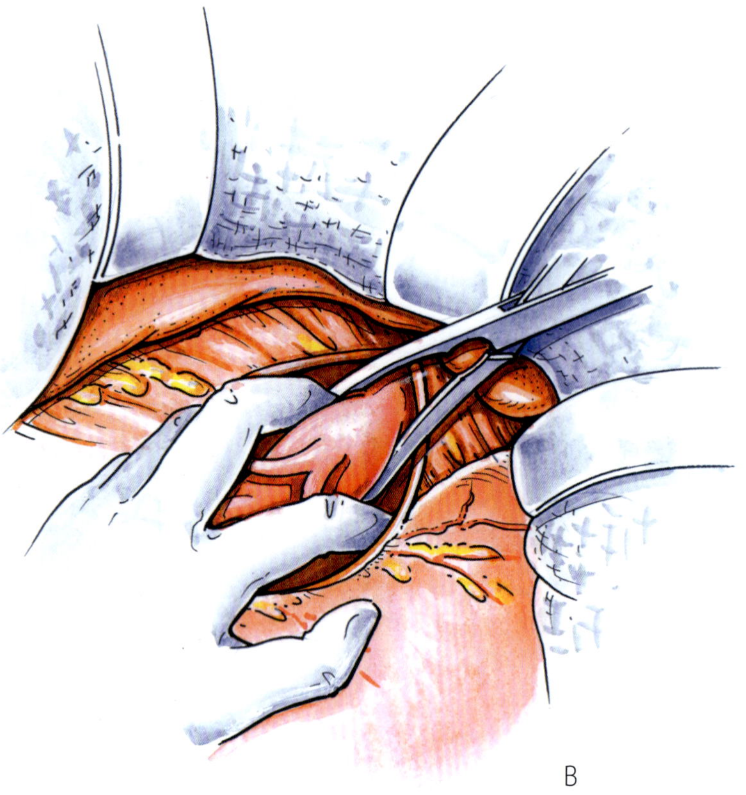

B. 切开后腹膜显露动脉瘤。腹主动脉瘤近端和双侧髂动脉钳夹阻断。

B. Aneurysm is exposed after a retroperitoneal incision. Clamps are placed on the proximal abdominal aortic aneurysm and bilateral iliac artery for occlusion.

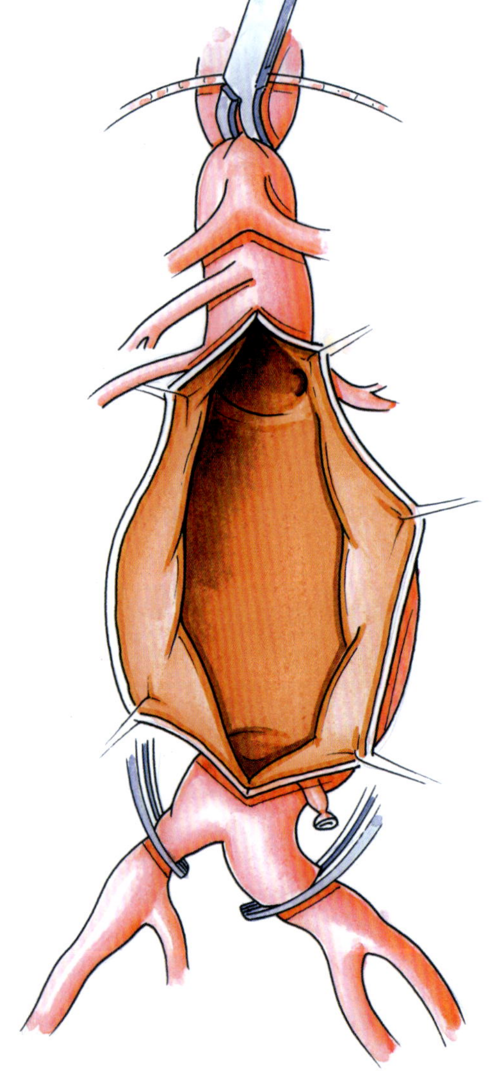

C. 腹主动脉前壁纵行切开动脉瘤，切口上端略超过肾动脉开口水平。

C. A longitudinal incision is made on the anterior wall of the abdominal aorta with the upper end of the incision slightly above the level of the renal artery ostium.

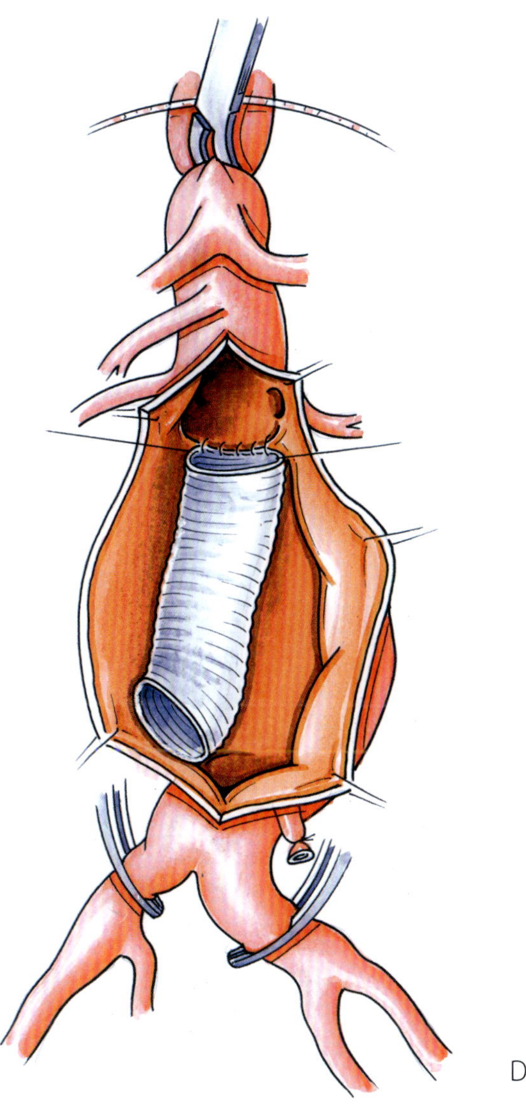

D. 选择合适口径的人工血管做近端吻合，后壁缝合要缝在肾动脉开口下方。确保吻合口近端的双侧肾动脉开口通畅。

D. An appropriate artificial vessel is used for proximal anastomosis, and the posterior wall is sutured below the opening of the renal artery. Ensure patency of the opening of the bilateral renal artery proximal to the anastomotic site.

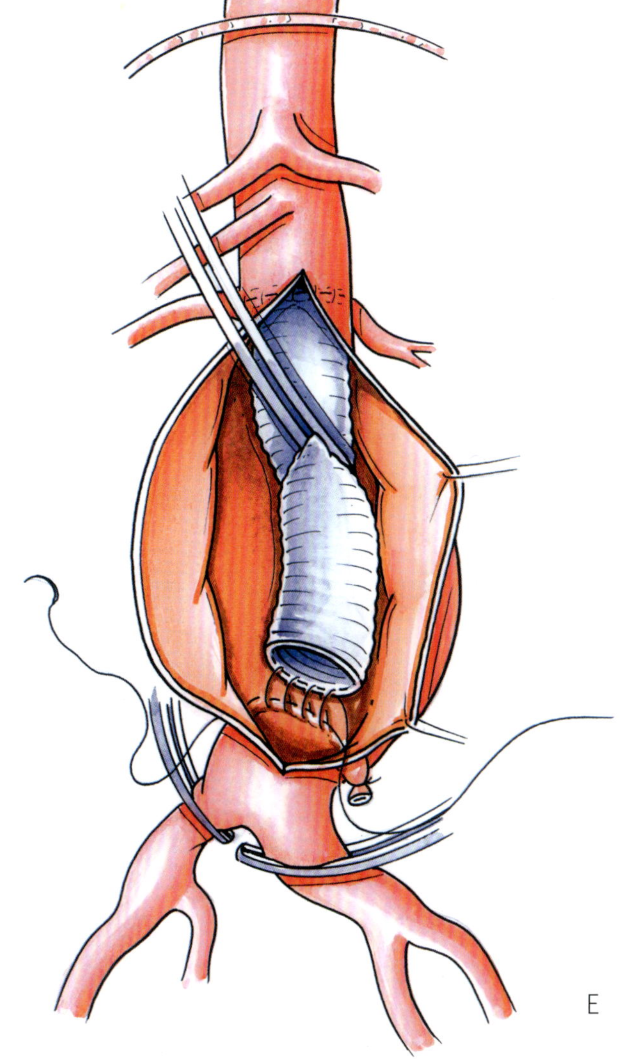

E. 人工血管另一端与远端腹主动脉端端吻合。

E. The other end of the graft is anastomosed end-to-end to the distal abdominal aorta.

第 七 节　主动脉内膜破裂
Section 7　Aortic Intimal Rupture

图 4-7-1　直视人工血管置换术
Figure 4-7-1　Open aorta graft replacement

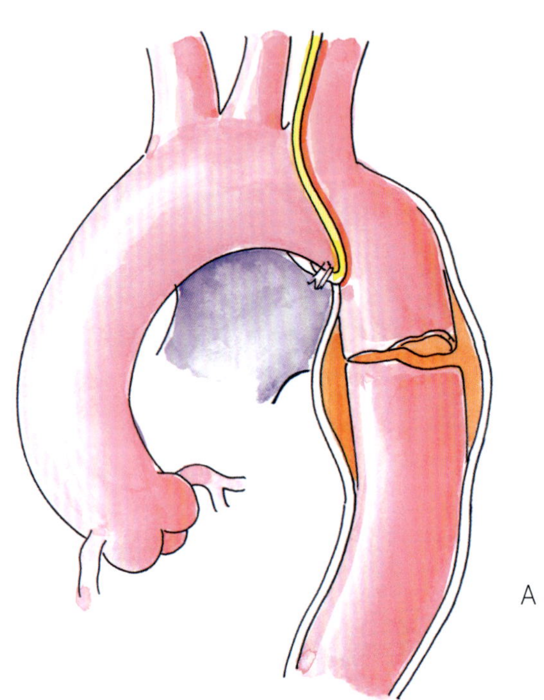

A. 胸降主动脉内膜破裂，局部壁间血肿形成。

A. Intimal rupture of the descending thoracic aorta complicated with local intramural hematoma.

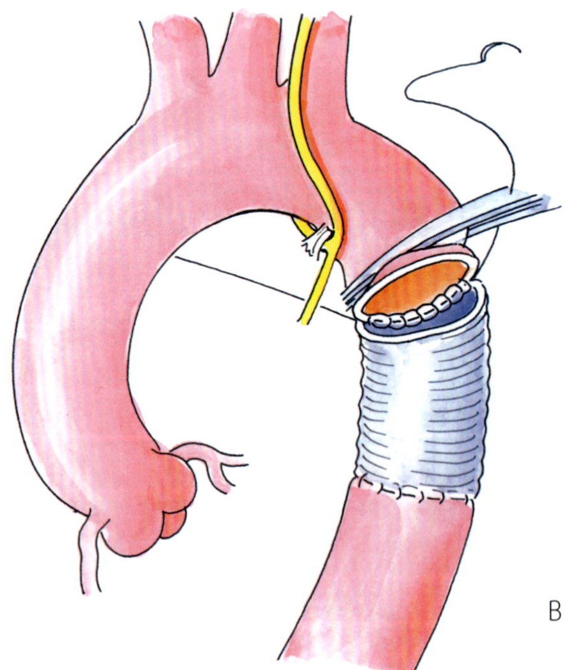

B. 在血肿两端正常降主动脉处钳夹阻断，切除血肿段降主动脉。人工血管与降主动脉远端做端端吻合，然后做近端吻合。

B. Clamp the normal descending aorta at both ends of the hematoma and resect the segment with hematoma. Make an end-to-end anastomosis of the artificial vessel to the distal end of descending aorta, and then proximal anastomosis.

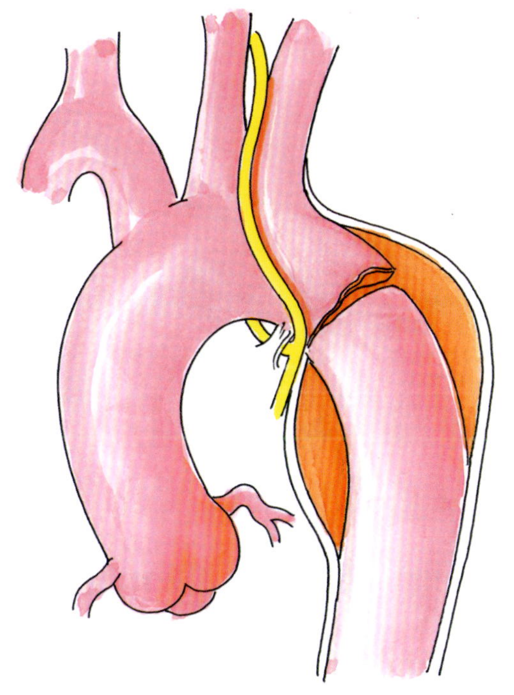

C

C. 胸降主动脉内膜破裂，长段壁间血肿形成。

C. Intimal tear of the descending thoracic aorta with a long-segmental intramural hematoma.

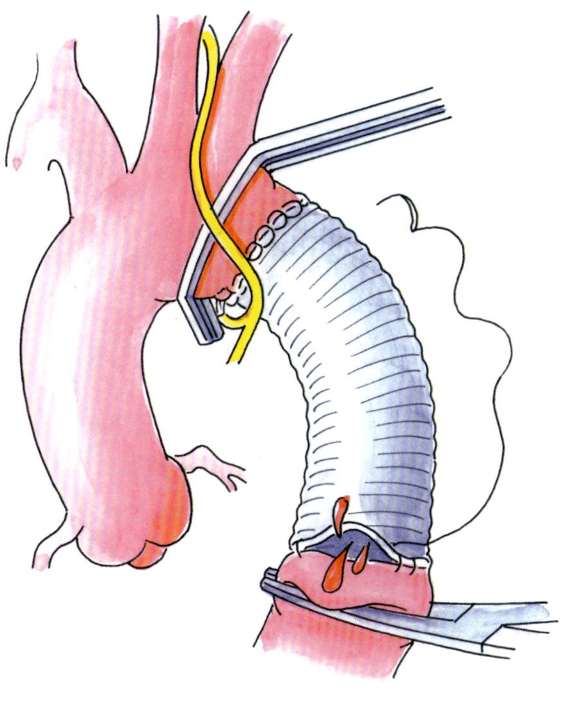

D

D. 在血肿两端正常降主动脉处钳夹阻断，切除血肿段降主动脉。人工血管与降主动脉近端做端端吻合，然后做远端吻合，结扎前人工血管排气。

D. Clamp the normal descending aorta at both ends of the hematoma and resect the segment with hematoma. Make an end-to-end anastomosis of the artificial blood vessel to the proximal end of the descending aorta, and then distal anastomosis. Ventilate the graft before ligation.

第八节　霉菌性主动脉瘤
Section 8　Mycotic Aortic Aneurysm

图 4-8-1　血管内支架植入及肠瘘后霉菌性主动脉瘤
Figure 4-8-1　Mycotic aortic aneurysm following endograft implantation and intestinal fistula

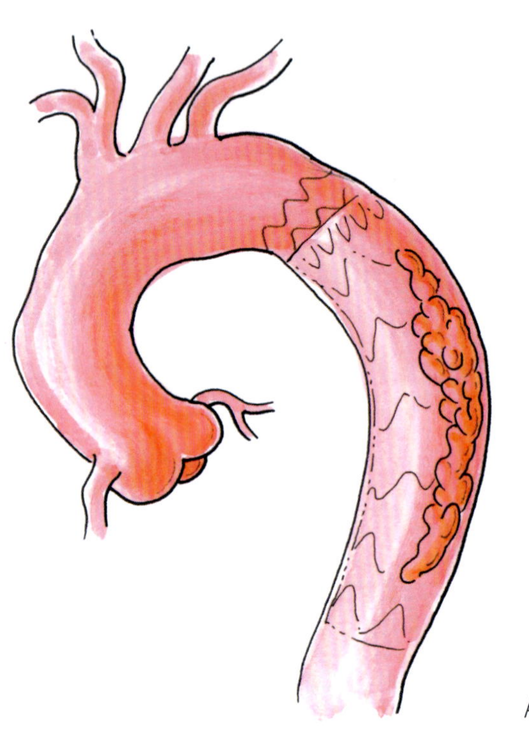

A. 胸降主动脉血管内支架植入后发生霉菌性主动脉瘤。
A. Mycotic aortic aneurysm secondary to endograft implantation of the descending thoracic aorta.

B. 在原植入血管内支架两端正常降主动脉处钳夹阻断，连同血管内支架一并切除该段降主动脉。采用同种异体主动脉与降主动脉近端做端端吻合。
B. Clamp the normal descending aorta at both ends of the endovascular stent implantation, and remove that portion of the descending aorta with its endovascular stent. End-to-end anastomosis is performed between an aorta allograft and the proximal end of the descending aorta.

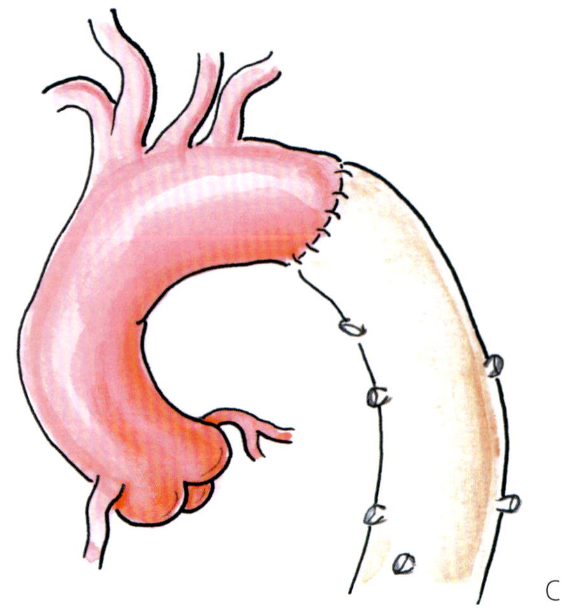

C. 同种异体主动脉与降主动脉远端做端端吻合。
C. End-to-end anastomosis is performed between the distal ends of the allograft and the descending aorta.

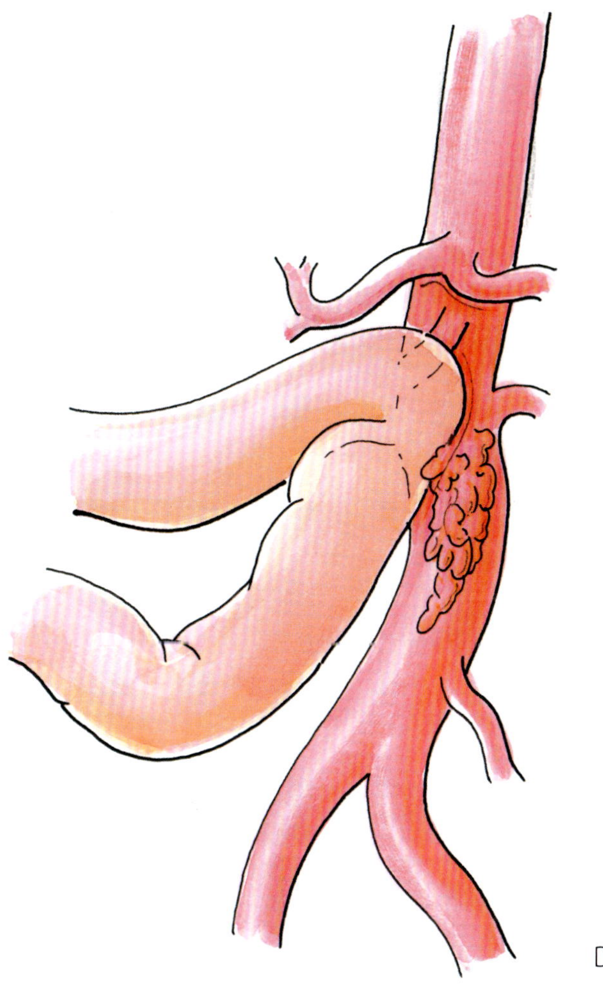

D. 空肠瘘后腹主动脉霉菌性主动脉瘤。

D. Mycotic aortic aneurysm in the abdominal aorta following jejunal fistula.

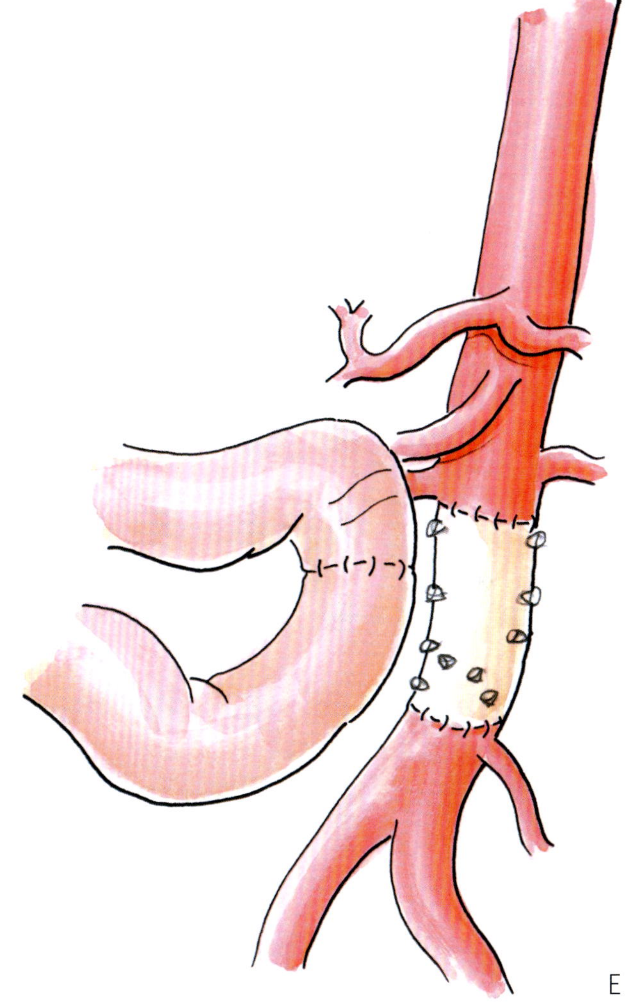

E. 切除该段降腹主动脉，植入同种异体主动脉重建腹主动脉。肠瘘处行空肠切除端端吻合。

E. This segment of the descending abdominal aorta is resected, and an allograft is implanted to reconstruct the abdominal aorta. Jejunectomy is performed at the site of the intestinal fistula with end-to-end anastomosis.

图 4-8-2 直视修补椎间盘炎导致的主动脉假性动脉瘤

Figure 4-8-2 Open repair for aortic pseudoaneurysm caused by spondylodiscitis

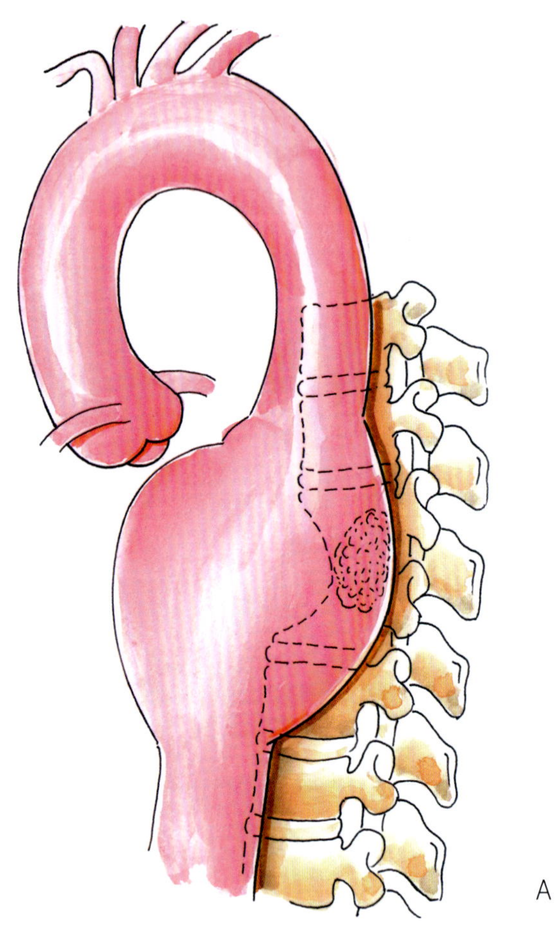

A. 胸椎椎间盘炎侵犯邻近的主动脉导致胸降主动脉假性动脉瘤形成。

A. Thoracic spondylodiscitis invades the adjacent aorta, resulting in descending thoracic aortic pseudoaneurysm.

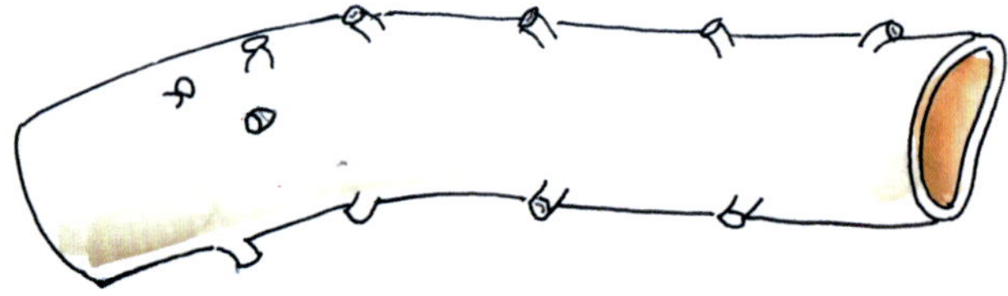

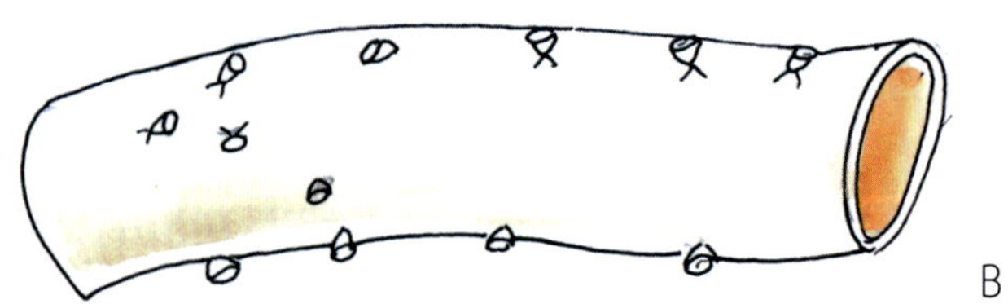

B. 选择合适口径的同种异体主动脉。

B. Choose an appropriate aorta allograft.

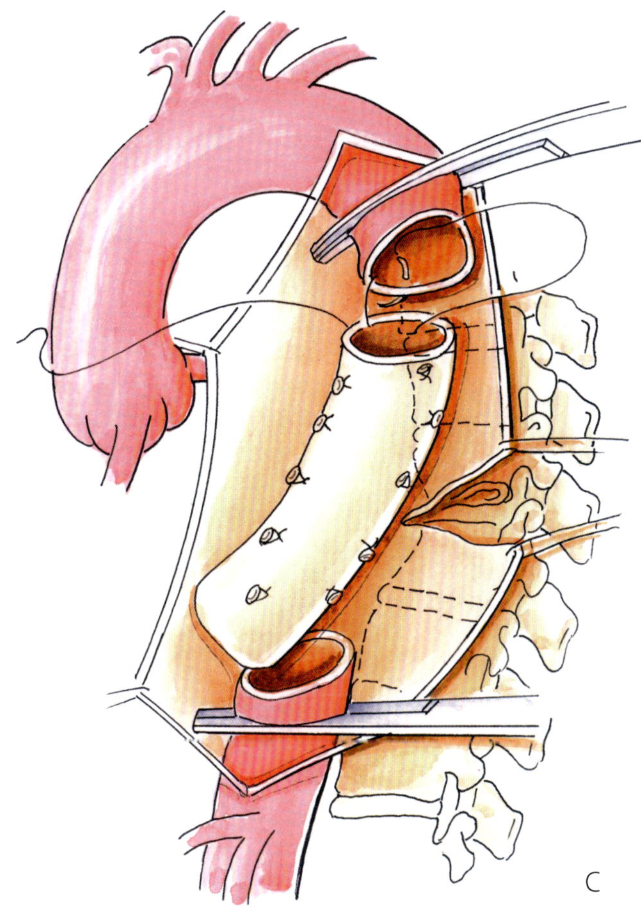

C. 在假性动脉瘤两端正常降主动脉处钳夹阻断，切除该段降主动脉，胸椎椎间盘炎处彻底清创。采用同种主动脉移植置换该段降主动脉。

C. Place clamps the normal descending aorta at both ends of the pseudoaneurysm, excise this portion of the descending aorta, and thoroughly debride the thoracic spondylodiscitis. The descending aorta is replaced with an aorta allograft.

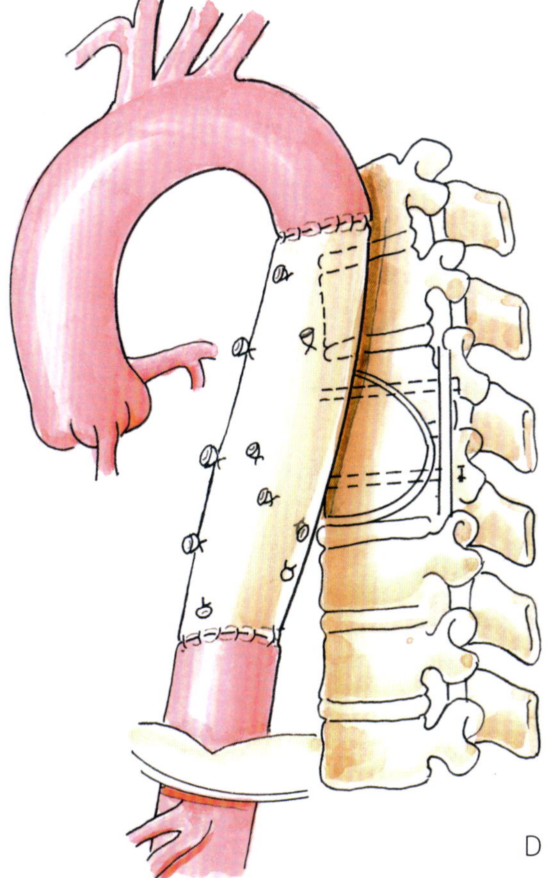

D. 胸椎内固定加固。

D. Thoracic internal fixation and reinforcement.

第九节　主动脉杂交手术
Section 9　Hybrid Aorta Surgery

图 4-9-1　杂交修补远段主动脉弓和降主动脉瘤
Figure 4-9-1　Hybrid repair for distal segment of aortic arch and descending aortic aneurysm

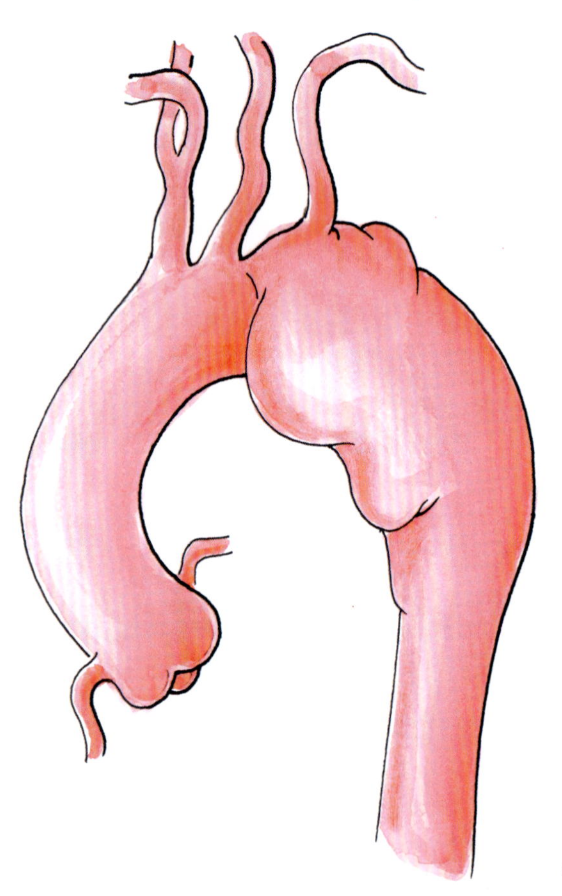

A. 远段主动脉弓和降主动脉瘤，累及左锁骨下动脉开口。
A. The distal segment of the aortic arch and the descending aortic aneurysm, involving the ostium of the left subclavian artery.

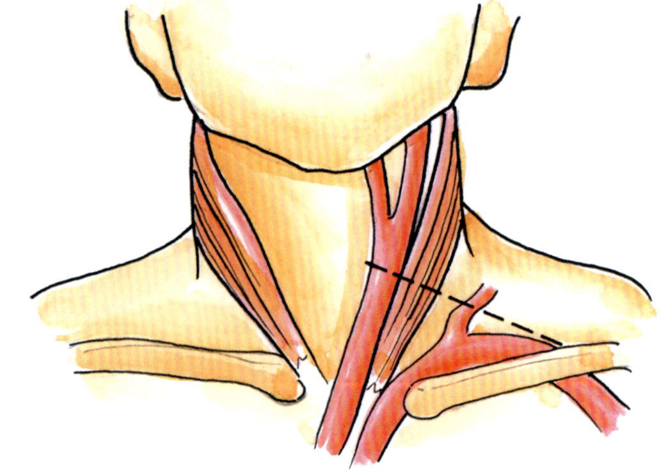

B. 左锁骨上切口。
B. Make a left supraclavicular incision.

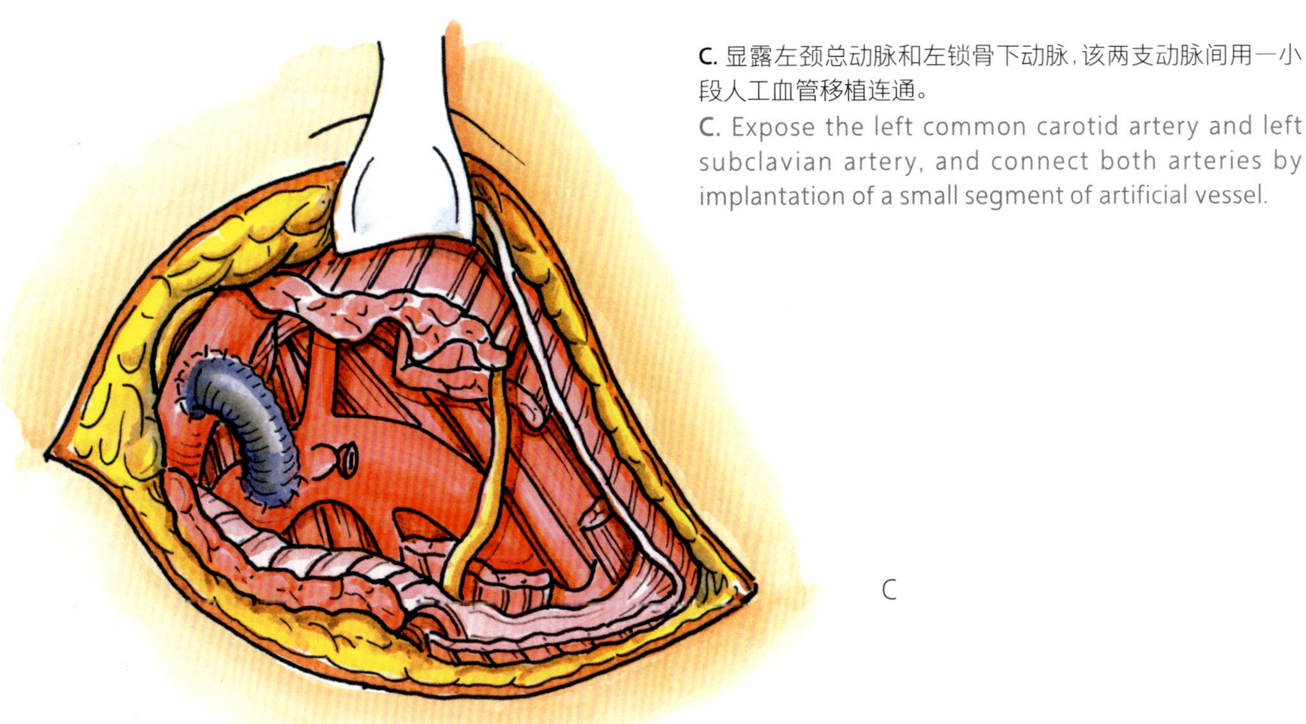

C. 显露左颈总动脉和左锁骨下动脉，该两支动脉间用一小段人工血管移植连通。

C. Expose the left common carotid artery and left subclavian artery, and connect both arteries by implantation of a small segment of artificial vessel.

C

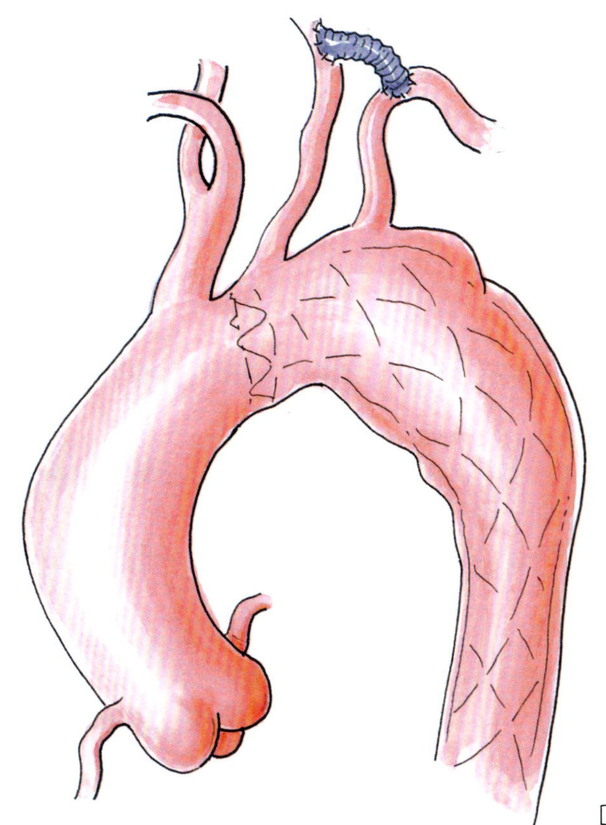

D. 经股动脉介入植入主动脉内支架，其近端锚定于左颈总动脉开口和左锁骨下动脉开口之间，支架覆盖左锁骨下动脉开口。左锁骨下动脉由人工血管桥供血。

D. A stent is implanted into the aorta via the femoral artery. With its proximal end anchored between the ostia of the left common carotid artery and the left subclavian artery, the stent covers the ostium of the left subclavian artery. The blood is supplied to the left subclavian artery by a bridging artificial vessel.

D

图 4-9-2 杂交修补主动脉弓和降主动脉瘤

Figure 4-9-2 Hybrid repair for aortic arch and descending aortic aneurysm

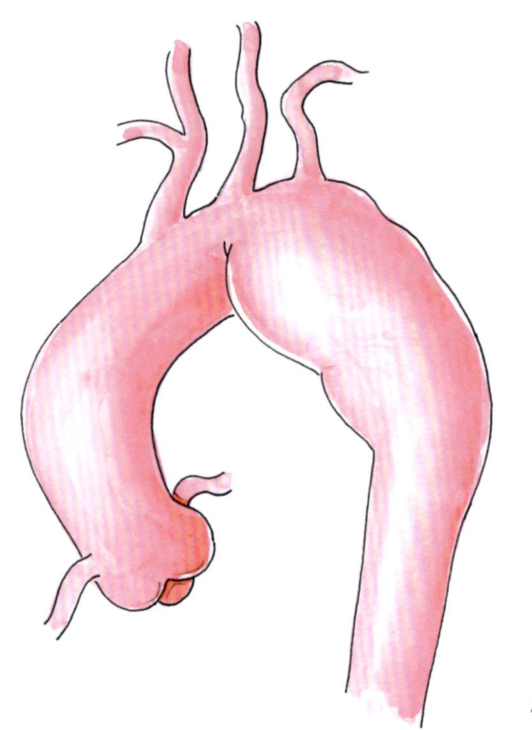

A. 主动脉弓和降主动脉瘤，累及左锁骨下动脉和左颈总动脉开口。

A. Aortic arch and descending aortic aneurysm involves the left subclavian artery and the ostium of the left common carotid artery.

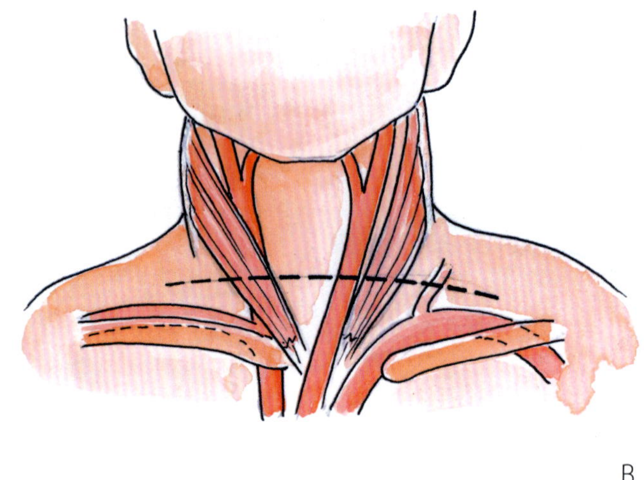

B. 颈部横切口并向左延长到左锁骨上。

B. A transverse neck incision is created and extended left to the left clavicle.

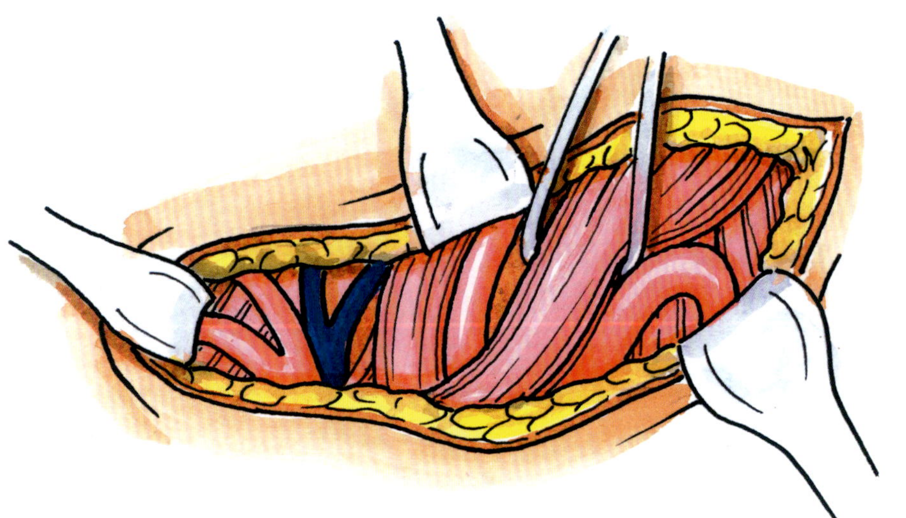

C. 显露头臂干、左颈总动脉和左锁骨下动脉。

C. Expose the brachiocephalic trunk, left common carotid artery, and left subclavian artery.

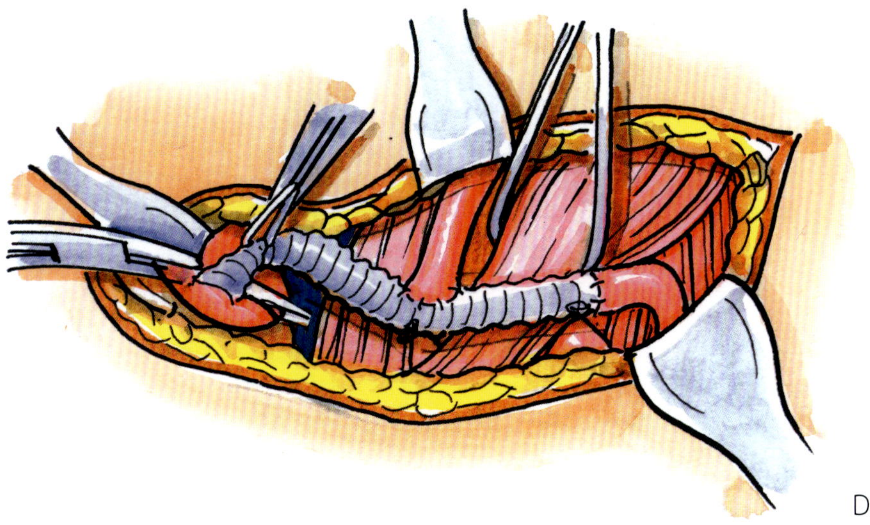

D. 切断左锁骨下动脉，近侧断端缝扎，远侧断端与人工血管端端吻合。切断左颈总动脉，近侧断端缝扎，远侧断端与人工血管侧壁开口端侧吻合。人工血管的另一端与头臂干侧壁开口端侧吻合。

D. The left subclavian artery is transected, its proximal stump sutured, and the distal stump anastomosed to a artificial vessel in an end-to-end fashion. The left common carotid artery is transected with its proximal stump sutured and distal stump anastomosed to the opening of the artificial vessel using end-to-side anastomosis. The other end of the graft is sutured to the opening of the lateral wall of the brachiocephalic trunk with end-to-side anastomosis.

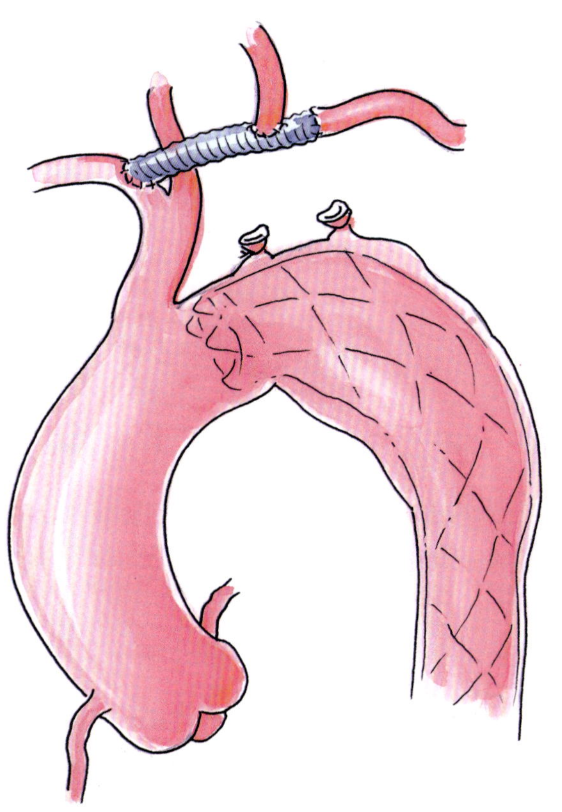

E. 经股动脉介入植入主动脉内支架，其近端锚定于头臂干开口和左颈总动脉开口之间，支架覆盖左颈总动脉开口和左锁骨下动脉开口。左颈总动脉和左锁骨下动脉由人工血管桥供血。

E. An intra-aortic stent is implanted through the femoral artery. With its proximal end anchored between the ostia of the brachiocephalic trunk and the left common carotid artery, the stent covers the ostia of the left common carotid artery and the left subclavian artery. The blood is supplied to the left common carotid artery and left subclavian artery by a bridging artificial vessel.

图 4-9-3 一期杂交修补胸主动脉瘤
Figure 4-9-3 One-stage hybrid repair for thoracic aortic aneurysm

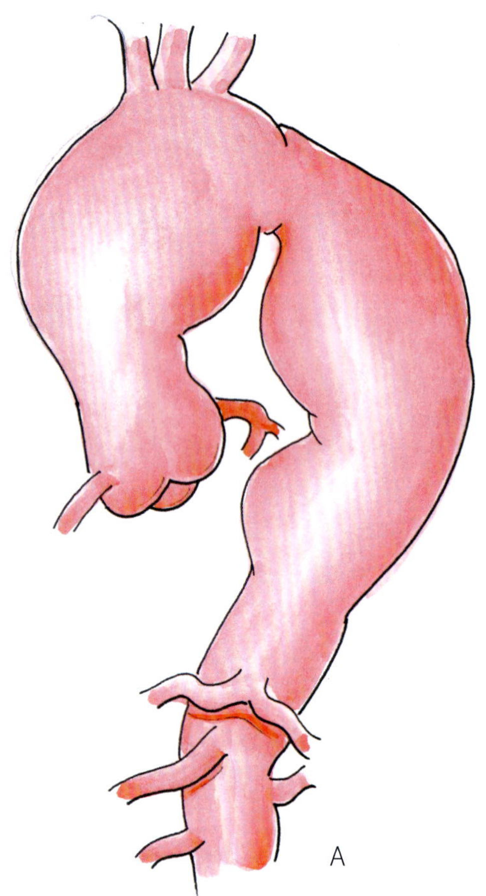

A. 主动脉梭形动脉瘤，病变广泛，起自升主动脉近端止于胸降主动脉末端。

A. A fusiform aortic aneurysm with extensive lesions originates from the proximal ascending aorta to the distal descending thoracic aorta.

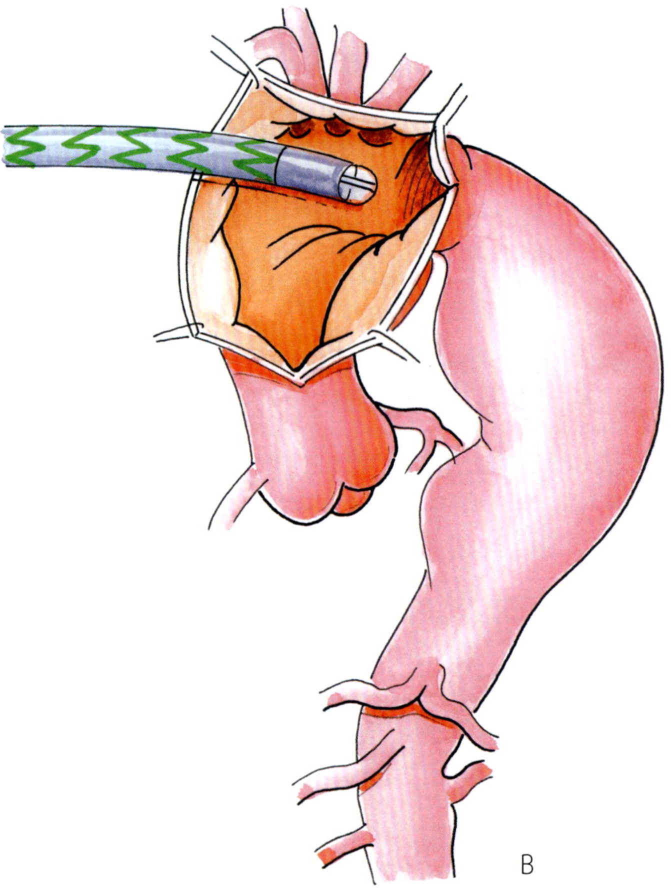

B. 深低温停循环，切开远段升主动脉，切口向主动脉弓延长至弓降部。经主动脉切口向降主动脉植入主动脉内支架。

B. Under deep hypothermia circulatory arrest, an incision is placed on the distal segment of the ascending aorta and extended toward the aortic arch to the descending arch. An intra-aortic stent graft is implanted into the descending aorta through an aortic incision.

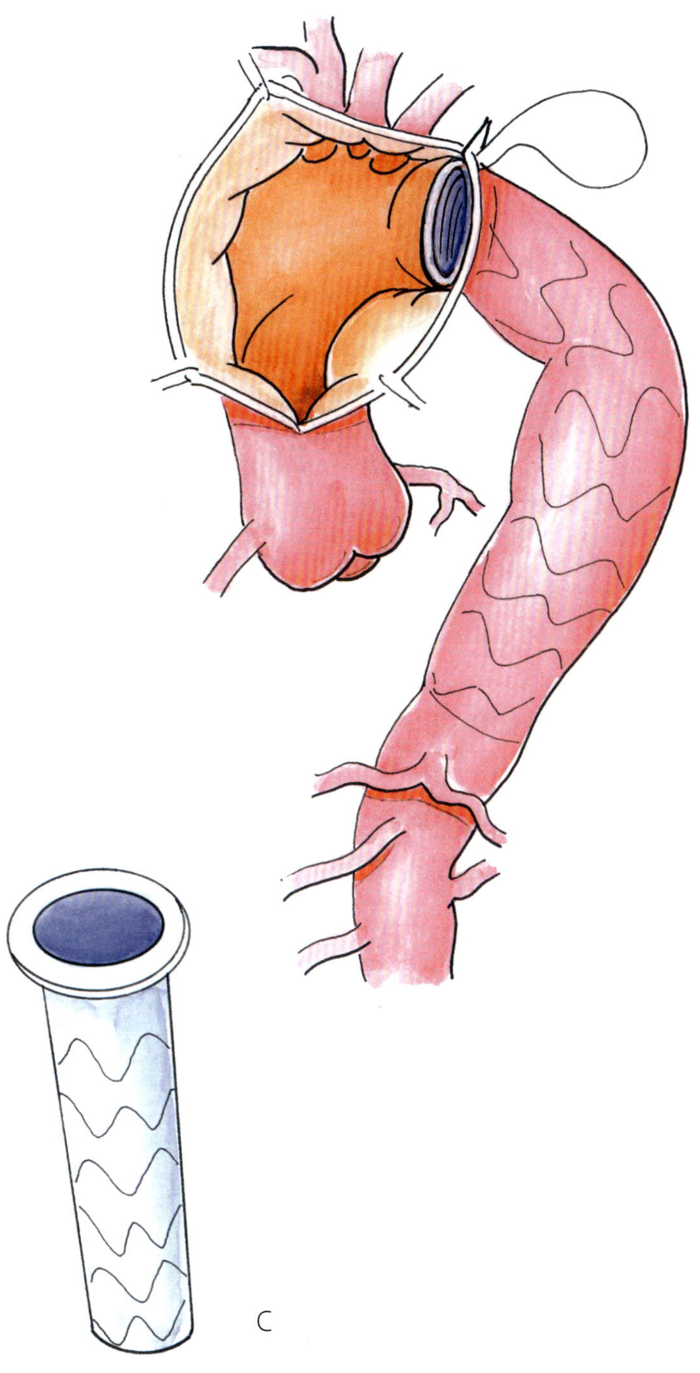

C. 将主动脉内支架近端缝合圈与降主动脉缝合。

C. Suture the proximal suture loop of the intra-aortic stent to the descending aorta.

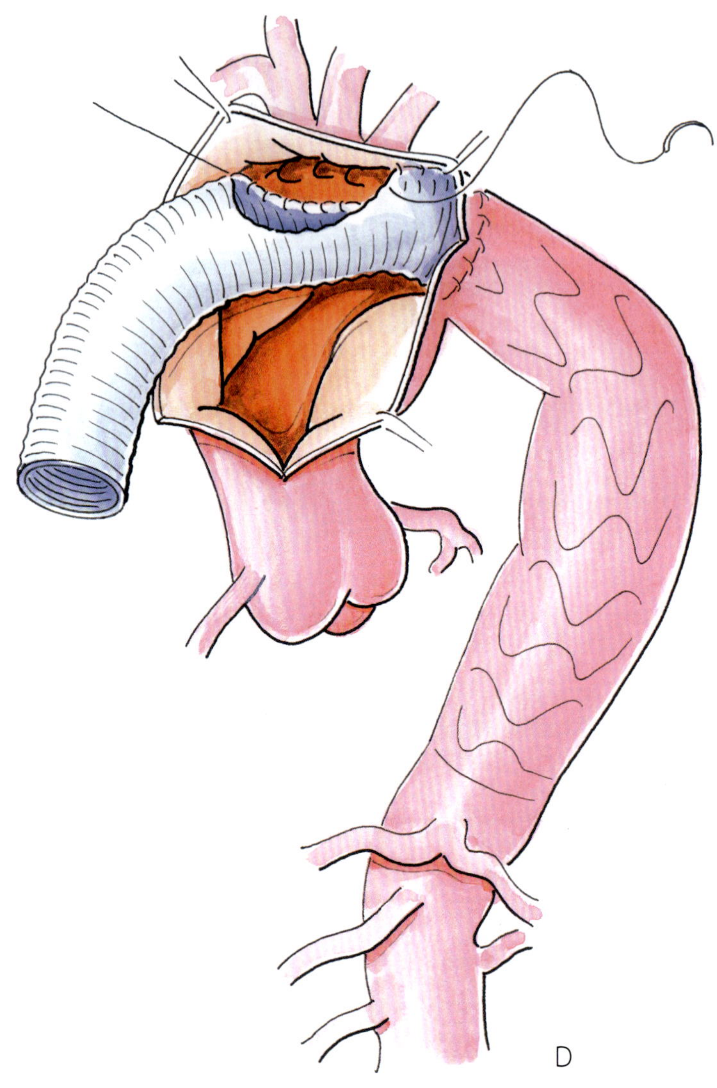

D. 选择合适口径的人工血管与降主动脉及主动脉内支架端端吻合。人工血管顶部椭圆形开窗，与包含三个头臂动脉开口的主动脉弓顶部吻合。

D. An appropriate artificial vessel is utilized for end-to-end anastomosis to the descending aorta and the intra-aortic stent. With an oval window made on its roof, the artificial vessel is anastomosed to the roof of the aortic arch containing three brachiocephalic artery ostia.

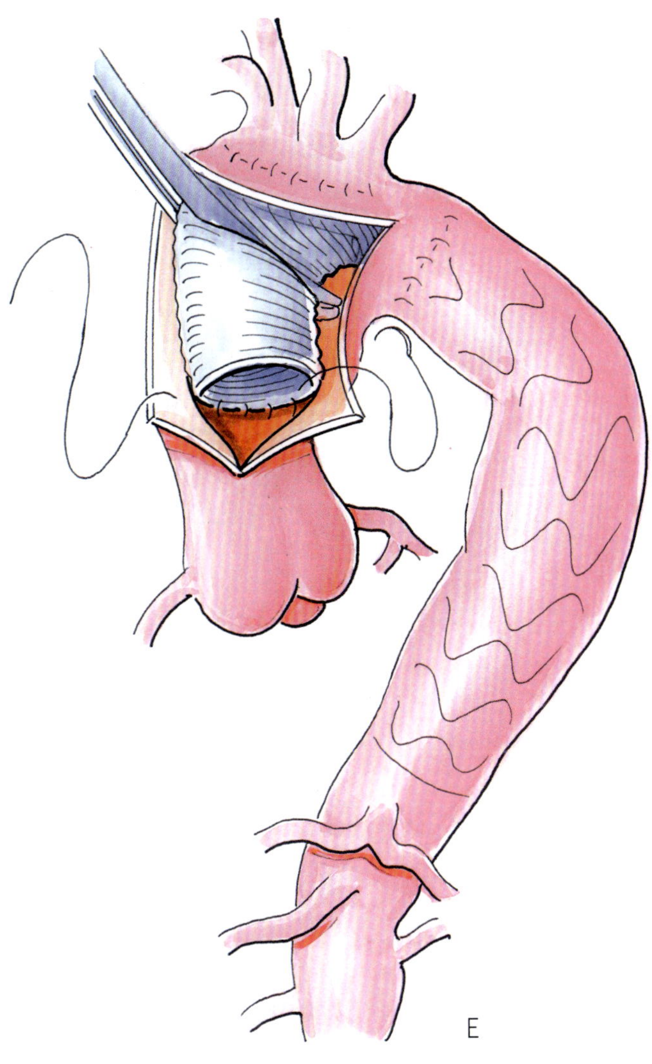

E. 在深低温停循环下完成远端和弓顶的吻合后，恢复体外循环，在体外循环下将人工血管另一端与升主动脉端端吻合。

E. After anastomosis between the distal end and the arch roof under deep hypothermic circulatory arrest, extracorporeal circulation is resumed, and the other end of the artificial vessel is sutured to the ascending aorta in an end-to-end fashion.

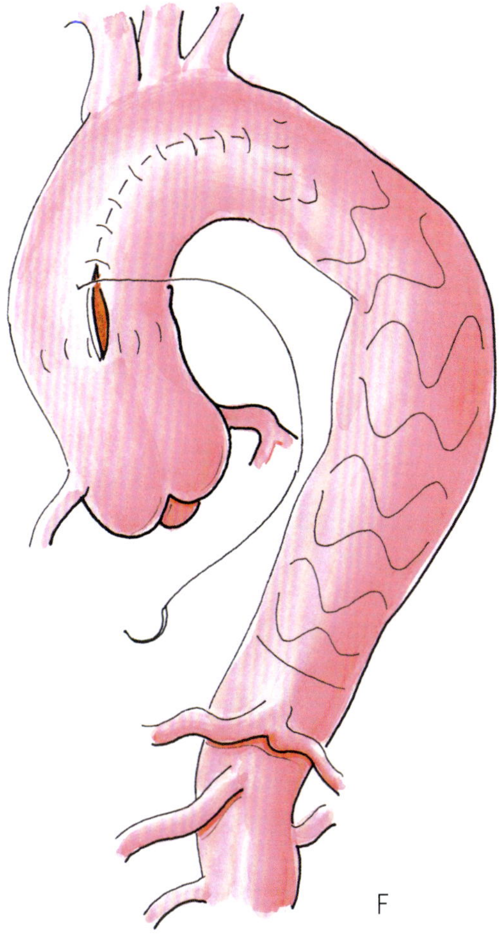

F. 剪除多余的动脉瘤壁，缝合包埋人工血管。

F. The excess aneurysm wall is cut off, and the artificial vessel is sutured and embedded.

图 4-9-4 一期杂交修补胸主动脉瘤伴主动脉瓣关闭不全

Figure 4-9-4 One-stage hybrid repair for thoracic aortic aneurysm with aortic valve insufficiency

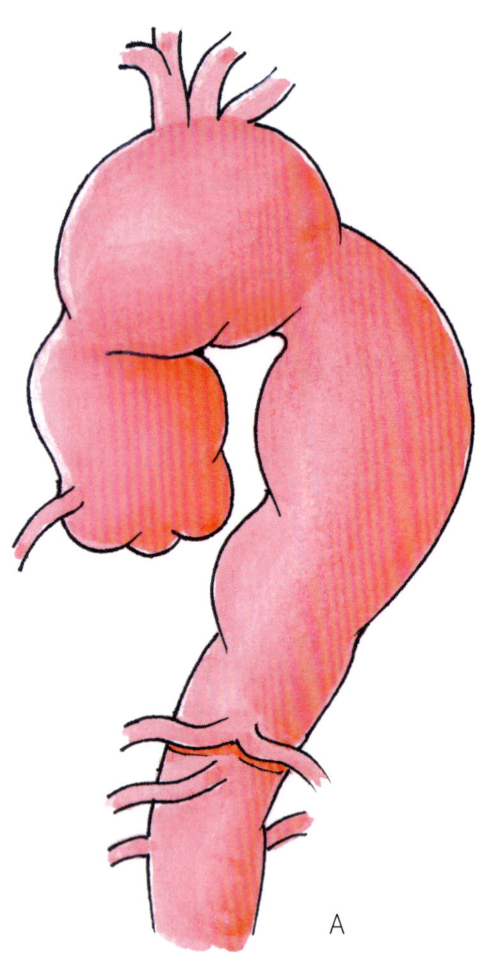

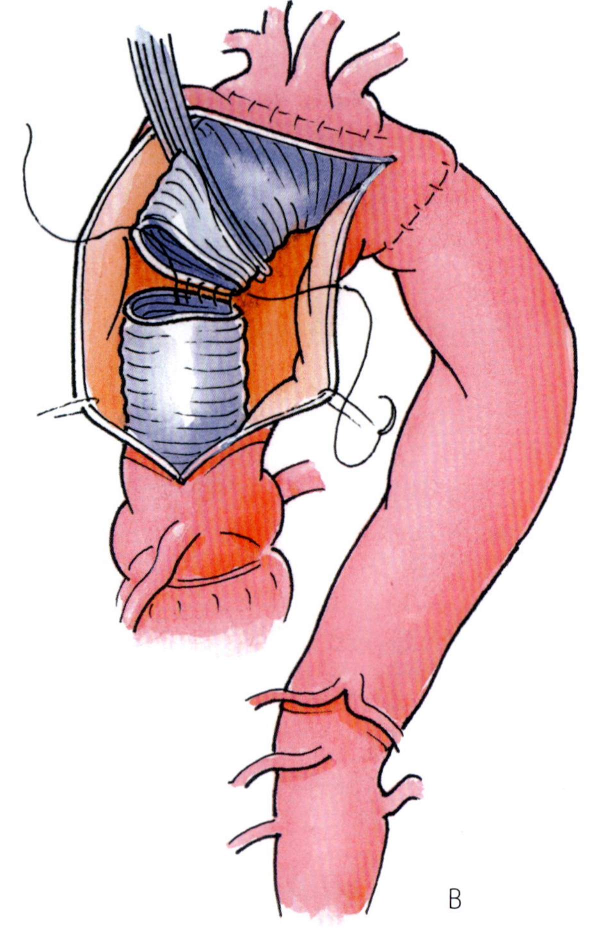

A. 主动脉梭形动脉瘤，病变广泛，起自升主动脉近端止于胸降主动脉末端，同时合并主动脉瓣关闭不全。

A. A fusiform aortic aneurysm with extensive lesions originates from the proximal ascending aorta to the distal descending thoracic aorta and is complicated with aortic insufficiency.

B. 深低温停循环下切开升主动脉和主动脉弓，直视向降主动脉植入主动脉内支架，再用一段人工血管完成远端和弓顶的吻合后，恢复体外循环。另取一带瓣外导管在体外循环下主动脉根部做 Bantall 手术。

B. Under deep hypothermic circulatory arrest, the ascending aorta and aortic arch are incised and an intra-aortic stent is implanted into the descending aorta under direct vision. The distal end and arch roof are anastomosed with a segment of the artificial vessel, and extracorporeal circulation is resumed. A composite valved conduit is used to perform the Bantall procedure on the aortic root under extracorporeal circulation.

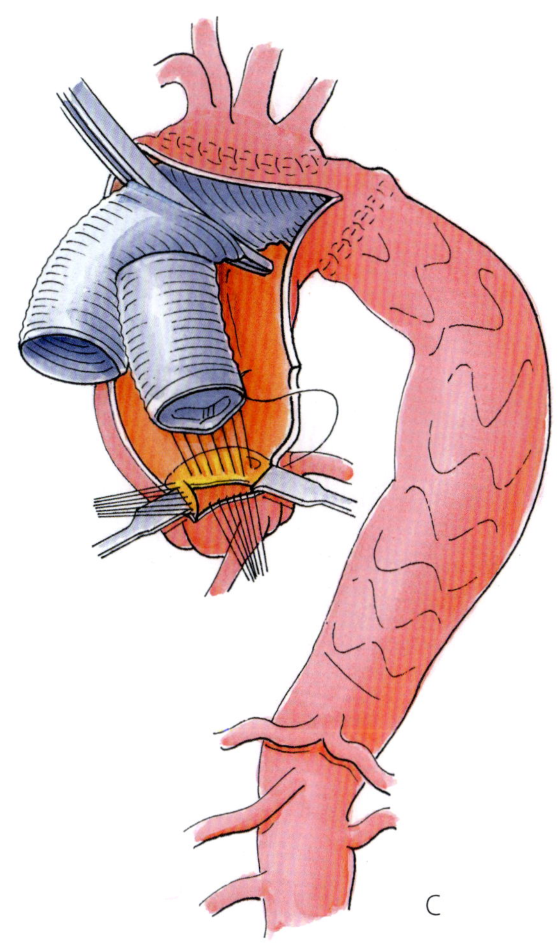

C. 将两人工血管端端吻合。

C. End-to-end anastomosis of the two grafts is made.

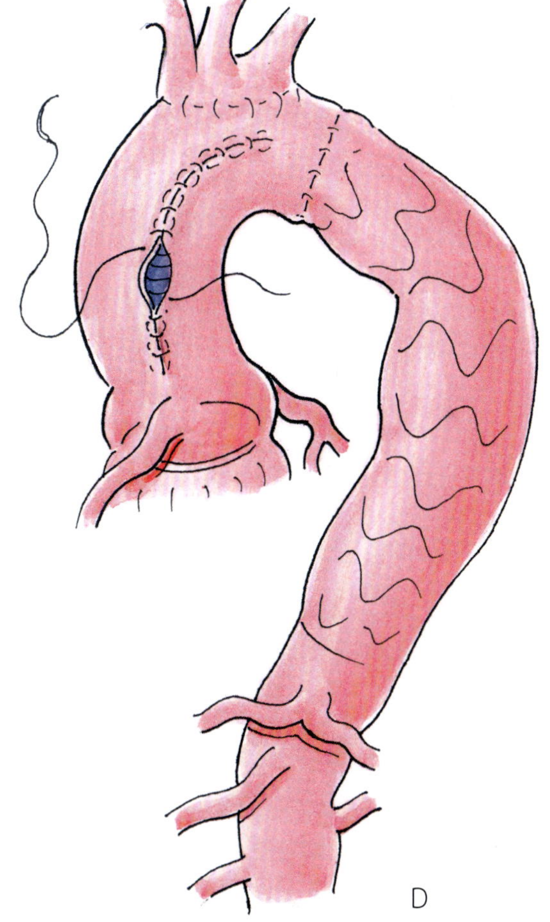

D. 剪除多余的动脉瘤壁，缝合包埋人工血管。

D. Cut off the redundant aneurysm wall; sew up and embed the grafts.

第五章
心律失常

Chapter 5
Arrhythmia

第 一 节　心动过缓和心脏起搏器

Section 1　Bradycardia and Pacemaker

图 5-1-1　心外膜起搏

Figure 5-1-1　Epicardial pacing

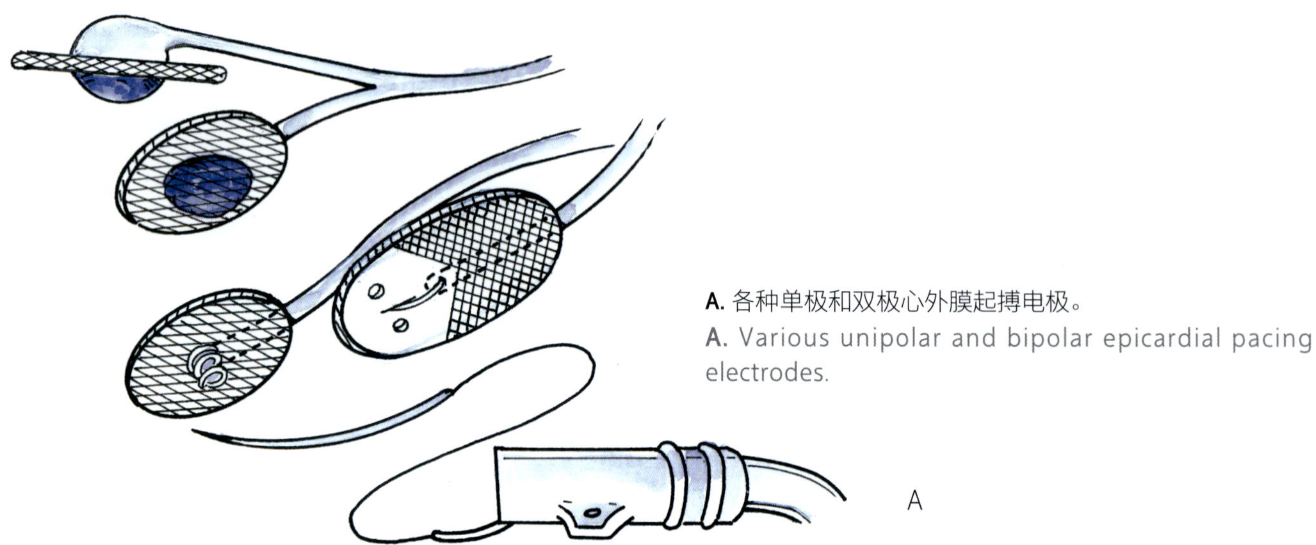

A. 各种单极和双极心外膜起搏电极。

A. Various unipolar and bipolar epicardial pacing electrodes.

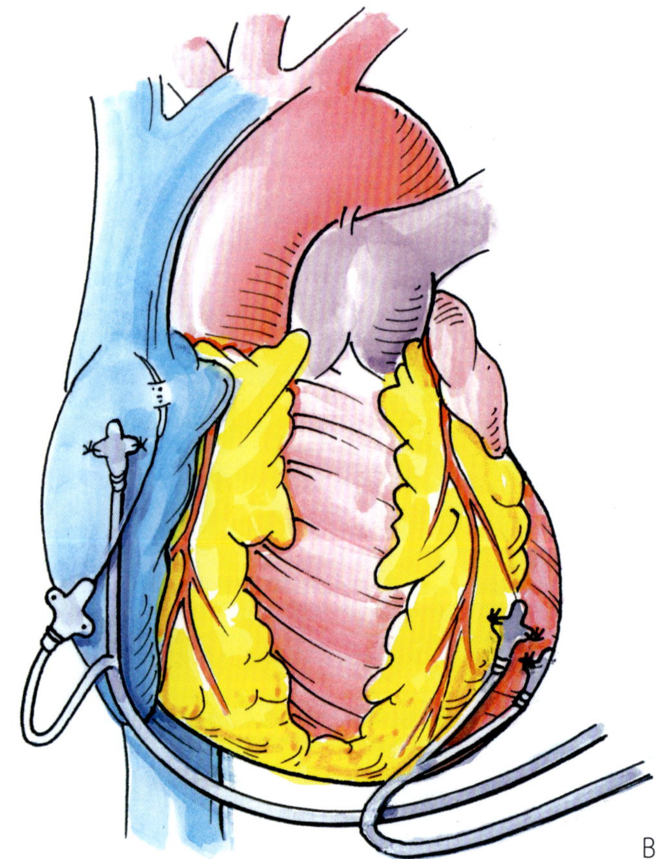

B. 心外膜起搏电极分别安置在右心房心外膜和左心室心尖区心外膜，缝线固定。

B. Epicardial pacing electrodes are placed on the epicardium of the right atrium and the epicardium in the left ventricle apex, respectively, and fixed with sutures.

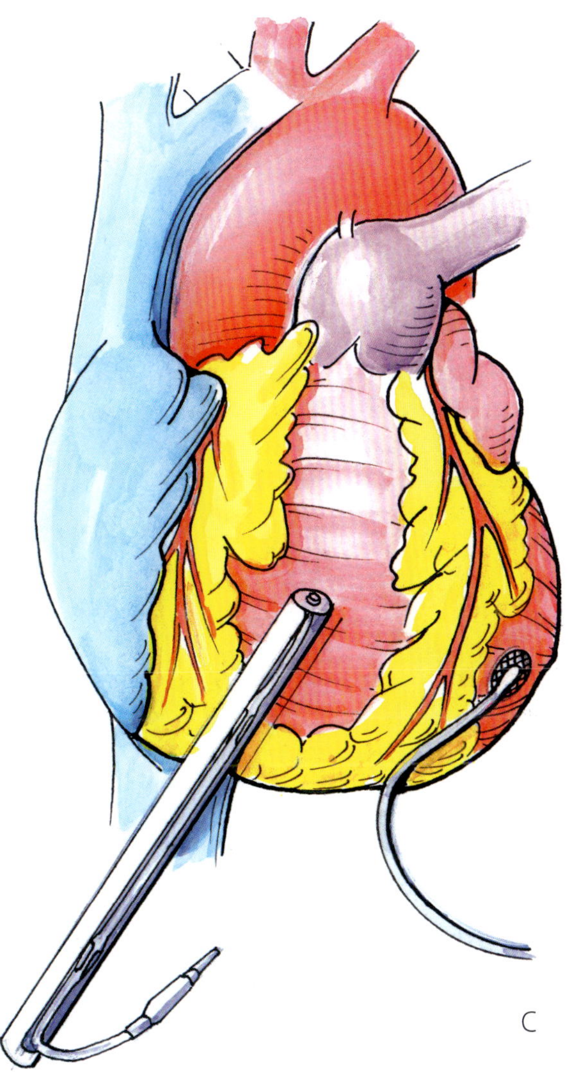

C. 心外膜起搏电极安置在左心室心尖区心外膜，另一电极安置在皮下或心包等软组织上。

C. One epicardial pacing electrode is placed on the epicardium in the left ventricle apex, and the other is placed on soft tissues such as the subcutaneous or pericardial tissues.

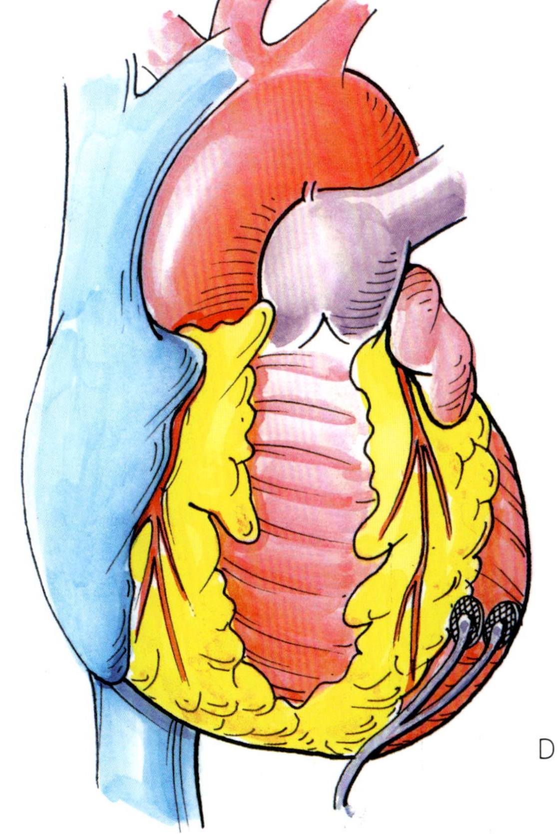

D. 心外膜起搏两电极均安置在左心室心尖区心外膜。

D. Both epicardial pacing electrodes are placed on the epicardium of the left ventricular apex.

图 5-1-2　经胸起搏器植入术
Figure 5-1-2　Transthoracic approach for placement of pacemaker

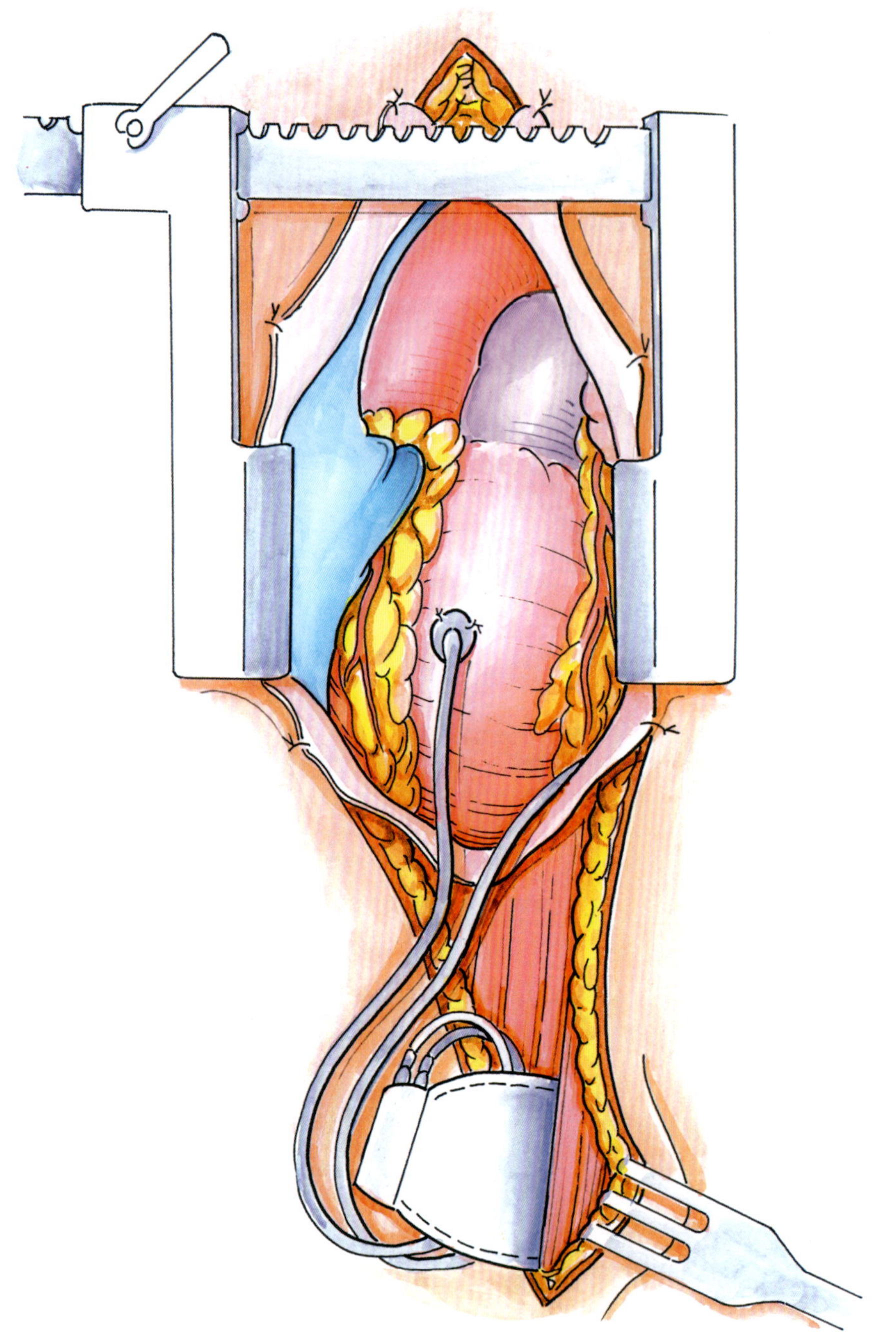

A

A. 胸骨正中切口。切开心包后分别在右心室表面和左心室表面安装心外膜起搏电极，缝线固定。起搏电极导线在心包切口下部引出，与植入式起搏器连接。

A. A median sternotomy is performed. After a pericardiotomy, the epicardial pacing electrodes are placed on the right ventricle surface and the left ventricle surface, respectively, and secured with sutures. The pacing electrode lead is drawn out of the lower pericardial incision to be connected to the implantable pacemaker.

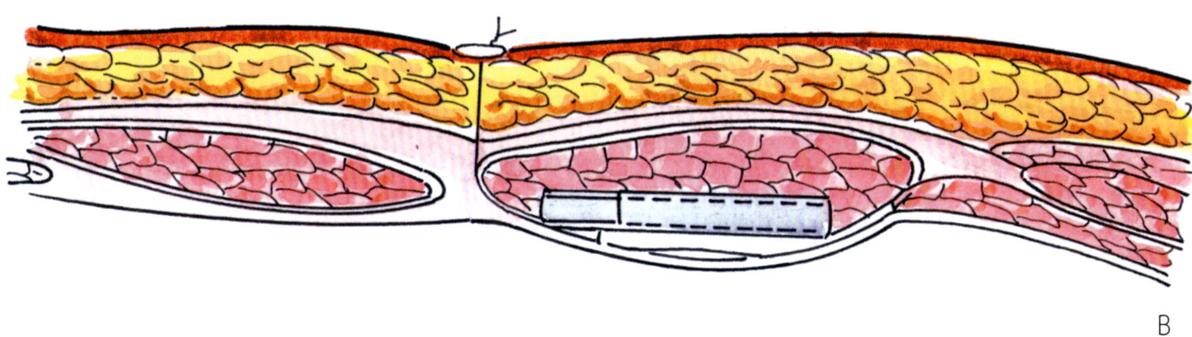

B. 切开左侧腹直肌前鞘，将植入式起搏器埋入腹直肌后方。关闭切口。

B. Incise the anterior sheath of the left rectus abdominis to embed the implantable pacemaker behind the rectus abdominis. Close the incision.

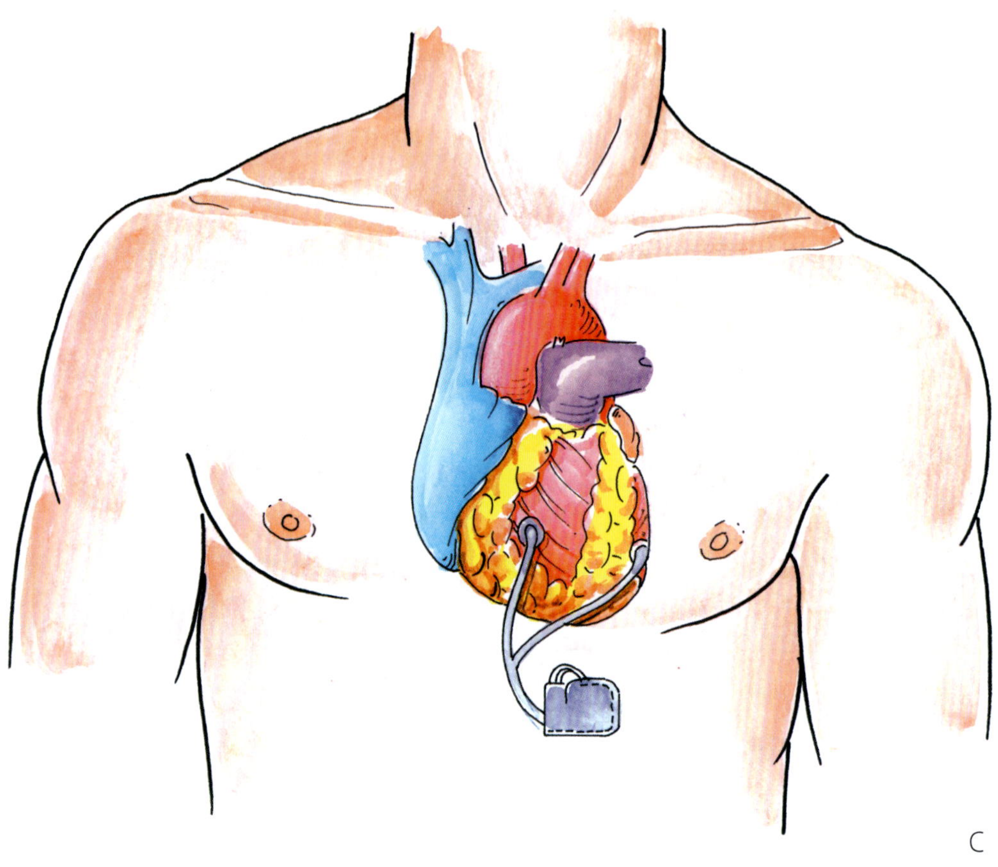

C. 植入式心外膜永久起搏器安装完成。

C. An implantable permanent epicardial pacemaker is installed.

第 二 节 心房颤动的外科治疗
Section 2 Surgical Treatment of Atrial Fibrillation

图 5-2-1 **微创经胸心房颤动消融术（Wolf 法）**

Figure 5-2-1 **Ablation of atrial fibrillation in minimally invasive thoracotomy (Wolf procedure)**

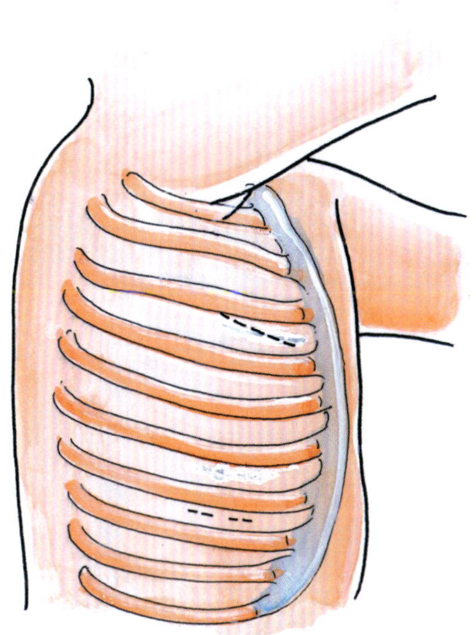

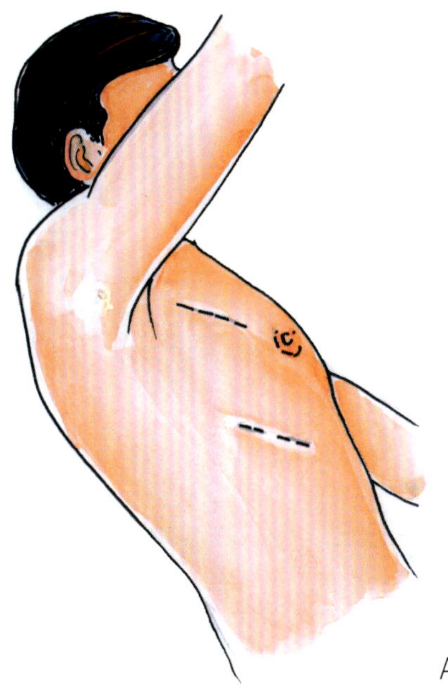

A

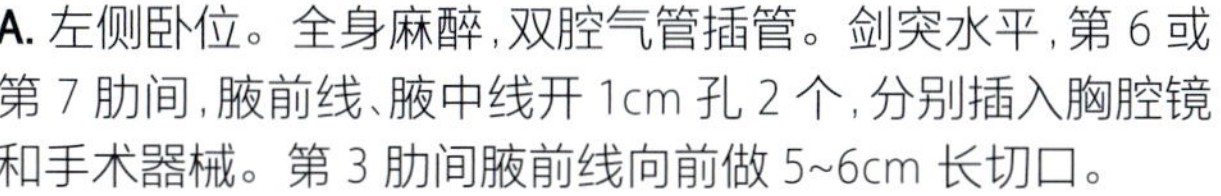

A. 左侧卧位。全身麻醉，双腔气管插管。剑突水平，第 6 或第 7 肋间，腋前线、腋中线开 1cm 孔 2 个，分别插入胸腔镜和手术器械。第 3 肋间腋前线向前做 5~6cm 长切口。

A. In the left lateral decubitus position, the patient undergoes bicaval and endotracheal intubation under general anesthesia. Make the two 1 cm holes in the sixth or seventh intercostal space on the anterior axillary line and the midaxillary line at the level of the xiphoid process, through which thoracoscopic and surgical instruments are inserted, respectively. An incision of 5-6 cm is made anteriorly at the third intercostal space in the anterior axillary line.

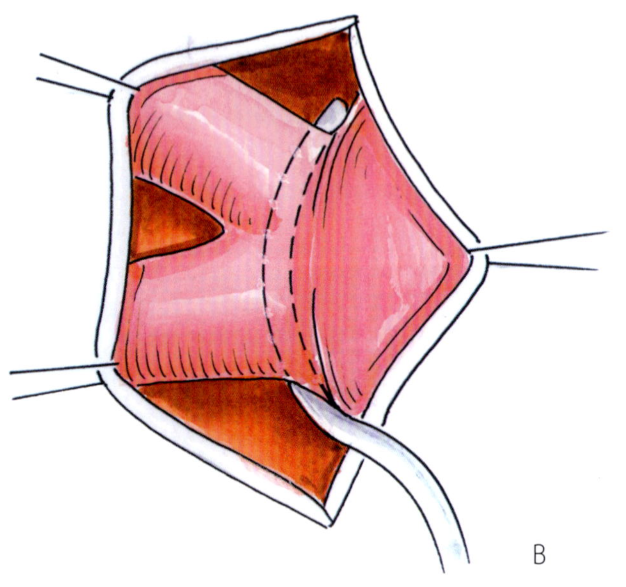

B. 膈神经前 2cm 纵行切开心包，心包悬吊线经胸壁引出，显露房间沟部位。心包内用分离器由下往上钝性分离右上、下肺静脉。

B. The pericardial suspension line is brought out through the chest wall to expose the interatrial groove after a longitudinal pericardiotomy 2 cm anterior to the phrenic nerve. The right superior and inferior pulmonary veins are separated bluntly from bottom to top in the pericardium by using a separator.

C. 套入双极射频消融钳，钳夹住靠近肺静脉口的左房组织即肺静脉前庭，做环右肺静脉消融。关闭心包切口，留置胸腔引流管，鼓肺缝合右胸切口。

C. Introduce the bipolar radiofrequency ablation forceps to clamp the pulmonary vein vestibule (the left atrial tissue close to the pulmonary vein ostium) and perform circumferential right pulmonary vein ablation. Close the pericardial incision, place the thoracic drainage tube, inflate the lung and suture the right thoracic incision.

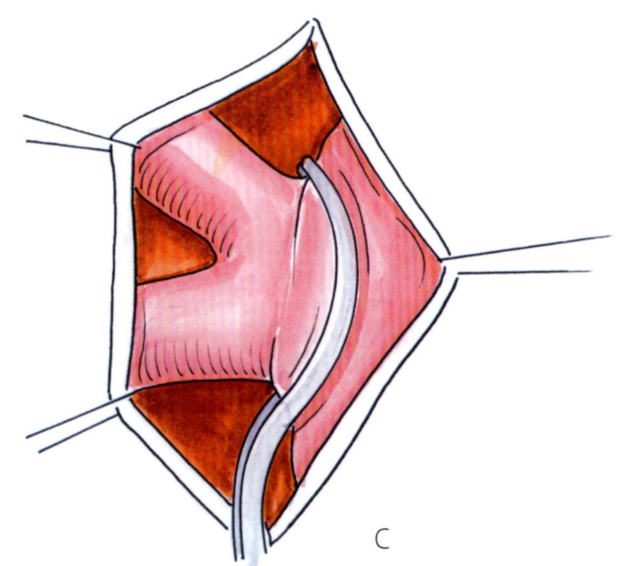

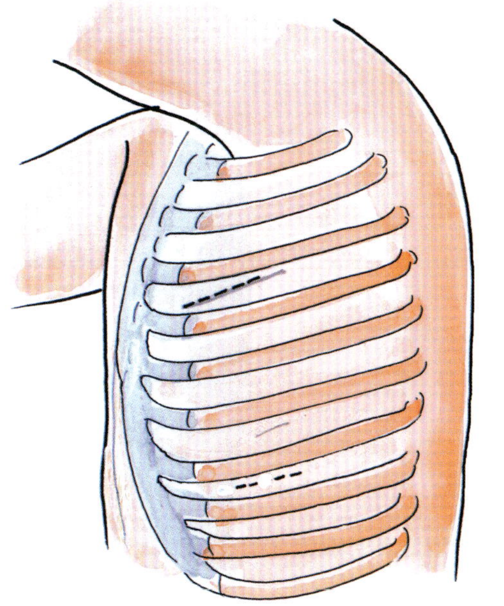

D. 改右侧卧位，切口与右胸相仿，进入心包腔心脏左侧。

D. With the patient in the right lateral decubitus position, a left thoracotomy, similar to the right thoracotomy, is performed to enter the left side of the heart in the pericardial cavity.

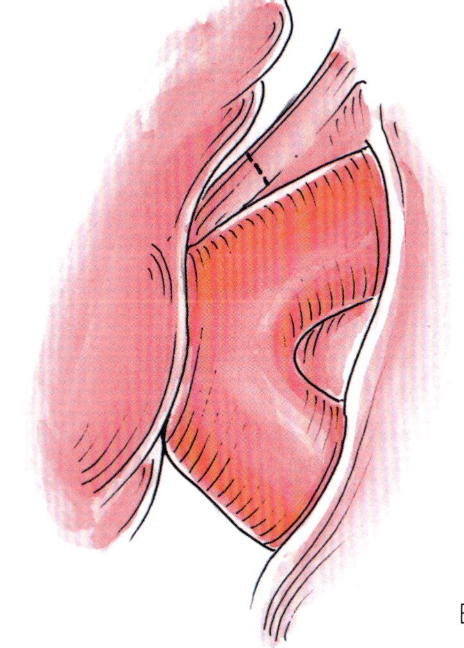

E. 先在左上肺静脉上方、左肺动脉前电凝切断 Marshall 韧带。

E. First, the Marshall ligament is resected with electrocoagulation above the left upper pulmonary vein and anterior to the left pulmonary artery.

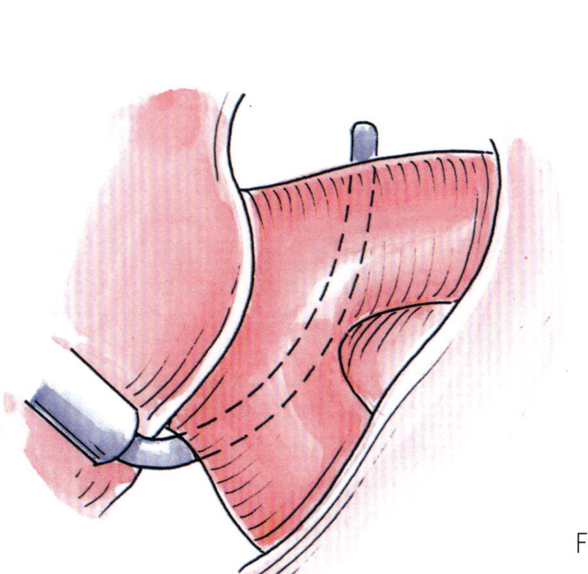

F. 用分离器由下往上钝性游离左上、下肺静脉。

F. The left superior and inferior pulmonary veins are bluntly dissociated with a separator from bottom to top.

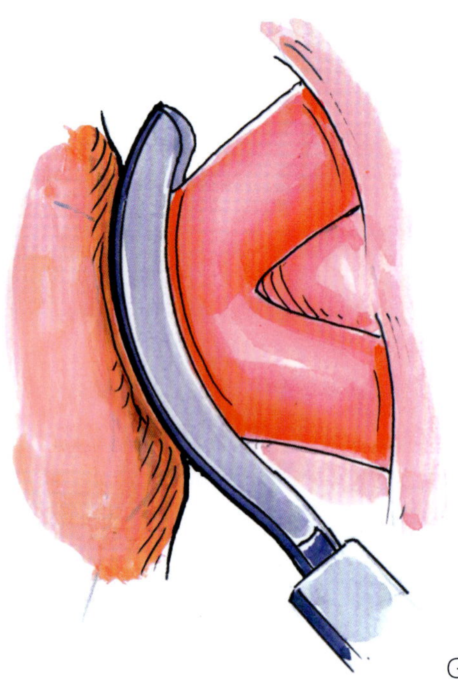

G. 套入双极射频消融钳，钳夹住靠近肺静脉口的左房组织，做环左肺静脉消融。

G. Insert the bipolar radiofrequency ablation forceps, clamp the left atrial tissue proximal to the pulmonary vein ostium, and perform circumferential left pulmonary vein ablation.

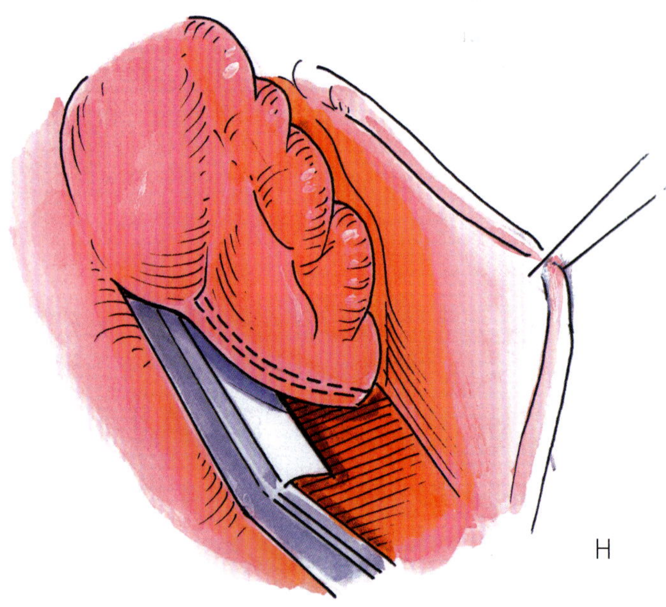

H. 插入切割缝合器，做左心耳切除。留置胸腔引流管，鼓肺缝合右胸切口。

H. Insert the "cut-and-sew" device to resect the left atrial appendage. Place the thoracic drainage tube, inflate the lung and suture the right thoracic incision.

图 5-2-2 心脏直视手术时伴行心房颤动消融术
Figure 5-2-2 Ablation of atrial fibrillation in concomitant open heart surgery

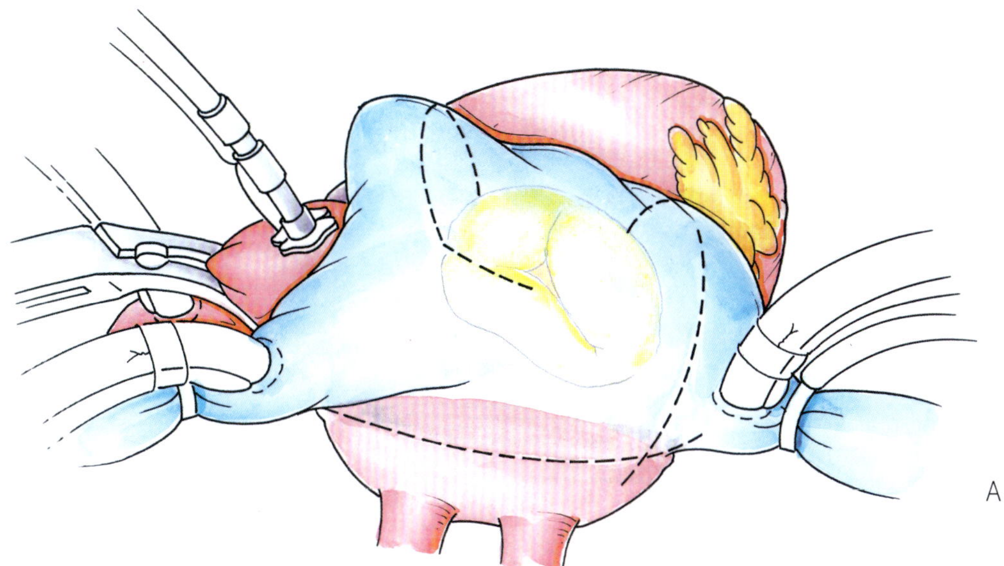

A. 建立体外循环。右心耳虚线示右心耳处消融线。右心房下部虚线和房间沟处虚线为右心房和左心房拟切开处。

A. Establish extracorporeal circulation. The dotted line at the right atrial appendage indicates the ablation line at the right atrial appendage. The dotted lines at the inferior part of the right atrium and the interatrial groove indicate the intended incisions in the right and left atria.

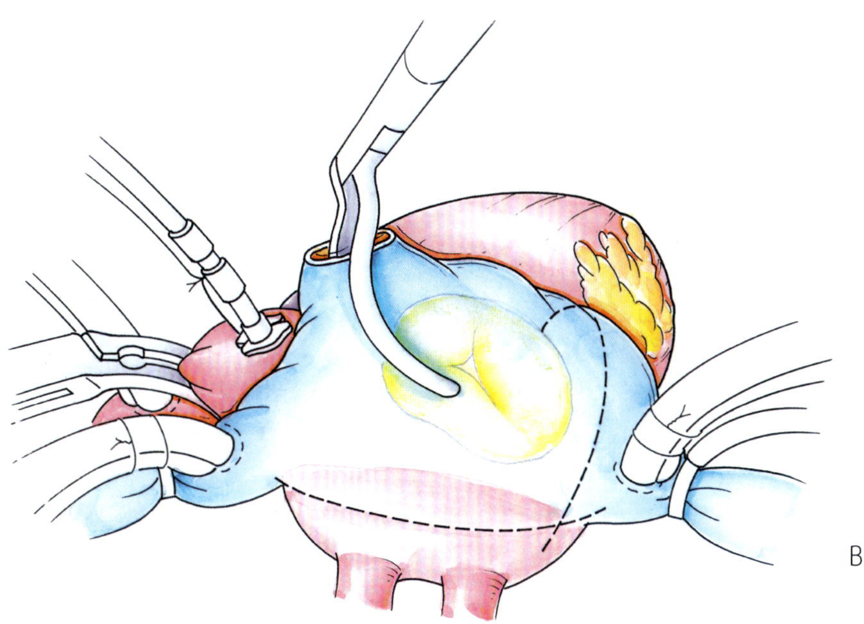

B. 右心耳切除，双极消融夹插入做右心房壁透壁消融。

B. The right atrial appendage is resected, and a bipolar ablation clamp is inserted to perform transmural ablation of the right atrial wall.

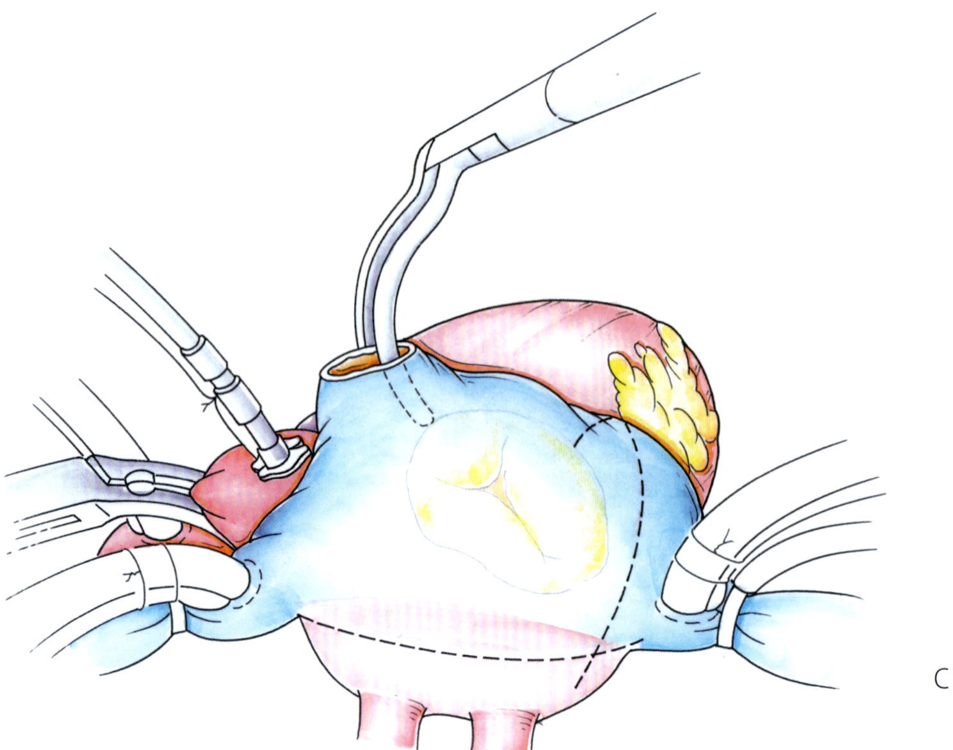

C. 双极消融夹经右心耳做另一侧右心房壁透壁消融，该消融线要到达三尖瓣环前-隔交界处。

C. Perform transmural ablation at the other side of the right atrial wall through the right atrial appendage by using the bipolar ablation clamp, with the ablation line traveling onto the anterior-septal commissure of the tricuspid annulus.

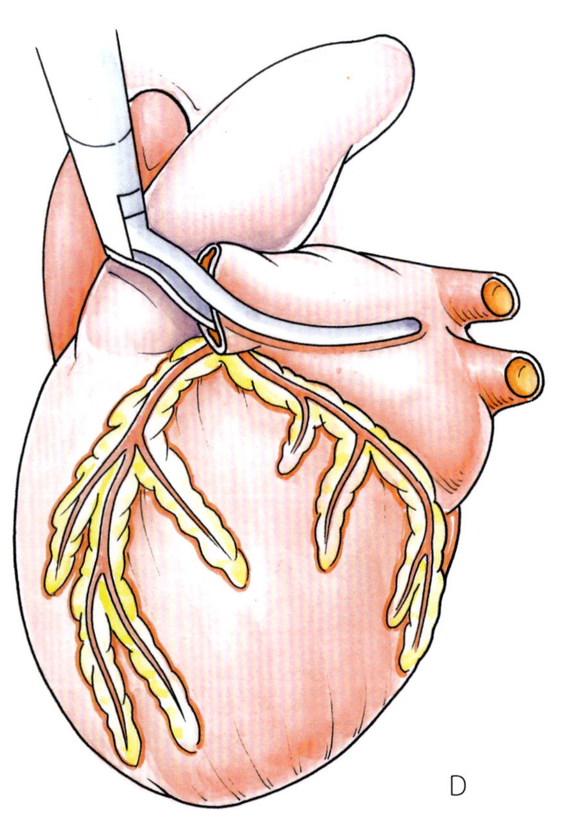

D. 经房间沟纵行切开左心房，切除左心耳，双极消融夹经左心耳插入做左心房后壁透壁消融。

D. A left atriotomy is performed longitudinally through the atrial groove to resect the left atrial appendage. The bipolar ablation clamp is inserted into the left atrial posterior wall through the left atrial appendage for transmural ablation.

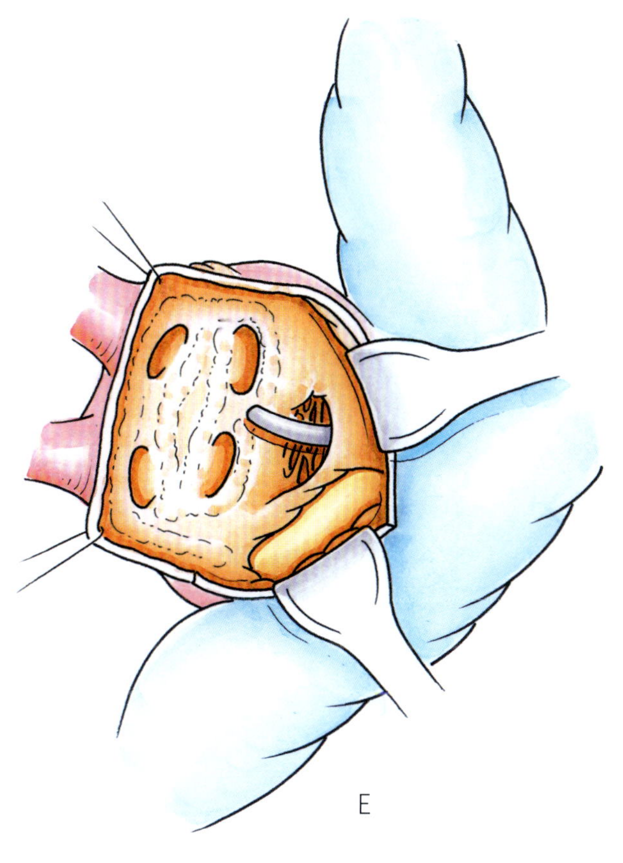

E. 左心房后壁消融线要到达左上肺静脉附近，与后续的环左肺静脉的消融线相连。

E. The left atrial posterior wall ablation line should reach near the left upper pulmonary vein and be connected to the subsequent circumferential left pulmonary vein ablation line.

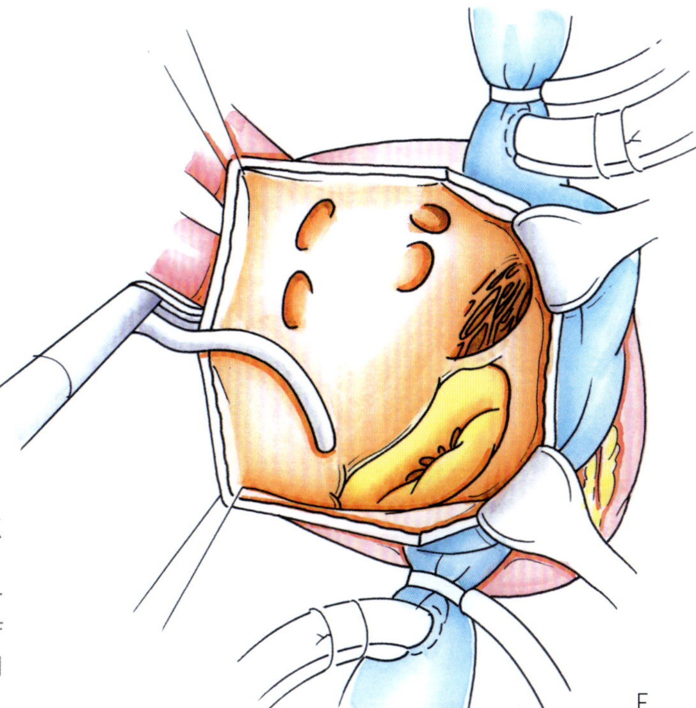

F. 左心房切口下部插入双极消融夹直至二尖瓣后瓣环中点做透壁消融。

F. A bipolar ablation clamp is inserted from the lower part of the left atrial incision until the midpoint of the posterior mitral annulus to perform transmural ablation.

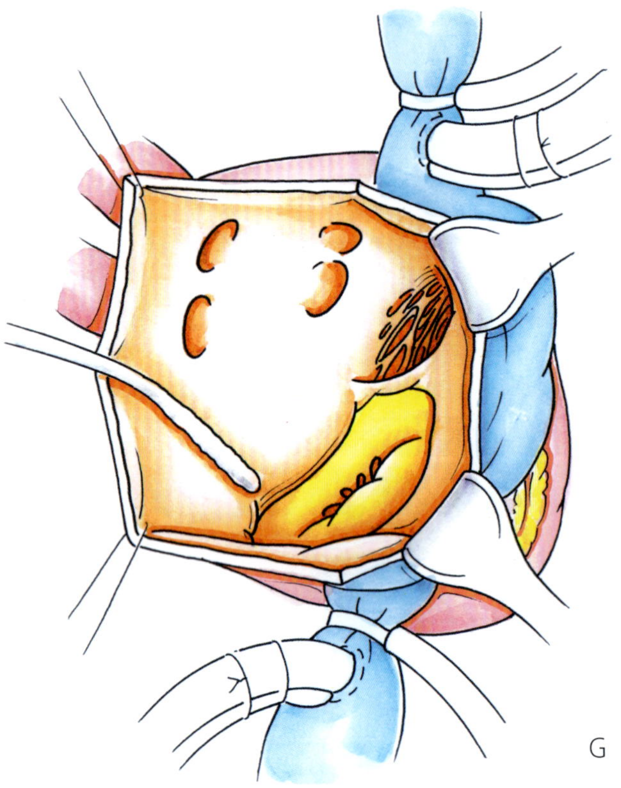

G. 消融线顶端二尖瓣环处做冰冻处理。

G. The mitral annulus at the top of the ablation line is frozen.

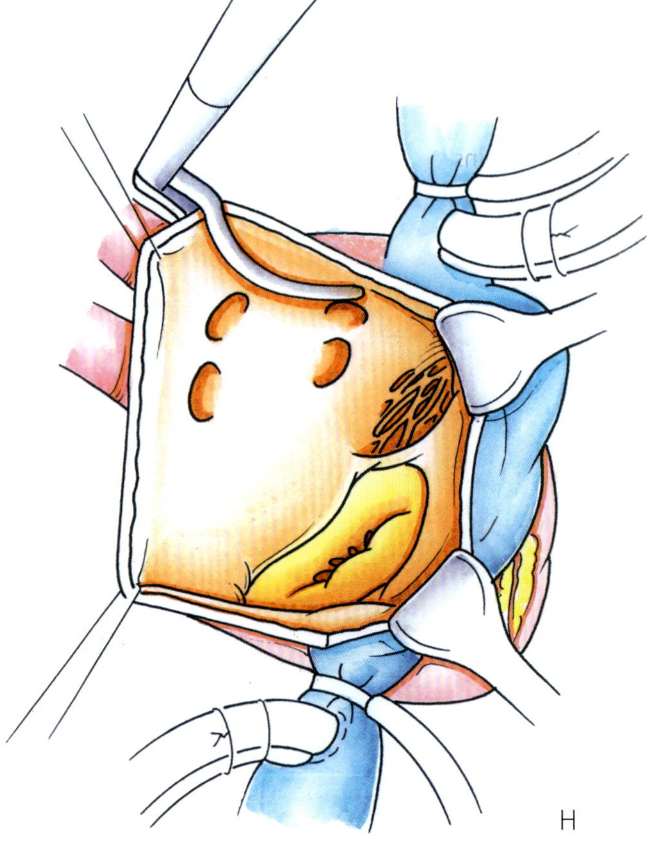

H. 左心房切口上部插入双极消融夹做左房顶透壁消融。

H. A bipolar ablation clamp is inserted into the upper part of the left atrial incision for the left atrial roof transmural ablation.

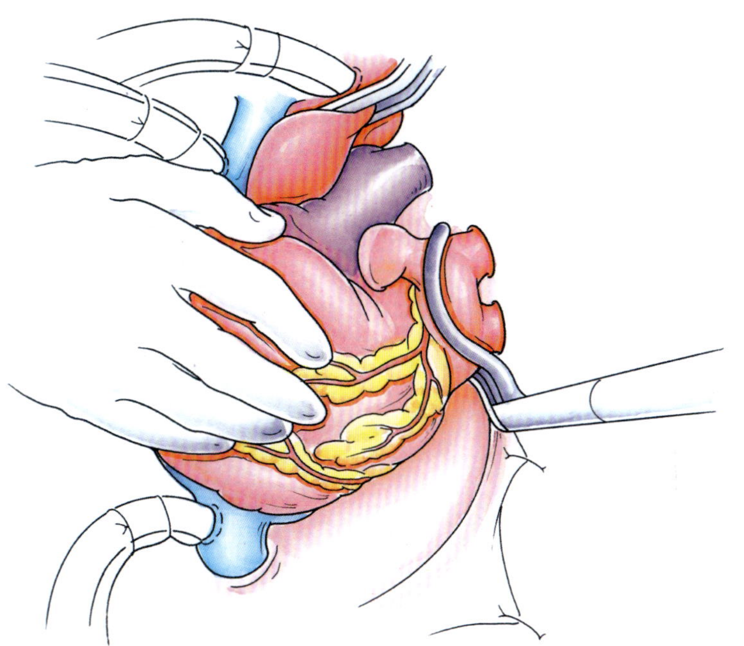

I. 抬起心脏，游离左肺静脉，双极消融夹跨过左上、下肺静脉，在左心房后壁上做环肺静脉消融。

I. Lift the heart and free the left pulmonary vein to perform circumferential pulmonary vein ablation on the left atrial posterior wall with the bipolar ablation clamp crossing the left superior and inferior pulmonary veins.

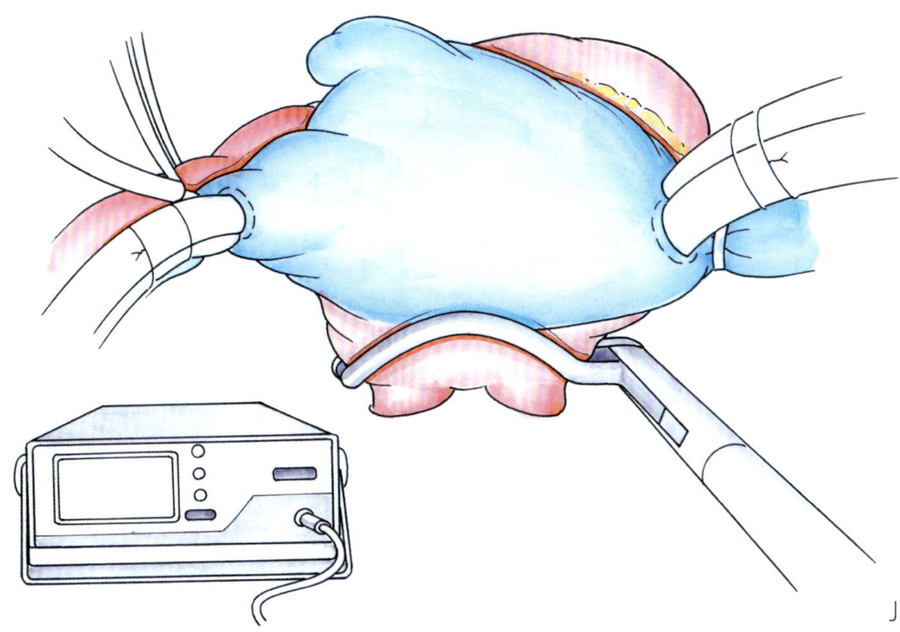

J. 游离右肺静脉，双极消融夹跨过右上、下肺静脉做左心房后壁的透壁消融，形成环右肺静脉的消融线。

J. Free the right pulmonary vein. The bipolar ablation clamp, which crosses the right superior and inferior pulmonary veins, is used to perform transmural ablation of the left atrial posterior wall to form the ablation line of the circumferential right pulmonary vein.

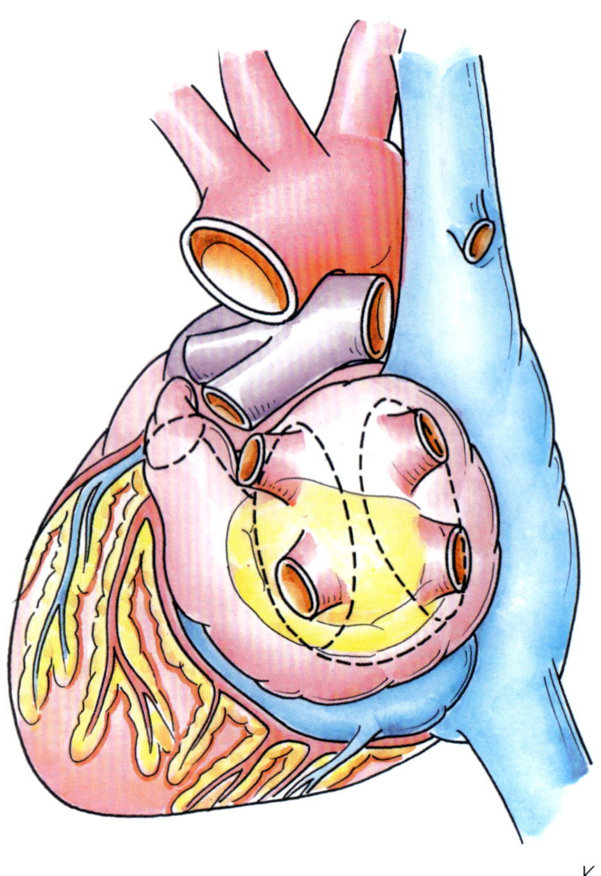

K. 虚线示左心耳和左心房后壁消融线。

K. The dotted line at the left atrial appendage and the left atrial posterior wall indicates the ablation line.

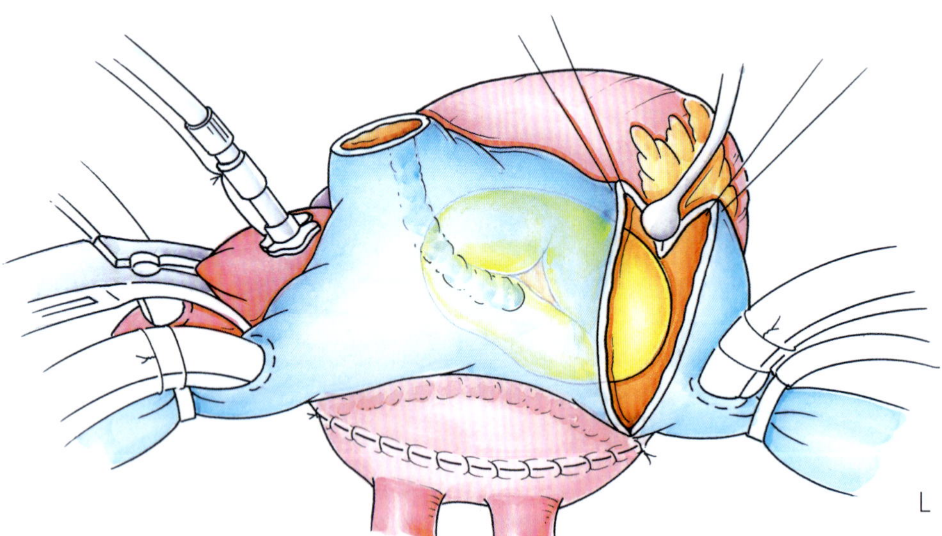

L. 缝合房间沟切口，关闭左心房。横行切开右心房。单极消融笔做右心房切口内端到三尖瓣环前-后瓣交界处的透壁消融。

L. Close the left atrium by suturing the interatrial groove incision. Perform the right atriotomy transversely. Perform the transmural ablation from the inner end of the right atrial incision to the anterior-posterior commissure of the tricuspid annulus using a unipolar ablation pen.

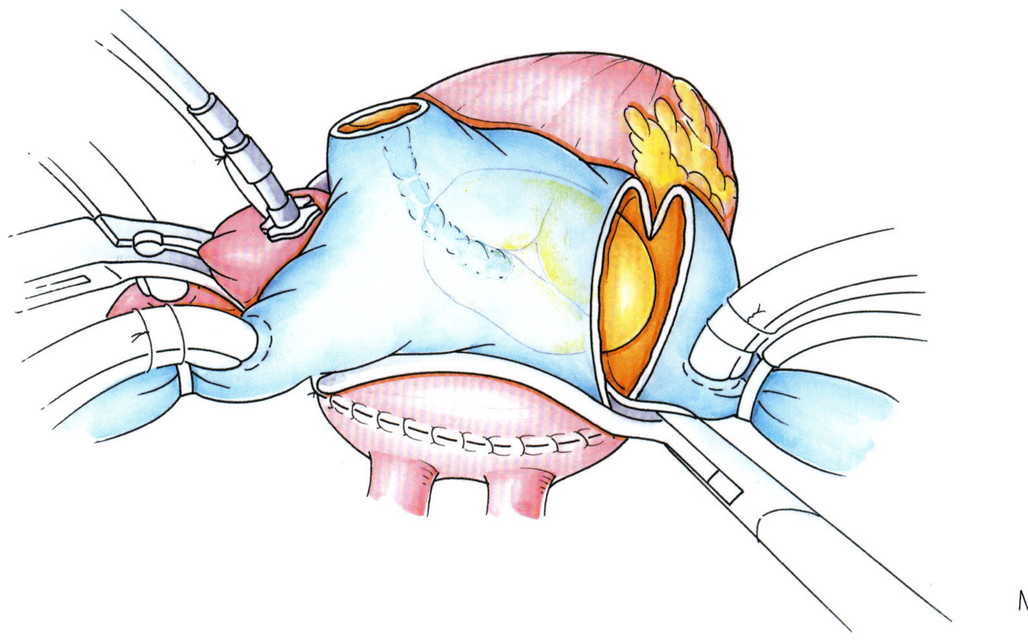

M. 双极消融夹做右心房切口外端到上腔静脉口的消融线。该消融线尽量靠后，贴近房间沟，以避免损伤窦房结。

M. The bipolar ablation clamp is employed to create an ablation line from the outer end of the right atrial incision to the superior vena cava ostium. The ablation line is created as posteriorly as possible and close to the interatrial groove to avoid injury to the sinus node.

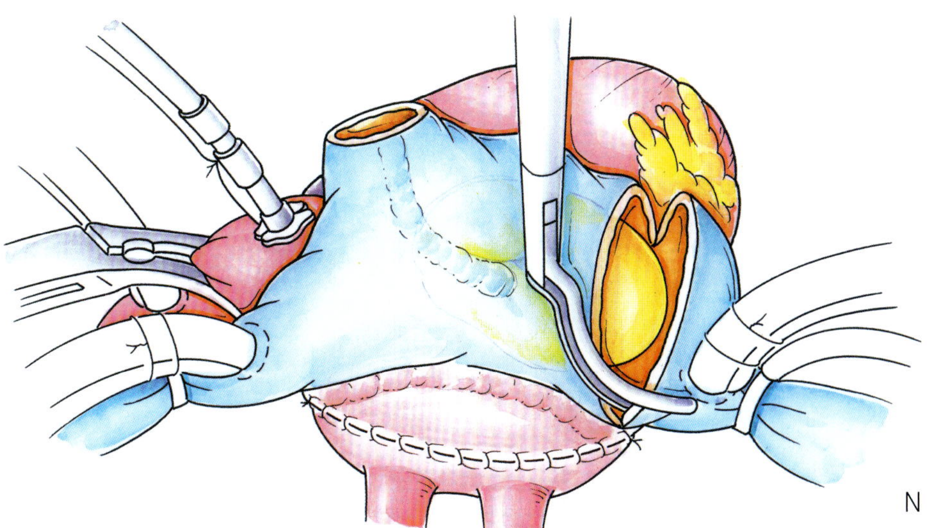

N. 双极消融夹做右心房切口外端到下腔静脉口的消融线。消融完成。

N. The bipolar ablation clamp is used to make the ablation line from the outer end of the right atrial incision to the inferior vena cava ostium. Ablation is completed.

图 5-2-3 Cox 迷宫Ⅳ型手术
Figure 5-2-3 Cox-maze Ⅳ procedure

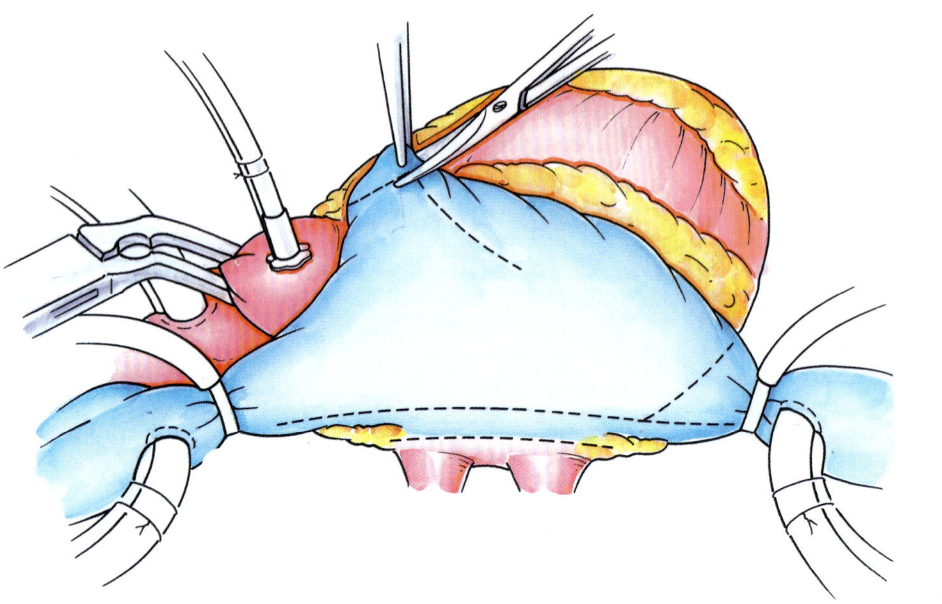

A. 体外循环下心脏停搏。切除右心耳。

A. Under extracorporeal circulation and cardiac arrest, the right atrial appendage is excised.

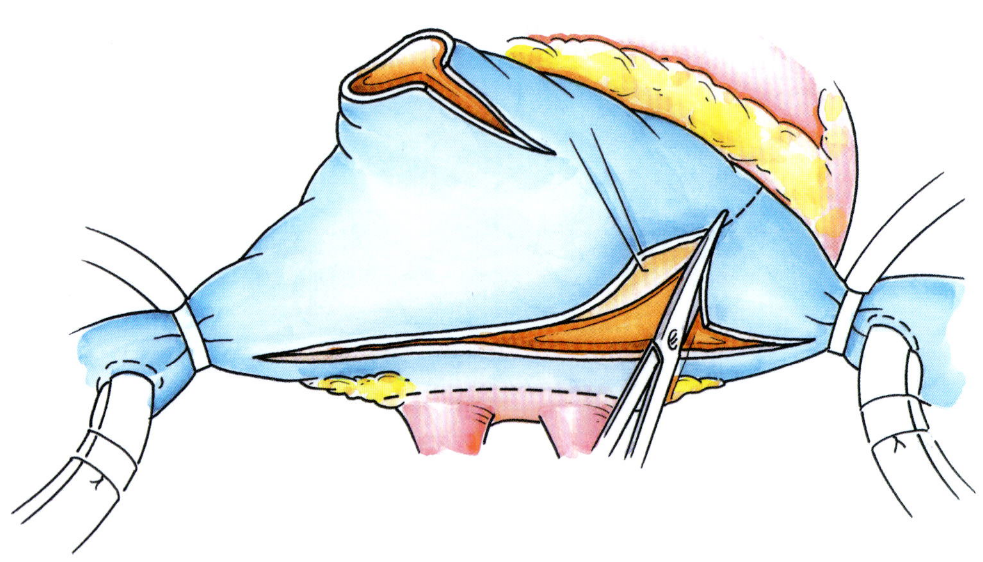

B. 右心耳切口右侧壁的中点开始向右心房切开 2~3cm。右心房侧壁纵行切开，切口两端直至上、下腔静脉开口。该纵切口应尽量靠后，以避免损伤窦房结。右心房下部再横行切开，切口外端与右心房纵切口相连，内端切至房室沟。

B. The right atrium is incised 2-3 cm from the middle point of the right lateral wall of the right atrial appendage incision. The right atrium lateral wall is longitudinally incised, with its both ends proceeding to the superior and inferior vena cava ostia. This longitudinal incision should be made as far back as possible to avoid injury to the sinus node. The lower part of the right atrium is transversely incised, with the outer end of the incision connected to the longitudinal incision of the right atrium, and the inner end incised into the atrioventricular groove.

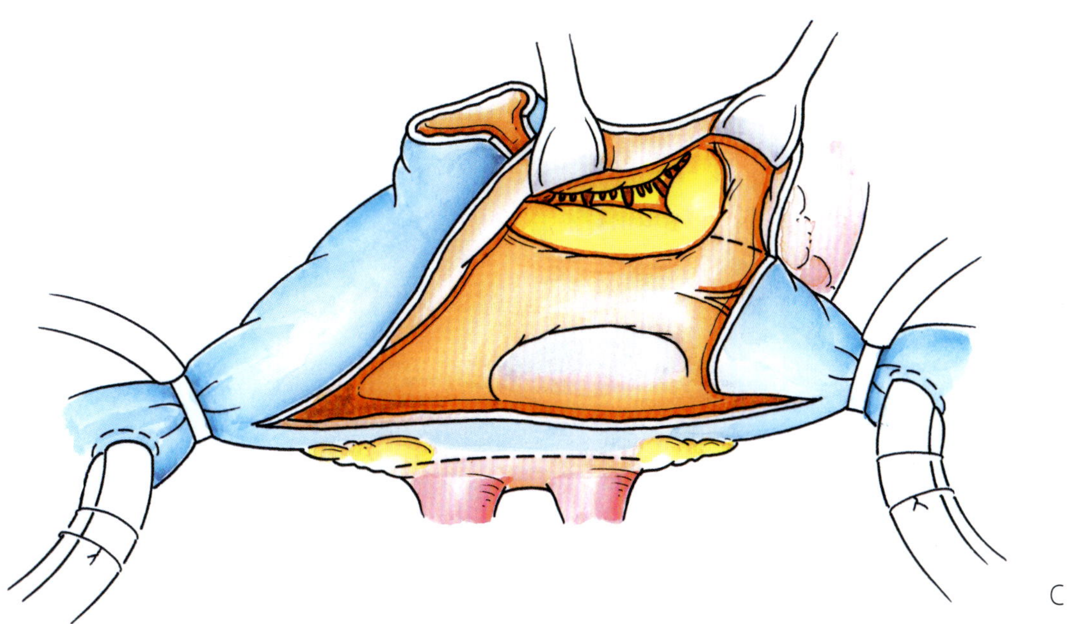

C. 继续将右心房横切口的内端由房室沟至三尖瓣环切开，切开必须是心房壁全层，不得遗留任何心房肌纤维。

C. Continue to cut the inner end of the right atrial transverse incision from the atrioventricular groove to the tricuspid annulus. Note that the atrial wall must be incised in full-thickness, leaving no atrial muscle fibers.

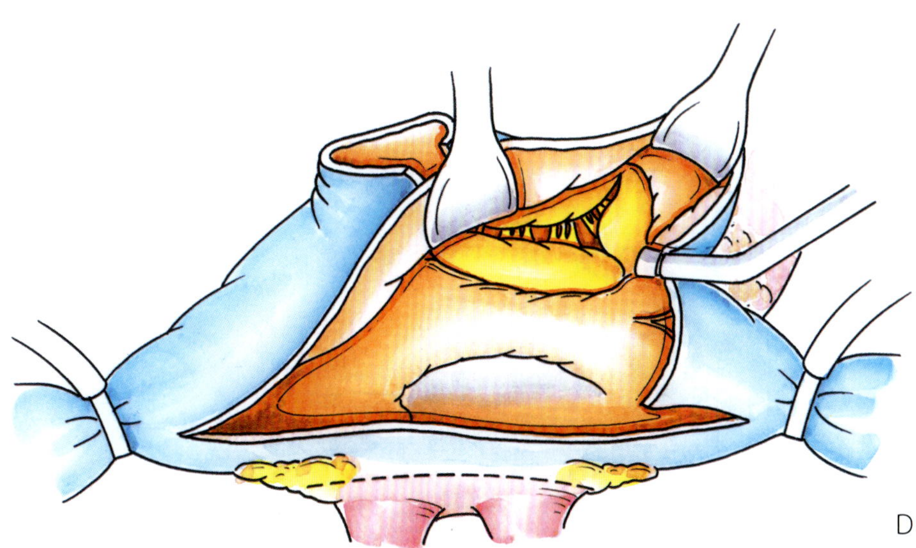

D. 右心房横切口的顶端三尖瓣环处做冰冻处理。

D. Freeze the apical tricuspid annulus of the right atrial transverse incision.

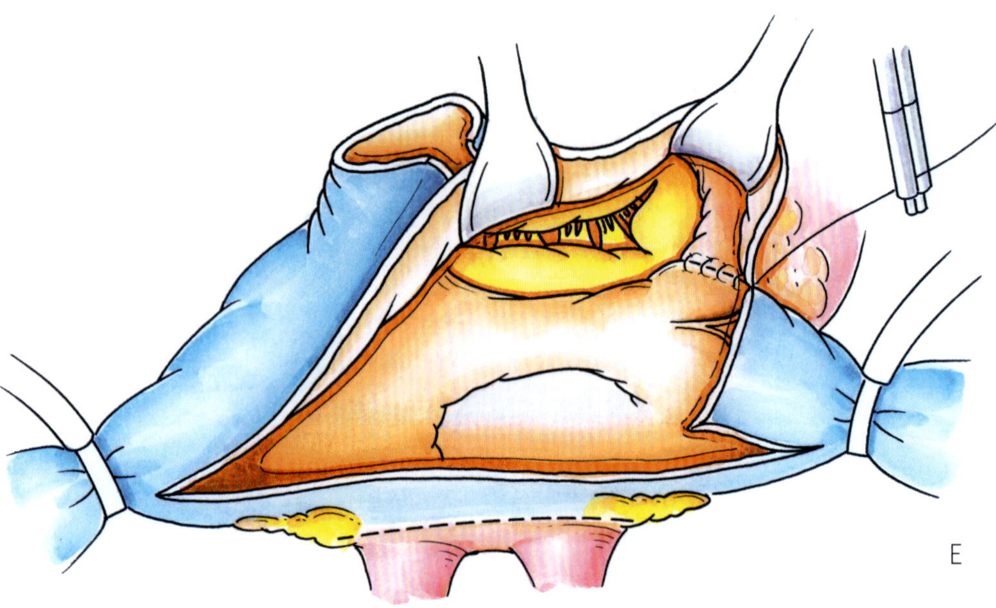

E. 从三尖瓣开始缝合部分右心房横切口，以避免因牵拉而撕破。

E. The right atrium transverse incision is partially sutured from the tricuspid valve to avoid tearing due to traction.

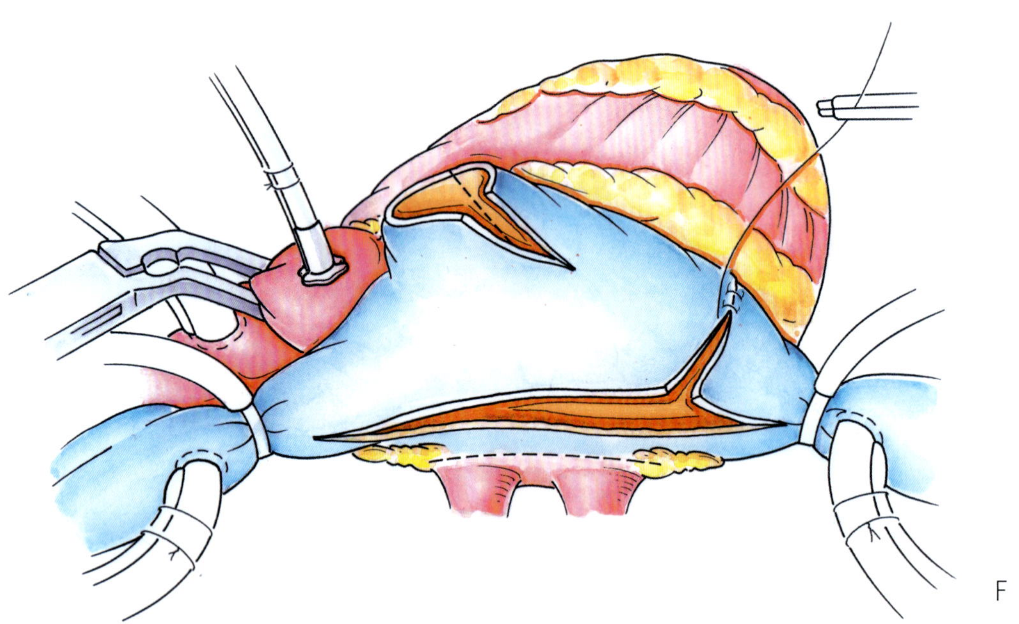

F. 右心耳切口左侧壁向房室沟方向切开。

F. The left lateral wall incision at the right atrial appendage is made toward the atrioventricular groove.

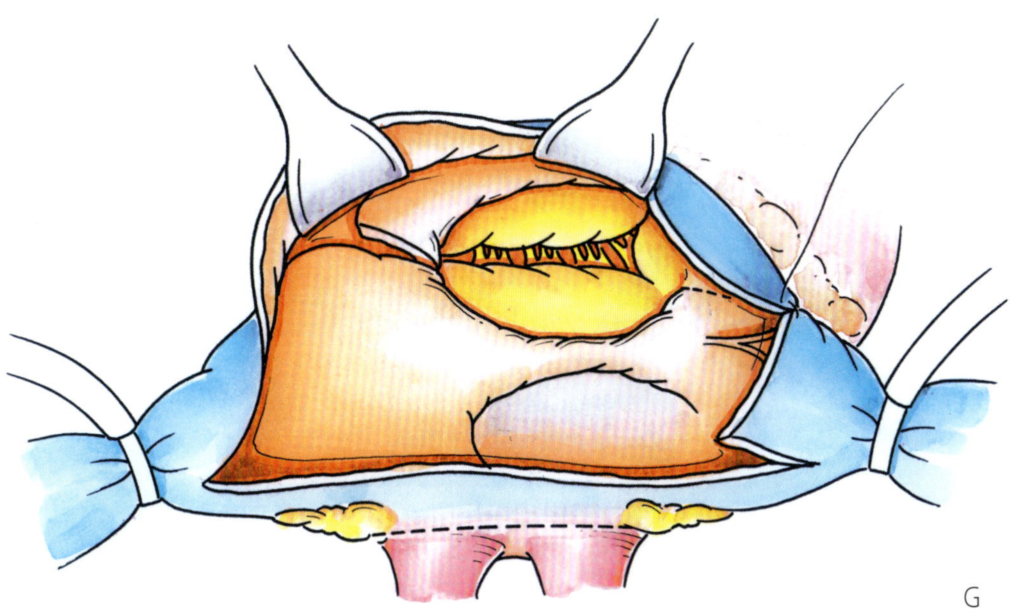

G. 右心耳左侧壁切口继续全层切开至三尖瓣环。
G. The left lateral wall incision at the right atrial appendage requires a full-thickness incision to the tricuspid annulus.

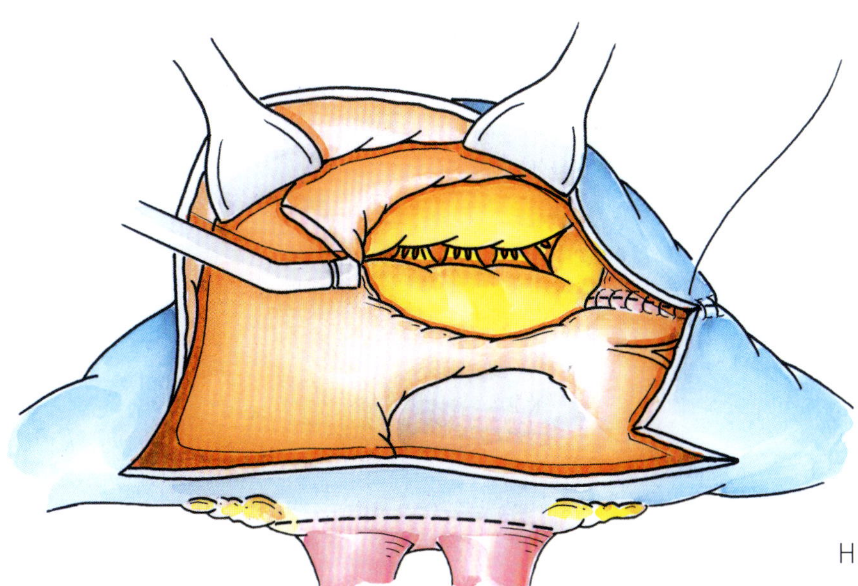

H. 在三尖瓣环处做冰冻处理。
H. Freeze the tricuspid annulus.

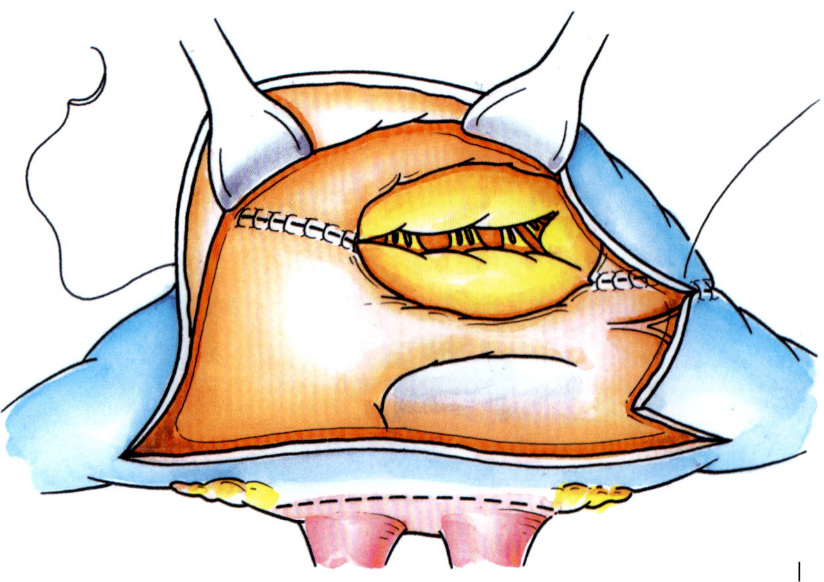

I. 缝合右心耳到三尖瓣环的右心房切口。
I. Suture the right atrial incision from the right atrial appendage to the tricuspid annulus.

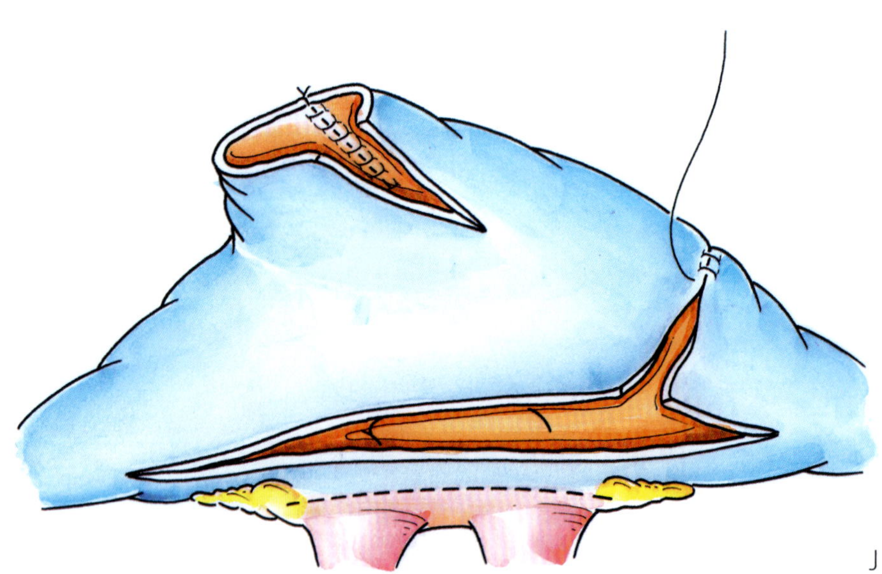

J. 右心房切口全部完成，大部分切口保持敞开以利后续操作。
J. The right atrium incisions are all completed, most of which are kept exposed to facilitate subsequent operations.

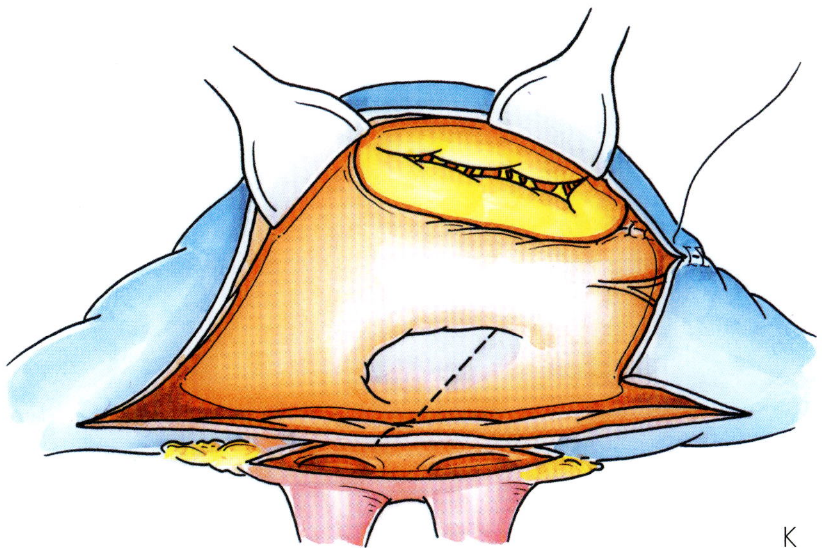

K. 经房间沟纵行切开左心房。

K. The left atrium is incised longitudinally through the interatrial groove.

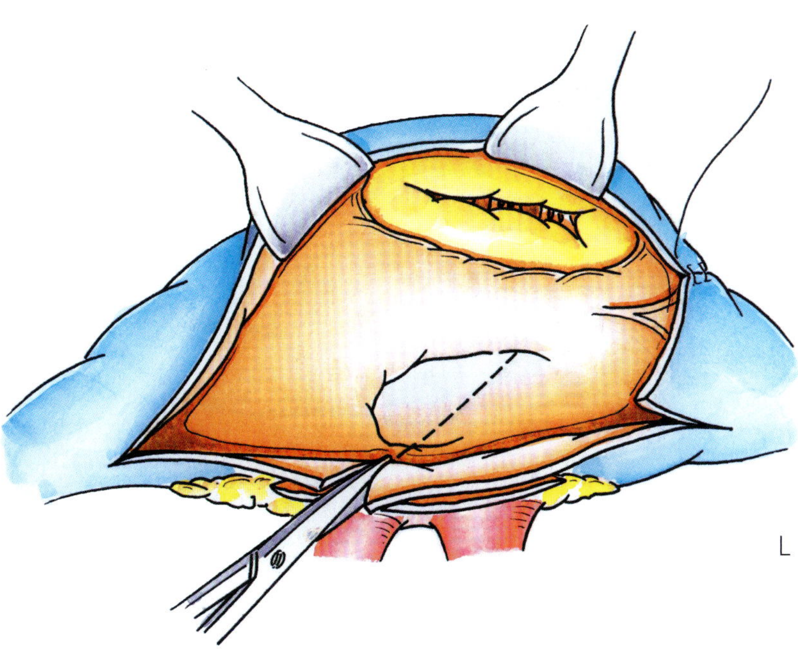

L. 准备做房间隔切口。

L. Prepare to make an atrial septal incision.

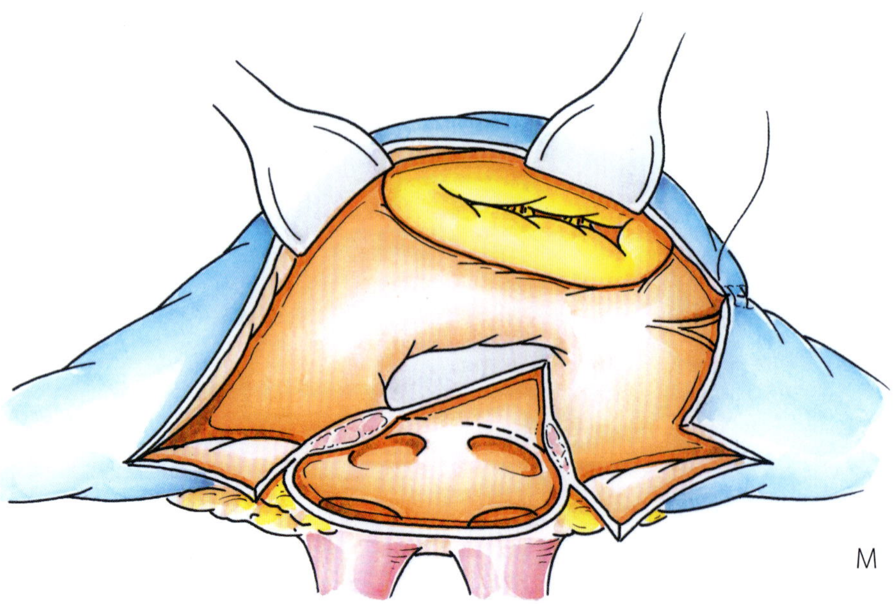

M. 由右心房纵切口和左心房纵切口中上部开始向下斜行剪开房间隔，继续剪开卵圆窝直至卵圆窝前缘。

M. The atrial septum is incised obliquely downward from the middle and upper aspects of the right and left atrial longitudinal incisions. Proceed to incise the fossa ovalis until the anterior margin of the fossa ovalis.

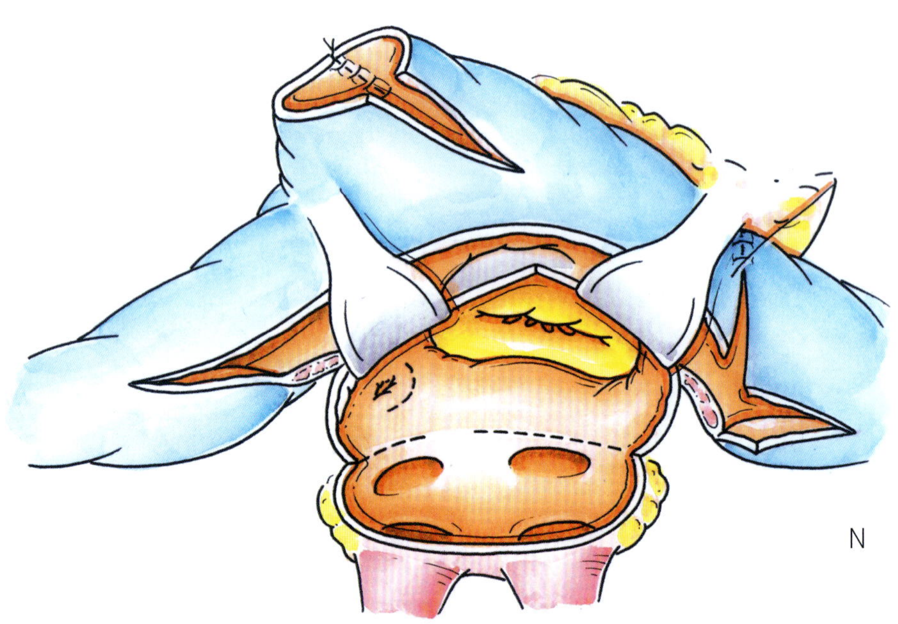

N. 心房拉钩拉开房间隔，显露左心房。将左心房切口两端延长，形成环绕肺静脉开口的切口。在左肺静脉和左心耳之间保留一小块左心房后壁不切开，以方便以后的缝合。在左心房下部做横行全层切开，该切口起自左心房外下方环肺静脉切口，止于二尖瓣后瓣环中点。切口顶端二尖瓣环处做冰冻处理。

N. The atrial retractor pulls apart the atrial septum, revealing the left atrium. Extend both ends of the left atrium incision to form an incision surrounding the pulmonary vein opening. A small piece of the left atrial posterior wall is left intact between the left pulmonary vein and the left atrial appendage to facilitate subsequent sutures. A transverse full-thickness incision is made in the lower part of the left atrium, starting from the lateral inferior circumferential pulmonary vein incision of the left atrium and ending at the midpoint of the posterior mitral annulus. The mitral valve annulus at the top of the incision is frozen.

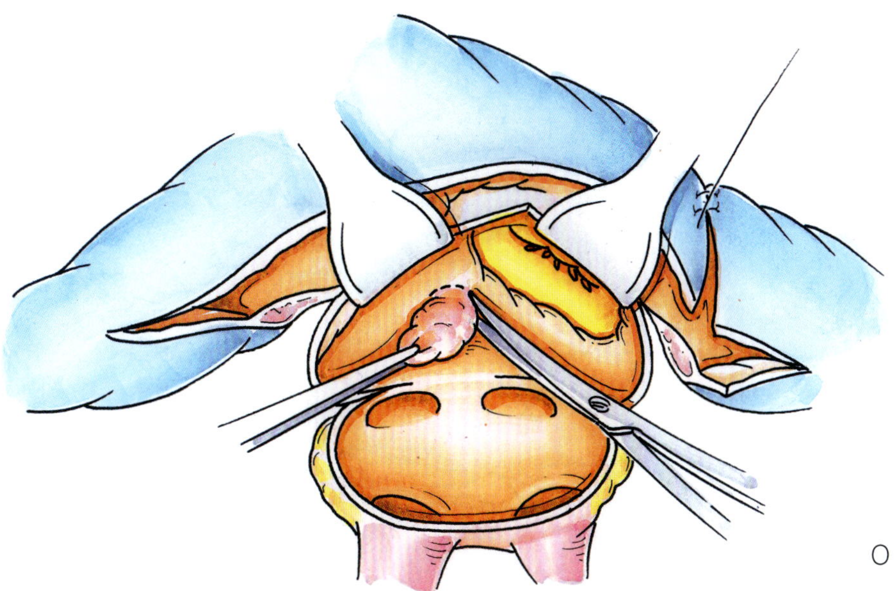

O. 左心耳内翻，基底部切除左心耳，注意保护其下方通过的冠状动脉回旋支。

O. The left atrial appendage is inverted to be excised at the base. Take care to protect the circumflex coronary artery passing thereunder.

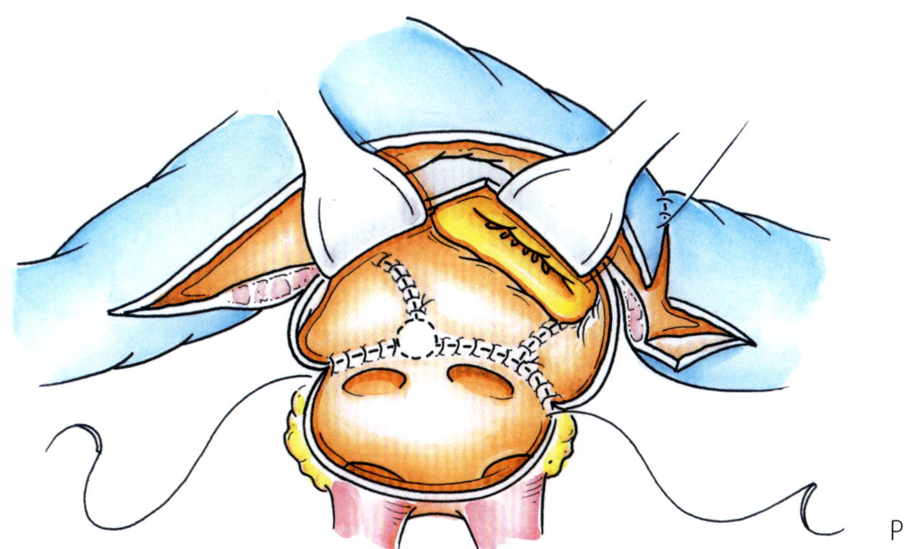

P. 在左心房内缝合左心耳，缝合左心房左侧的切口，均为单纯连续缝合。在左心耳切口与左心房环肺静脉切口之间未切开处做冰冻处理，将三个切口端连接起来。

P. With simple continuous sutures, the left atrial appendage is sutured in the left atrium, and the incision on the left side of the left atrium is sutured. Freeze the uncut part between the left atrial appendage incision and the left atrial circumferential pulmonary vein incision, and the three cut edges are connected.

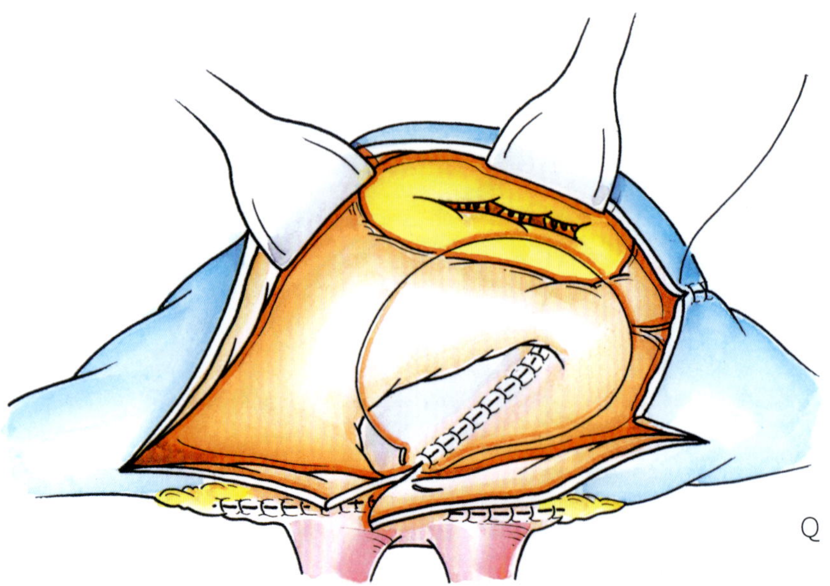

Q. 继续缝合左心房环肺静脉切口，缝合房间隔横切口。左心房关闭。
Q. Continue to suture the left atrial circumferential pulmonary vein incision and the atrial septal transverse incision. Close the left atrium.

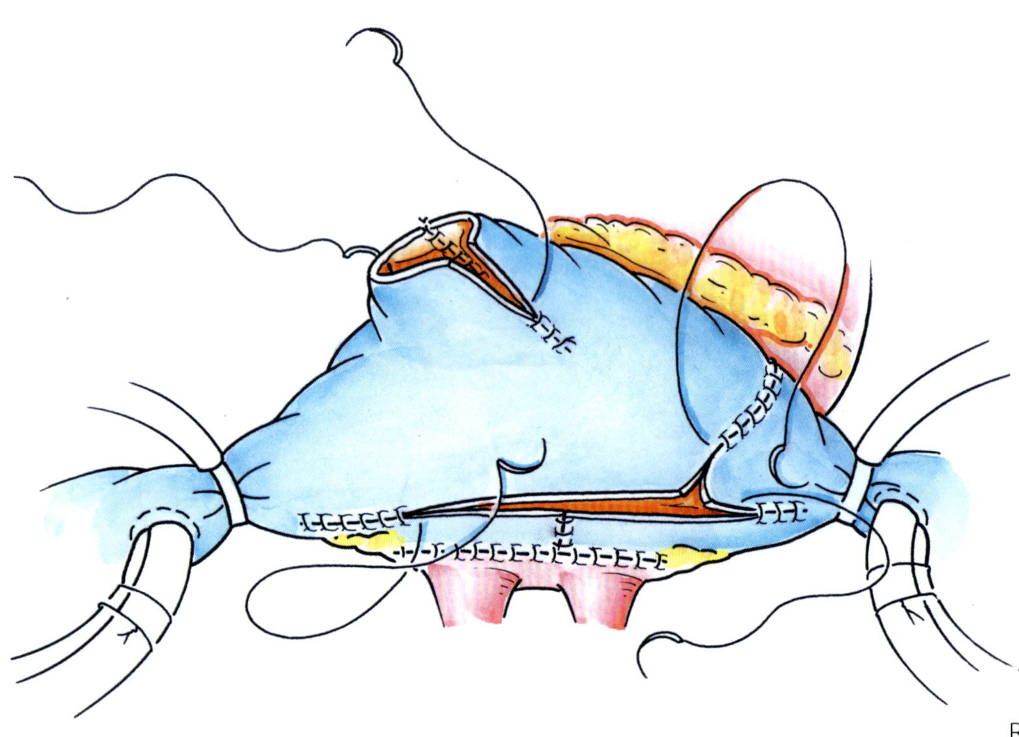

R. 缝合右心房诸切口和右心耳切口。
R. Suture right atrial incisions and right atrial appendage incision.

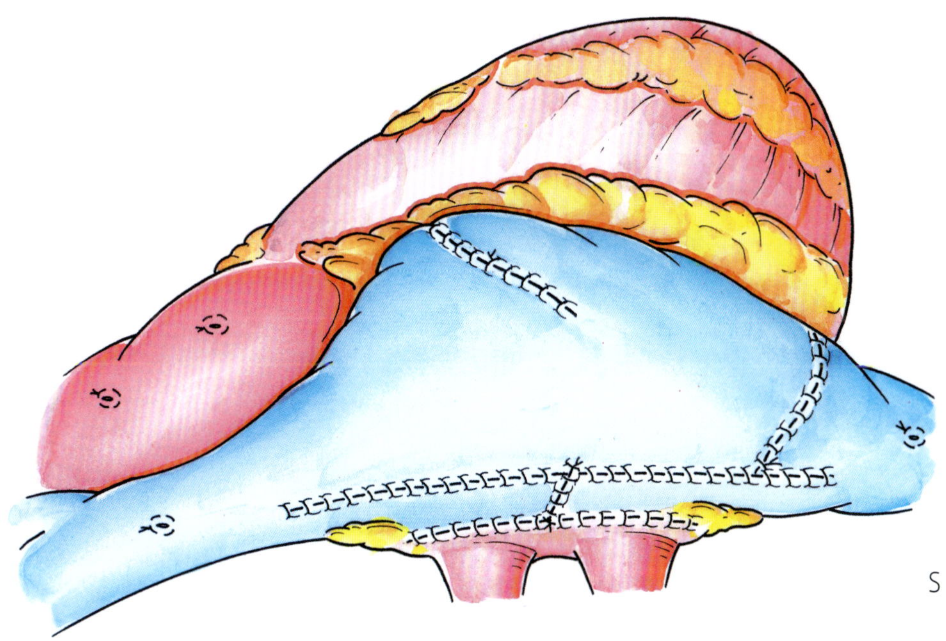

S. 缝合完成。撤除体外循环。

S. The suture is complete, and the extracorporeal circulation is weaned off.

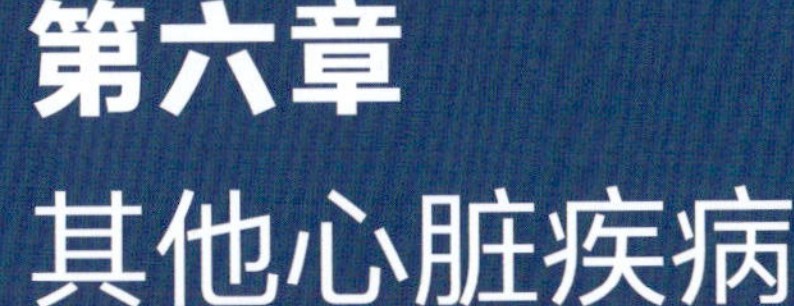

第六章 其他心脏疾病

Chapter 6 Other Cardiac Diseases

第一节　肺栓塞和肺动脉血栓清除术
Section 1　Pulmonary Embolism and Pulmonary Artery Embolectomy

图 6-1-1　肺动脉血栓清除术
Figure 6-1-1　Pulmonary artery embolectomy

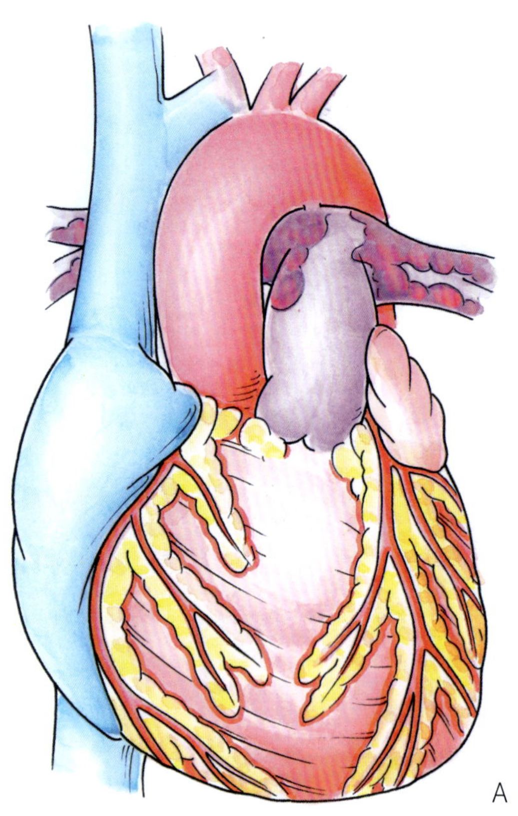

A. 肺动脉及左、右肺动脉血栓形成。

A. Pulmonary artery and thrombosis in the left and right pulmonary arteries.

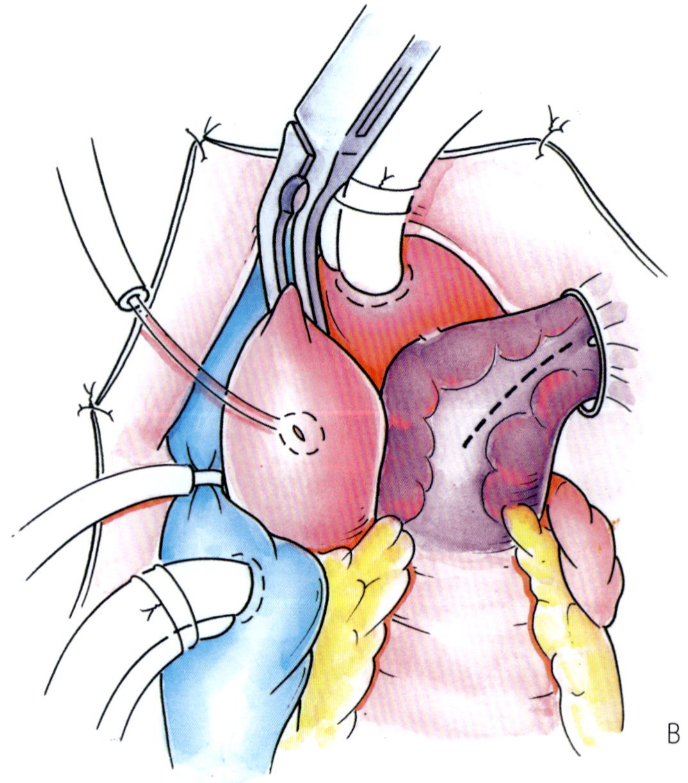

B. 建立体外循环，阻断升主动脉心脏停搏后，在肺动脉前壁做纵行切口并延伸至左肺动脉心包内段。

B. After establishing extracorporeal circulation and clamping the ascending aorta to induce cardiac arrest, a longitudinal incision is made in the anterior wall of the pulmonary artery and extended to the left pulmonary artery segment in the pericardium.

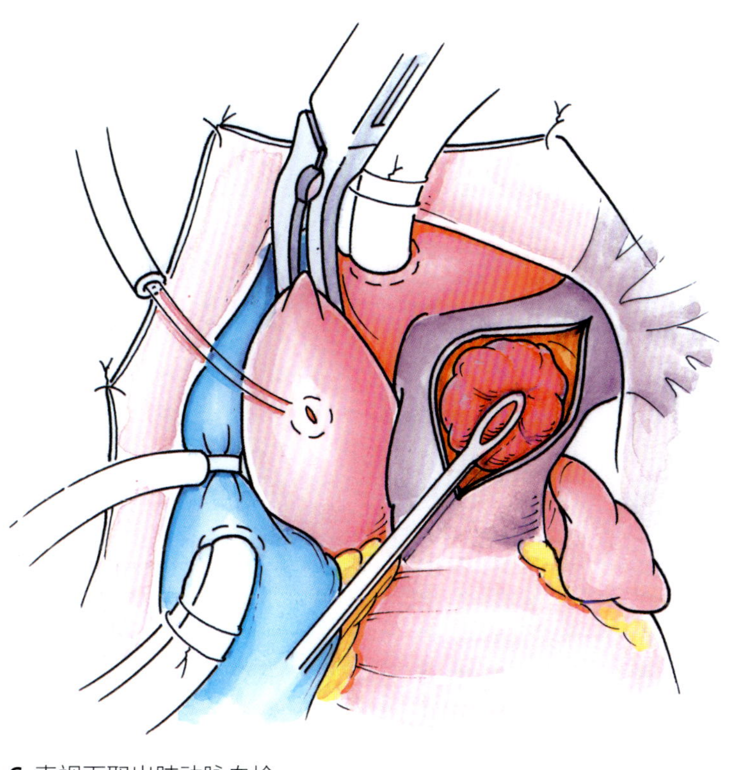

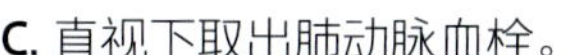

C. 直视下取出肺动脉血栓。

C. Pulmonary artery thrombus is removed under direct vision.

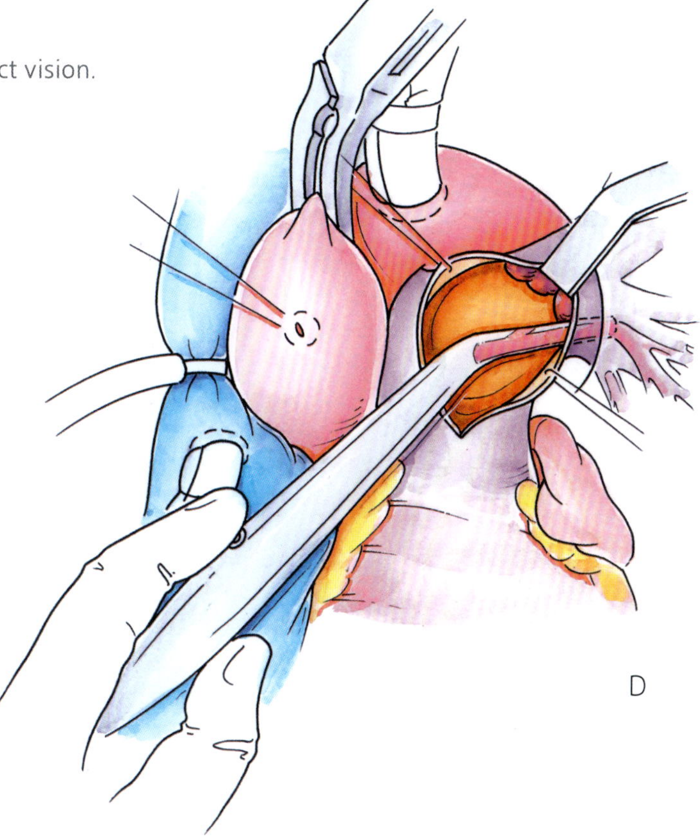

D. 深入左肺动脉，取出左肺动脉及其分支内的血栓。

D. Go deep into the left pulmonary artery and remove the thrombus within the left pulmonary artery and its branches.

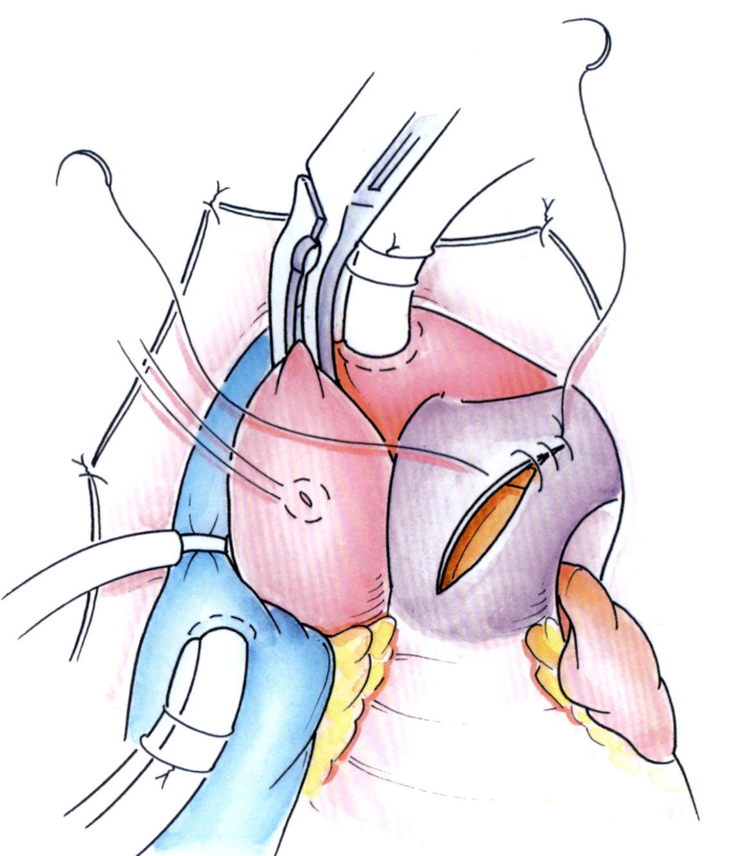

E. 缝合肺动脉及左肺动脉切口。

E. Suture the incisions in the pulmonary artery and the left pulmonary artery.

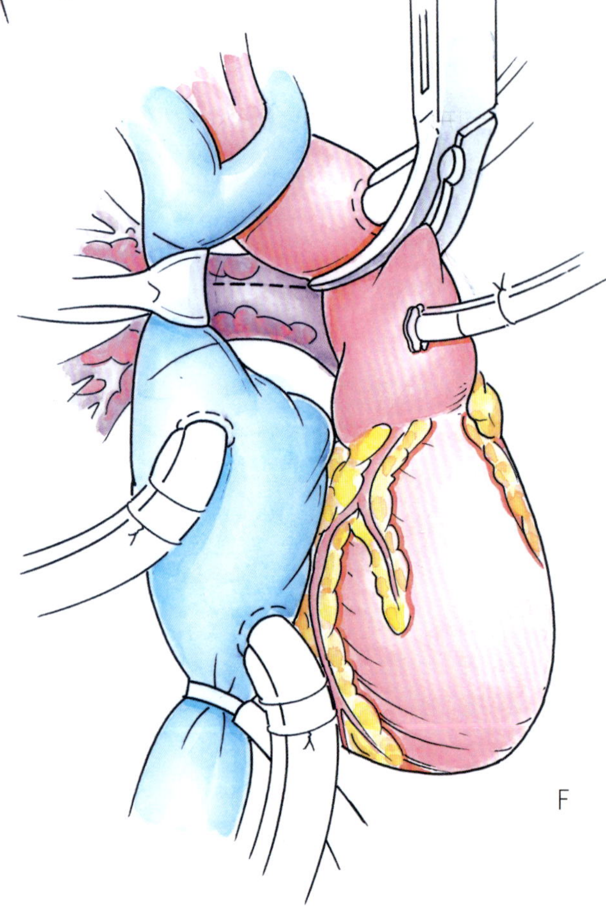

F. 向左牵开升主动脉，显露右肺动脉。

F. Retract the ascending aorta towards the left to expose the right pulmonary artery.

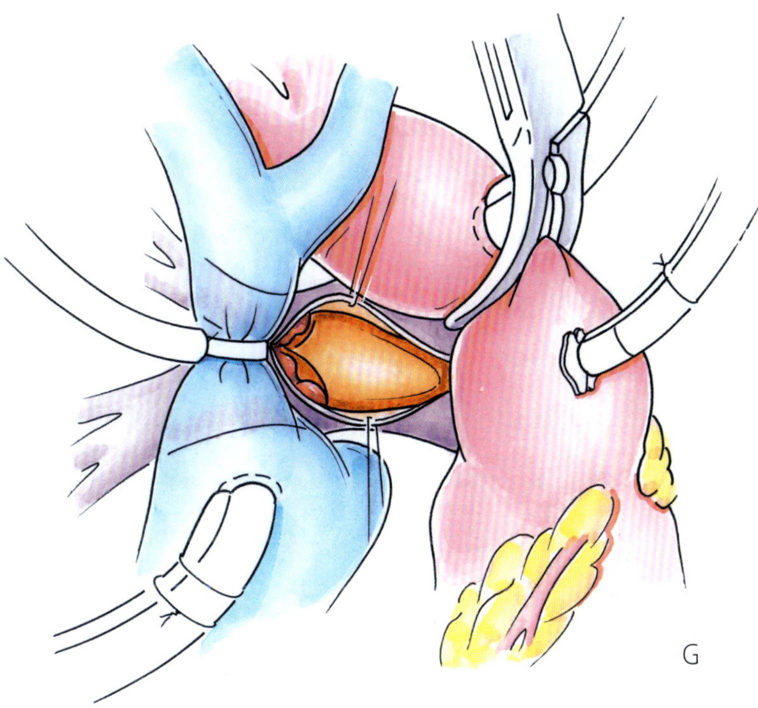

G. 横行切开右肺动脉，取出其中的血栓

G. Make a transverse incision into the right pulmonary artery to remove the thrombus within it.

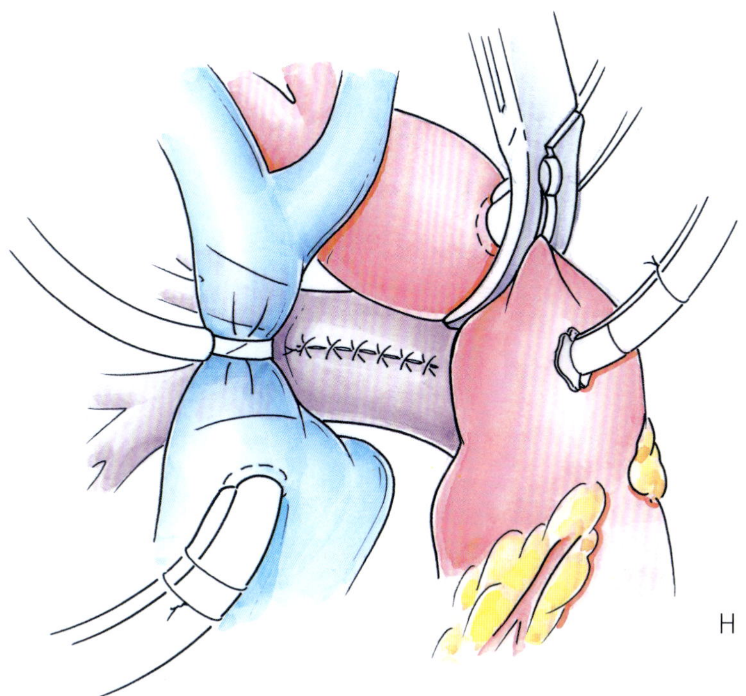

H. 缝合右肺动脉切口。

H. Suture the right pulmonary artery incision.

图 6-1-2　抗血栓夹植入术
Figure 6-1-2　Implantation of antithrombotic clip

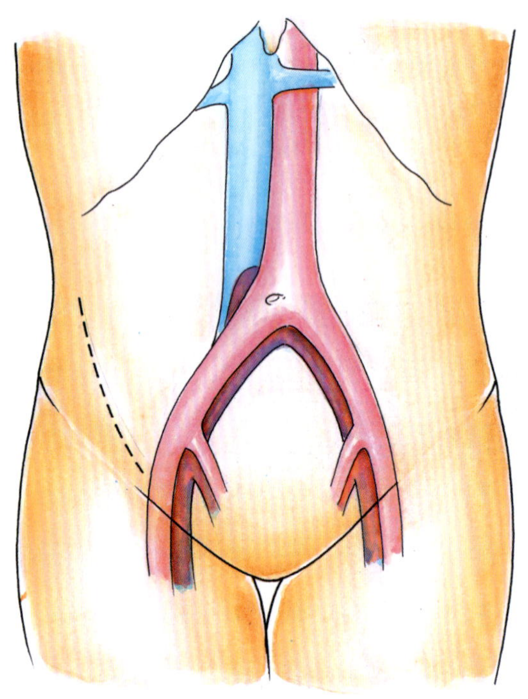

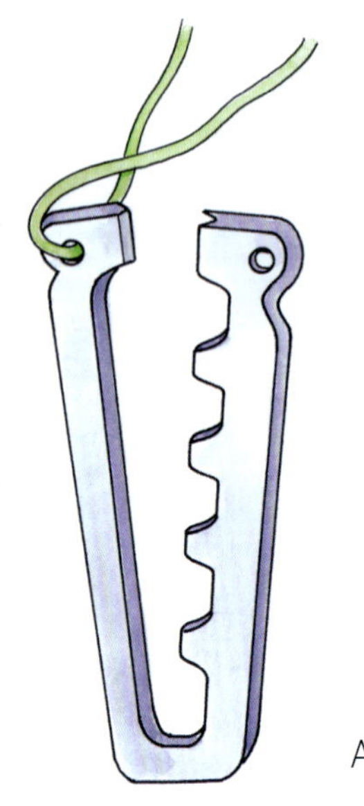

A. 右下腹斜切口。
A. An oblique incision is made into the right inferior abdomen.

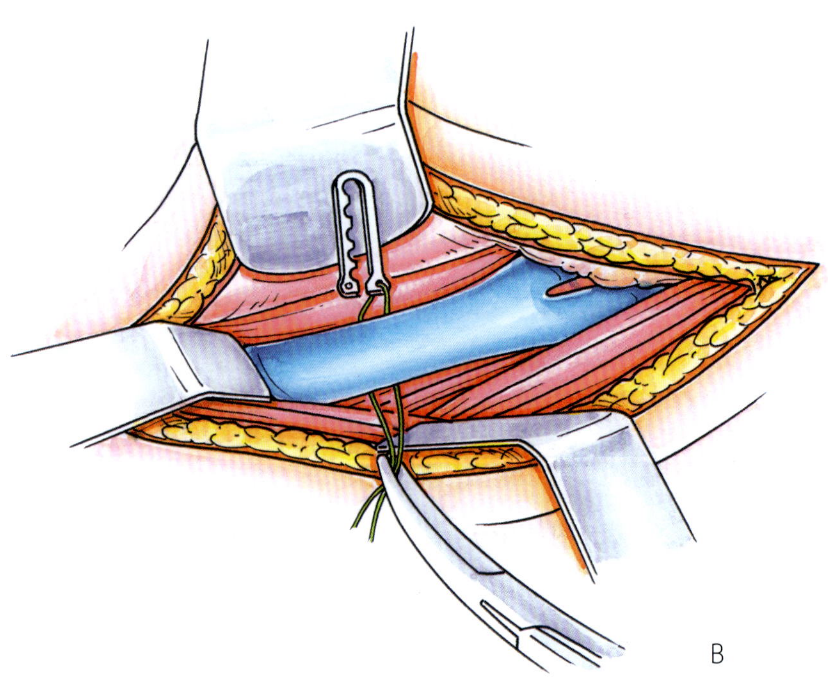

B. 腹膜外显露右髂静脉。
B. Expose the right iliac vein outside the peritoneum.

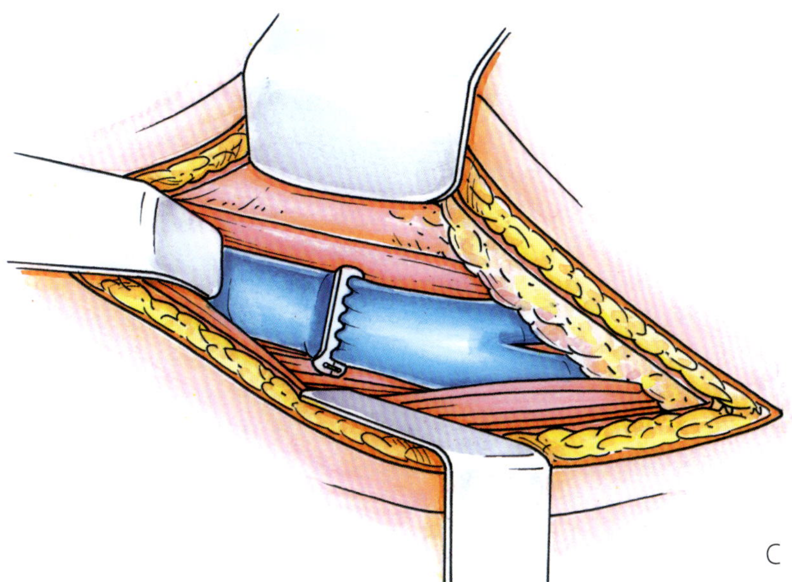

C. 右髂静脉游离后置入抗血栓夹。
C. Antithrombotic clips are placed after dissociating the right iliac vein.

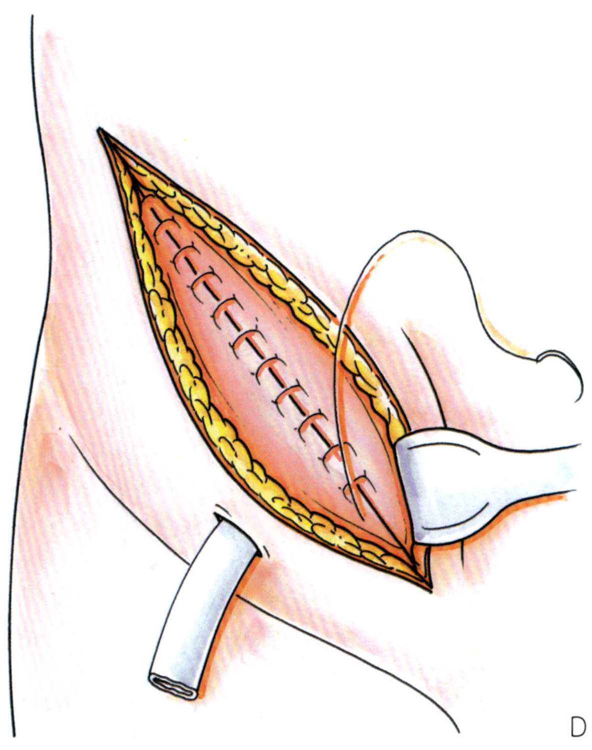

D. 腹腔留置引流条后逐层缝合腹壁切口。
D. The abdominal wall incision is sutured layer by layer after the draining strip is placed in the abdominal cavity.

第 二 节　心脏肿瘤（黏液瘤）
Section 2　Cardiac Tumor (Myxoma)

图 6-2-1　左心房黏液瘤摘除术
Figure 6-2-1　Left atrial myxoma resection

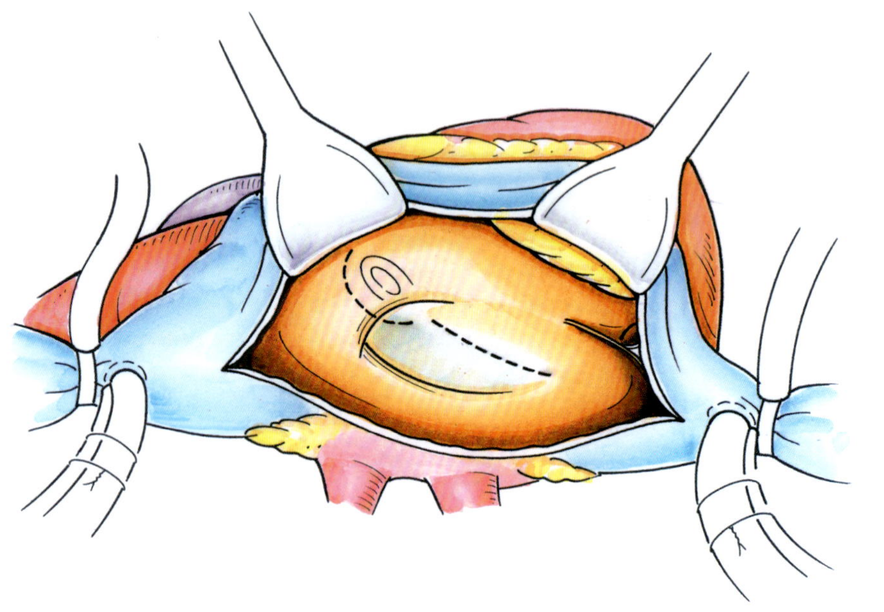

A

A. 体外循环下心脏停搏，纵行切开右心房。

A. A right atriotomy is longitudinally performed with extracorporeal circulation and cardiac arrest.

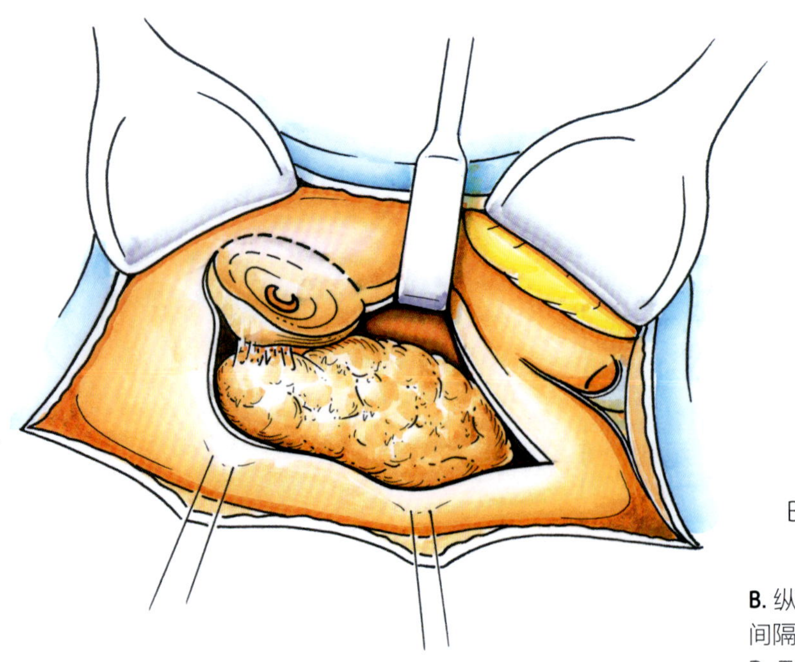

B

B. 纵行切开卵圆窝，沿黏液瘤的蒂部切除其附着的房间隔。

B. The fossa ovalis is incised longitudinally, and the attached atrial septum is resected along the pedicle of the myxoma.

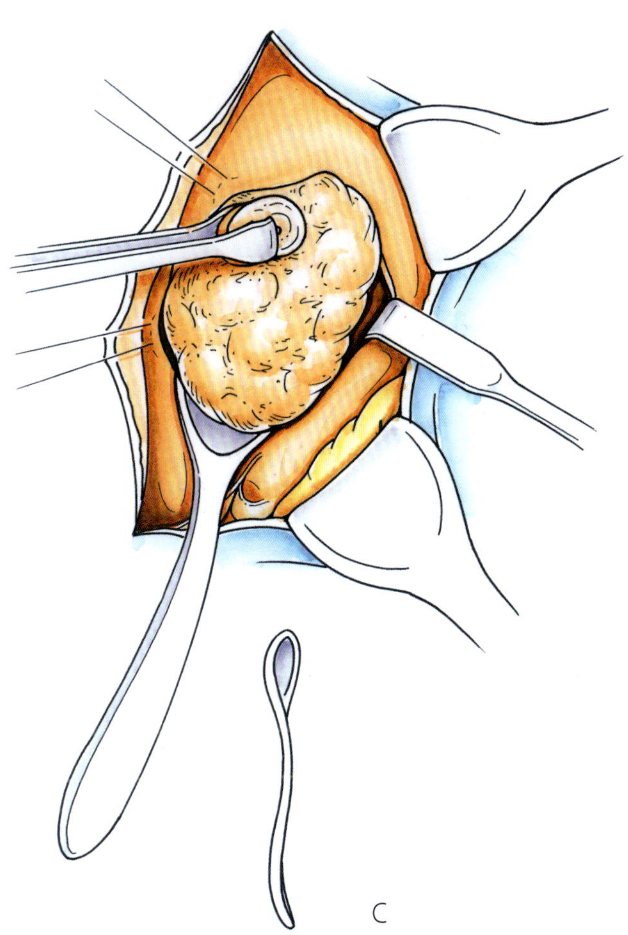

C. 从左心房完整取出黏液瘤。

C. The myxoma is completely removed from the left atrium.

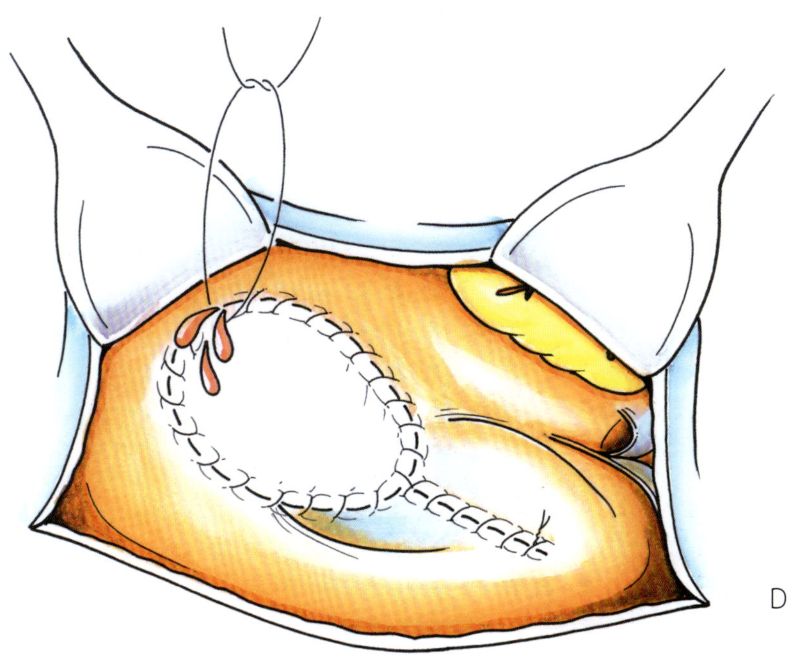

D. 补片修补房间隔。

D. A patch is used to repair the atrial septum.

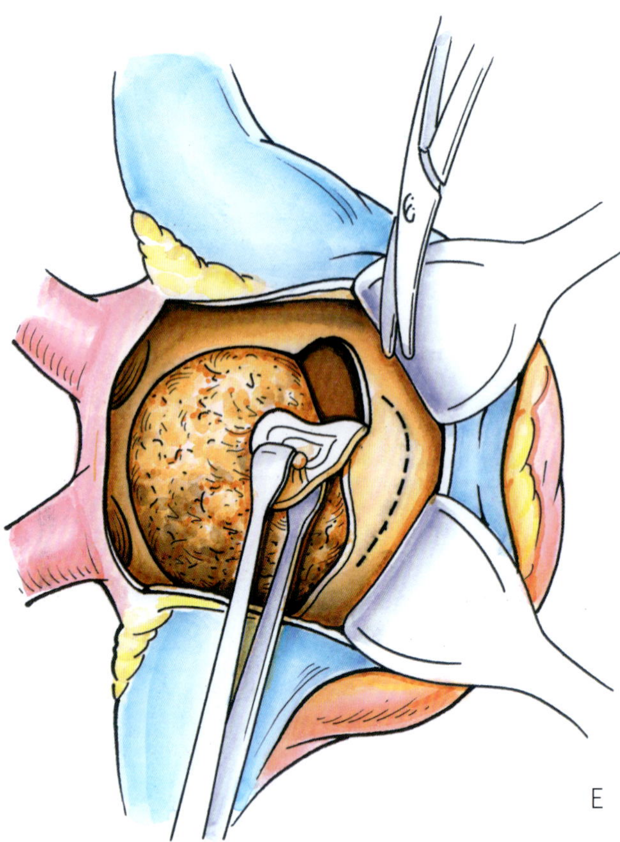

E. 巨大左心房黏液瘤右心房切口难以取出时，在房间沟加做左心房切口，向右扩大房间隔切口，取出黏液瘤。

E. When the left atrial myxoma is too giant to remove through the right atrium incision, make an additional incision into the left atrium in the interatrial groove, and expand the atrial septum incision toward the right to remove the myxoma.

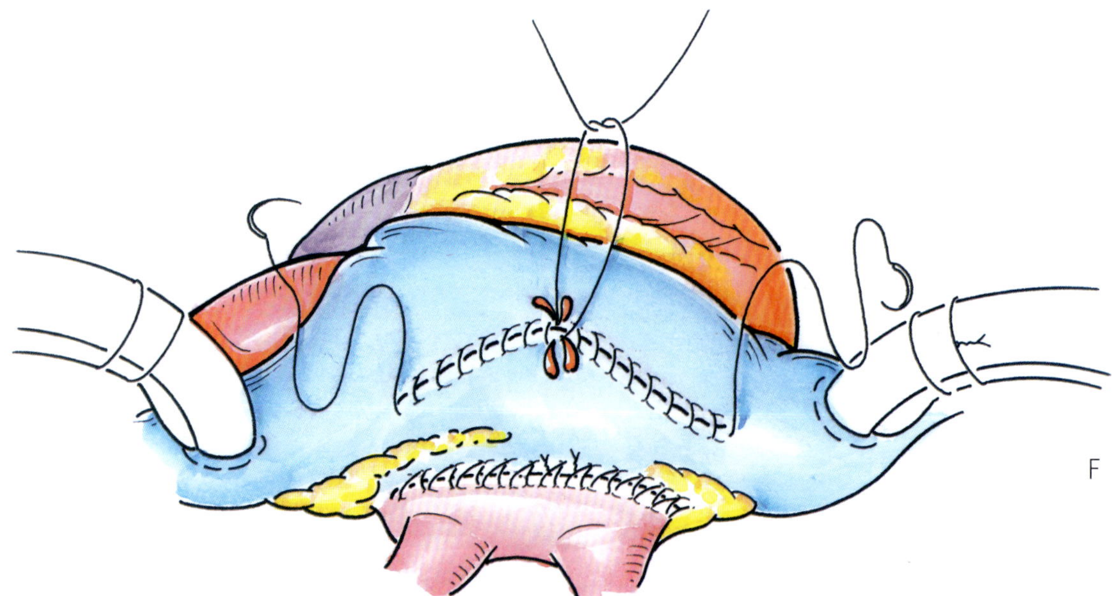

F. 修补房间隔，分别缝合左、右心房切口。

F. Repair the atrial septum and suture the left and right atrium incisions respectively.

第三节 心包疾病
Section 3 Pericardial Disease

图 6-3-1 心包切开引流术
Figure 6-3-1 Pericardiotomy for drainage

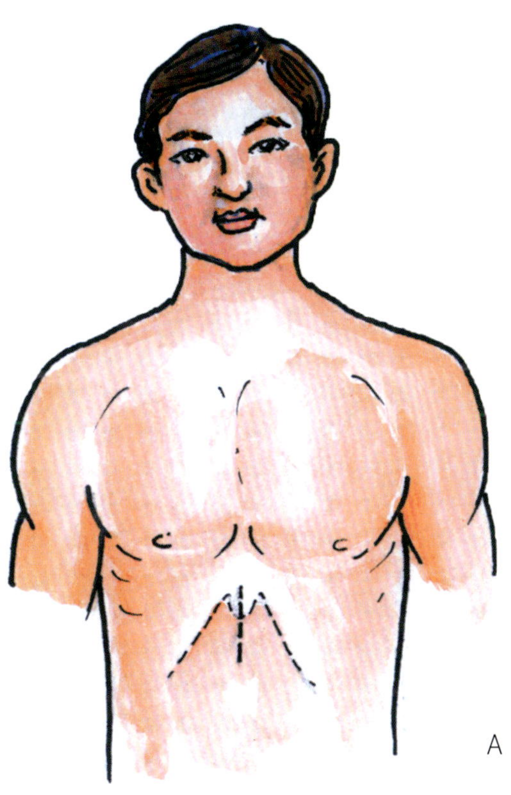

A

A. 局部麻醉下，剑突下纵行切口。
A. Make a longitudinal incision under the xiphoid process under local anesthesia.

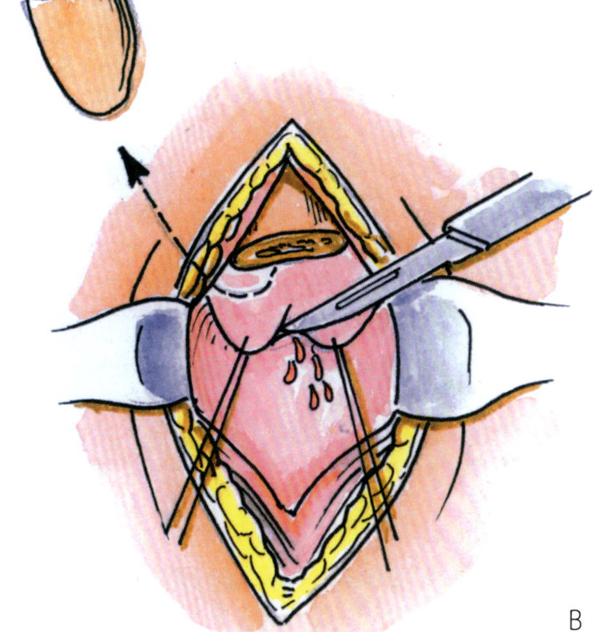

B

B. 切除剑突，向后上分离显露心包。心包缝牵引线提起后切开心包。
B. Excise the xiphoid process and separate upward and backward to expose the pericardium. Traction lines are sewn to the pericardium, to lift the pericardium for a pericardiotomy.

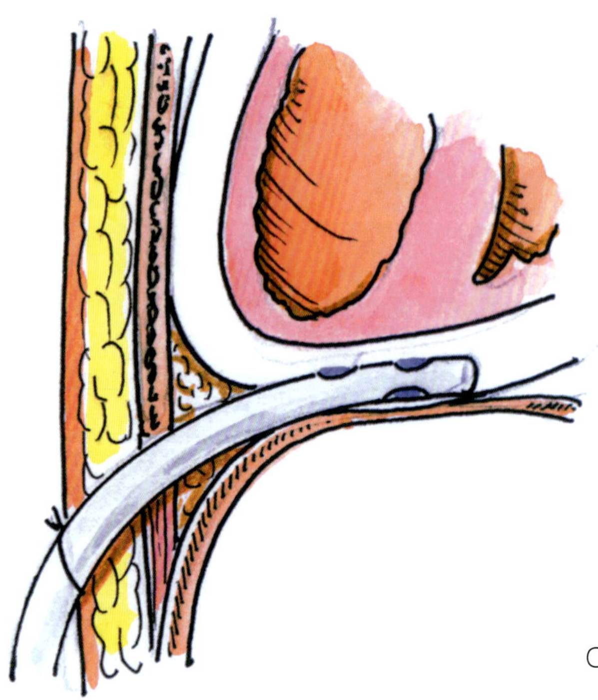

C. 插入心包引流管至心脏膈面，引流管经切口引出接水封瓶。

C. Insert the pericardial drainage tube to the diaphragm surface of the heart, and the drainage tube is brought out through the incision and connected to a water-sealed bottle.

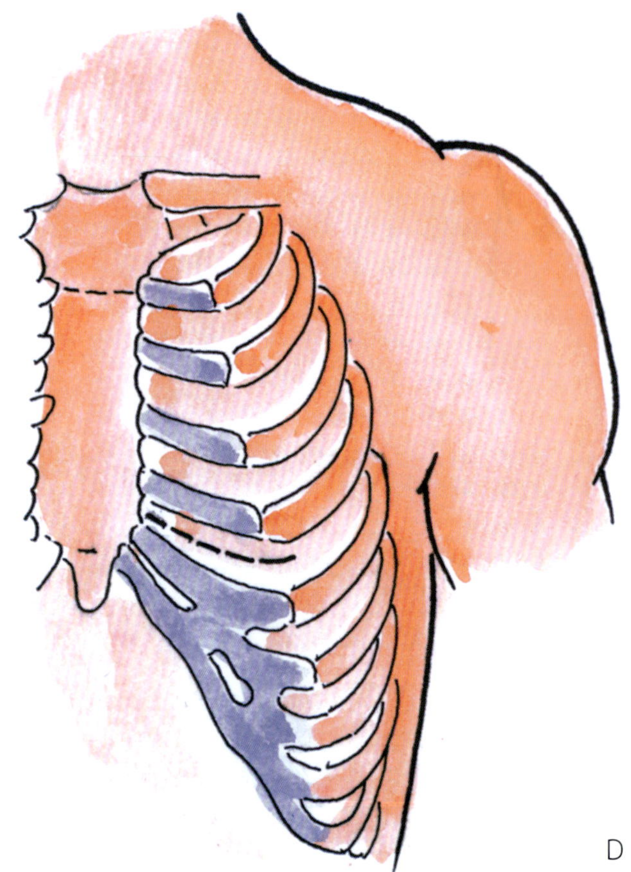

D. 另一引流途径是在胸骨左缘第 5 肋间切开。

D. Another way of drainage is to make an incision in the fifth intercostal space at the left border of the sternum.

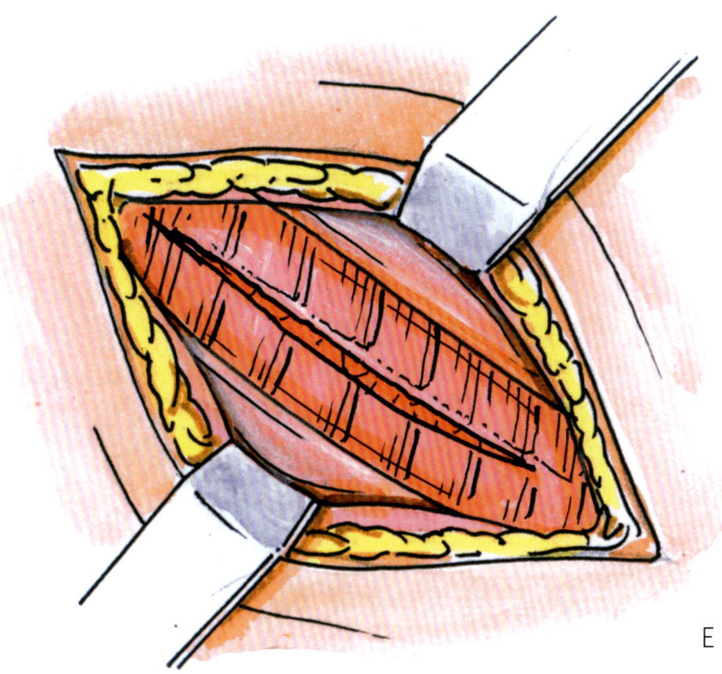

E. 由肋间进入胸腔。湿纱布挡开肺，心尖区切开心包，插入心包引流管。

E. Enter the thoracic cavity through the intercostal space. Use wet gauze to block the lungs, and perform a pericardiotomy in the apex to insert a pericardial drainage tube.

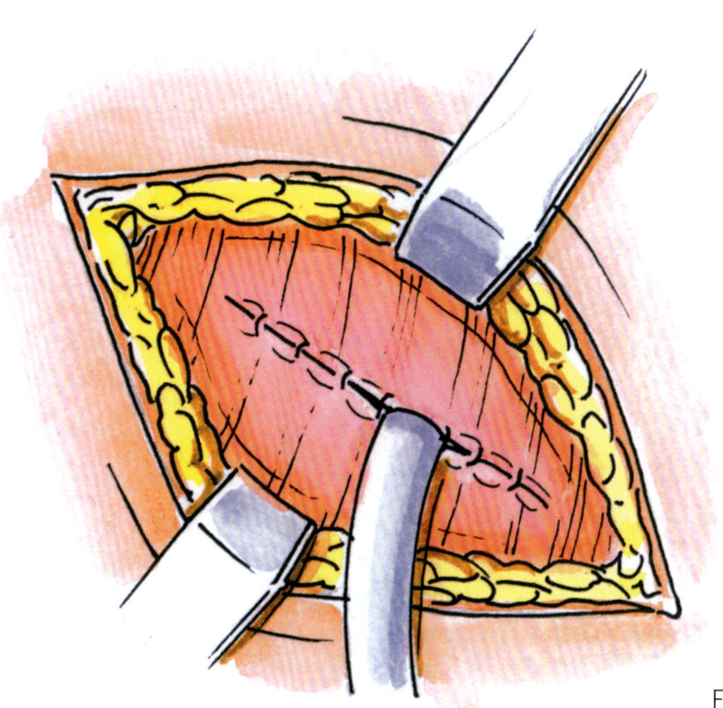

F. 逐层缝合切口，引流管接水封瓶。

F. The incision is sutured in layers, and the drainage tube is connected to a water-sealed bottle.

图 6-3-2　心包剥脱术
Figure 6-3-2　Pericardial decortication

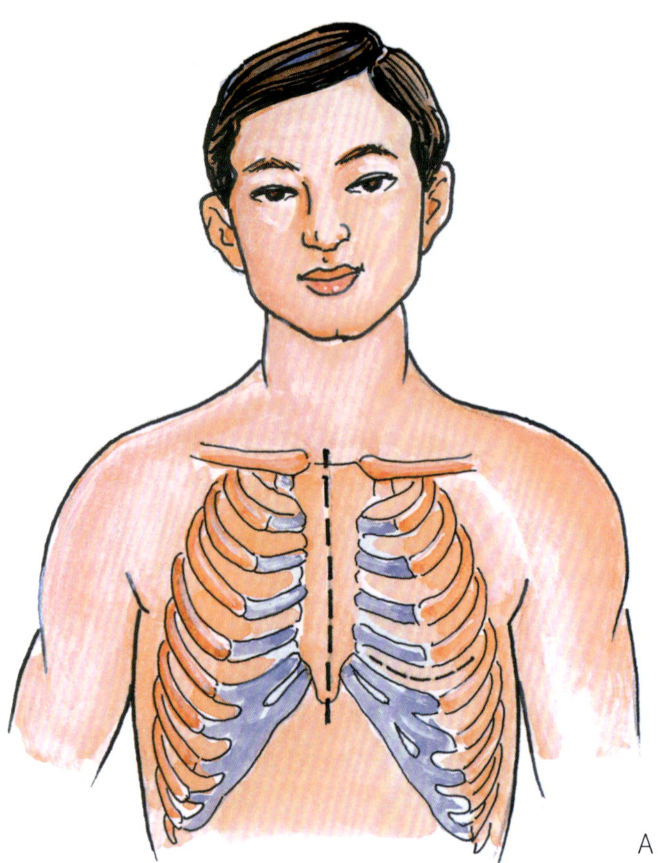

A

A. 缩窄性心包炎心包剥脱术的常用切口是胸骨正中切口或左胸前外侧第 5 肋间切口。

A. A median sternotomy or a left anterolateral thoracotomy at the fifth intercostal space is routinely performed in pericardial decortication for constrictive pericarditis.

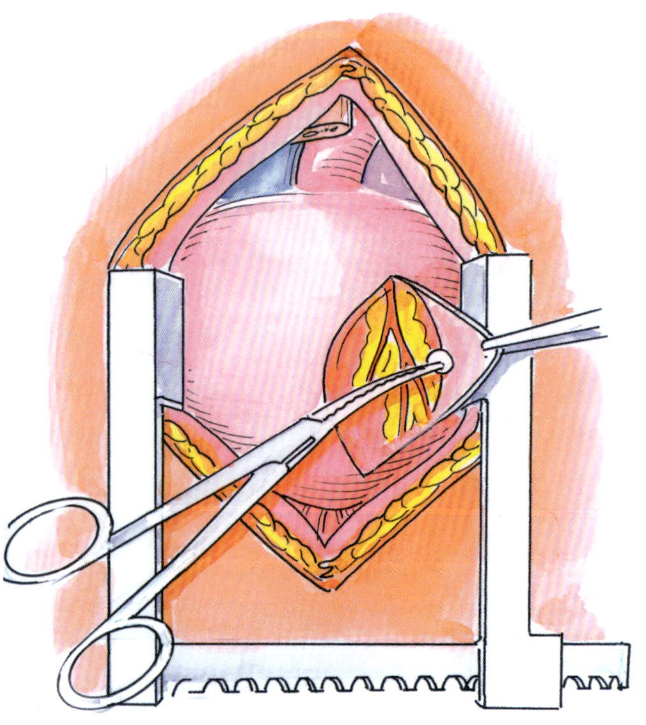

B

B. 胸骨正中切口，撑开胸骨。心尖区切开增厚的心包至心外膜。先解除左心室的缩窄，向左分离心包到左膈神经后。粘连疏松者可用钝性分离。

B. Perform median sternotomy to open the sternum. Cut the thickened pericardium in the apical area to the epicardium. The left ventricle constriction is first released, and the pericardium is separated to the left until behind the left phrenic nerve. Bluntly dissociate loose adhesions.

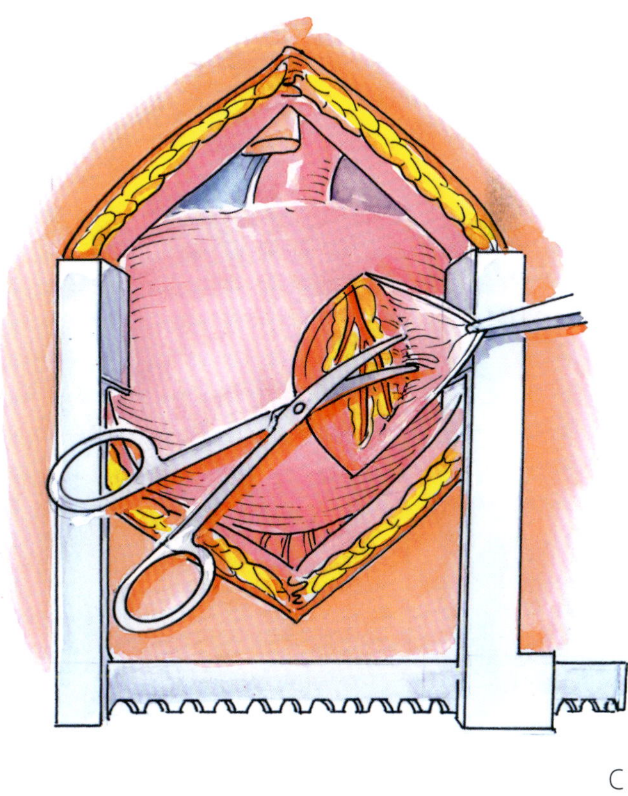

C

C. 多数情况粘连紧密，须用锐性分离，仔细地剪开或切开粘连。

C. Mostly, it is so deeply adherent that sharp separation is necessary. Cut the adhesion carefully.

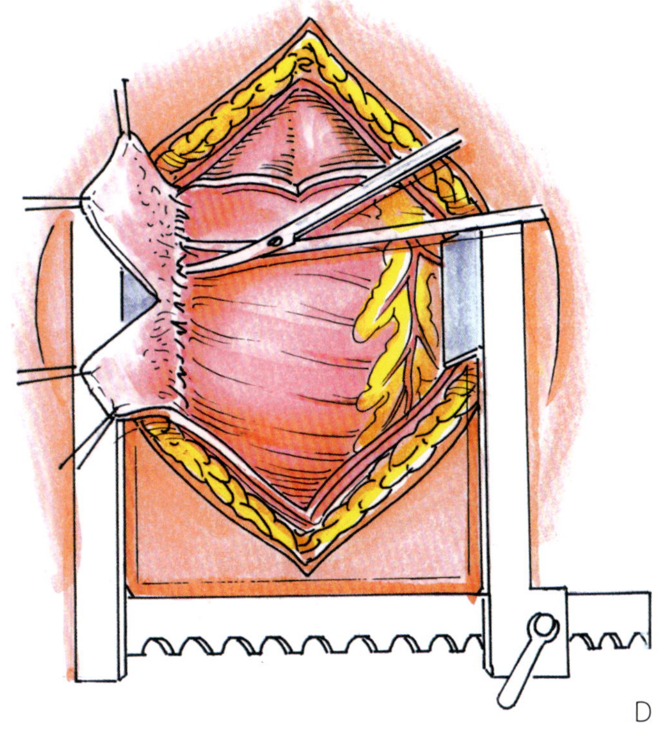

D

D. 左心室松解后再向右分离。先分离右心室流出道，然后右心室的前面和膈面。最后分离右心房，腔静脉入心脏处的环形瘢痕必须剪开松解。

D. The left ventricle is released and separated towards the right. Separate the right ventricular outflow tract first, and then the anterior and diaphragmatic surfaces of the right ventricle. Finally, the right atrium is dissociated, and the annular scar located at the junction of the vena cava and right atrium must be cut and loosened.

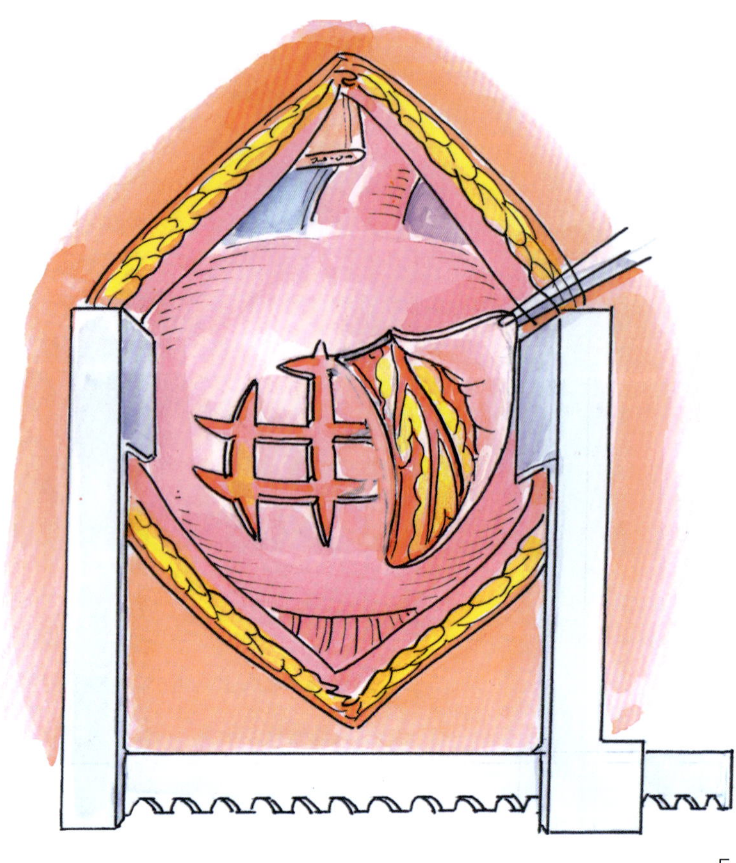

E

E. 对于嵌入心肌难以剥离的瘢痕，不必强行分离，岛状遗留即可。大片的嵌入性心包瘢痕，则须多处“十”字形切开，松解对心脏的缩窄束缚。
E. For scars embedded in the myocardium that are difficult to peel off, it is unnecessary to force the separation, and an island-shaped scar can be left. For large embedded pericardial scars, multiple cruciate incisions are required to loosen the constriction on the heart.

第四节 梗阻性肥厚型心肌病
Section 4 Hypertrophic Obstructive Cardiomyopathy

图 6-4-1 梗阻性肥厚型心肌病左心室流出道疏通术

Figure 6-4-1 Left ventricular outflow tract dredging for hypertrophic obstructive cardiomyopathy

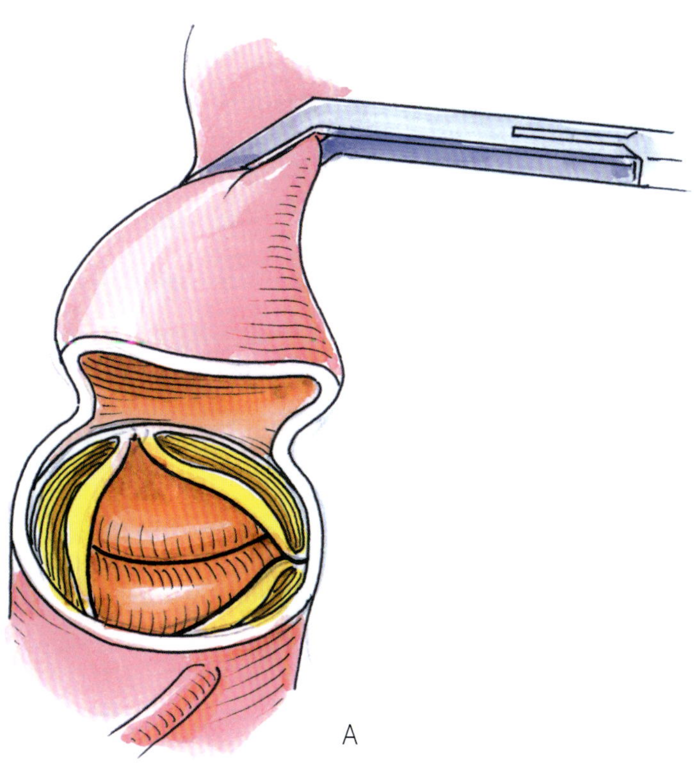

A. 主动脉横切口，切开主动脉。

A. A transverse aortotomy is made to open the aorta.

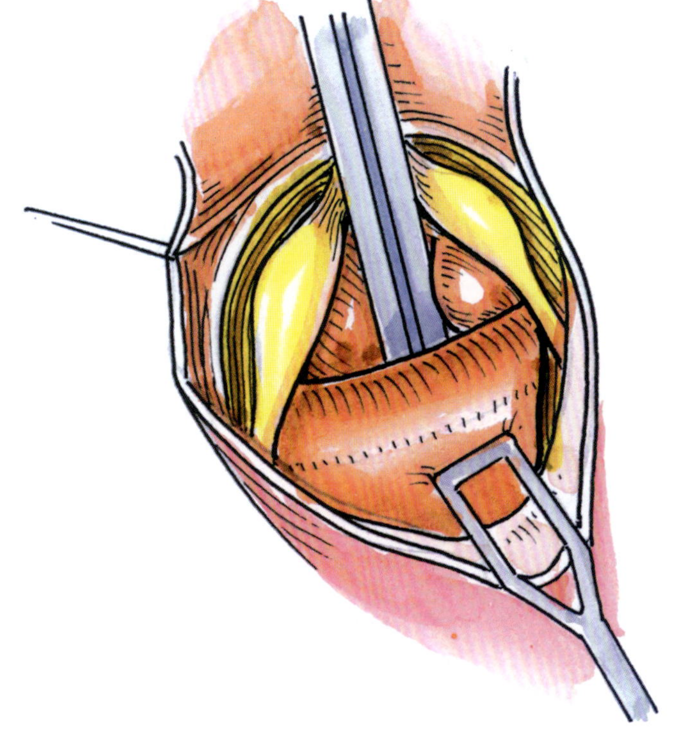

B. 主动脉右冠瓣叶向前牵开，显露其下肥厚的室间隔。手指经主动脉瓣口进入左心室流出道探明肥厚室间隔的范围。

B. The right coronary valve leaflet of the aorta is retracted anteriorly, exposing the hypertrophic ventricular septum underneath it. A finger enters the left ventricular outflow tract through the aortic valve orifice to detect the hypertrophic ventricular septum.

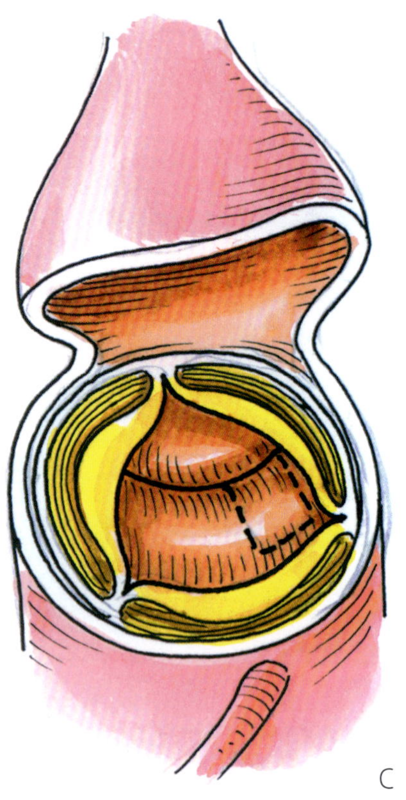

C. 右冠瓣靠近左、右冠瓣交界下方，距主动脉瓣环 2~3mm 处垂直向心室方向切入，切割的深度视室间隔肥厚的程度而定，为 15~20mm。切割长度贯穿左心室流出道，约 40mm。再在该切口右侧，相当于右冠瓣中点下方做一平行切开，深度和长度与室间隔第一个切口相同。

C. Under the right coronary valve, an incision is made perpendicularly to the ventricle at 2-3 mm from the aortic valve annulus, near the commissure of the left and right coronary valves. The incision depth, determined by the ventricular septal hypertrophy, is about 15-20 mm, and the incision length is about 40 mm, passing through the left ventricular outflow tract. On the right side of the incision, a parallel incision is made below the midpoint of the right coronary valve, with the same depth and length as the first incision in the interventricular septum.

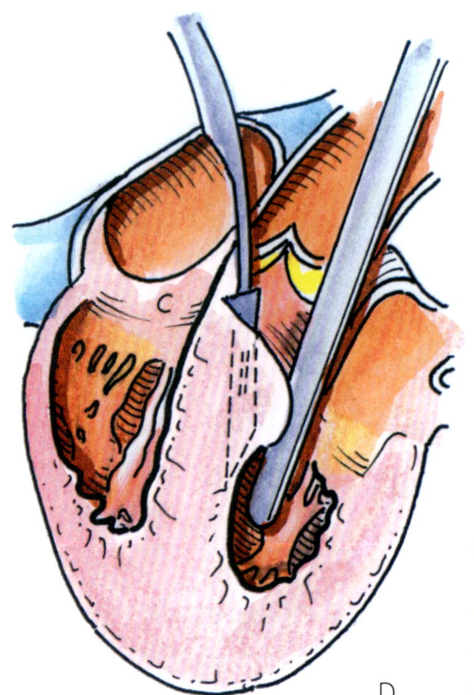

D. 将室间隔两切口之间的肥厚心肌切除，注意避免将室间隔切穿。

D. Excise the hypertrophic myocardium between the two septum incisions, taking care not to cut through the interventricular septum.

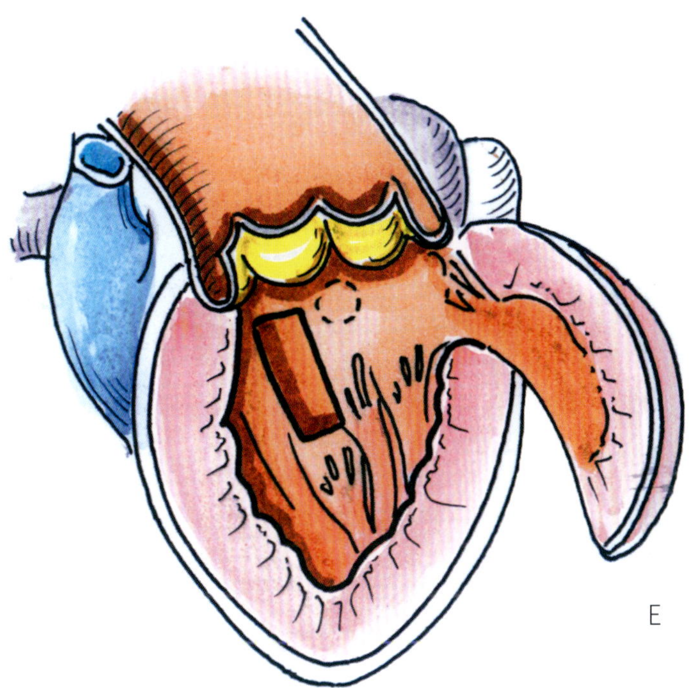

E. 右冠瓣右侧下方有房室束经过，注意避免损伤。

E. Take care to avoid injury to the atrioventricular bundle, which passes by the right inferior area of the right coronary valve.

E

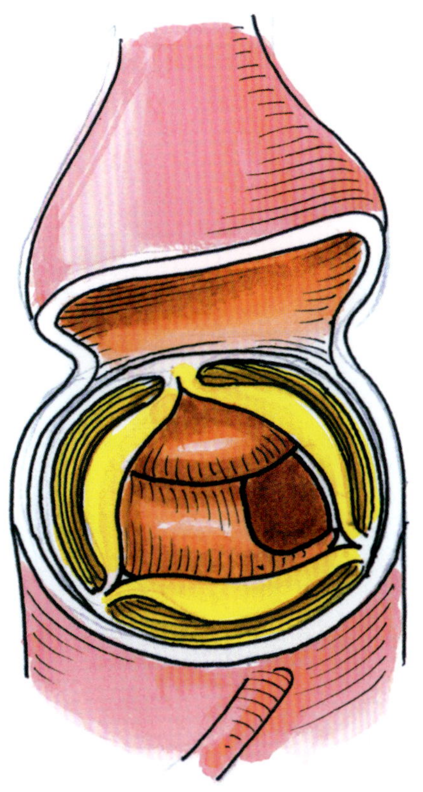

F. 左心室流出道部分心肌已切除，梗阻解除。

F. Part of the myocardium in the left ventricular outflow tract has been excised, and the obstruction is relieved.

F

第七章
心脏移植和肺移植

Chapter 7
Heart Transplantation and Lung Transplantation

第一节　原位心脏移植
Section 1　Orthotopic Heart Transplantation

图 7-1-1　摘取供心
Figure 7-1-1　Harvest of donor heart

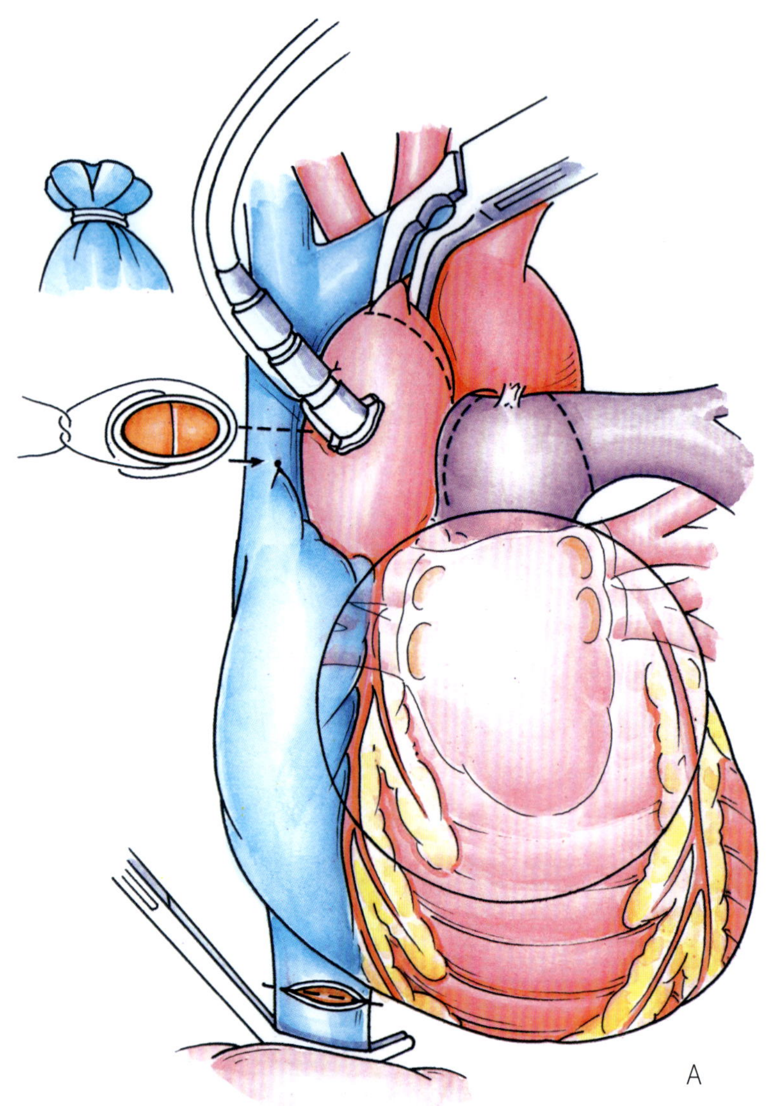

A. 供者胸骨正中切口，切除胸腺组织，切开两侧纵隔胸膜和心包。游离上腔静脉，近心端结扎后切断。游离升主动脉至无名动脉处，插入心肌保护液灌注针。游离下腔静脉，紧贴膈肌钳夹阻断下腔静脉，靠近阻断钳切断下腔静脉。左心耳顶端切开。升主动脉远端钳夹阻断，灌注心肌保护液。

A. A median sternotomy in the donor is performed to excise the thymus tissue and cut into the bilateral mediastinal pleura and the pericardium. Free the superior vena cava for ligation and transection at the end proximal to the heart. Free the ascending aorta to the innominate artery, and insert the cardioplegic solution perfusion needle. Free the inferior vena cava, block the inferior vena cava with the clamp immediately close to the diaphragm, and cut off the inferior vena cava close to the blocking clamp. Cut apart the top of the left atrial appendage. Block the distal ascending aorta with the clamp for cardioplegic solution perfusion.

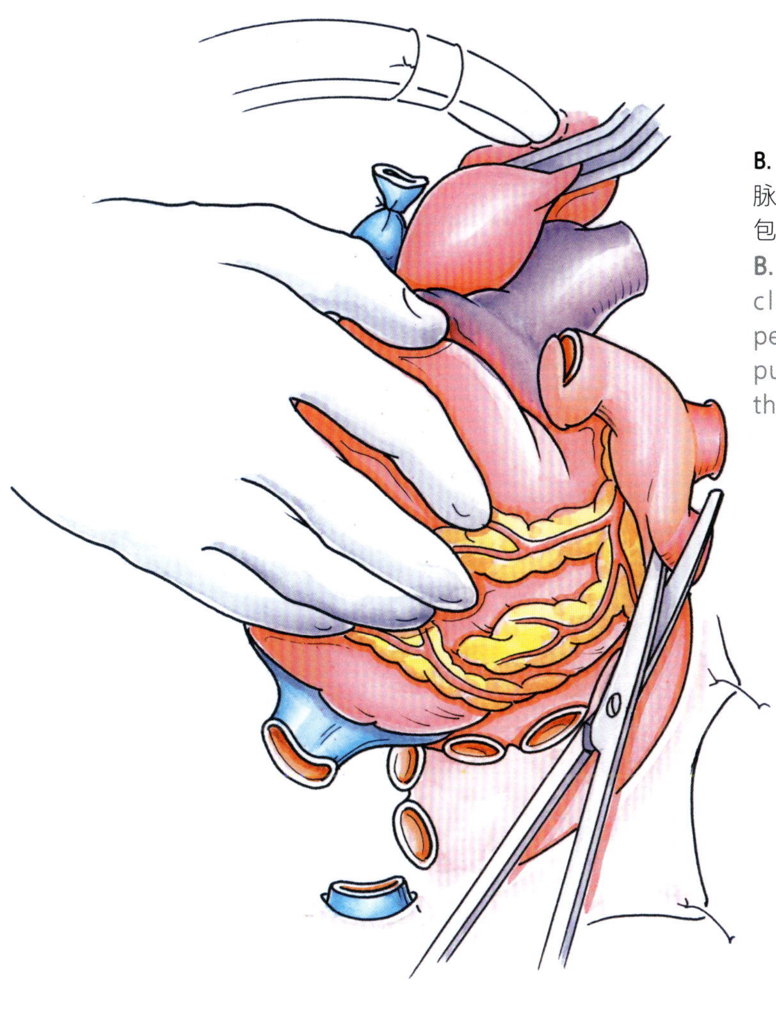

B. 心肌保护液灌注完成后，在阻断钳近端切断主动脉。游离并切断左、右肺动脉。托起心脏，紧贴心包剪断肺静脉。

B. Cut off the aorta proximal to the blocking clamp after the cardioplegic solution perfusion. Dissociate and cut the left and right pulmonary arteries. Hold up the heart to cut the pulmonary veins close to the pericardium.

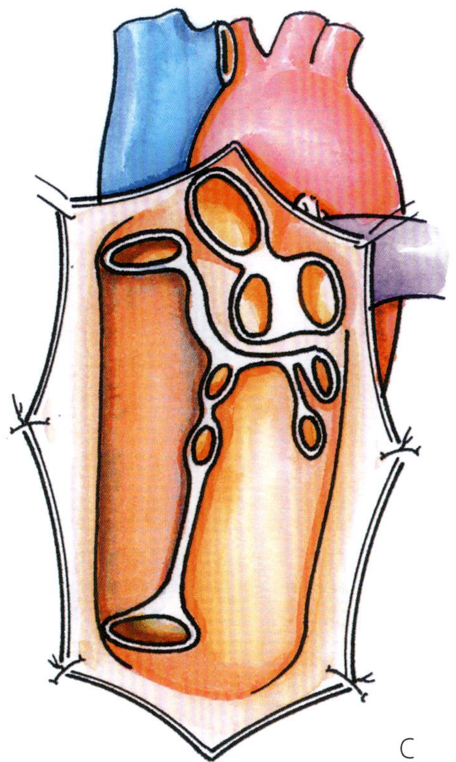

C. 供心从心包腔内取出。

C. The donor heart is harvested from the pericardial cavity.

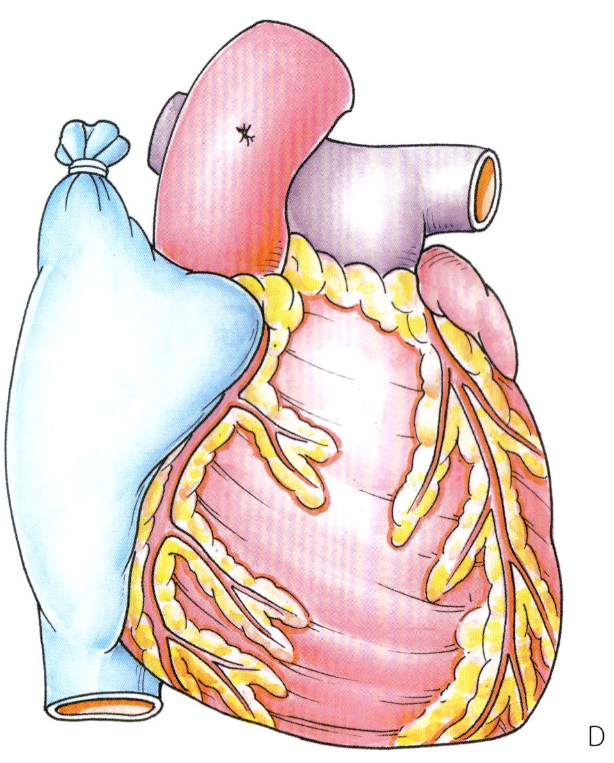

D. 缝合升主动脉灌注针孔。

D. Suture the perfusion pinholes in the ascending aorta.

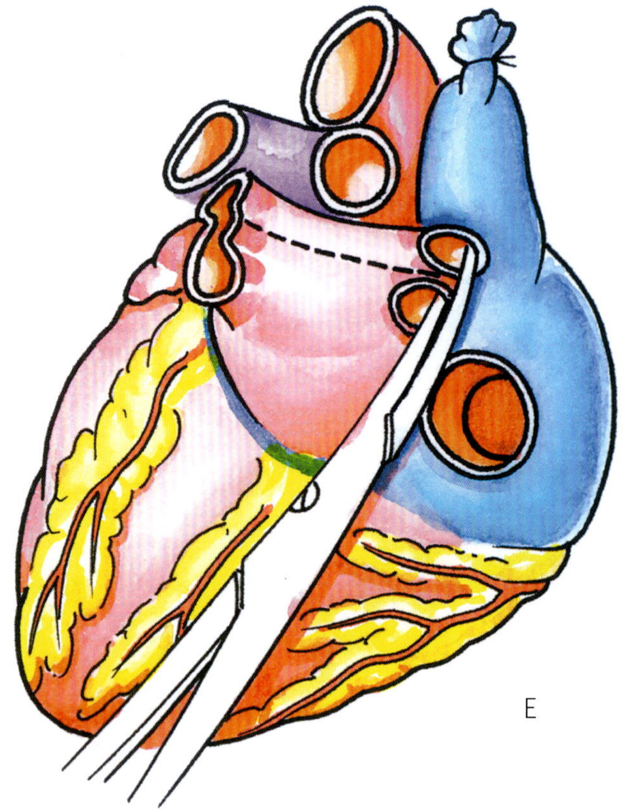

E. 分别纵行剪通供心左、右肺静脉上、下分支。然后横行剪开左心房后壁。供心处理完成。

E. The upper and lower branches of the left and right pulmonary veins are longitudinally cut through. The left atrial posterior wall is then transversely cut. The donor heart treatment is complete.

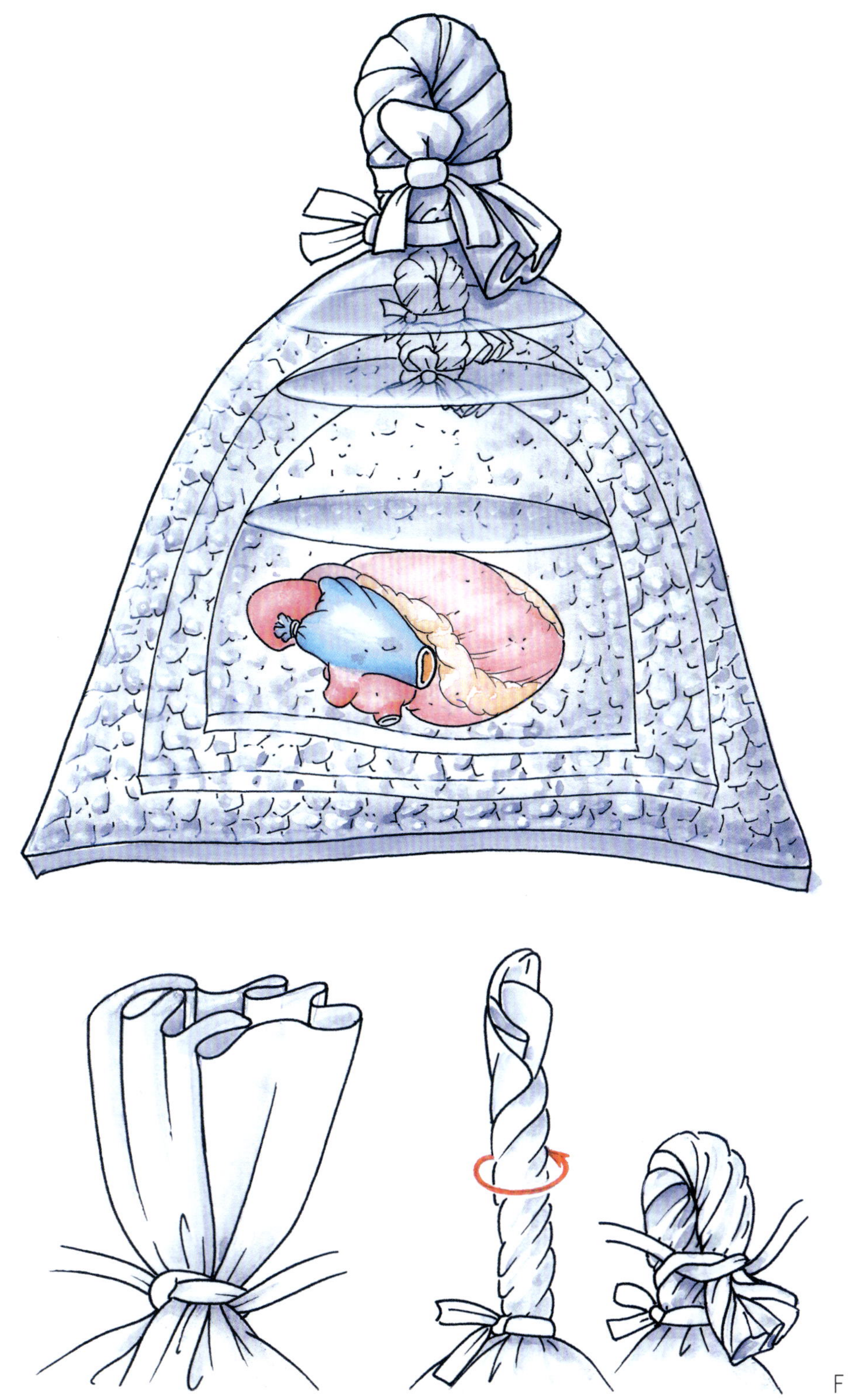

F. 将供心置入装有心肌保护液的无菌塑料袋内。外面再套两层装有冰块和心肌保护液的无菌塑料袋。每个塑料袋口均要妥善扎紧。

F. Place the donor heart in a sterile plastic bag filled with cardioplegic solution. Put another two layers of sterile plastic bags filled with ice cubes and cardioplegic solution on the outside. Fasten each plastic bag properly.

图 7-1-2　双心房移植法
Figure 7-1-2　Biatrial technique

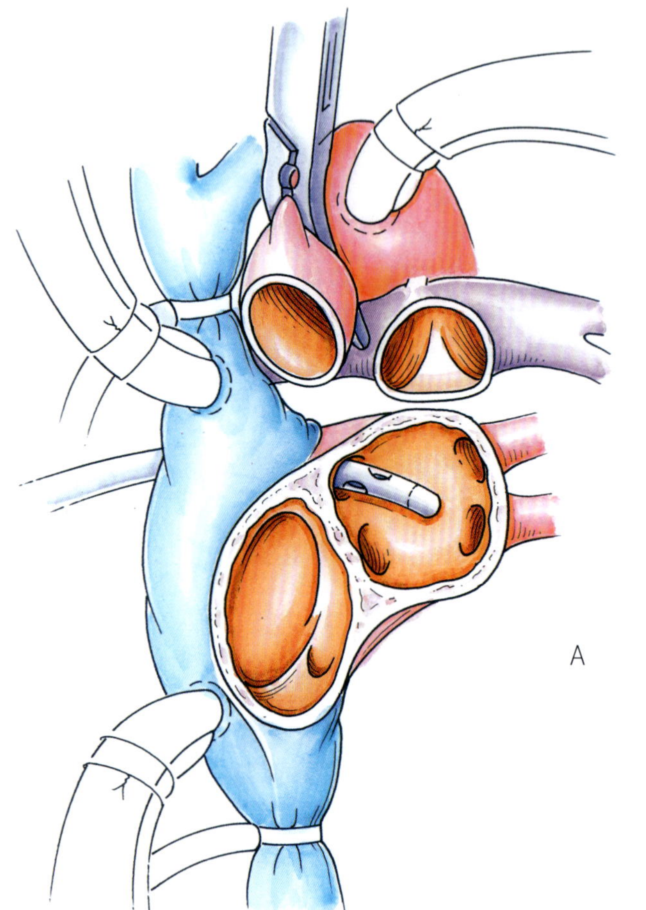

A. 受者升主动脉远端插供血管，上、下腔静脉分别插静脉引流管，右上肺静脉插左心减压管，建立体外循环。收紧上、下腔静脉束带，阻断主动脉。以先右心房、后左心房顺序，沿房室沟将心房、心室完全切断。靠近半月瓣切断主动脉和肺动脉。取出病心。

A. A arterial cannulation is inserted into the distal aspect of the recipient's ascending aorta, venous cannulas into the superior and inferior vena cava respectively, and a left cardiac venting catheter into the right superior pulmonary vein to establish extracorporeal circulation. Tighten the upper and inferior vena cava bands, and clamp the aorta. The connection between the atrium and the ventricle is completely cut off along the atrioventricular groove in the order of the right atrium first and then the left atrium. The aorta and the pulmonary artery close to the semilunar valve are cut off. The diseased heart is removed.

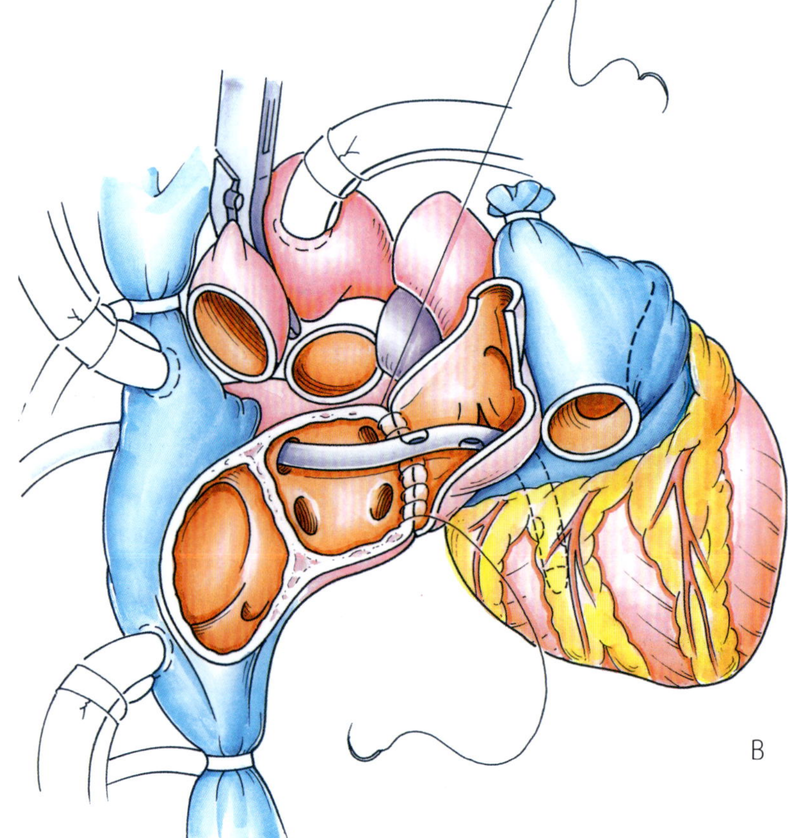

B. 将供心置入心包腔，首先吻合左心房。用双头针从左上肺静脉处开始，缝合到房间隔处 2 针会合结扎。

B. Place the donor heart into the pericardial cavity and anastomose the left atrium first. A double-armed suture starts from the left upper pulmonary vein to the interatrial septum, where the two sutures are ligated together.

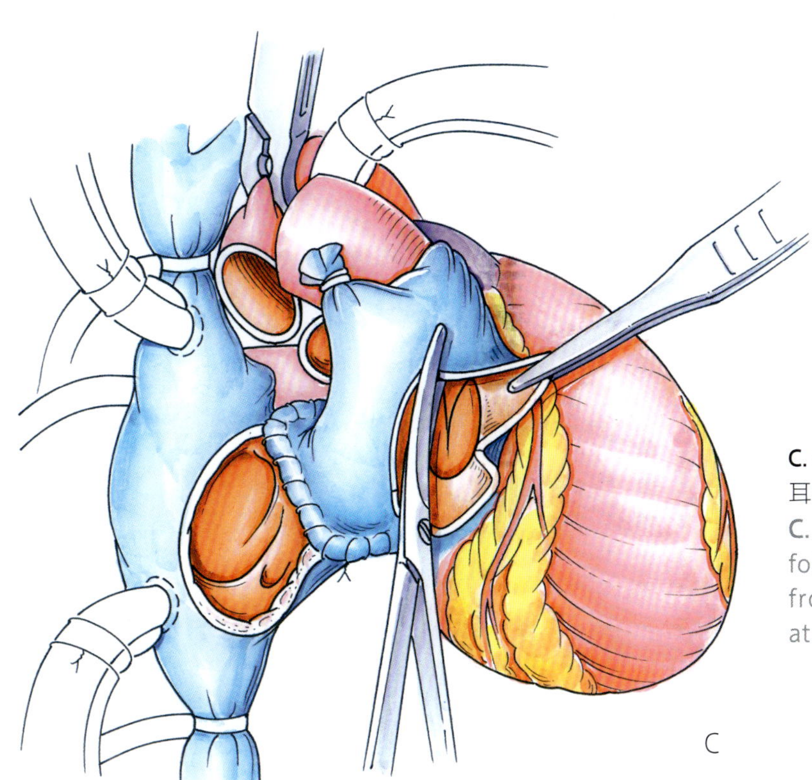

C. 继而吻合右心房。将供心自下腔静脉向右心耳方向切开部分右心房。

C. The anastomosis to the right atrium is followed. Part of the right atrium is incised from the inferior vena cava to the right atrial appendage.

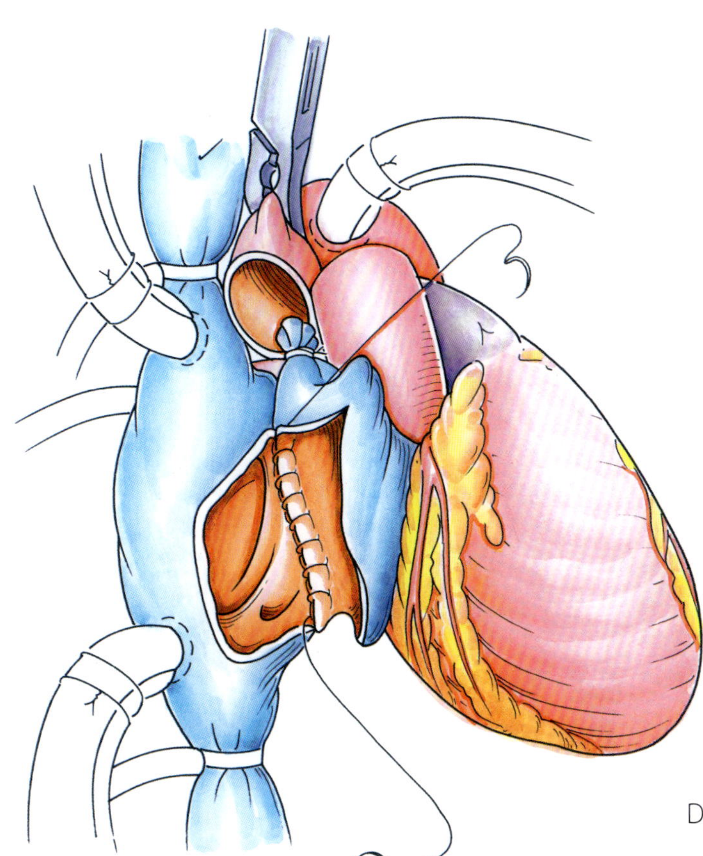

D. 双头针自后壁开始吻合右心房。

D. The right atrium is anastomosed from the posterior wall with a double-armed needle.

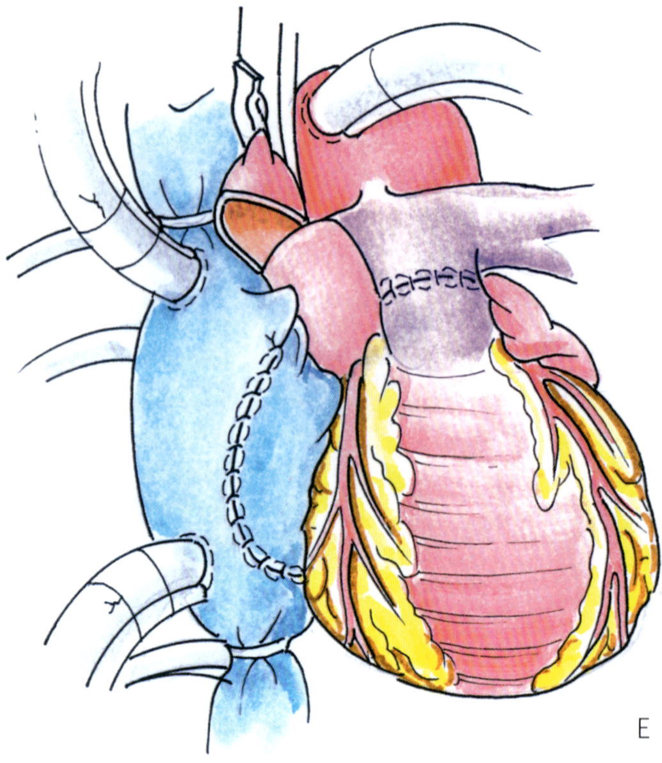

E. 缝合至右心房前壁结扎缝线。吻合肺动脉和主动脉。

E. Suture is proceeded to the right atrial anterior wall and ligated there. Perform the anastomosis of the pulmonary artery and the aorta respectively.

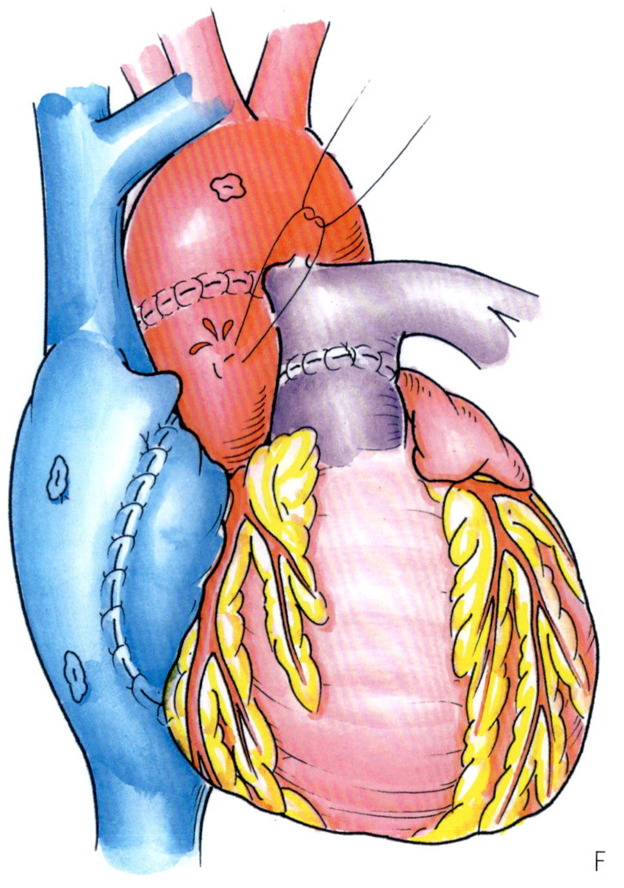

F. 吻合完成，升主动脉戳孔排气，开放循环心脏复跳，撤离体外循环。

F. After the anastomoses are completed, the ascending aorta is punctured to vent, the circulation is initiated, the heart re-beats and the extracorporeal circulation is weaned off.

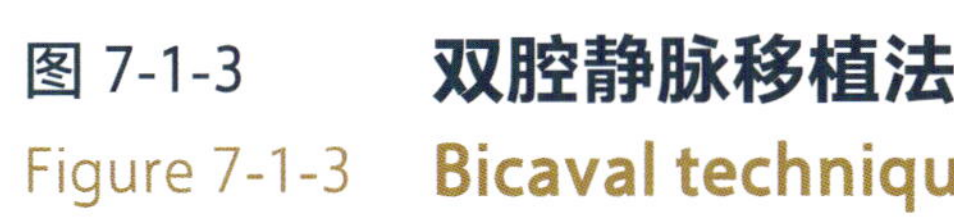

图 7-1-3　**双腔静脉移植法**
Figure 7-1-3　**Bicaval technique**

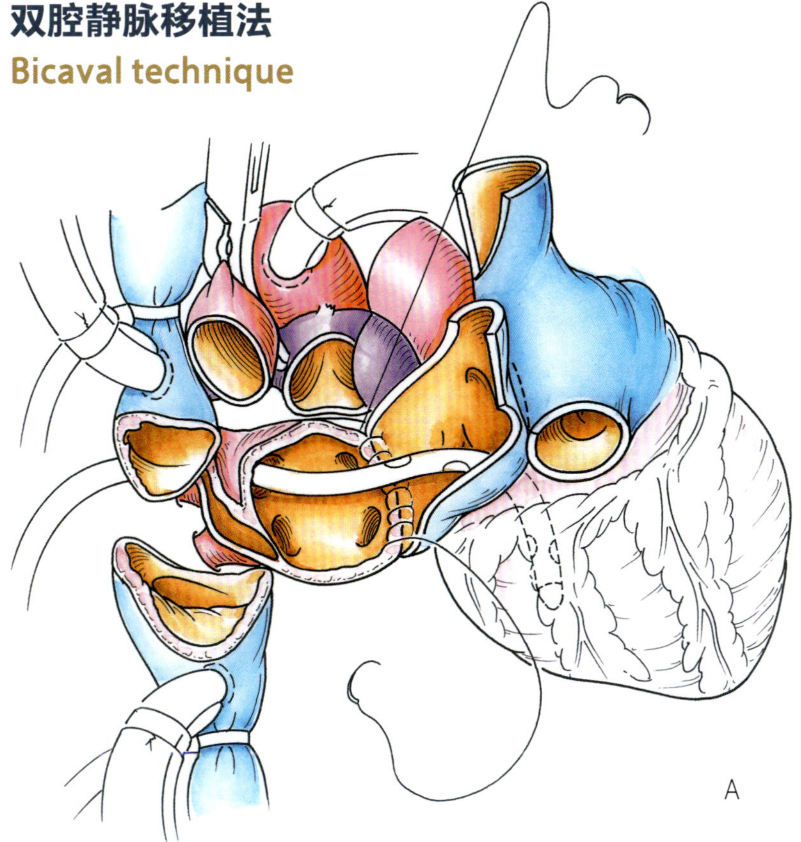

A. 沿房室沟将受者心房、心室完全切断。靠近半月瓣切断主动脉和肺动脉。取出病心。切除右心房壁，上、下腔静脉近心端均保留约 2cm 右心房壁以方便吻合。左心房吻合与双心房移植法相同。供心的上、下腔静脉剪开至右心房，以匹配受者相应吻合口的口径。

A. The recipient atria and ventricles are completely severed along the atrioventricular groove. The aorta and the pulmonary artery close to the semilunar valve are severed. Remove the diseased heart. The right atrium wall is excised, with about 2 cm of the right atrium wall left at the superior and inferior vena cava near the heart to facilitate anastomosis. The left atrium is anastomosed using the biatrial technique. The upper and inferior vena cava of the donor heart is cut to the right atrium to match the anastomotic diameter of the recipient.

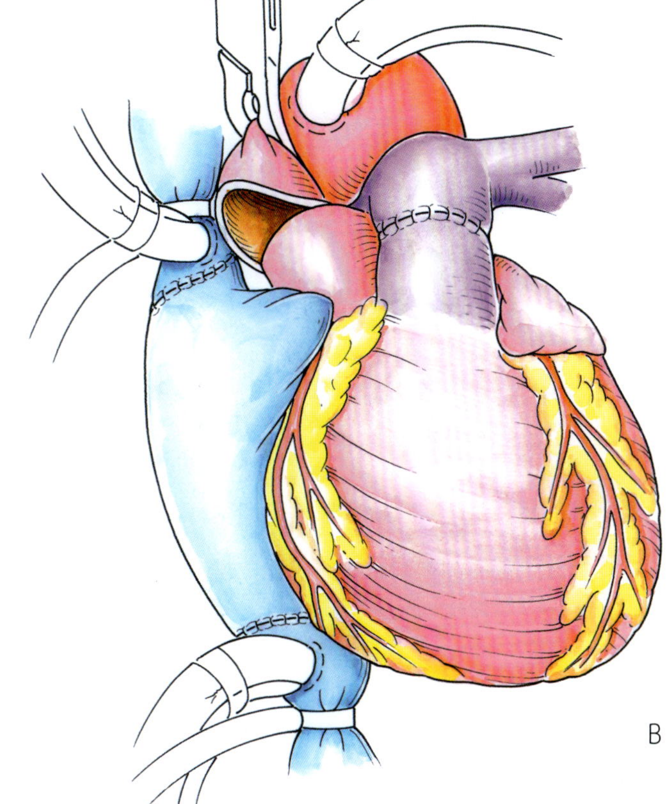

B. 继而按下腔静脉、上腔静脉、肺动脉和主动脉的顺序逐一吻合。

B. The inferior vena cava, the superior vena cava, the pulmonary artery, and the aorta are anastomosed in sequence.

第 二 节　心肺移植

Section 2　Heart-Lung Transplantation

图 7-2-1　获取供者心肺

Figure 7-2-1　Donor operation for heart-lung transplantation

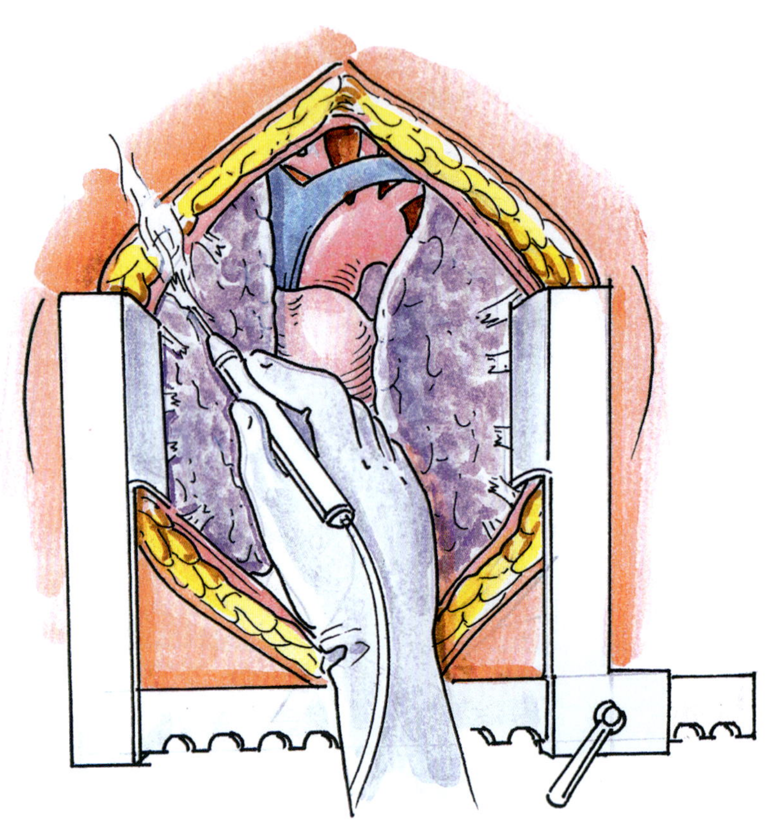

A. 供者胸骨正中切口，切除胸腺组织，切开两侧纵隔胸膜和心包，分离胸膜腔和心包腔粘连，切断下肺韧带。

A. A median sternotomy in the donor is performed to excise the thymus tissue and cut open the bilateral mediastinal pleura and the pericardium. Separate the pleural cavity and the pericardial cavity adhesions and sever the lower lung ligament.

A

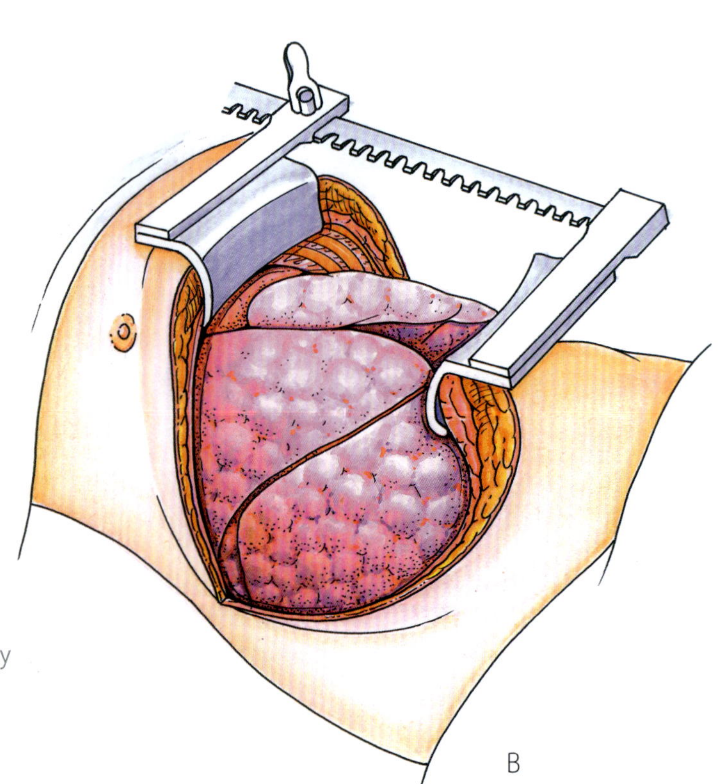

B. 亦可采用双侧胸部横断切口。

B. Bilateral thoracic transverse incisions may also be taken alternatively.

B

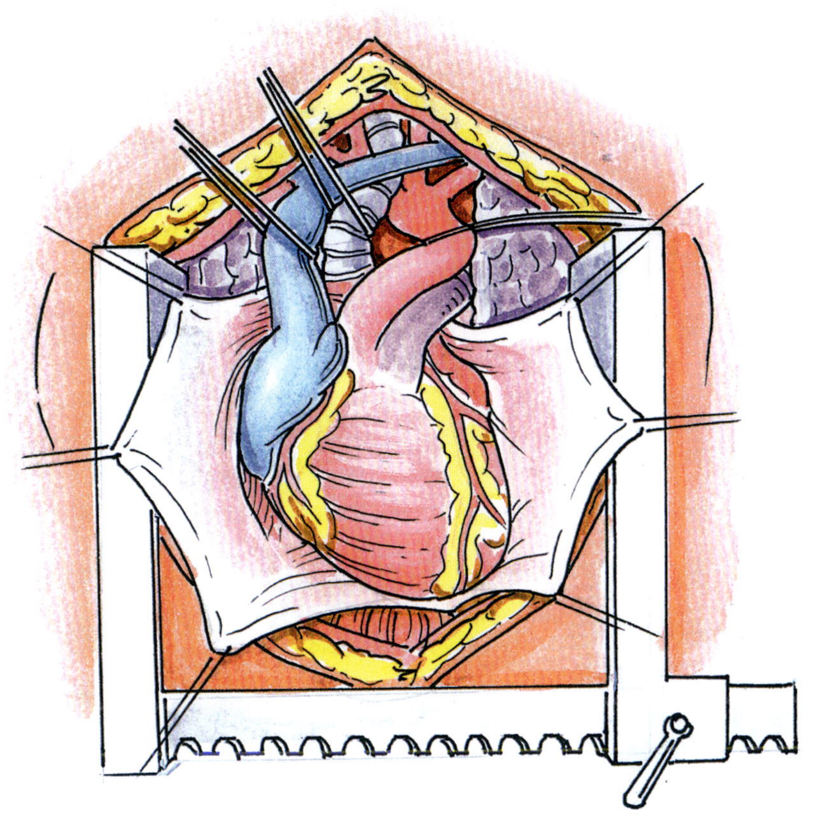
C

C. 游离上、下腔静脉。在升主动脉和上腔静脉间纵行切开心包，游离气管。

C. Dissociate superior and inferior vena cava. A longitudinal pericardiotomy is performed between the ascending aorta and the superior vena cava to dissociate the trachea.

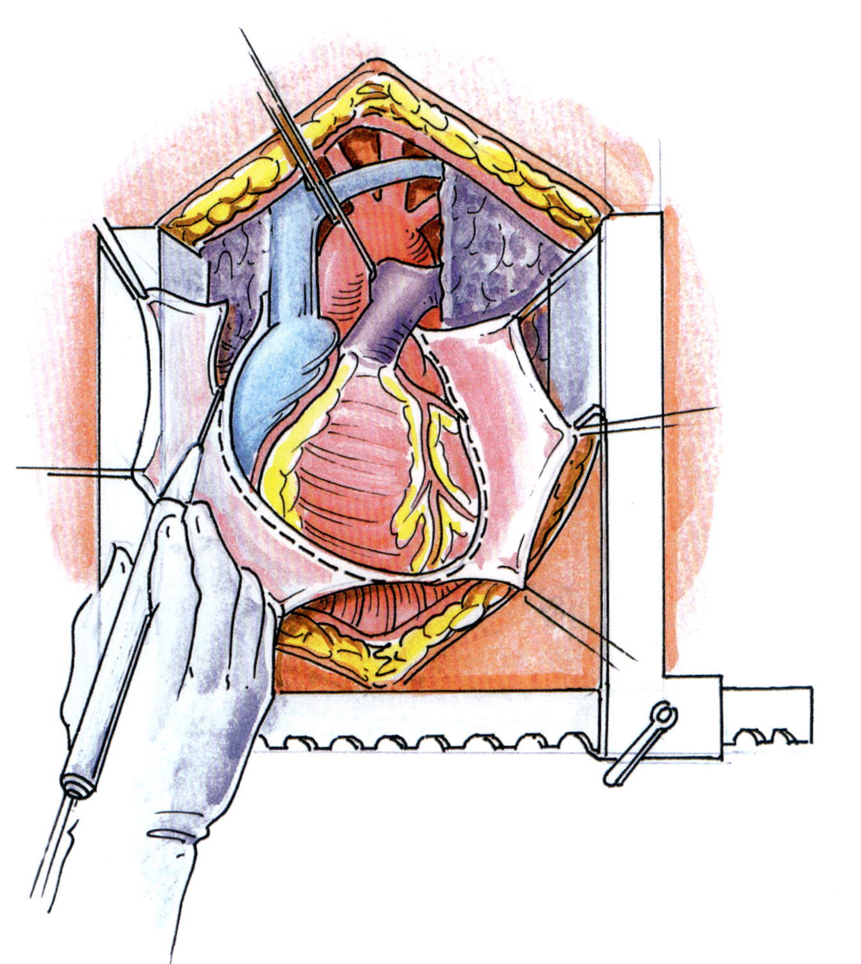
D

D. 切除心包。

D. Pericardiectomy.

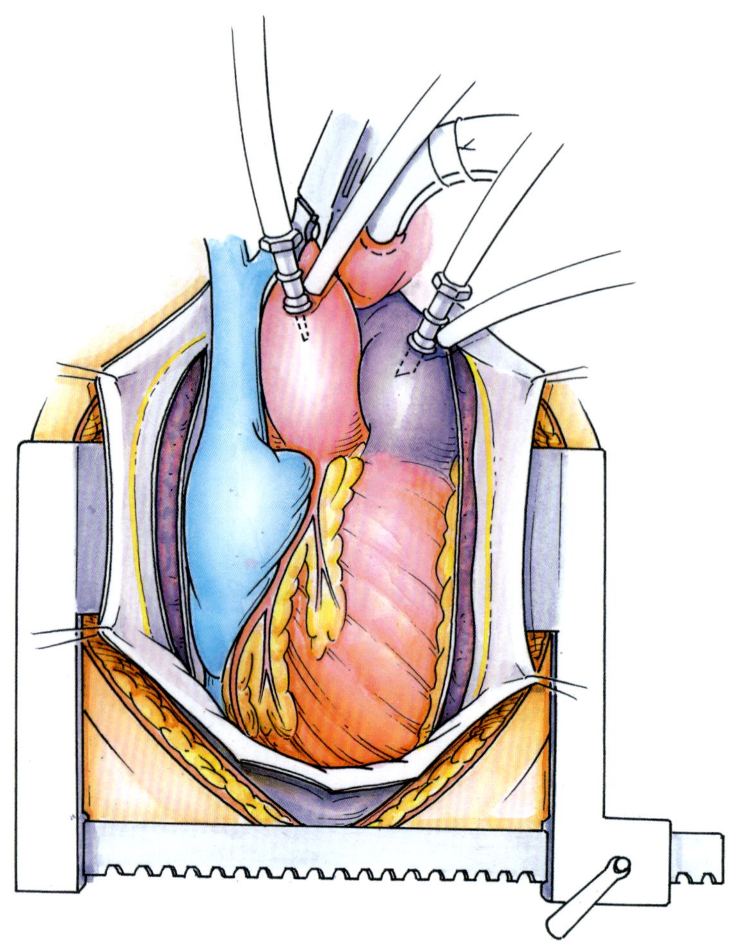

E. 升主动脉和肺动脉分别插保护液灌注管。升主动脉远端钳夹阻断，阻断钳远端切断主动脉。上腔静脉结扎后切断。下腔静脉在贴近膈肌处切断。气管在靠近环状软骨处切断。分别灌注心、肺保护液。

E. The ascending aorta and the pulmonary artery are inserted with a preservation solution perfusion tube, respectively. The ascending aorta at the distal end is blocked with the blocking clamp. The aorta is severed distal to the blocking clamp. The superior vena cava is ligated and severed. The inferior vena cava is severed close to the diaphragm. The trachea is severed near the cricoid cartilage. The cardioplegic solution is perfused into the heart and lung, respectively.

E

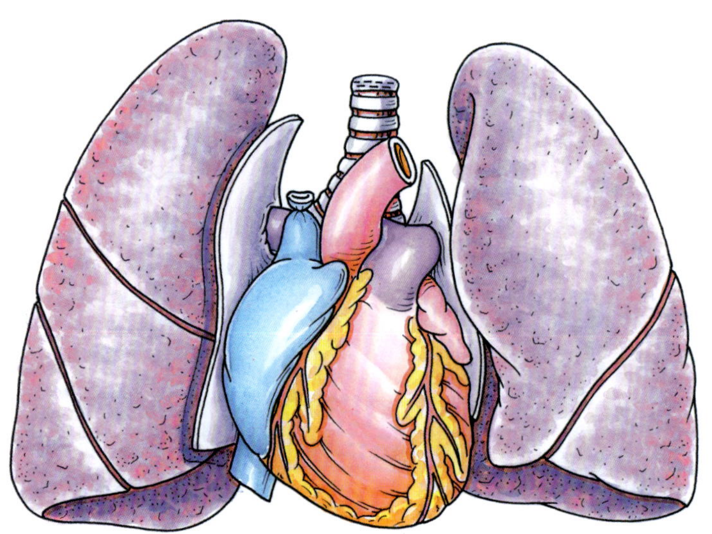

F. 供者心肺完整取出。

F. The donor heart and lung are taken out intact.

F

图 7-2-2　病心切除
Figure 7-2-2　Excision of diseased heart

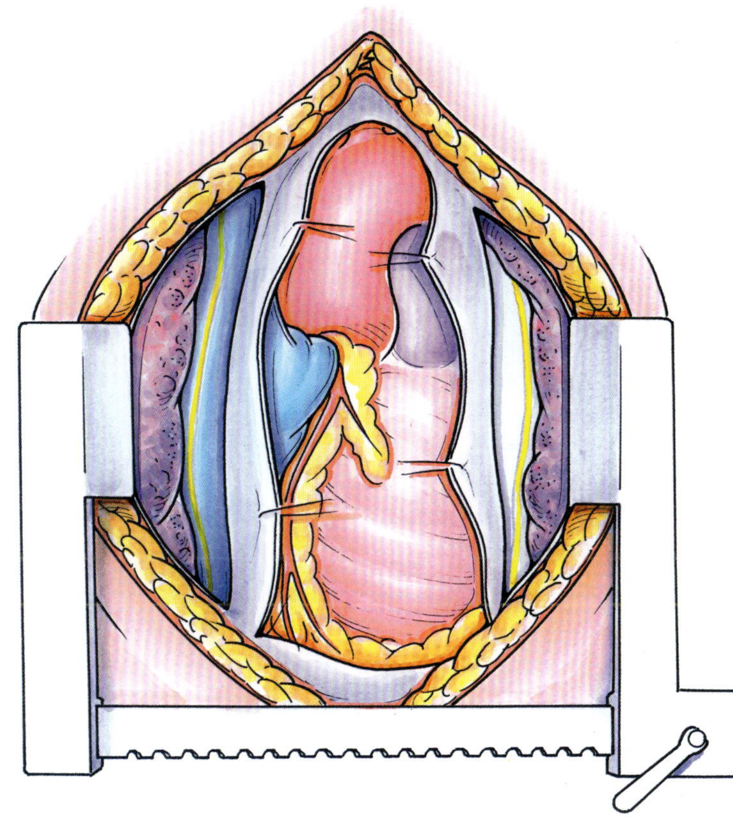

A. 受者胸骨正中切口，分离心包腔内粘连。
A. A median sternotomy is performed in the recipient to separate intrapericardial adhesions.

A

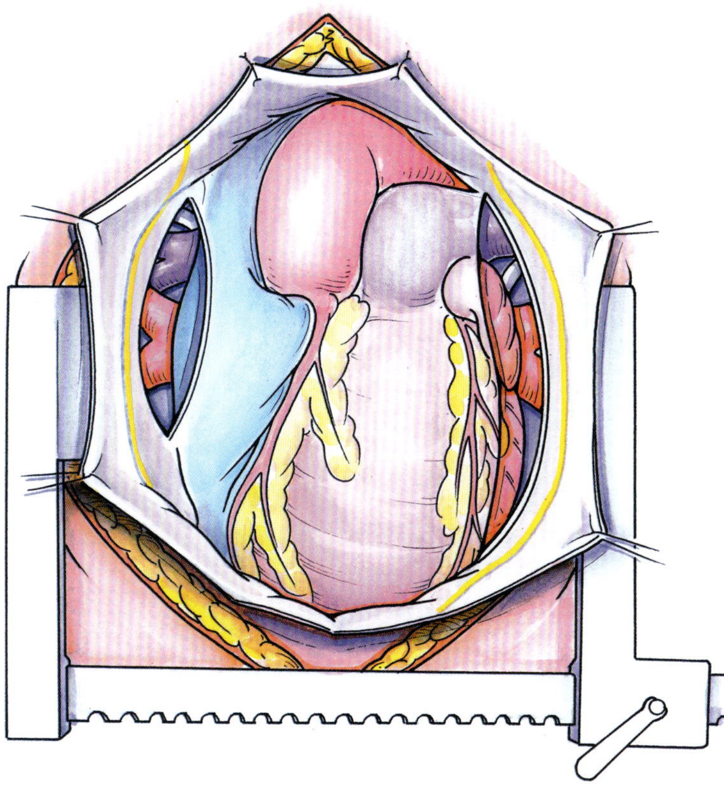

B. 心包内膈神经后方 1~2cm 纵行切开两侧纵隔胸膜。
B. The bilateral mediastinal pleura is longitudinally incised 1-2 cm posterior to the phrenic nerve in the pericardium.

B

C. 切除膈神经前面的心包。按双腔静脉移植法切除心脏，左心房后壁纵行剪开，将左、右肺静脉向两侧分离。两侧膈神经索带状保留。

C. The pericardium anterior to the phrenic nerve is excised. The heart is excised using the bicaval technique, the posterior wall of the left atrium is longitudinally cut, and the left and right pulmonary veins are separated to both sides. The bilateral phrenic cords are reserved in a band shape.

C

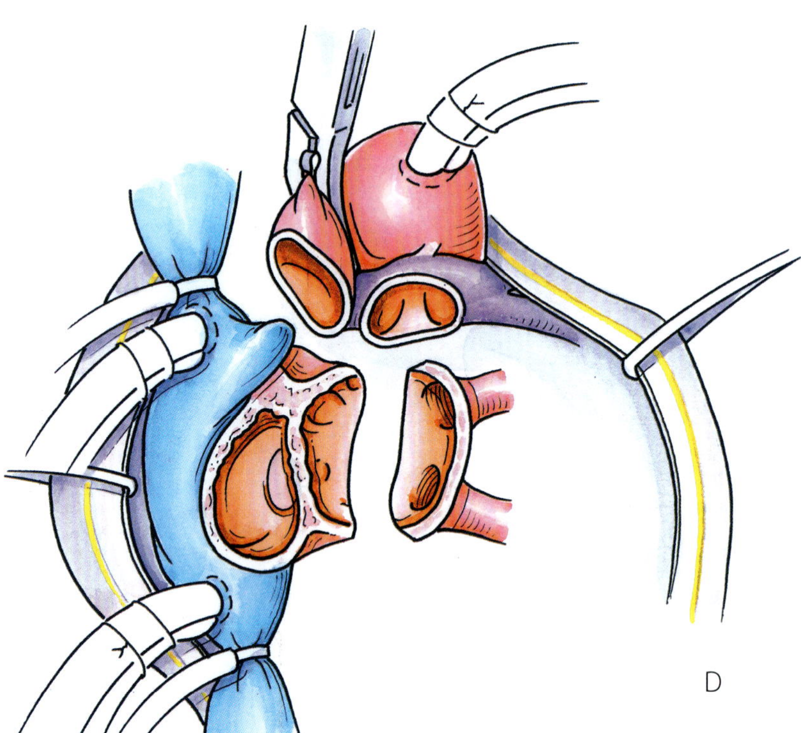

D. 也可按双心房移植法切除心脏，纵行剪开左心房后壁，将左、右肺静脉向两侧分离，两侧膈神经索带状保留。

D. Instead, the heart may be excised by using the biatrial technique, the left atrial posterior wall is longitudinally cut, the left and right pulmonary veins are separated to both sides, and the bilateral phrenic cords are reserved in a band shape.

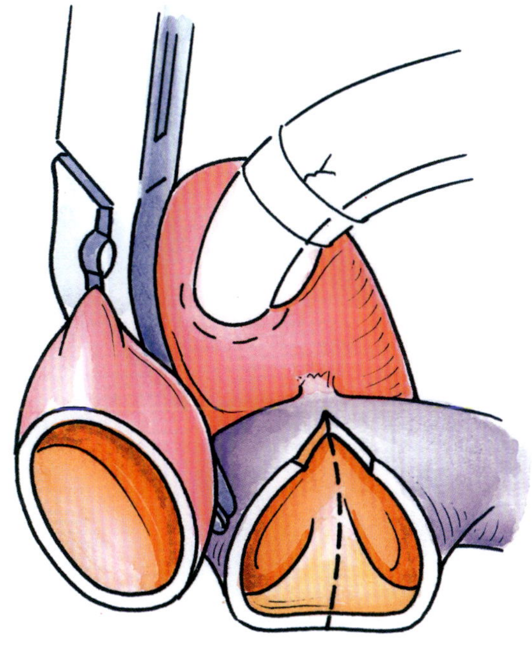

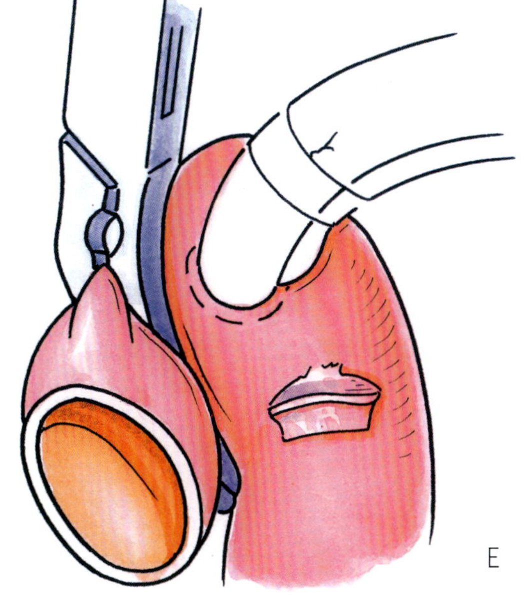

E. 剪除残存的肺动脉，动脉韧带处的肺动脉壁予以保留，以免损伤喉返神经。

E. The residual pulmonary artery is excised with the pulmonary artery wall at the arterial ligament left intact to avoid damaging the recurrent laryngeal nerve.

图 7-2-3　病肺切除
Figure 7-2-3　Excision of diseased lung

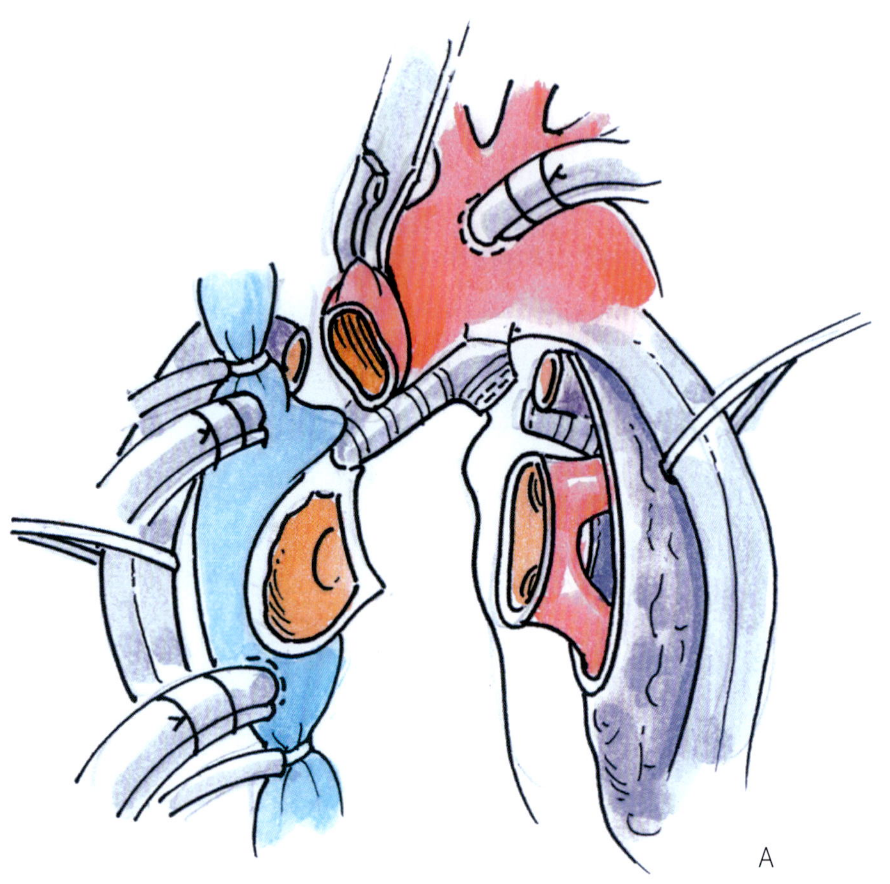

A. 切断左下肺韧带。游离肺门，显露左肺动脉予以切断，结扎支气管动脉，切断缝合左支气管。

A. The left inferior pulmonary ligament is severed. The hilum is dissociated to expose the left pulmonary artery to be severed. The bronchial artery is ligated. The left bronchus is severed and sutured.

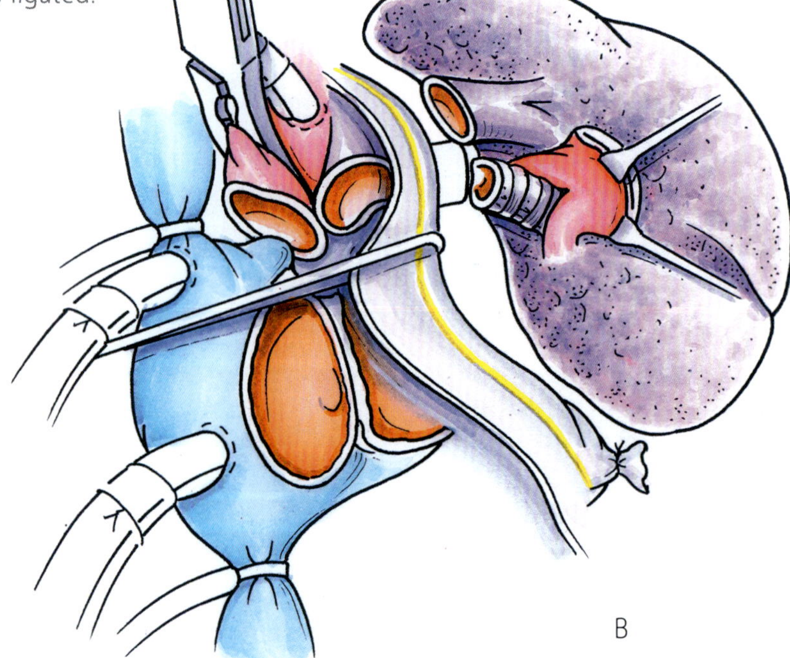

B. 取出左肺。

B. The left lung is taken out.

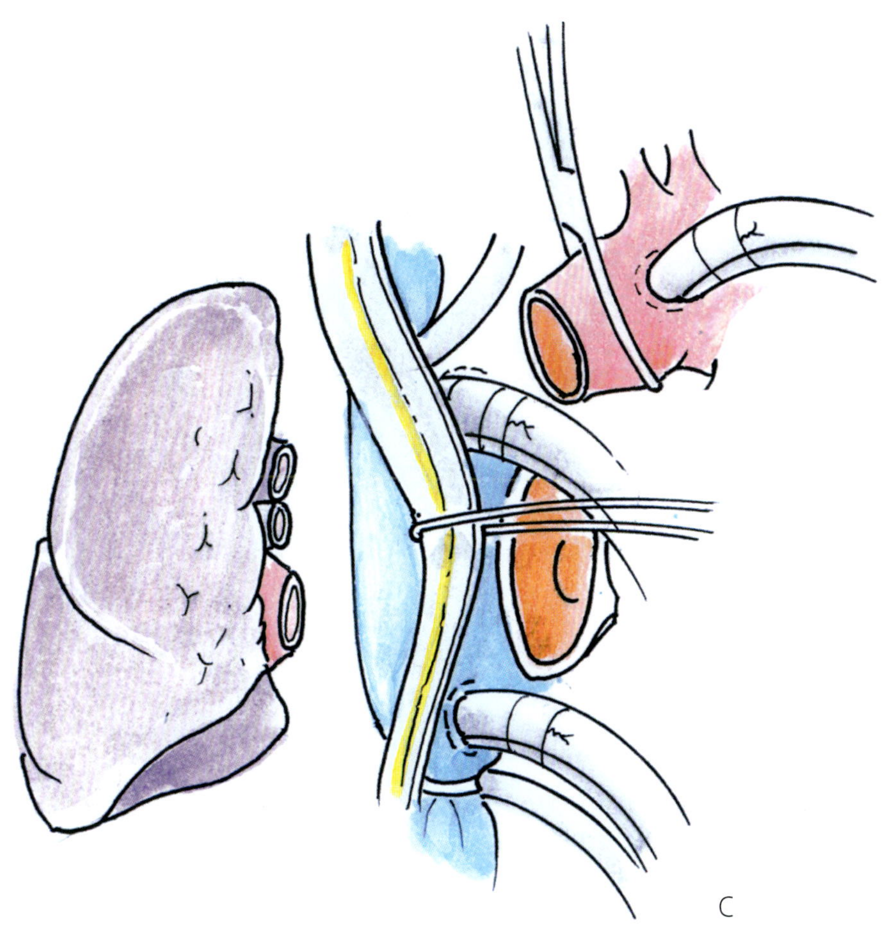

C. 同样方法切除右肺。

C. The right lung is resected similarly.

图 7-2-4　心肺移植

Figure 7-2-4　Heart-lung transplantation

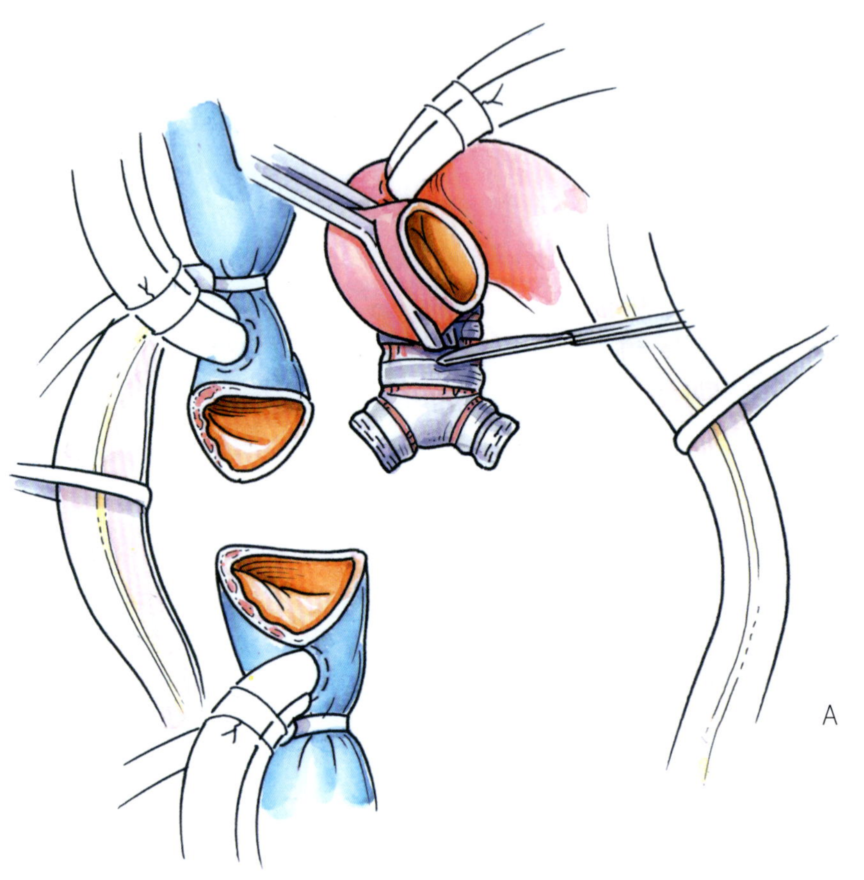

A. 隆突上方横行切断气管。

A. Transect the trachea above the carina.

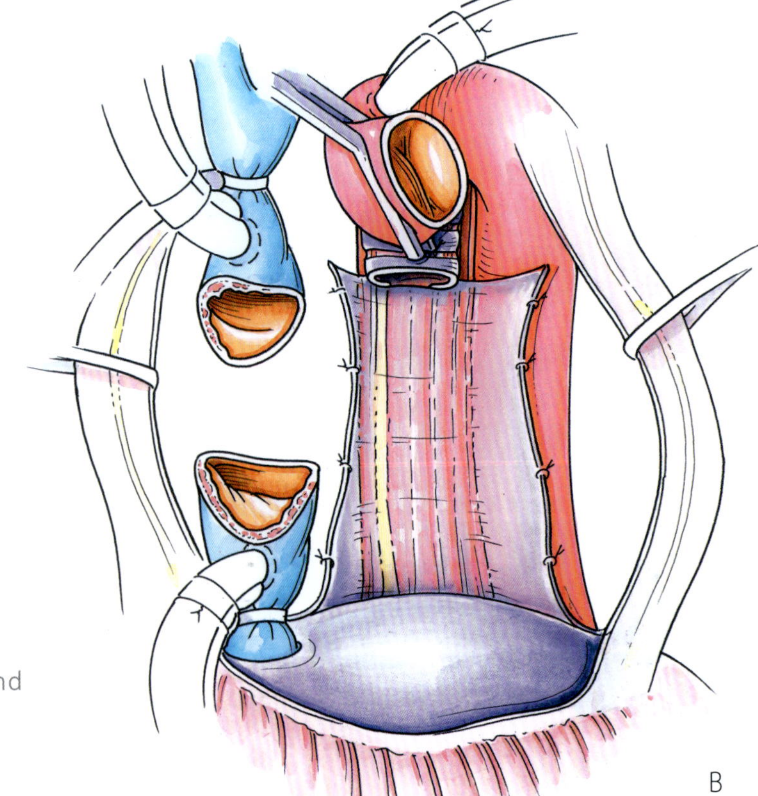

B. 膈神经和心脏后方的迷走神经均保护完好。

B. The phrenic nerve and vagus nerve behind heart are well protected.

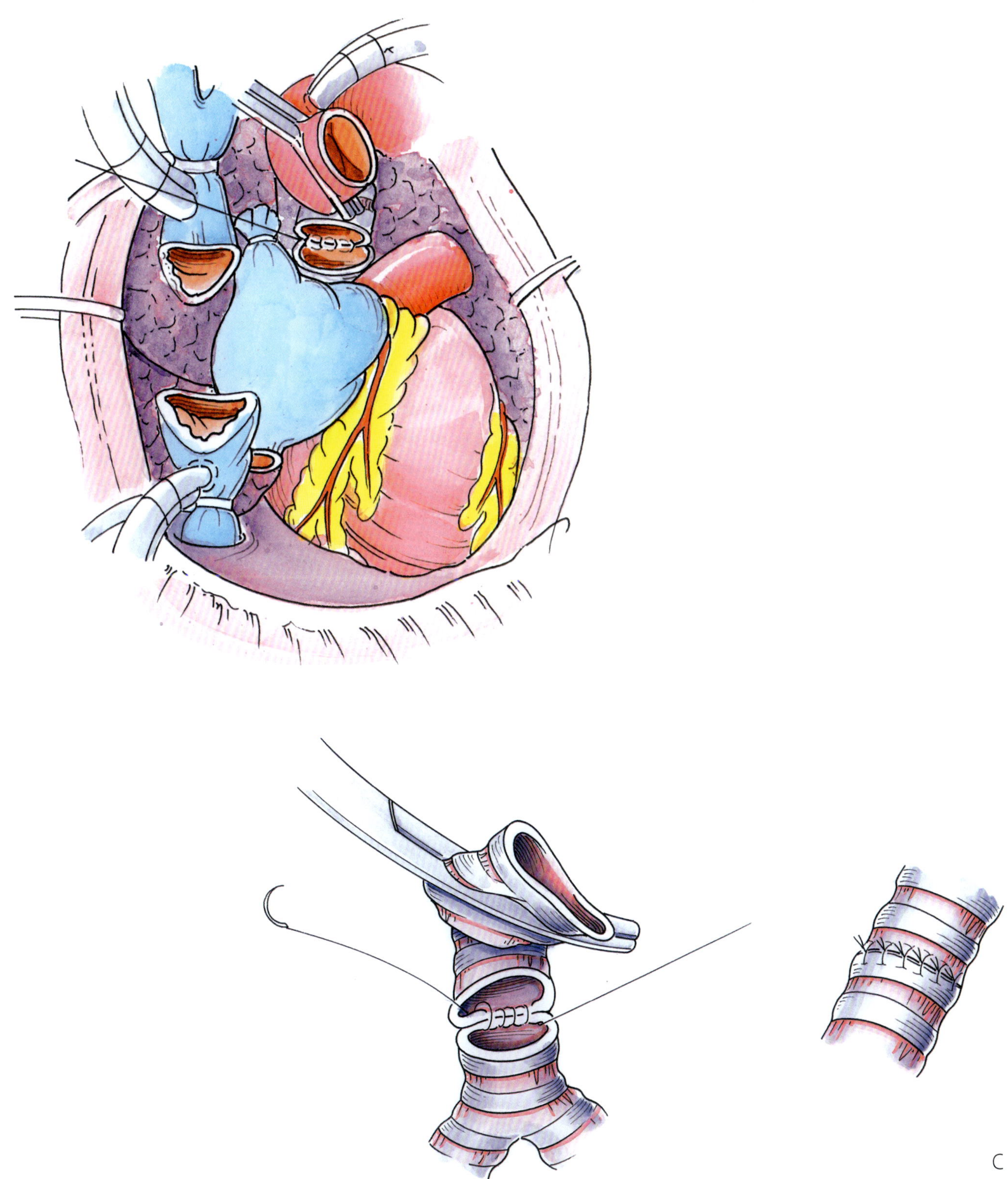

C. 将供者心肺置入。先端端吻合气管，从后壁开始缝，缝到前壁后打结，术野注入生理盐水检查气管吻合口，如有漏气予以缝合修补。

C. The donor heart and lung are placed. An end-to-end anastomosis is performed on the trachea, which is sutured from the posterior wall to the anterior wall, and then knotted. Physiological saline is injected into the surgical field to check the trachea anastomosis. If there is any air leakage, the trachea anastomosis is sutured and repaired.

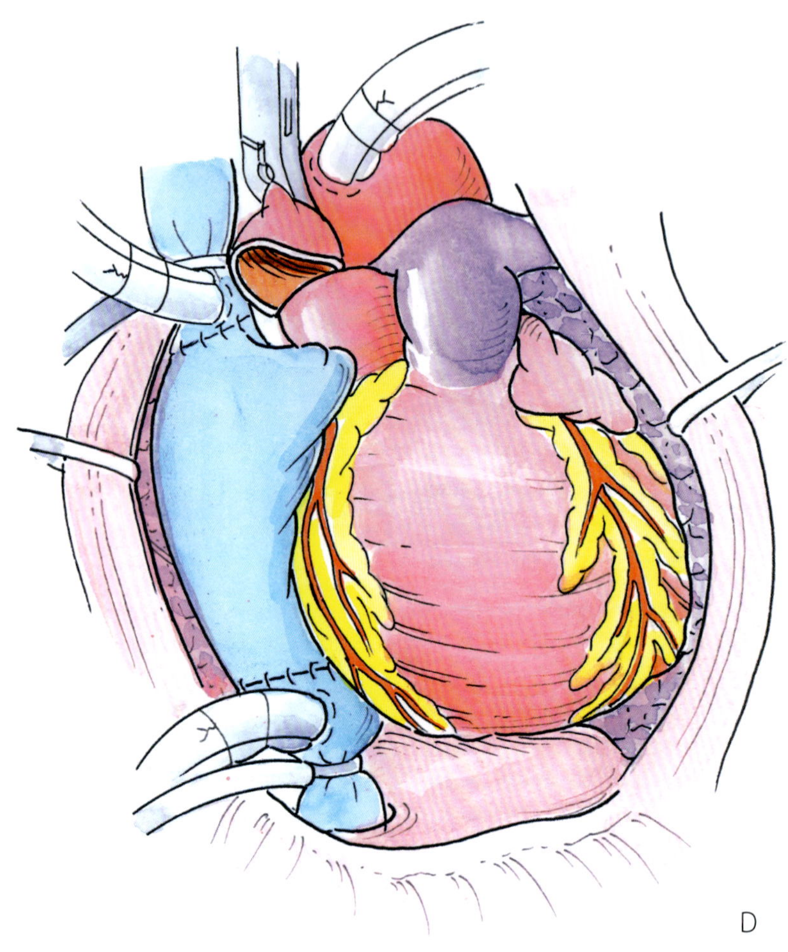

D. 吻合下腔静脉、上腔静脉，最后吻合升主动脉。

D. Anastomosis is performed on the inferior vena cava, the superior vena cava, and finally, the ascending aorta.

第三节 肺移植
Section 3 Lung Transplantation

图 7-3-1 肺移植切口
Figure 7-3-1 Incision for lung transplantation

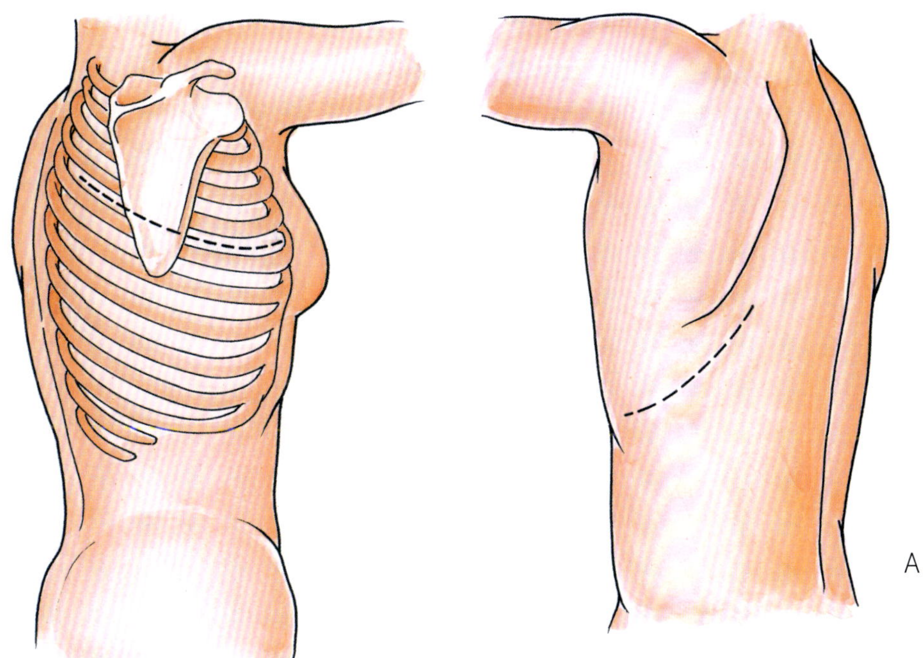

A. 胸部后外侧切口，适用于单肺移植。
A. Posterior lateral thoracotomy is indicated for single-lung transplantation.

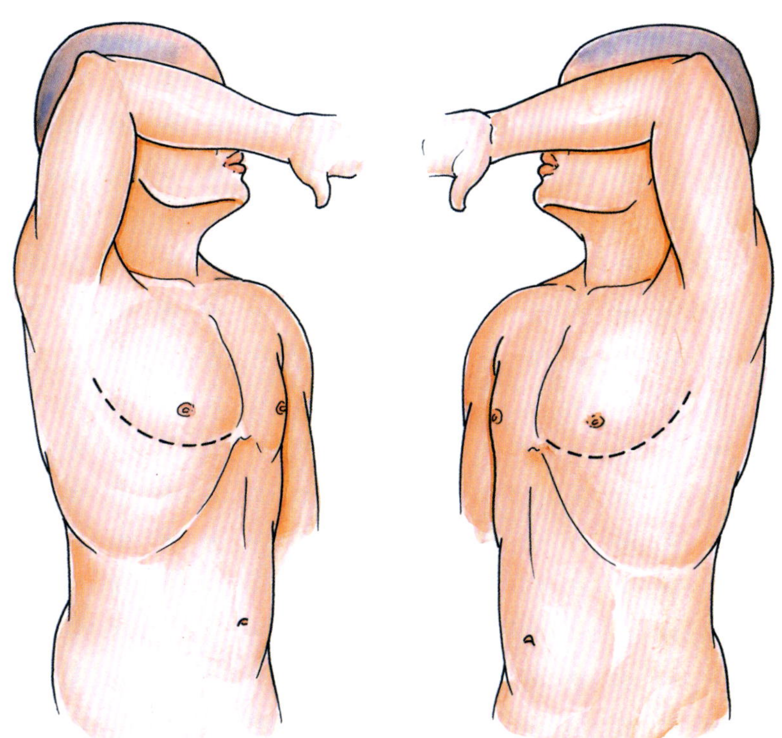

B

B. 胸部前外侧切口，适用于单肺移植。
B. Anterolateral thoracotomy is indicated for single-lung transplantation.

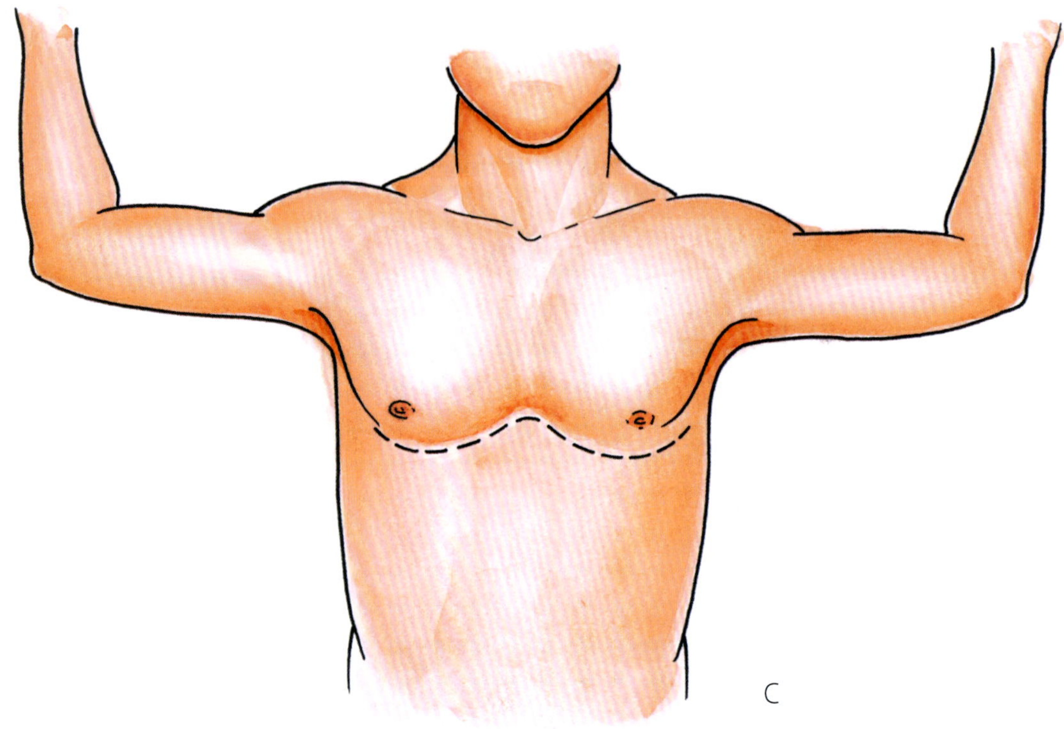

C. 双侧胸部横断切口，适用于双肺移植。
C. Bilateral transverse thoracotomy is indicated for bilateral lung transplantation.

图 7-3-2 气管插管
Figure 7-3-2 Tracheal intubation

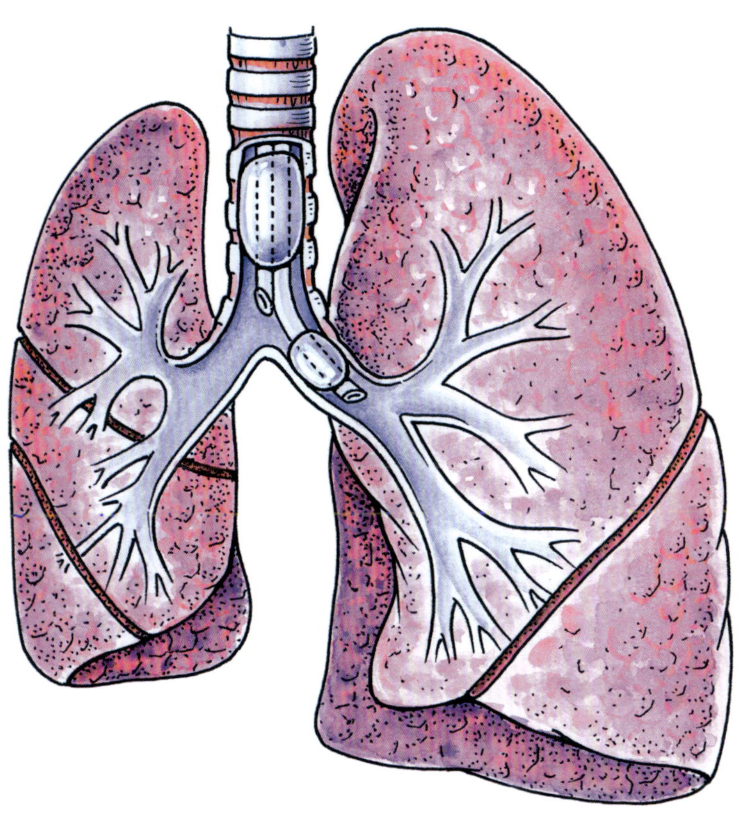

肺移植气管插管要用双腔管，以便术中单肺通气和良好的肺隔离。
Bicaval cannula is applied for lung transplantation to facilitate intraoperative single-lung ventilation and desirable lung isolation.

图 7-3-3　供肺准备
Figure 7-3-3　Preparation of donor lung

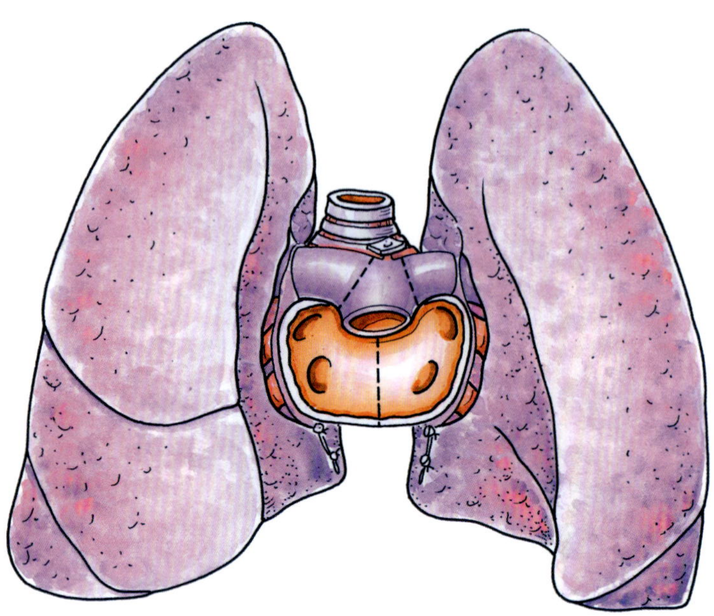

A

A. 供肺送到手术室后要进行裁剪，把左、右肺分开。其原则是肺动脉、肺静脉和支气管尽可能留长一些，以利吻合时进一步修剪。肺动脉在左、右肺动脉近心端剪断。左心房中部纵行剪开，将左、右肺静脉连同附着的左心房壁分开。

A. The donor lung is cut to separate the left and right lungs after being transported to the operating room. The guideline is to keep the pulmonary artery, the pulmonary vein, and the bronchi as long as possible to facilitate further trimming during anastomosis. The left and right pulmonary arteries are severed at the end proximal to the heart. The left and right pulmonary veins, together with the attached left atrial wall, are separated by a longitudinal cutting in the middle of the left atrium.

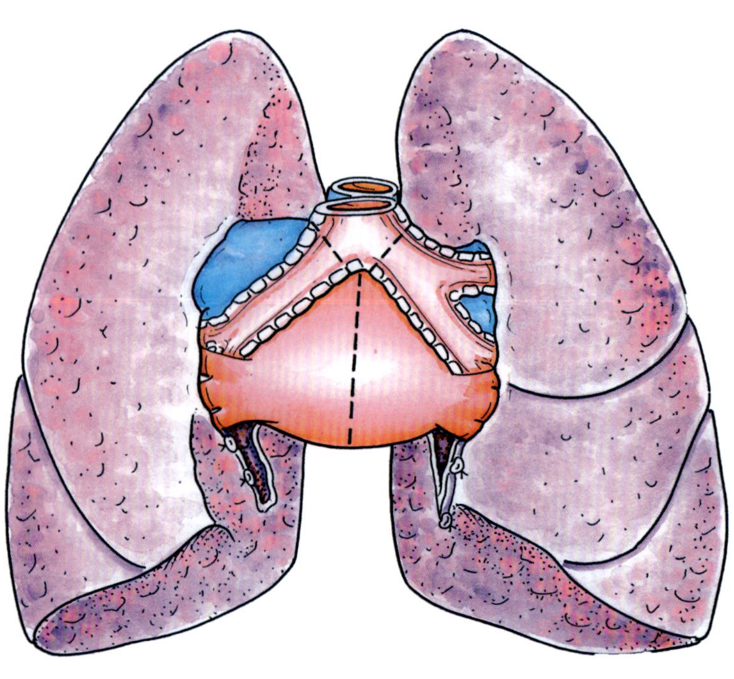

B

B. 左、右支气管在隆突处切断。

B. The left and right bronchi are cut off at the carina.

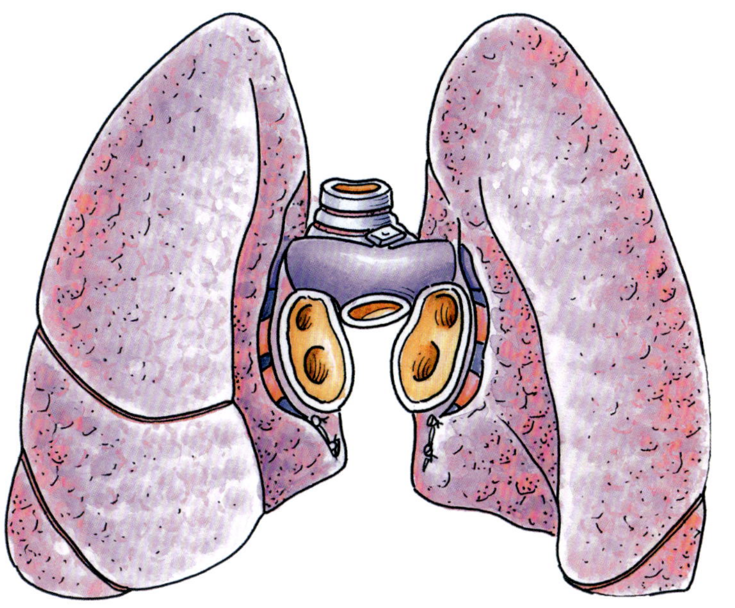

C. 左、右肺静脉分别形成一个带左心房的袖状补片。
C. The left and right pulmonary veins each form a cuff patch with the left atrium.

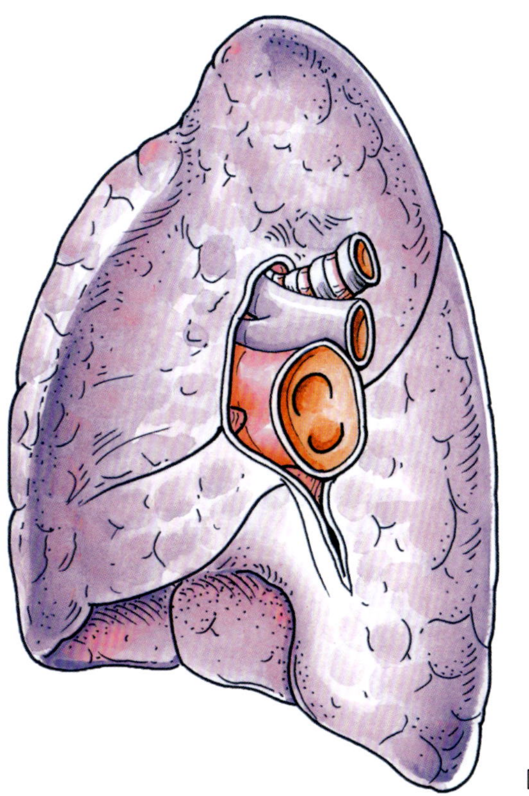

D. 准备完成的右肺。
D. The prepared right lung.

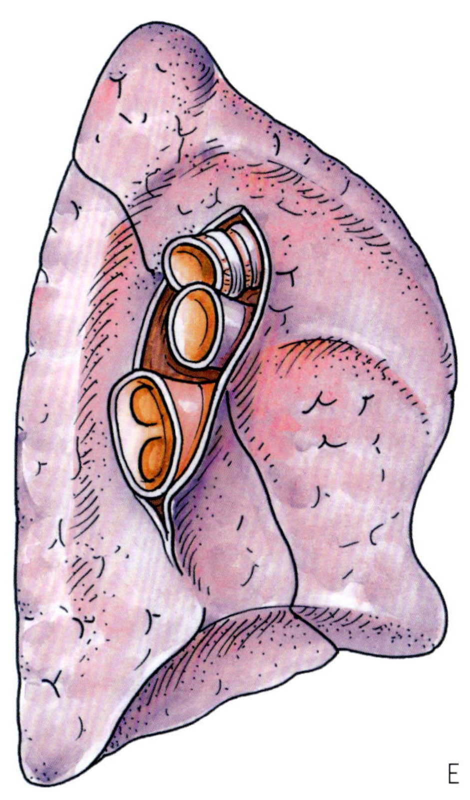

E. 准备完成的左肺。
E. The prepared left lung.

图 7-3-4　右病肺切除
Figure 7-3-4　Excision of right diseased lung

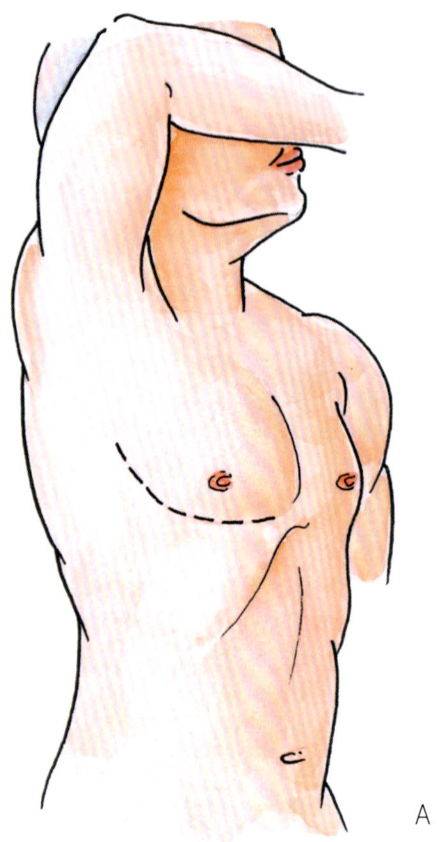

A. 仰卧位，右胸前外侧切口。

A. With the patient in the supine position, a right anterolateral thoracotomy is performed.

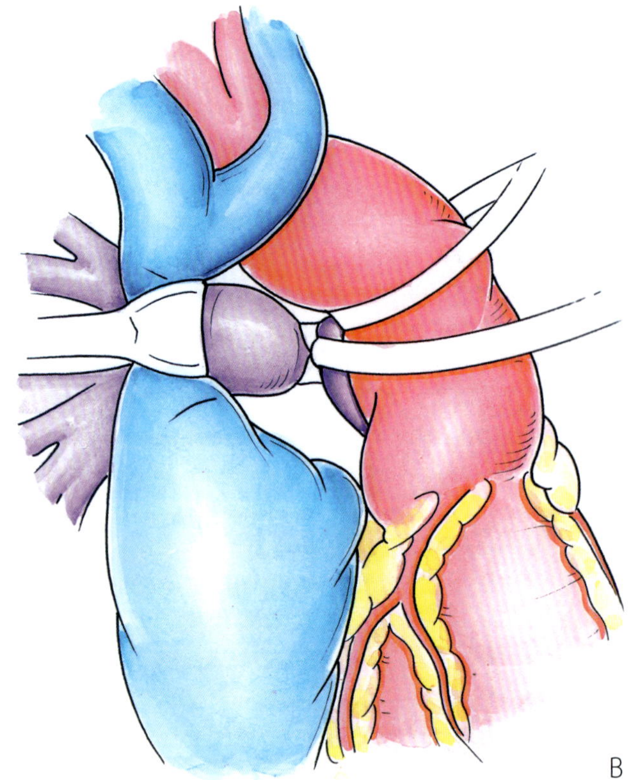

B. 膈神经前纵行切开心包，在上腔静脉和升主动脉之间游离右肺动脉，套纱带阻断右肺动脉。

B. Perform a longitudinal pericardiotomy anterior to the phrenic nerve. Separate the right pulmonary artery between the superior vena cava and the ascending aorta, and block the right pulmonary artery with a gauze band.

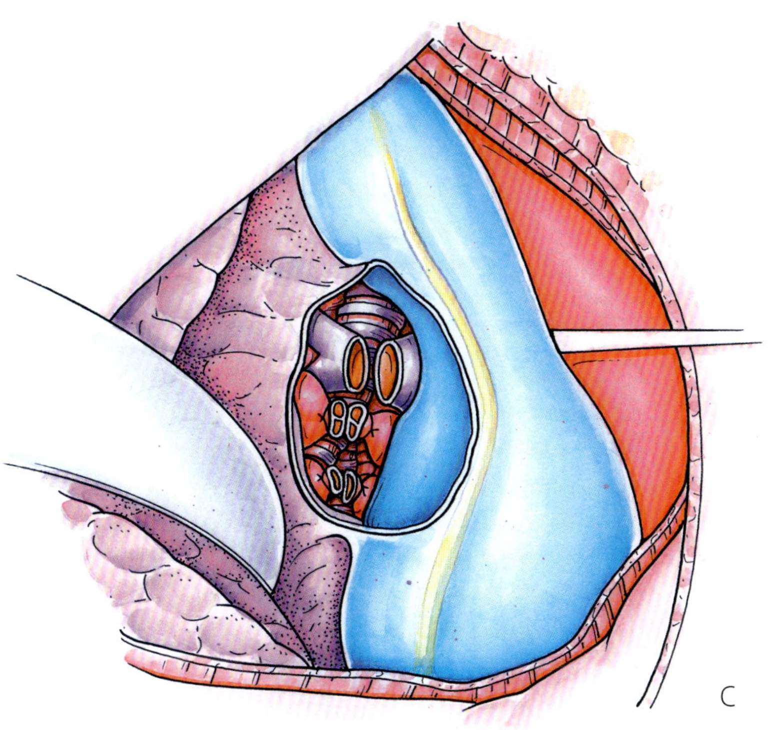

C. 膈神经后切开心包，分离肺门。游离右肺动脉远端并切断。游离右上、下肺静脉，两端结扎后切断。

C. Perform a pericardiotomy posterior to the phrenic nerve to dissociate the hilus. The distal right pulmonary artery is dissociated and severed. The right upper and lower pulmonary veins are dissociated, and both ends are severed after ligation.

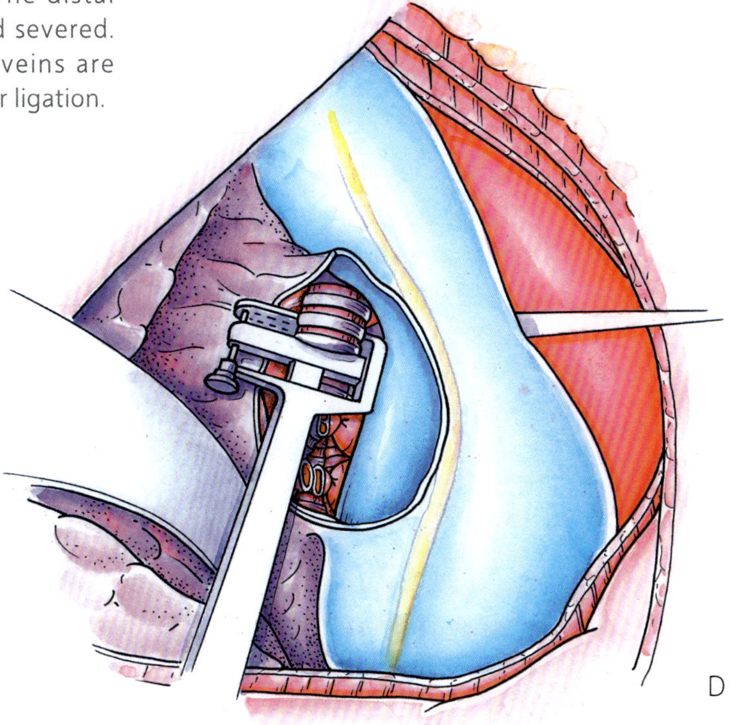

D. 右支气管在发出上叶支气管处切断。取出右肺。

D. The right bronchus is severed at the superior lobar bronchus. Remove the right lung.

图 7-3-5　右肺植入
Figure 7-3-5　Implantation of right lung

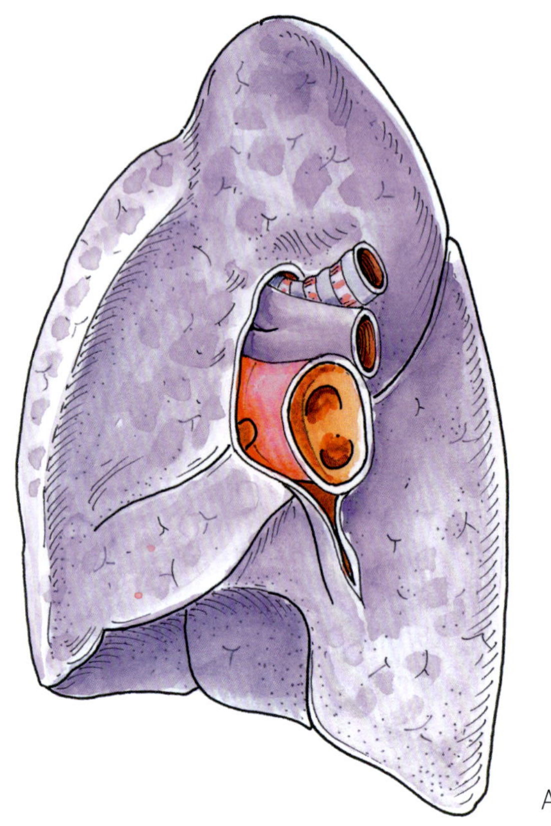

A. 供肺修剪完毕，置入胸腔。

A. The donor lung is trimmed and placed into the thoracic cavity.

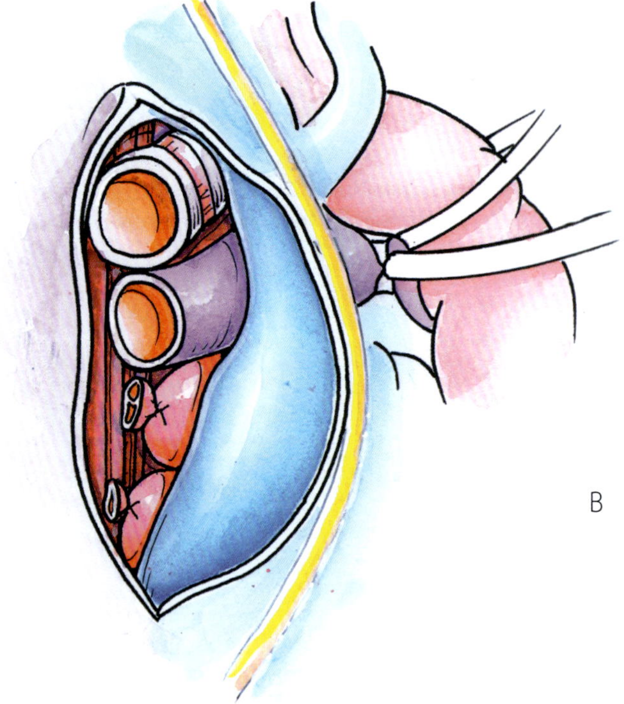

B. 受者肺门，从上到下依次是右支气管、右肺动脉，右上肺静脉和右下肺静脉。

B. The recipient hilus. In the order from top to bottom, they are the right bronchus, the right pulmonary artery, the right superior pulmonary vein, and the right lower pulmonary vein.

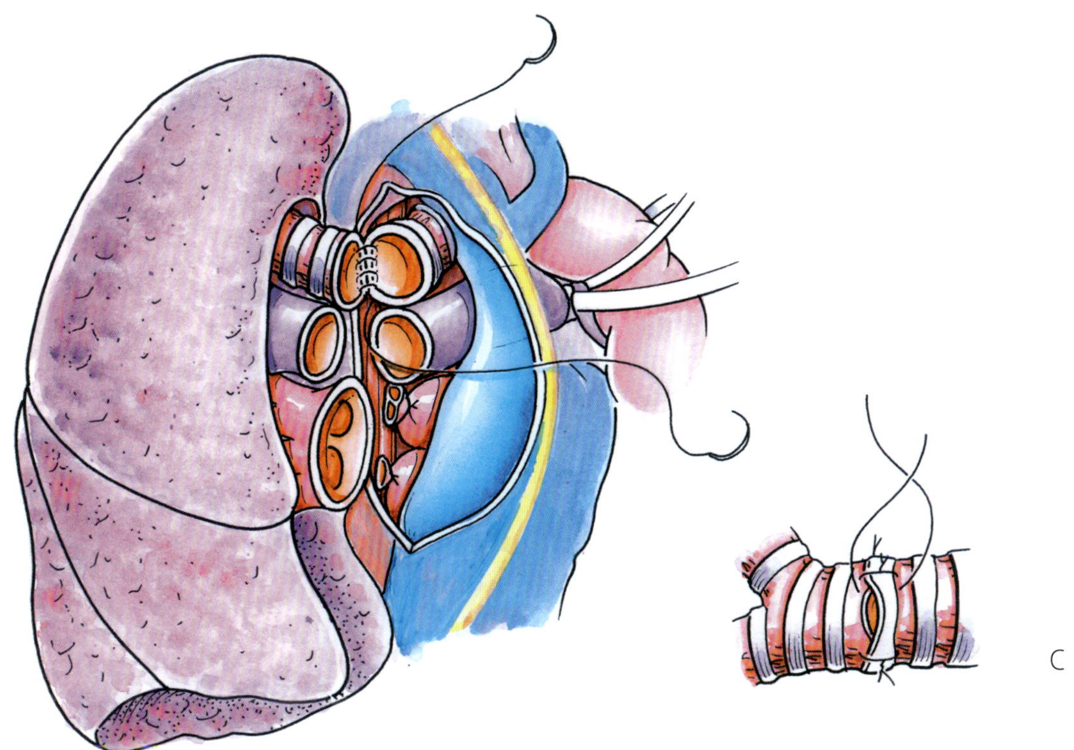

C. 先端端吻合支气管，从后壁缝起，缝到前壁打结。

C. The bronchus is end-to-end anastomosed, starting from the posterior wall to the anterior wall, and knotted.

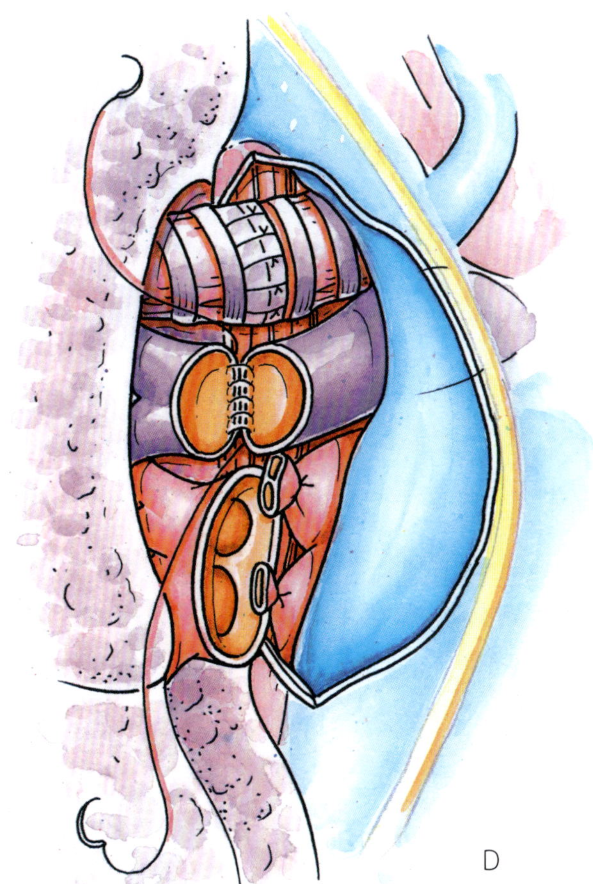

D. 端端吻合右肺动脉。

D. An end-to-end anastomosis is made onto the right pulmonary artery.

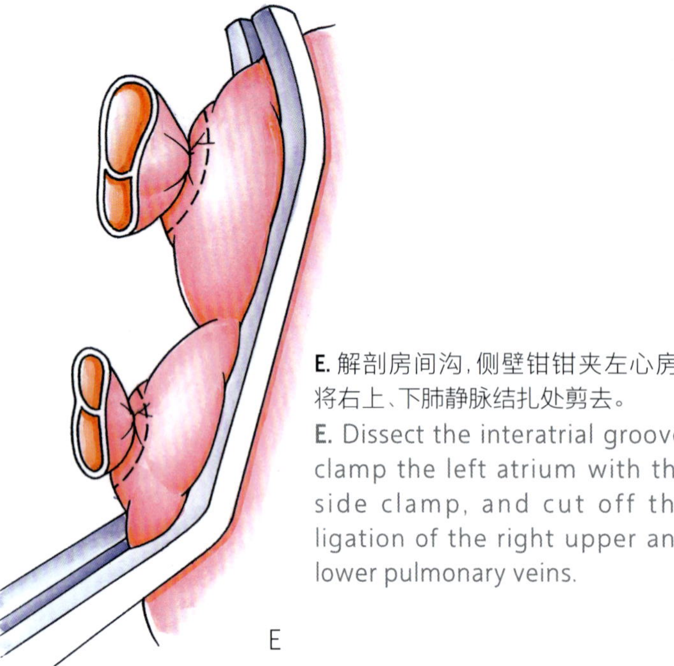

E. 解剖房间沟，侧壁钳钳夹左心房，将右上、下肺静脉结扎处剪去。

E. Dissect the interatrial groove, clamp the left atrium with the side clamp, and cut off the ligation of the right upper and lower pulmonary veins.

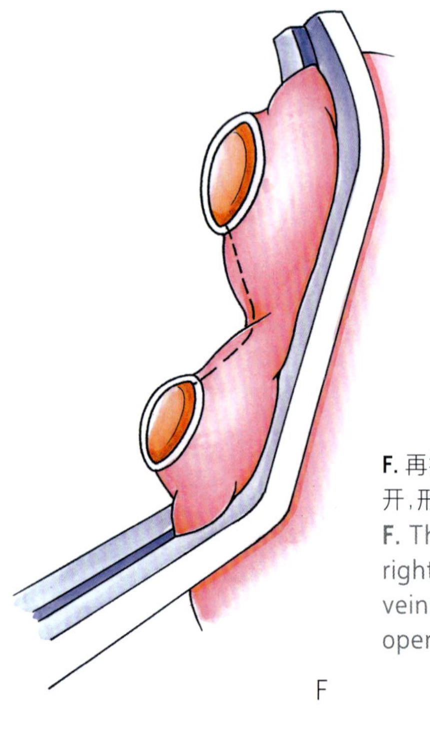

F. 再把右上、下肺静脉间的静脉壁剪开，形成左心房的一个单一开口。

F. The venous wall between the right upper and lower pulmonary veins is then cut to form a single opening in the left atrium.

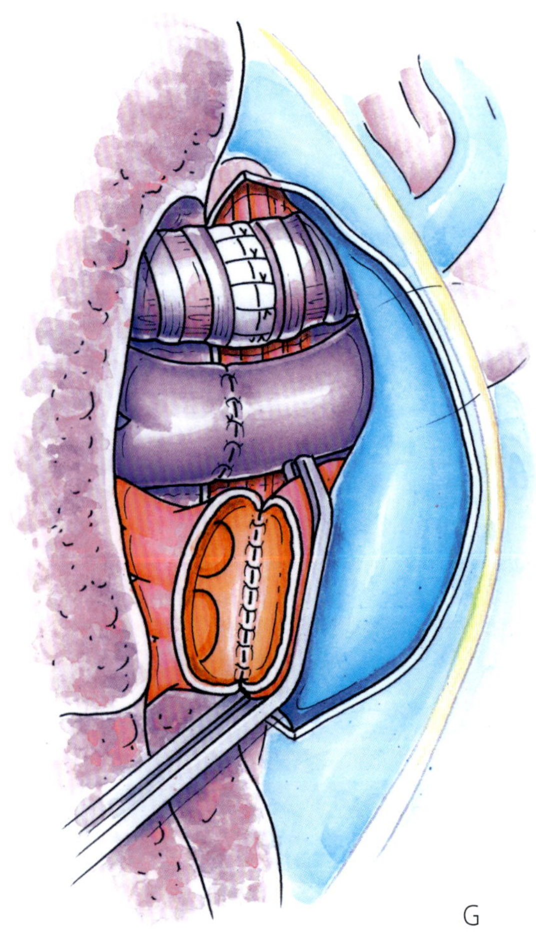

G. 将移植肺的肺静脉袖管与左心房开口吻合。

G. The pulmonary vein cuff of the donor lung is anastomosed to the left atrial opening.

图 7-3-6 左肺植入
Figure 7-3-6 Implantation of left lung

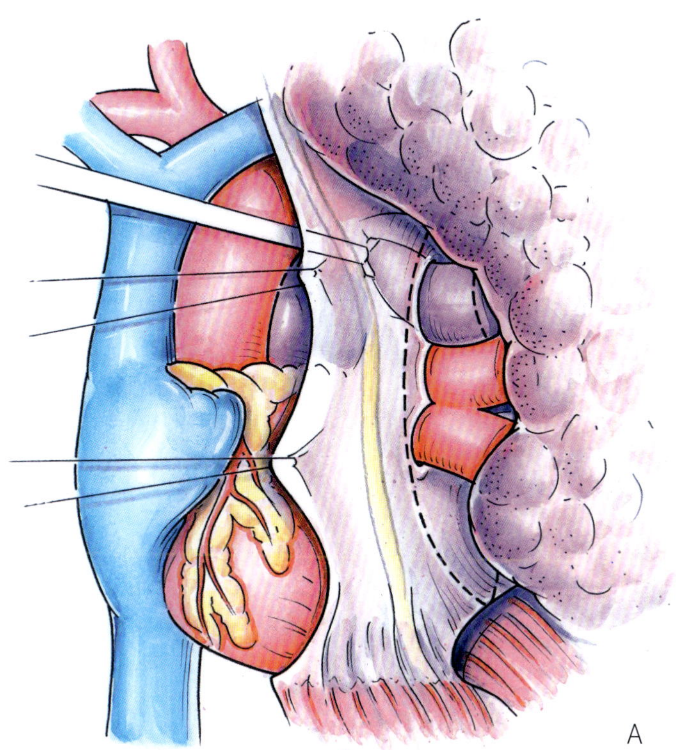

A. 解剖左肺门，于膈神经后切开心包。

A. The left hilus is dissected and a pericardiotomy is made posterior to the phrenic nerve.

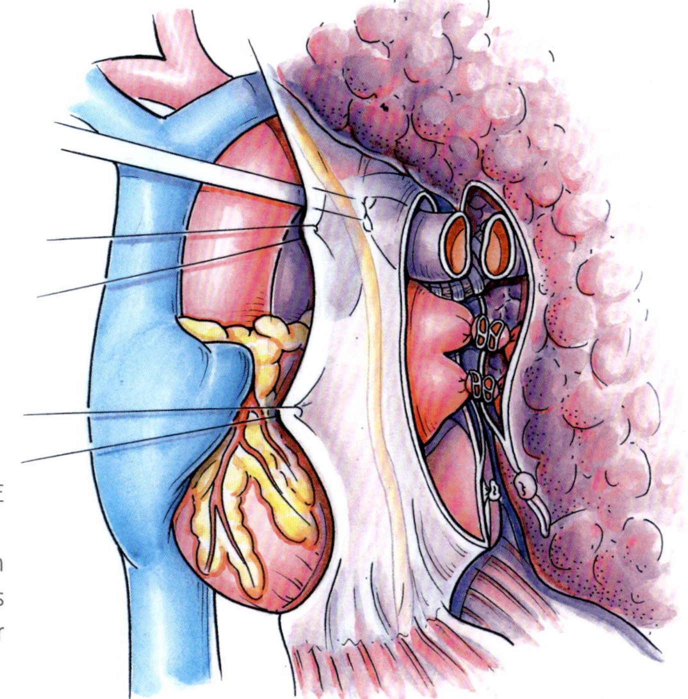

B. 心包内左肺动脉套束带，阻断左肺动脉后心包外切断左肺动脉，结扎切断左上、下肺静脉。

B. After the left pulmonary artery in the pericardium is banded and blocked, the left pulmonary artery is severed outside the pericardium, and the left upper and lower pulmonary veins are ligated and severed.

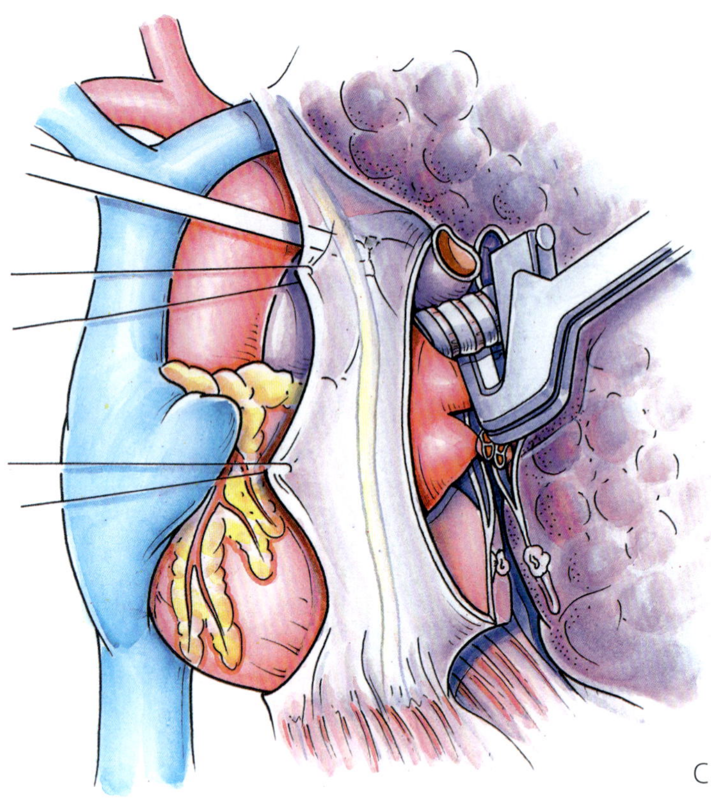

C. 切断左支气管，移除左肺。

C. Sever the left bronchus and remove the left lung.

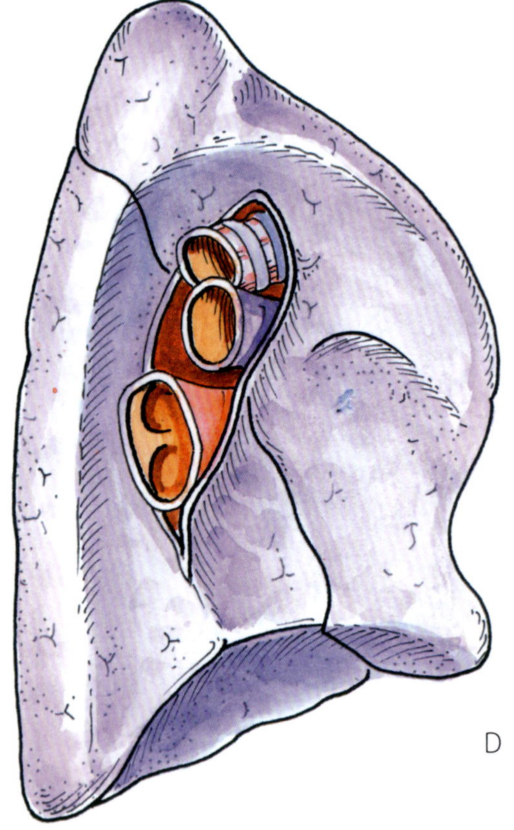

D. 供肺修剪完毕，从上到下依次是左支气管、左肺动脉和左上、下肺静脉袖管。

D. The donor lung is trimmed. In the order from top to bottom, they are the left bronchus, left pulmonary artery, and the cuffs of the left upper and lower pulmonary veins.

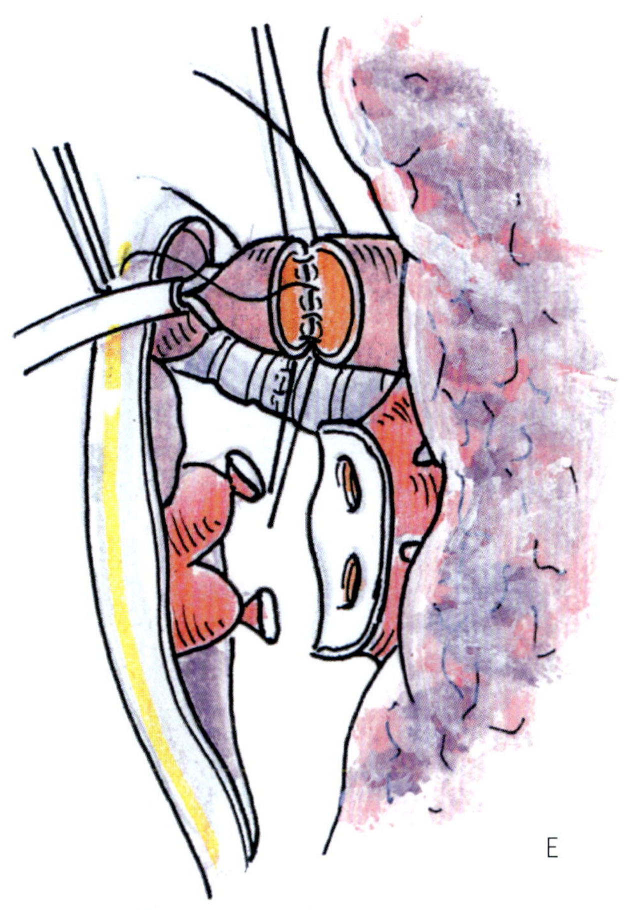

E. 先端端吻合左支气管，从后壁缝起，缝到前壁打结。然后端端吻合左肺动脉。

E. The left bronchus is end-to-end anastomosed, sutured from the posterior wall to the anterior wall to knot. The left pulmonary artery is then end-to-end anastomosed.

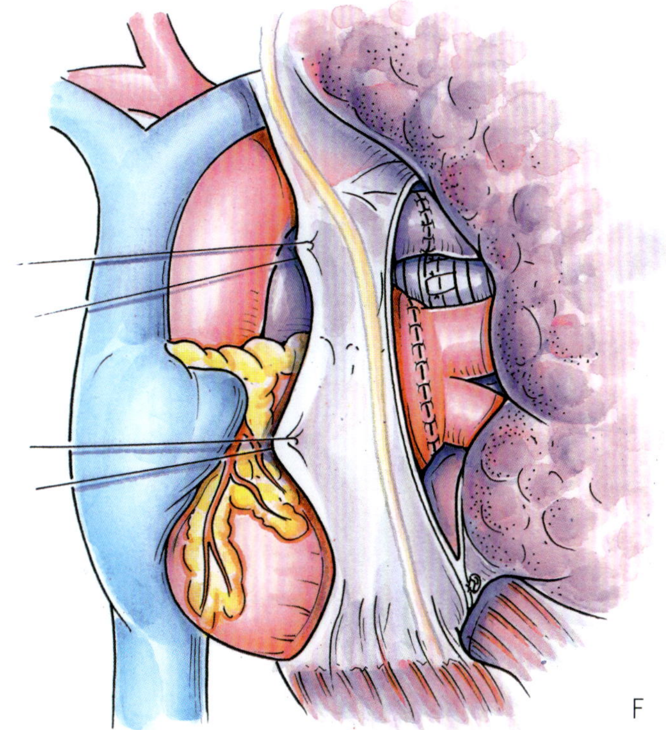

F. 用侧壁钳钳夹左心房，将左上、下肺静脉间的静脉壁剪开，形成左心房的单一开口，将移植肺的肺静脉袖管与左心房开口吻合。

F. With the left atrium side-clamped, the wall between the left upper and lower pulmonary veins is cut to form a single left atrium opening, which is anastomosed with the pulmonary vein cuff of the transplanted lung.

第 四 节　先天性心脏病的心脏移植

Section 4　Heart Transplantation for Congenital Heart Disease

图 7-4-1　左心发育不良综合征原位心脏移植

Figure 7-4-1　Orthotopic heart transplantation for hypoplastic left heart syndrome

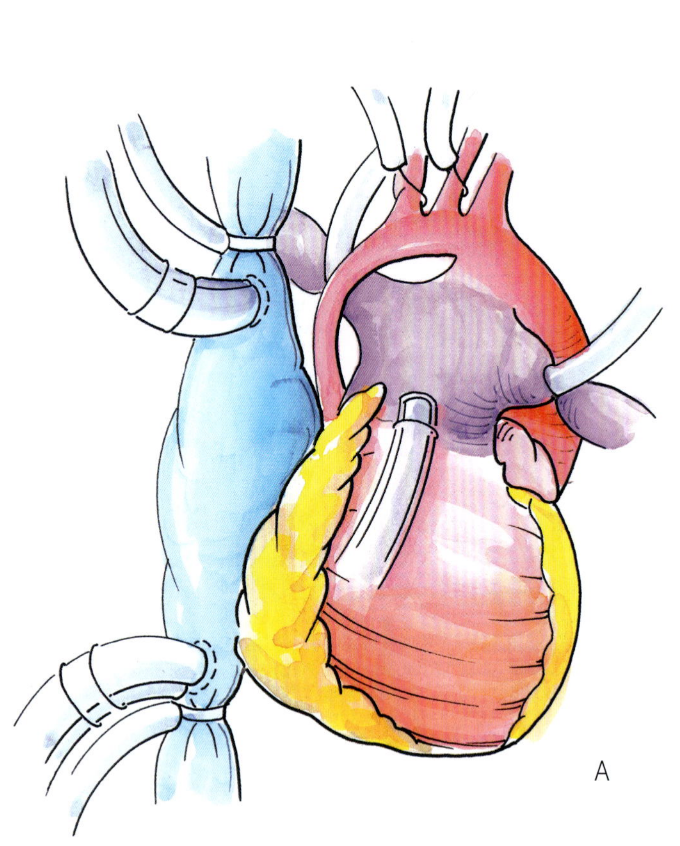

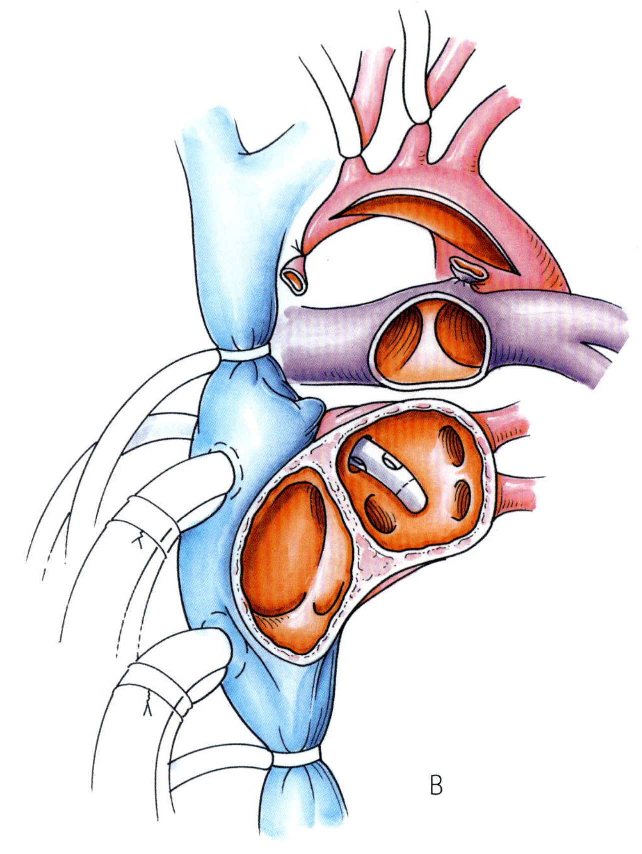

A. 切开左心发育不良综合征患者心包后见升主动脉和主动脉弓发育不良，巨大动脉导管未闭。上、下腔静脉插静脉引流管，肺动脉插引流管，股动脉插供血管，右上肺静脉插左心减压管。阻断上、下腔静脉和左、右肺动脉后开始体外循环。

A. Ascending aorta and aortic arch hypoplasia with a giant patent ductus arteriosus are found after pericardiotomy in patients with hypoplastic left heart syndrome. Venous draining cannulas are inserted into the superior and inferior vena cava. A draining cannula is inserted into the pulmonary artery, the arterial cannula is inserted into the femoral artery, and a left cardiac venting catheter is inserted into the right superior pulmonary vein. Extracorporeal circulation is initiated after blocking the superior and inferior vena cava and the left and right pulmonary arteries.

B. 按双心房移植法切除病心，阻断主动脉弓上方头臂分支，深低温停循环。切断动脉导管，肺动脉侧断端予以缝合。主动脉弓前下部横行切开。

B. The diseased heart is removed by using the biatrial technique, after the brachiocephalicus above the aortic arch is blocked and the circulation is discontinued at deep hypothermia. The ductus arteriosus is cut and the cut end on the pulmonary artery side is sutured. The anterior inferior aortic arch is transversely incised.

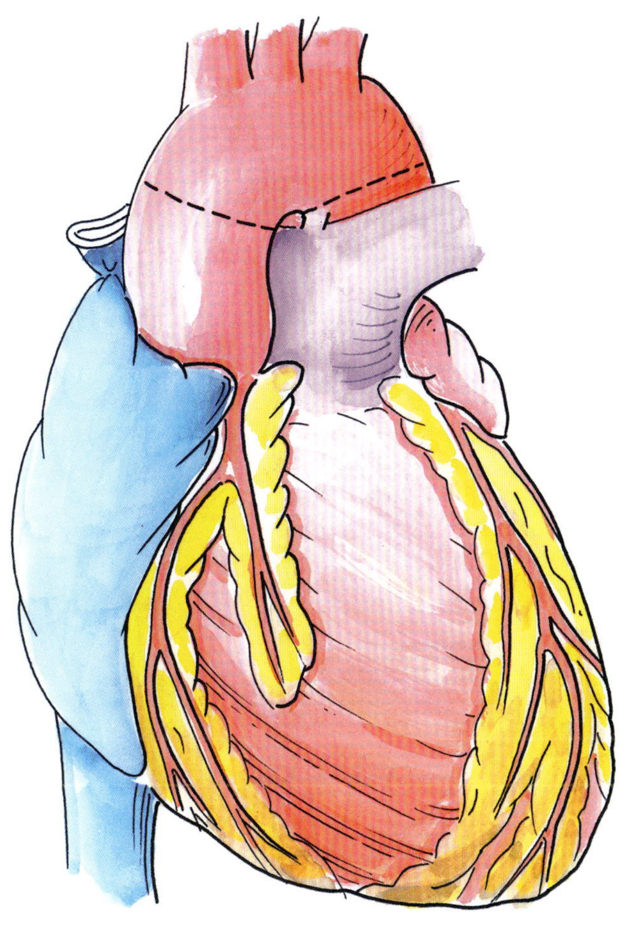

C. 将供心的主动脉弓自升主动脉中段至降主动脉起始段截下。

C. The aortic arch of the donor heart is severed from the middle segment of the ascending aorta to the initial segment of the descending aorta.

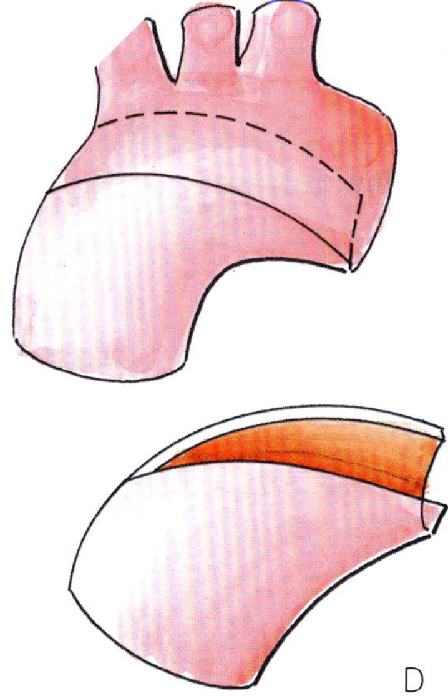

D. 修剪截下的主动脉弓，斜行将主动脉弓顶连同三大分支剪去，使该段主动脉远端开口匹配受者主动脉弓的切口。

D. Trim the sectioned aortic arch and obliquely cut off the top of the aortic arch together with the three major branches so that the distal opening of this aorta segment can be anastomosed to the incision of the recipient aortic arch.

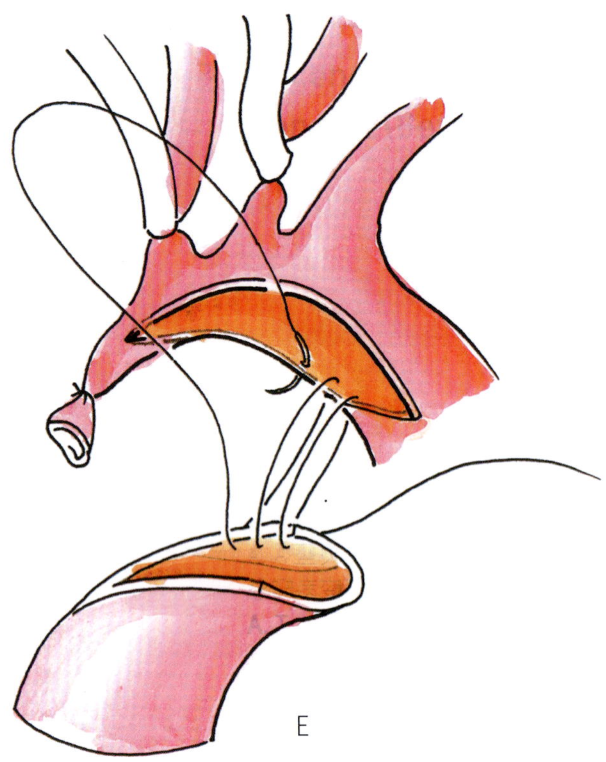

E. 将修剪好的供者主动脉段与受者主动脉弓吻合，扩大受者主动脉弓的直径。

E. The trimmed donor aortic segment is anastomosed to the recipient aortic arch to enlarge the diameter of the recipient aortic arch.

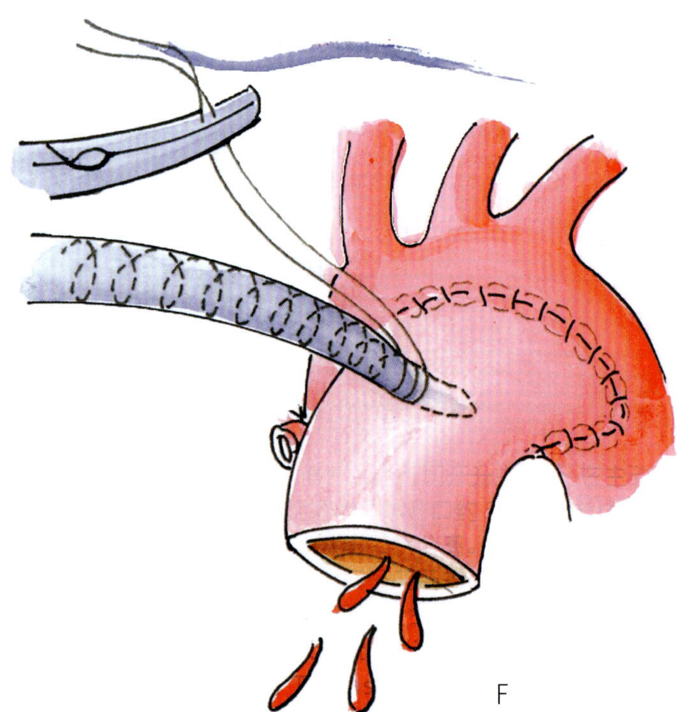

F. 在已吻合上的供者主动脉段上插入供血管。

F. Insert the arterial cannula into the anastomosed donor aortic segment.

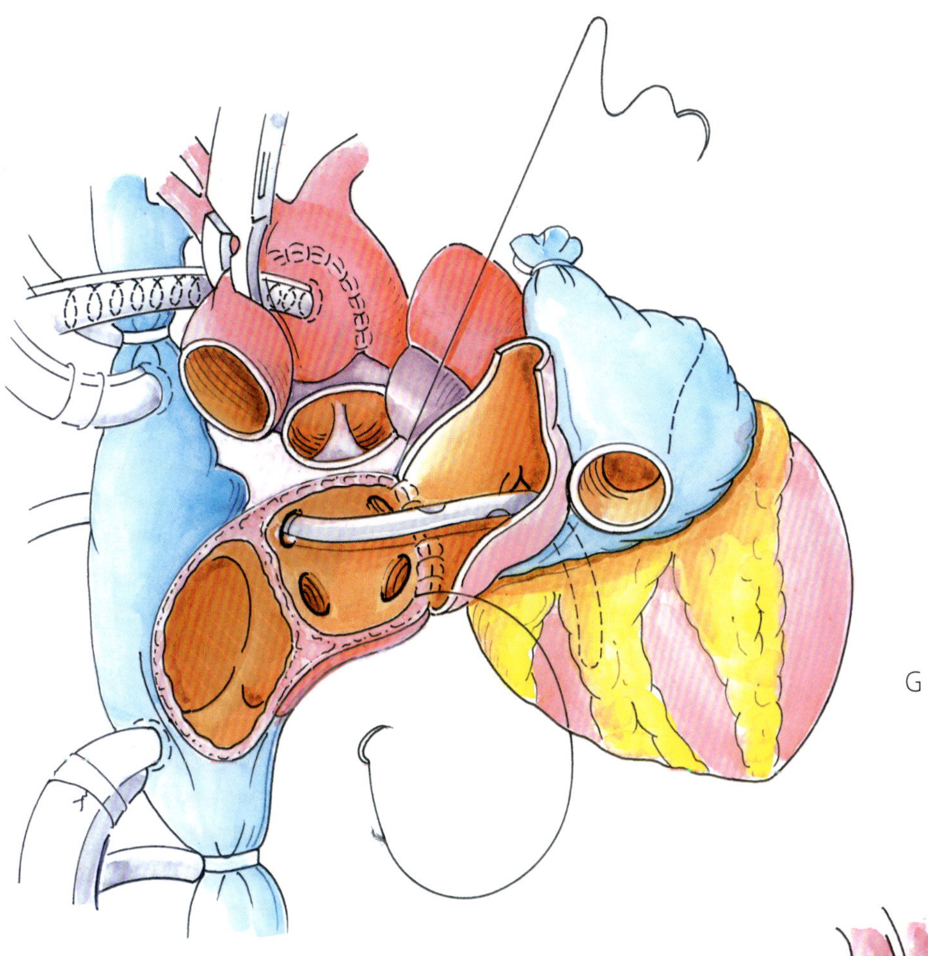

G. 排气后阻断钳钳夹主动脉，恢复体外循环，复温的同时按双心房移植法做心脏原位移植。

G. After de-airing, clamp the aorta with the blocking clamp, restore extracorporeal circulation, and perform orthotopic heart transplantation using the biatrial technique during rewarming.

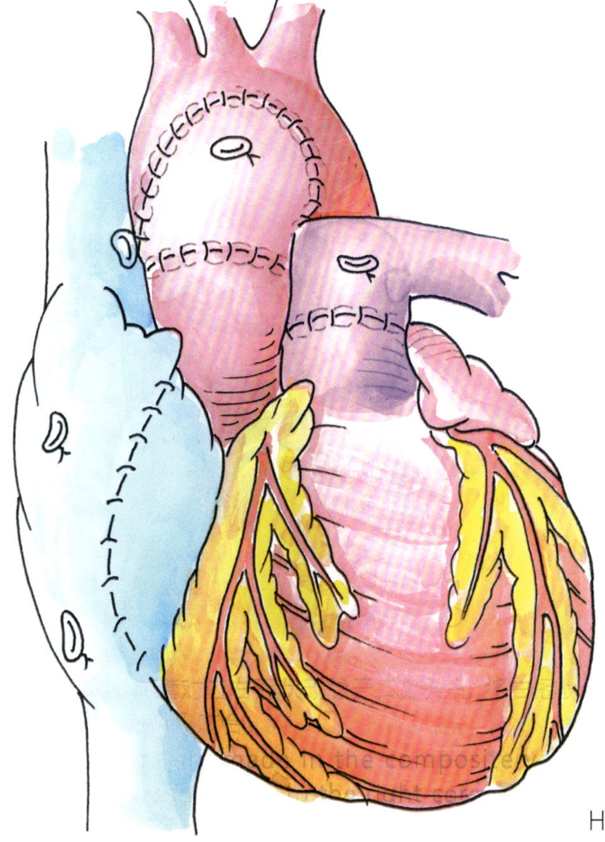

H. 移植完成。

H. The transplantation is completed.

图 7-4-2 Mustard/Senning 手术后原位心脏移植（双腔静脉移植法）

Figure 7-4-2 Orthotopic heart transplantation underwent Mustard/Senning procedure (bicaval technique)

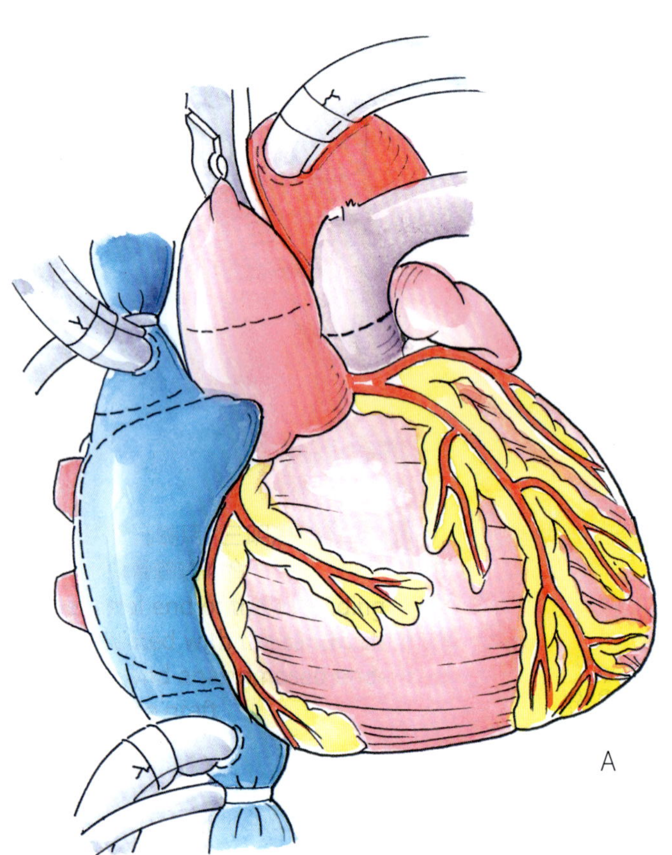

A. 上、下腔静脉分别插静脉引流管，升主动脉插供血管，建立体外循环。近心端切断肺动脉和升主动脉。

A. Insert the venous cannula into the superior and inferior vena cava respectively, and insert the arterial cannula into the ascending aorta to establish extracorporeal circulation. The pulmonary artery and the ascending aorta are severed at the site proximal to the heart.

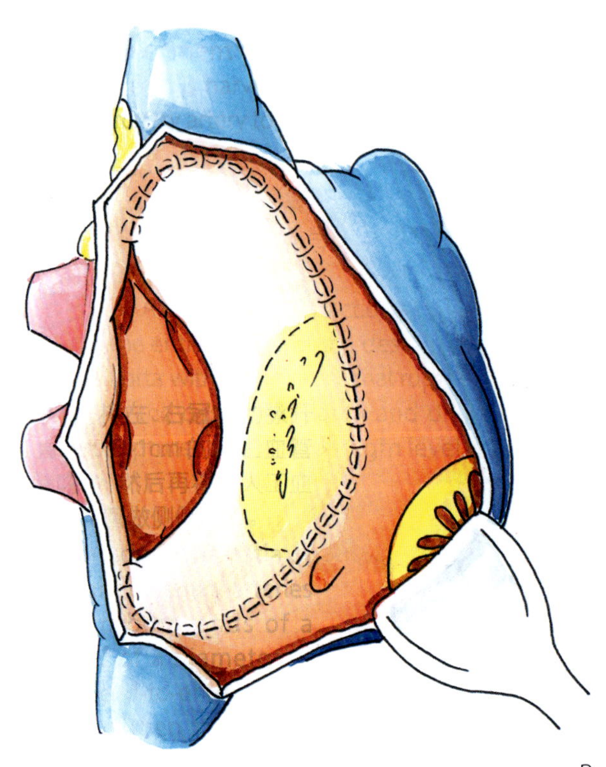

B. 原 Mustard 手术病例，房间沟处纵行切开左心房，见左肺静脉左侧和房间隔前缘之间的原 Mustard 手术心房内补片。

B. For patients who have undergone the Mustard operation, the left atriotomy is longitudinally performed at the atrial groove, exposing the intra-atrial patch previously used in the Mustard operation between the left side of the left pulmonary vein and the anterior border of the atrial septum.

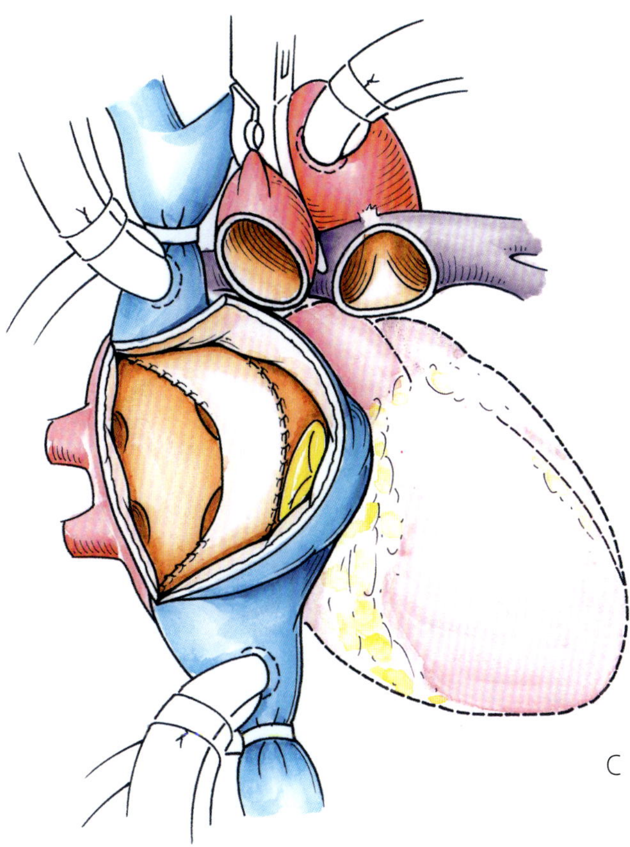

C. 沿缝合线拆除原 Mustard 手术心内补片，注意勿损伤左心房后壁。

C. Remove the intra-atrial patch previously used in the Mustard operation along the stitches, avoiding injury to the left atrial posterior wall.

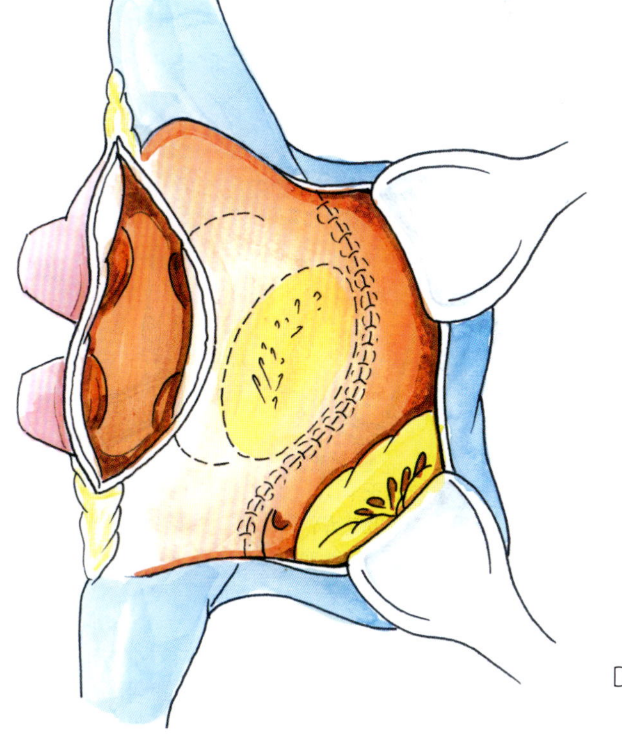

D. 对于 Senning 手术后患者，沿右心房和左心房的原缝合线处切开，见原 Senning 手术时右心房右侧壁缝至房间隔前缘。

D. For patients who have undergone the Senning procedure, cut along the prior sutures of the right and left atria to expose the stitches from the right lateral wall of the right atrium to the anterior border of the atrial septum in the Senning procedure.

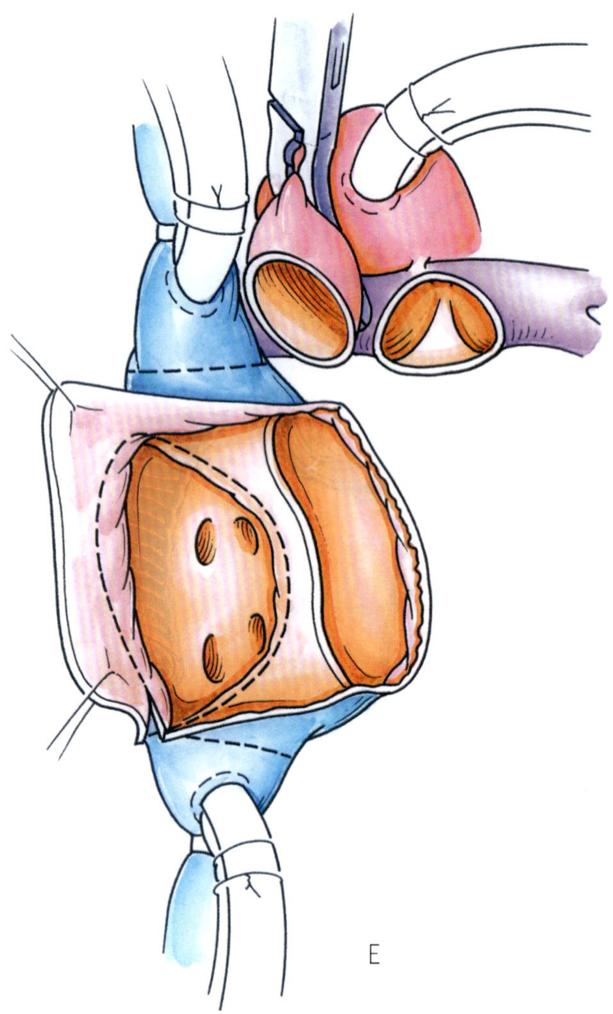

E. 将原 Senning 手术右心房右侧壁和房间隔前缘的缝合线全部剪开。

E. Cut off all sutures between the right lateral wall of the right atrium and the anterior border of the atrial septum in the previous Senning procedure.

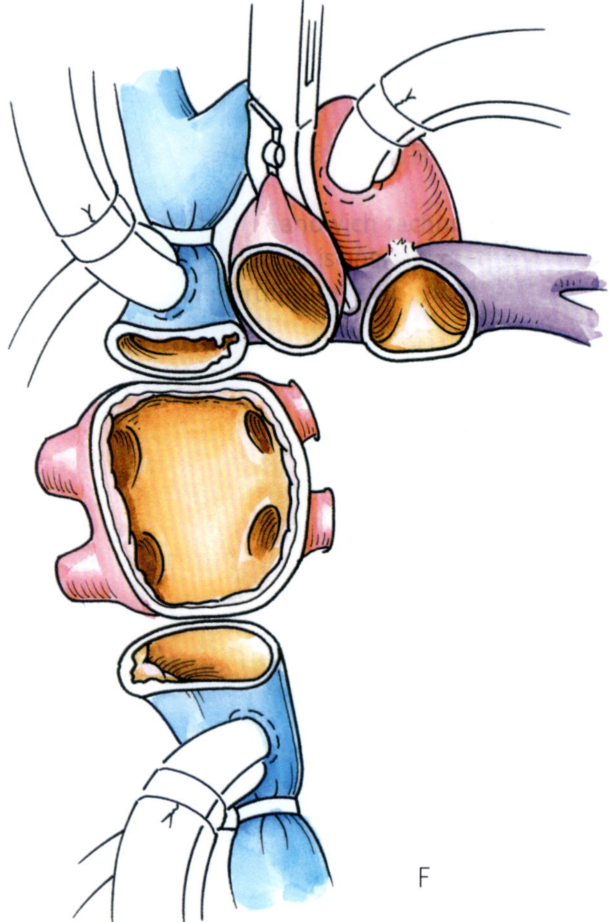

F. 按双腔静脉移植法切断上、下腔静脉，上、下腔静脉近心端各带一段心房袖，以利吻合。沿房室沟心房侧切下心脏，左心房壁大部分保留。

F. The superior and inferior vena cava are severed using the bicaval technique with a segment of the atrial cuff respectively reserved near the heart to facilitate anastomosis. The heart is cut along the atrial side of the atrioventricular groove, leaving most of the left atrial wall intact.

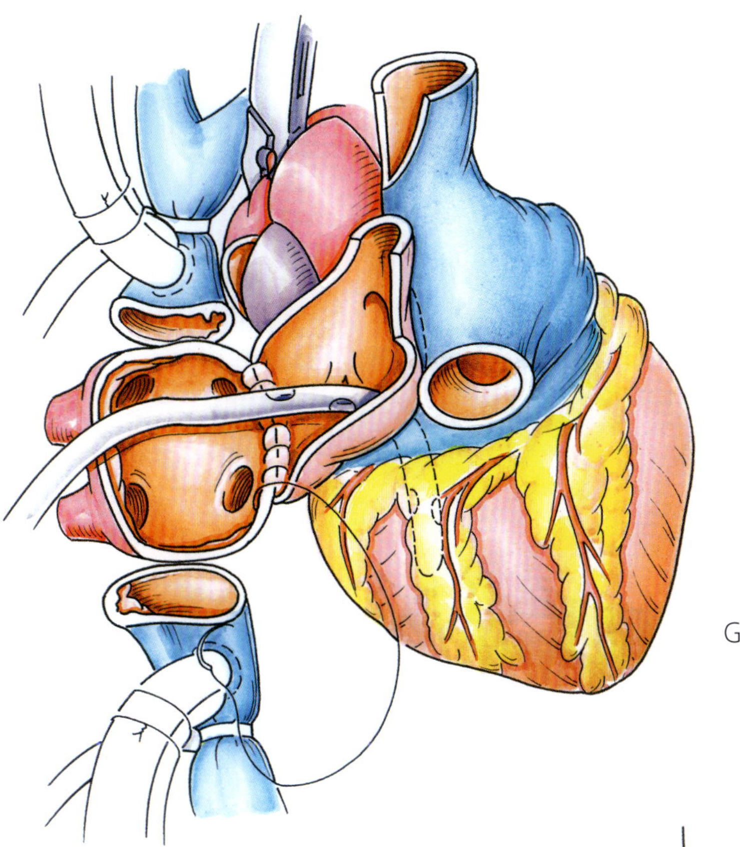

G. 将供心和受者的左心房连续缝合吻合。

G. The donor heart and the left atrium of the recipient are continuously sutured and anastomosed.

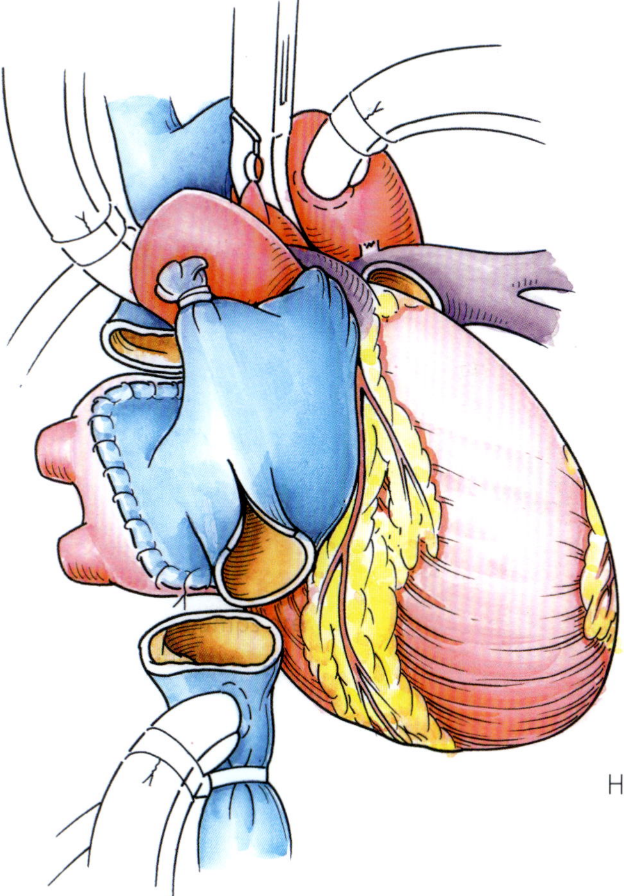

H. 左心房吻合完成，结扎缝线。

H. The left atrium anastomosis is completed, and the sutures are ligated.

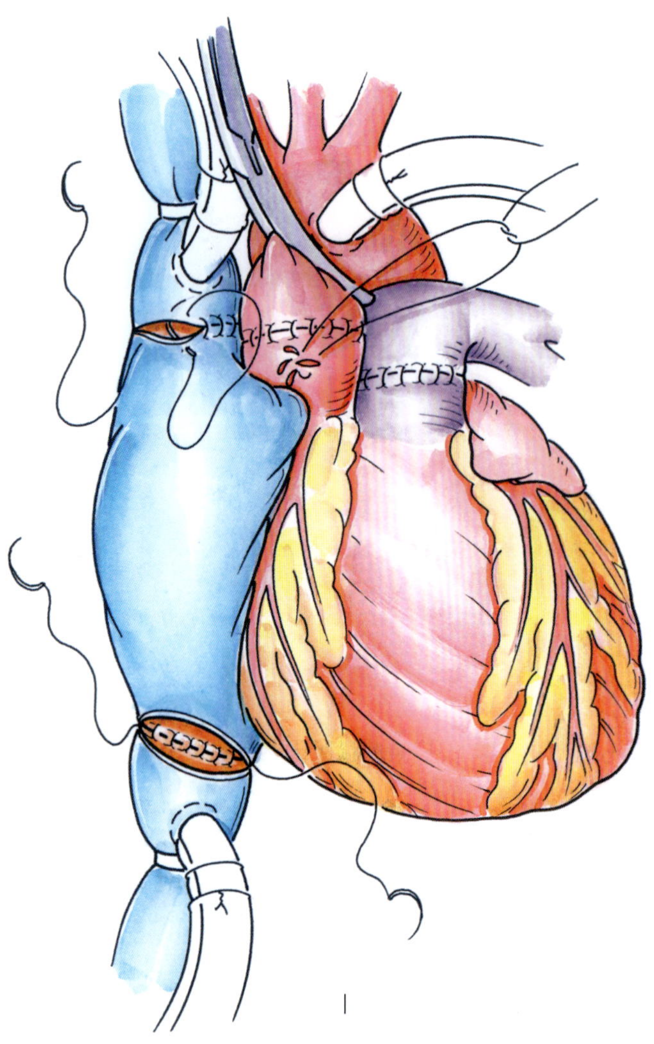

I. 依次吻合主动脉、肺动脉、下腔静脉和上腔静脉。

I. The aorta, the pulmonary artery, the inferior vena cava, and the superior vena cava are anastomosed successively.

图 7-4-3　Mustard/Senning 手术后原位心脏移植（双心房移植法）

Figure 7-4-3　Orthotopic heart transplantation underwent Mustard/Senning procedure (biatrial technique)

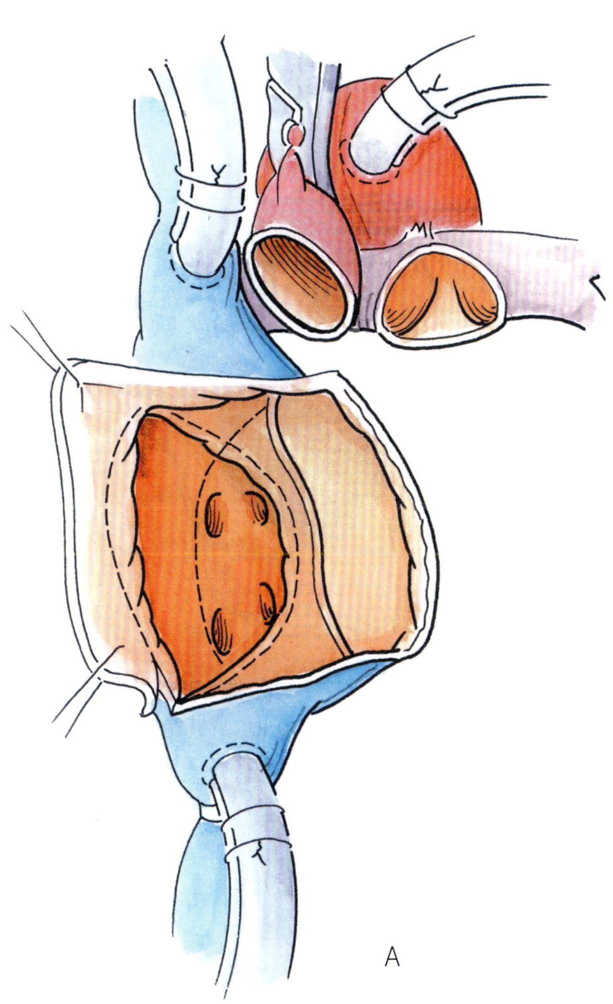

A. 离断升主动脉和肺动脉，切除心室，保留心房完整。纵行切开右心房，拆除原 Mustard 手术或 Senning 手术补片或心房内缝线。

A. The ascending aorta and pulmonary artery are severed, and the ventricles are excised, leaving the atria intact. The right atrium is incised longitudinally, and the patch or intra-atrial suture in prior Mustard or Senning procedure is removed.

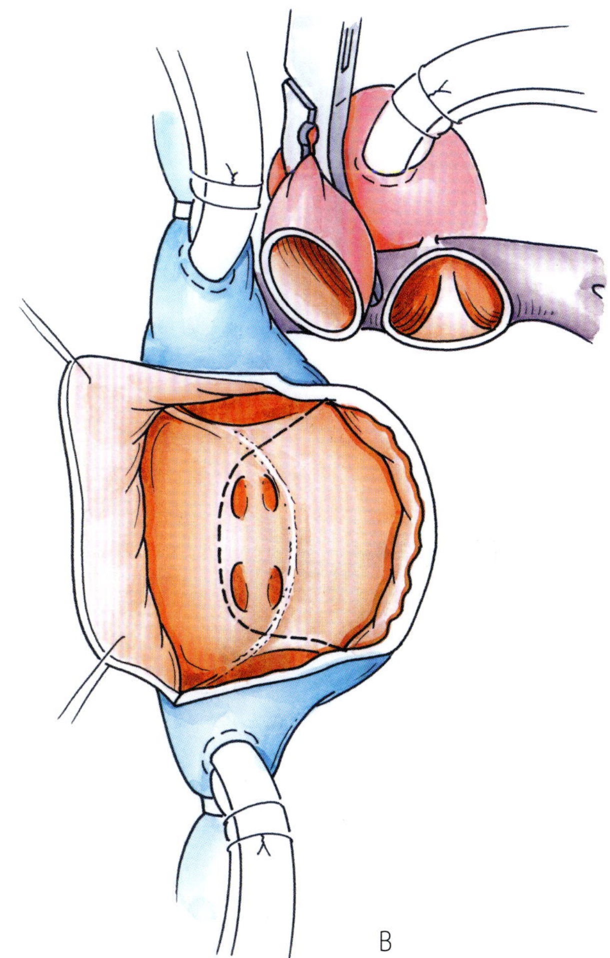

B. 左、右心房贯通后用补片重建房间隔，虚线为准备缝入新补片的位置。

B. As the chambers of the left and right atria are connected, the interatrial septum is reconstructed with a new patch. The dotted line indicates the site where the new patch is proposed to be sewn.

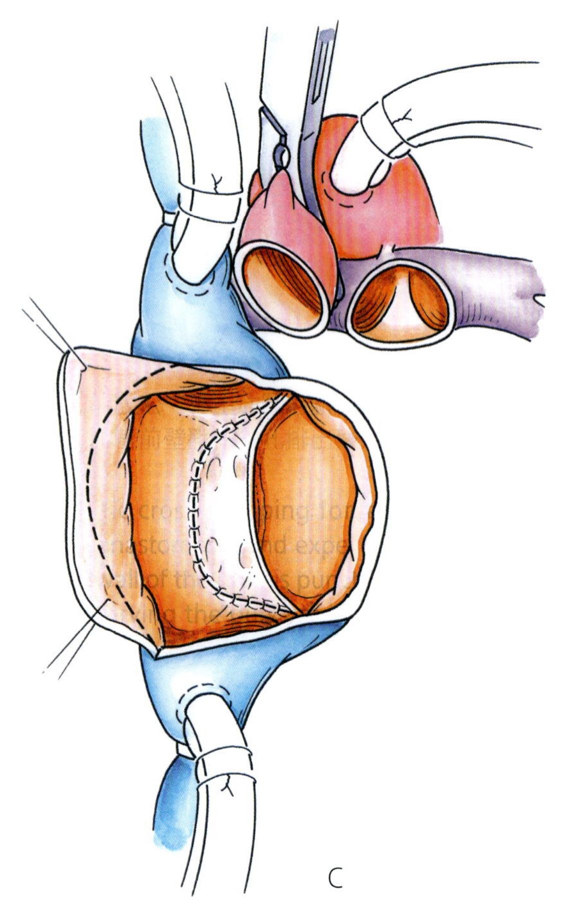

C. 补片由右肺静脉右侧开始缝入，两头分别缝到心房切口，补片左侧形成新的左心房，肺静脉汇入其中。补片右侧为右心房，腔静脉汇入其中。

C. The patch is sutured from the right side of the right pulmonary vein with the two ends sewn to the atrial incision respectively. The left side of the patch forms a new left atrium, into which the pulmonary vein flows. On the right side of the patch is the right atrium, into which the vena cava runs.

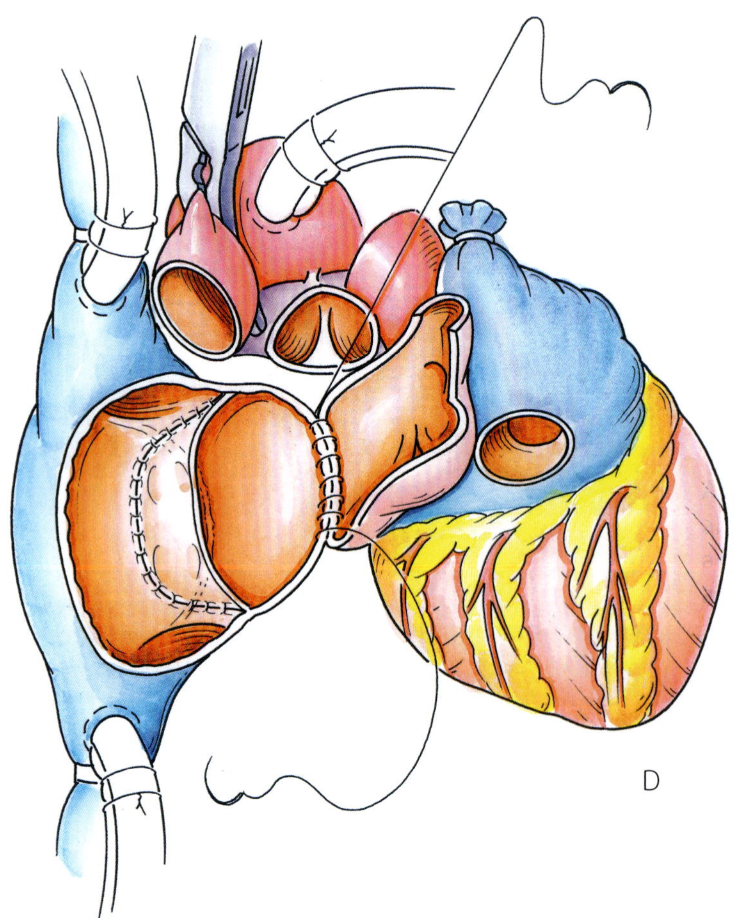

D. 将供心左心房与新构成的左心房吻合。继而吻合右心房、肺动脉和主动脉。

D. The donor left atrium is anastomosed to the newly constructed left atrium. The right atrium, the pulmonary artery, and the aorta are then anastomosed.

图 7-4-4 内脏反位的原位心脏移植

Figure 7-4-4 Orthotopic heart transplantation for patient with situs inversus viscerum

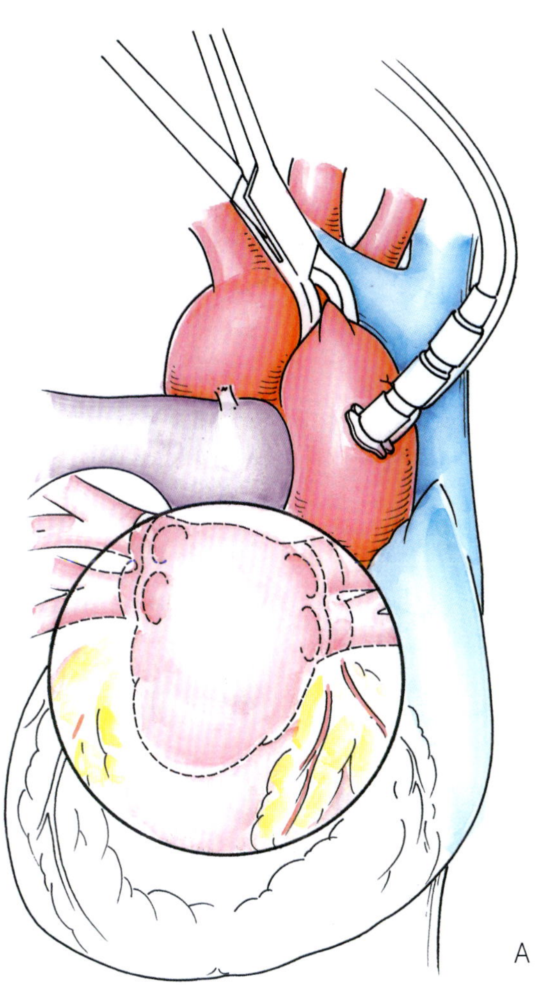

A. 内脏反位，上、下腔静脉位于心脏左侧，两大动脉升主动脉在左、肺动脉在右，心尖朝向右下方。

A. With situs inversus viscerum, the superior and inferior vena cava are located on the cardiac left side, the ascending aorta is left-sided, the pulmonary artery is right-sided, and the cardiac apex points to the lower right.

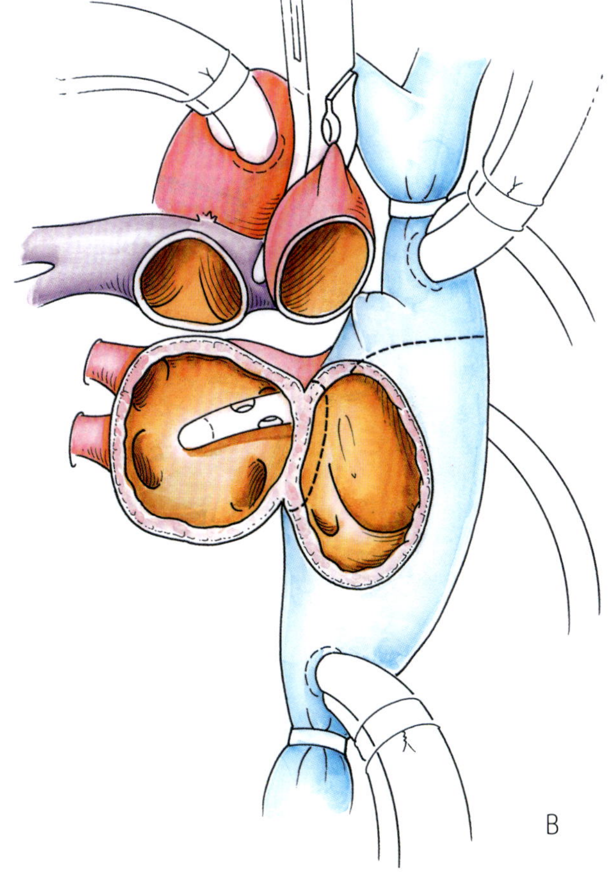

B. 建立体外循环，按双心房移植法将心脏切除。

B. Following extracorporeal circulation, the heart is removed using the biatrial technique.

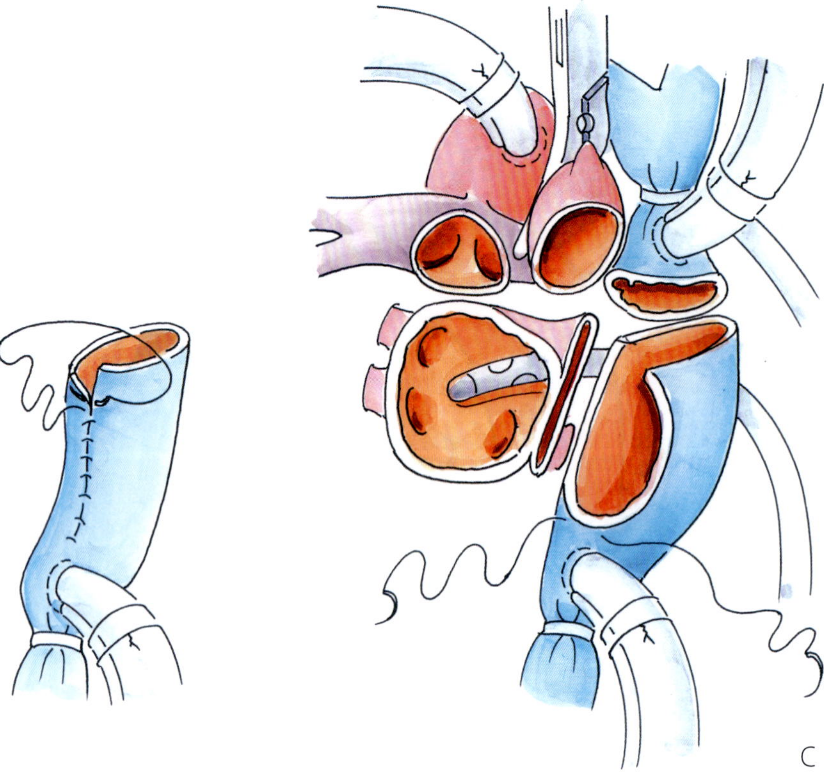

C. 将右心房从左心房上切下，保留左心房的完整。右心房的上部横断，中下部的右心房壁缝成管状，形成下腔静脉的延长。

C. Cut the right atrium from the left atrium, leaving the left atrium intact. The upper part of the right atrium is transected, and the right atrium wall in the lower middle part is sutured into a tube, forming an extension of the inferior vena cava.

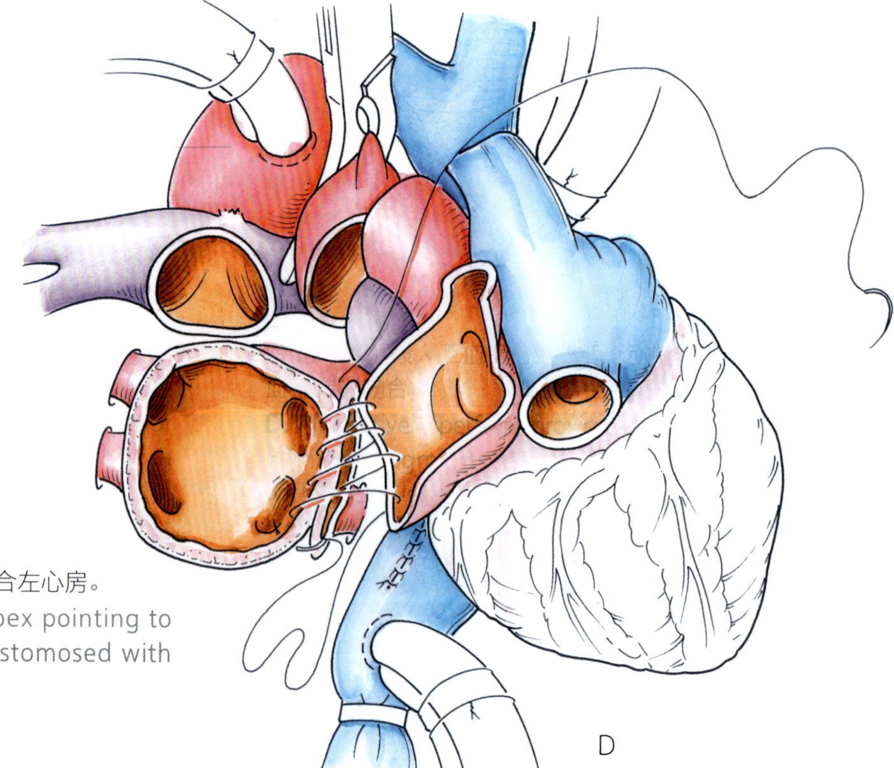

D. 置入供心，心尖朝左下方。连续缝合吻合左心房。

D. Place the donor heart with the apex pointing to the lower left. The left atrium is anastomosed with continuous sutures.

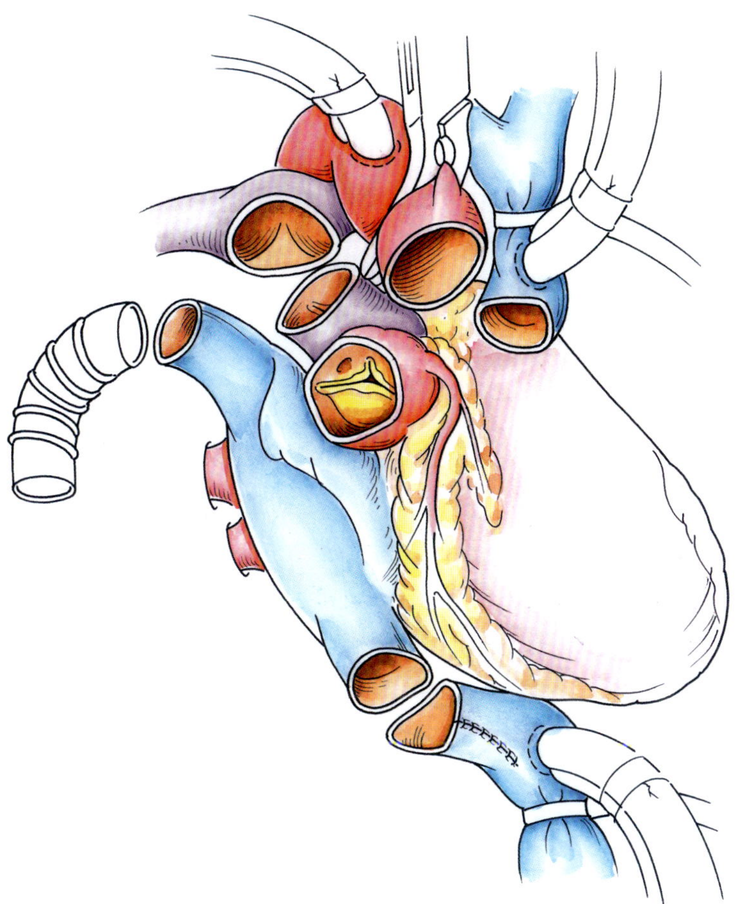

E. 下腔静脉及其心房缝成的延长管拉到右侧与供心下腔静脉吻合。

E. The extension tube sutured from the inferior vena cava and the atrium is pulled to the right side to be anastomosed to the donor inferior vena cava.

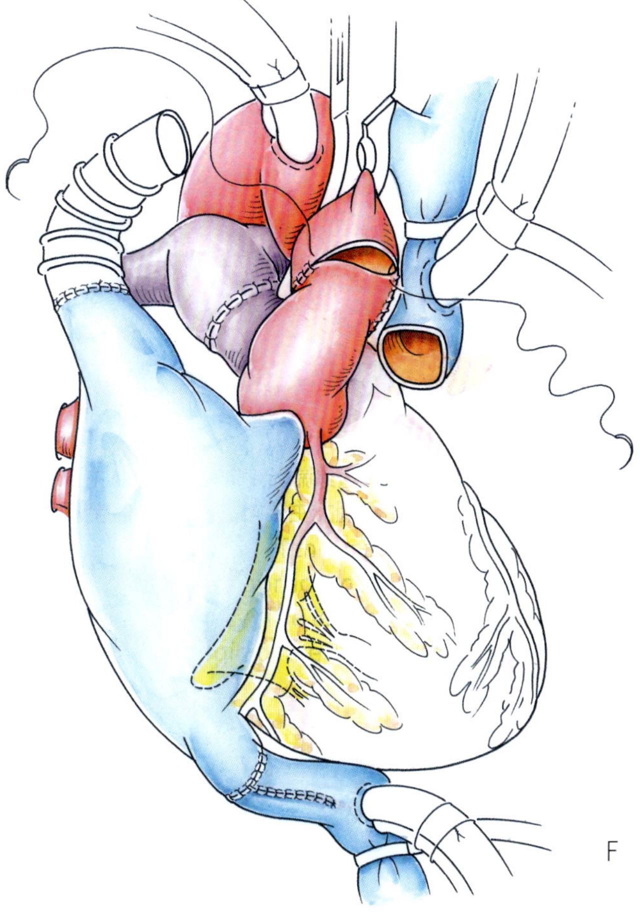

F. 先后吻合肺动脉和主动脉。取一段带垫圈的人工血管作为桥血管，从主动脉前跨过，将上腔静脉与供心上腔静脉连接。人工血管与供心上腔静脉端端吻合。

F. Perform the pulmonary artery anastomosis, which is followed by the aorta anastomosis. A segment of the artificial blood vessel with a support frame as a bridge crossing the front of the aorta connects the superior vena cava to the donor superior vena cava. The artificial blood vessel is end-to-end anastomosed to the donor superior vena cava.

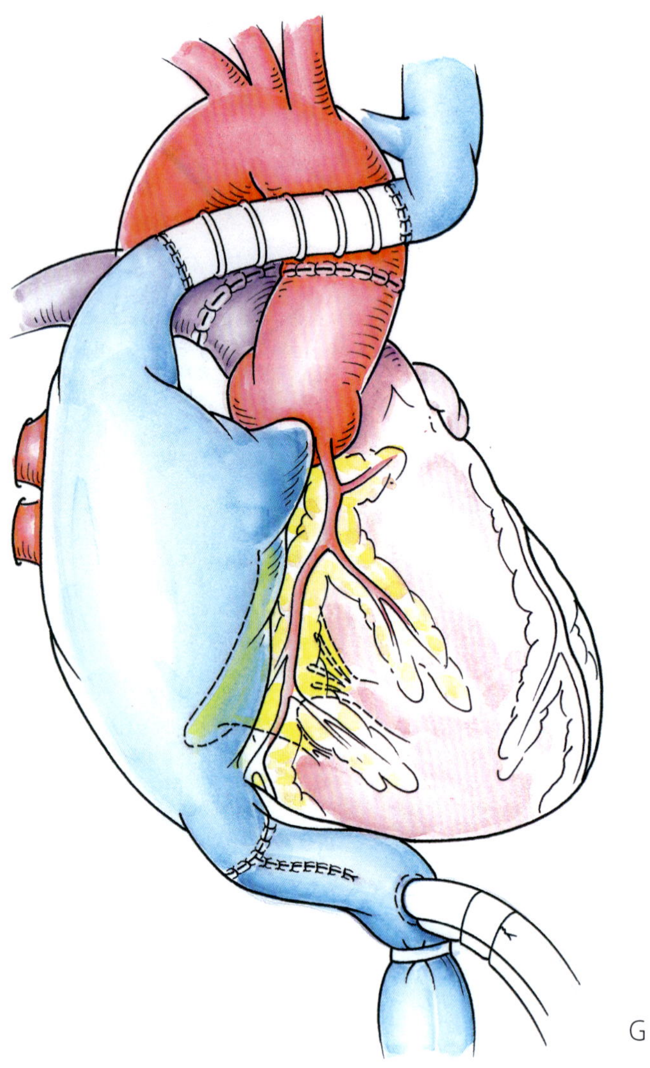

G. 最后将人工血管经主动脉前方延至左侧，与受者上腔静脉吻合。

G. Finally, the artificial blood vessel, extending to the left side through the front of the aorta, is anastomosed to the recipient superior vena cava.

图 7-4-5　外导管全腔静脉肺动脉连接术后原位心脏移植

Figure 7-4-5　Orthotopic heart transplantation underwent total cavopulmonary connection with external tunnel

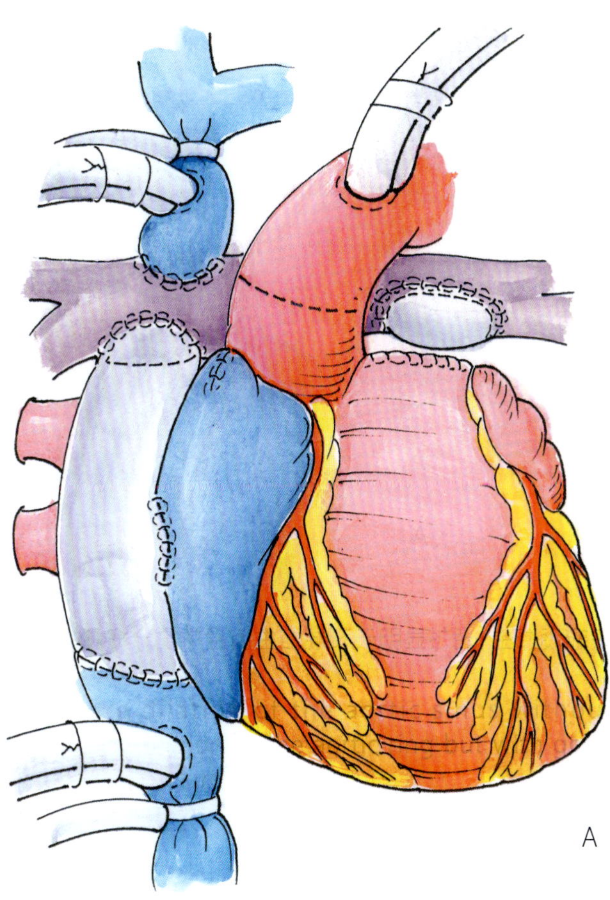

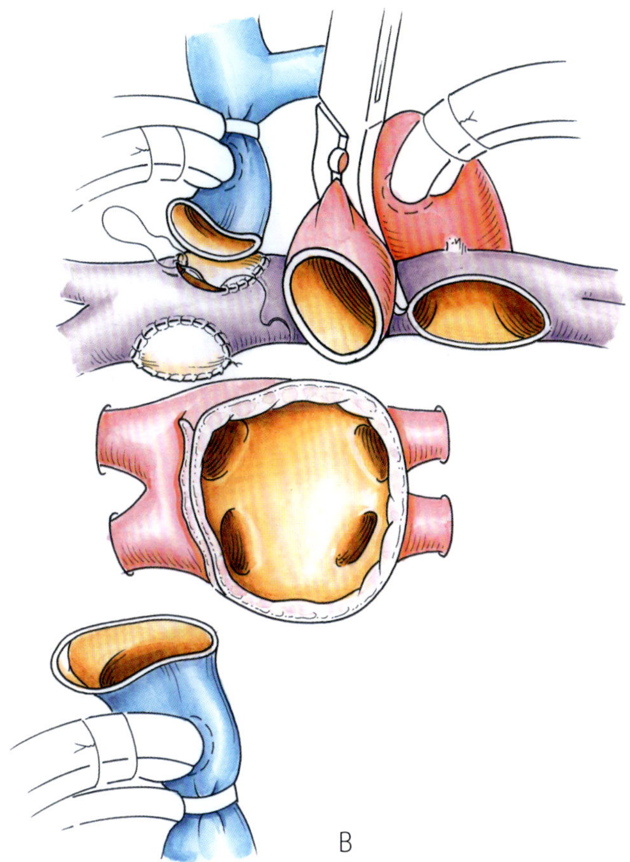

A. 上、下腔静脉分别插静脉引流管，升主动脉插供血管，建立体外循环。

A. Insert venous draining cannula into the superior and inferior vena cava respectively, and insert the arterial cannula into the ascending aorta to establish extracorporeal circulation.

B. 将原腔肺连接的外导管予以拆除。补片修补右肺动脉与外导管吻合处的开口。拆除上腔静脉与右肺动脉的吻合，遗留开口亦用补片修补。离断升主动脉。原肺动脉总干切断处补片予以拆除。在左心房沿房室沟切除心脏。

B. Remove the external tunnel used in the prior cavopulmonary connection. The patch repairs the ostium where the right pulmonary artery is anastomosed with the external tunnel. Anastomosis of the superior vena cava to the right pulmonary artery is undone with the residual ostium repaired with a patch. The ascending aorta is severed. Remove the patch where the primary trunk of the prior pulmonary artery is sectioned. The heart is excised along the atrioventricular groove in the left atrium.

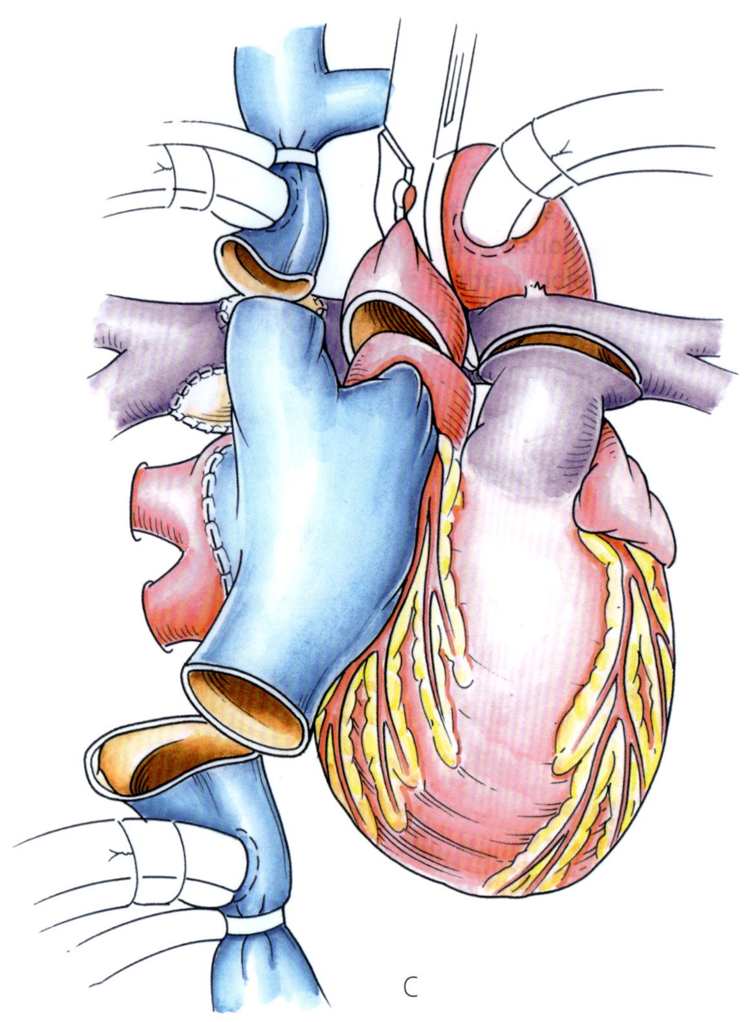

C. 置入供心，吻合左心房后再依次吻合下腔静脉、上腔静脉、主动脉和肺动脉。
C. After the donor heart is placed, the left atrium is anastomosed, followed by the sequential anastomoses of the inferior vena cava, the superior vena cava, the aorta, and the pulmonary artery.

图 7-4-6 大动脉转位原位心脏移植

Figure 7-4-6 Orthotopic heart transplantation for transposition of great arteries

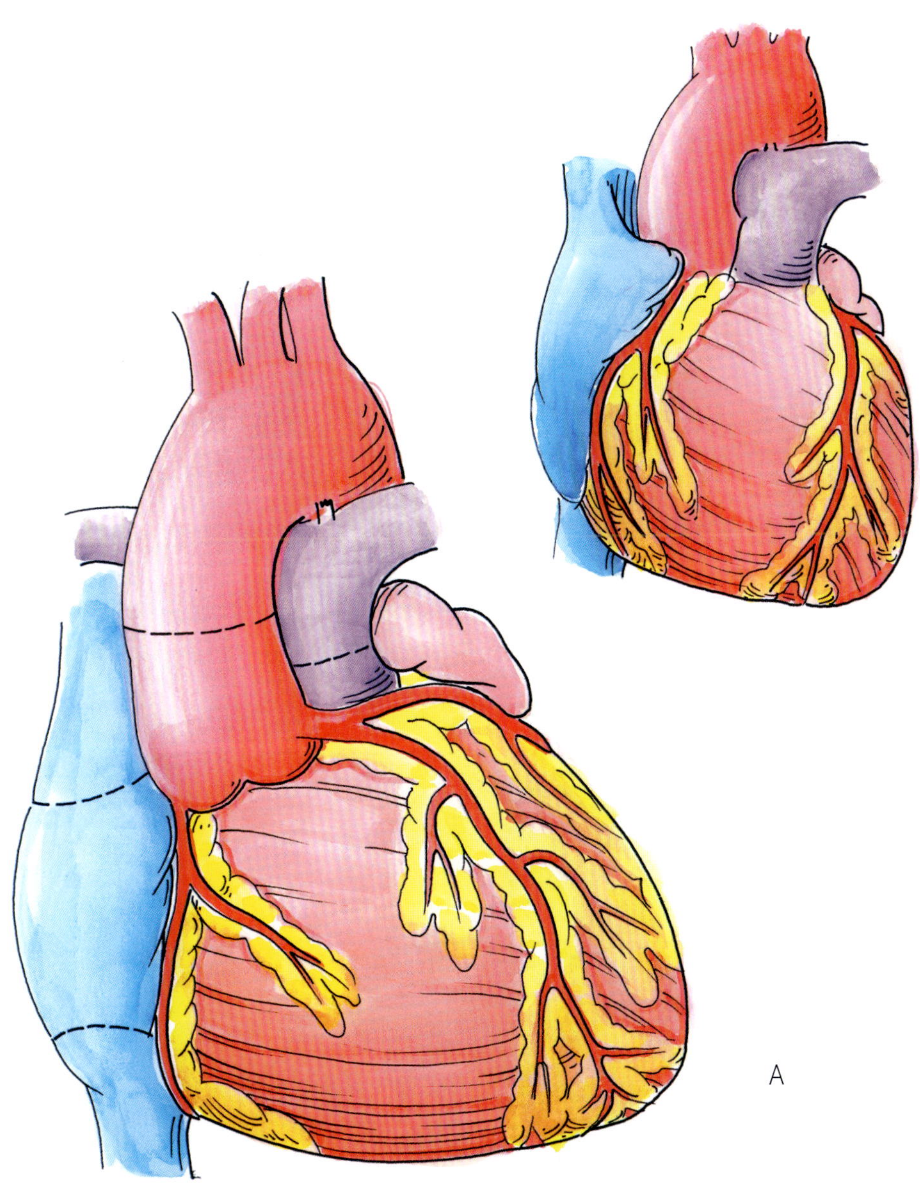

A. 打开心包后检查心脏。按双腔静脉移植法切除心脏。

A. Perform a pericardiotomy for a heart examination. Use the bicaval technique to excise the heart.

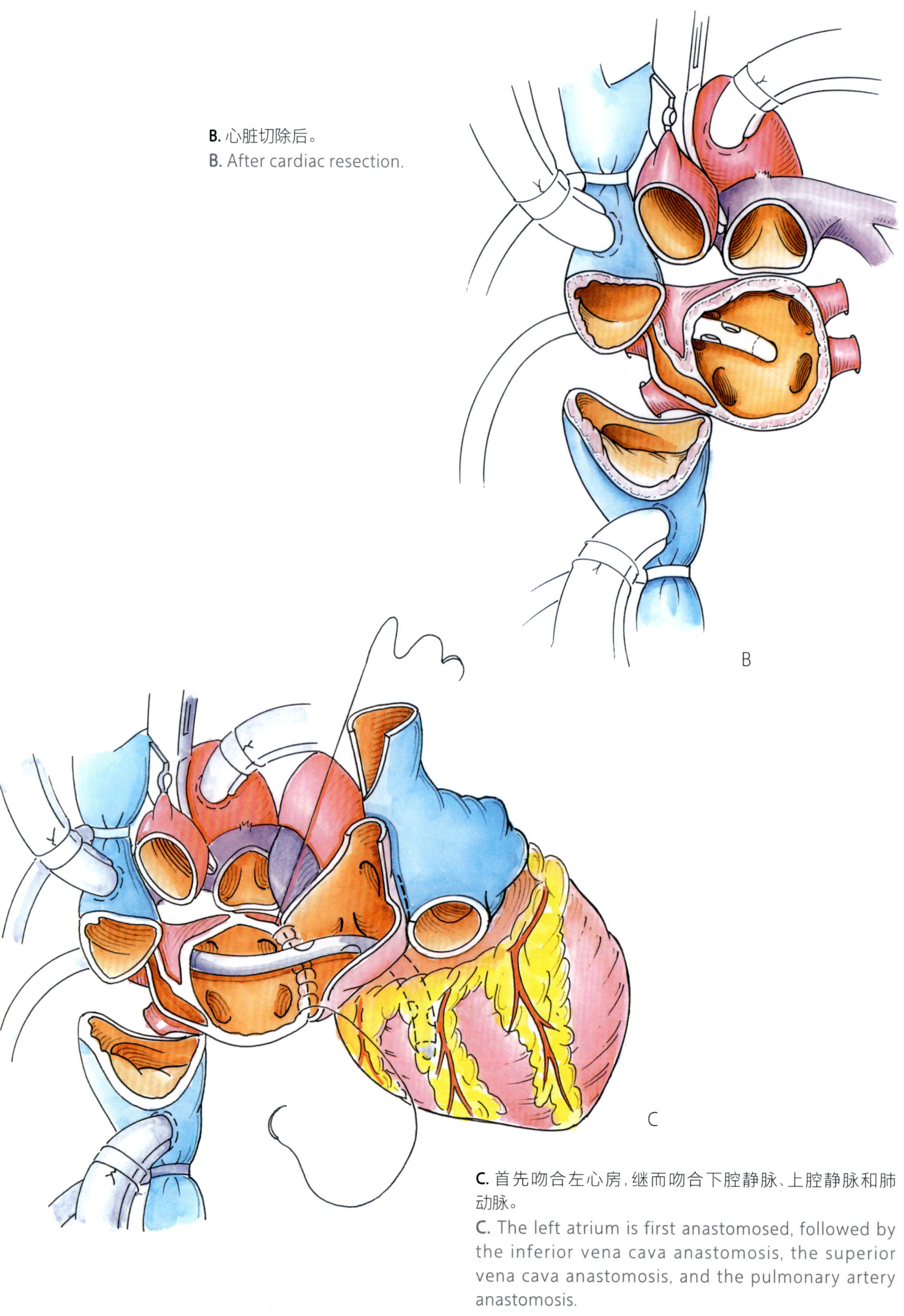

B. 心脏切除后。

B. After cardiac resection.

C. 首先吻合左心房，继而吻合下腔静脉、上腔静脉和肺动脉。

C. The left atrium is first anastomosed, followed by the inferior vena cava anastomosis, the superior vena cava anastomosis, and the pulmonary artery anastomosis.

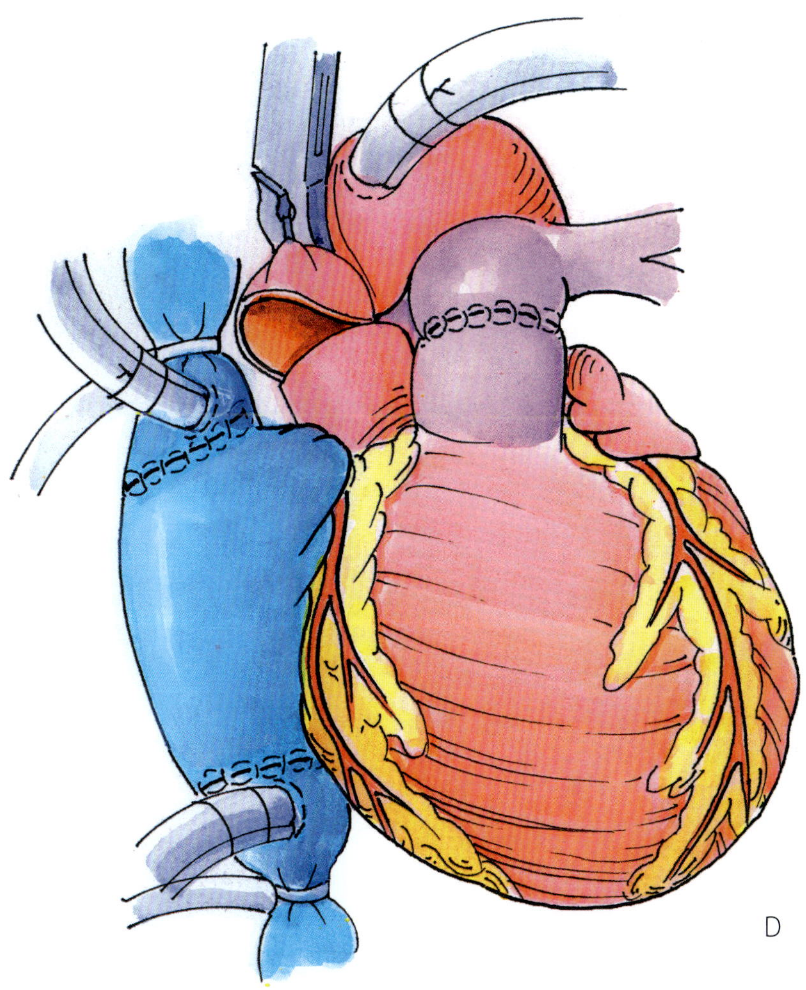

D. 最后吻合主动脉。

D. The aorta is finally anastomosed.

第八章
机械辅助循环

Chapter 8
Mechanical Circulatory Support

第一节　主动脉内球囊反搏
Section 1　Intra-Aortic Balloon Pump

图 8-1-1　经股动脉插入
Figure 8-1-1　Transfemoral insertion

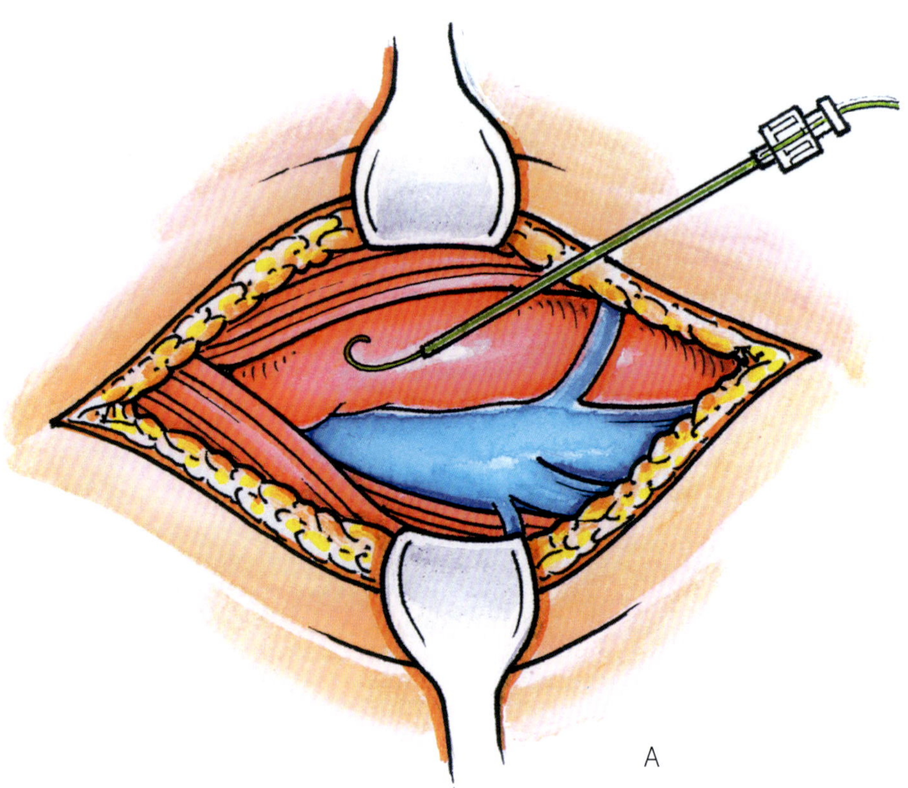

A. 腹股沟切口，显露股动脉。动脉穿刺针刺入股动脉，经穿刺针将导引钢丝送入股动脉。

A. An inguinal incision is made to expose the femoral artery. The guidewire is introduced into the femoral artery via the needle, which is punctured into the femoral artery.

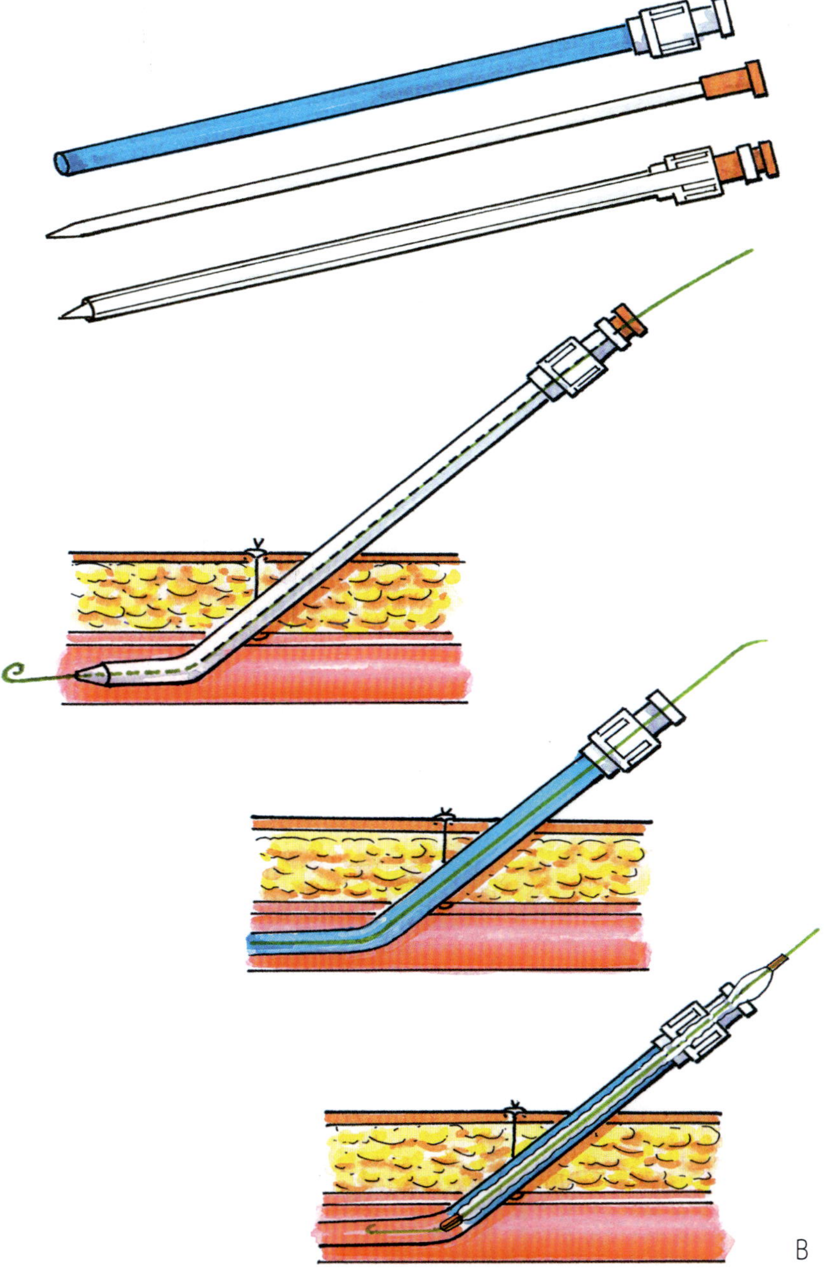

B. 亦可直接经皮穿刺股动脉。退出穿刺针后，先循导引钢丝插入扩张管扩张股动脉穿刺孔，然后插入鞘管。

B. The femoral artery can also be percutaneously punctured. After withdrawing the needle, insert the dilation tube following the guidewire to expand the femoral artery puncture hole, and then insert the sheath.

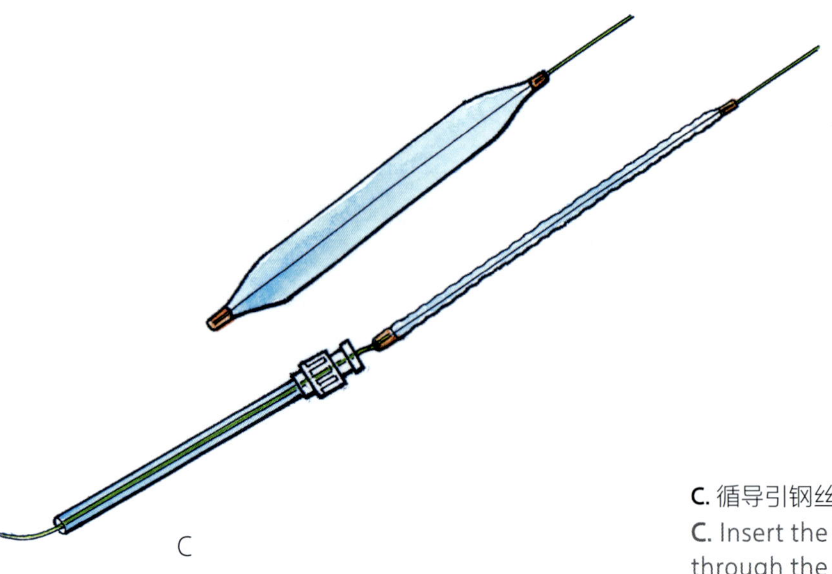

C. 循导引钢丝经鞘管插入球囊导管。

C. Insert the balloon catheter following the guidewire through the sheath.

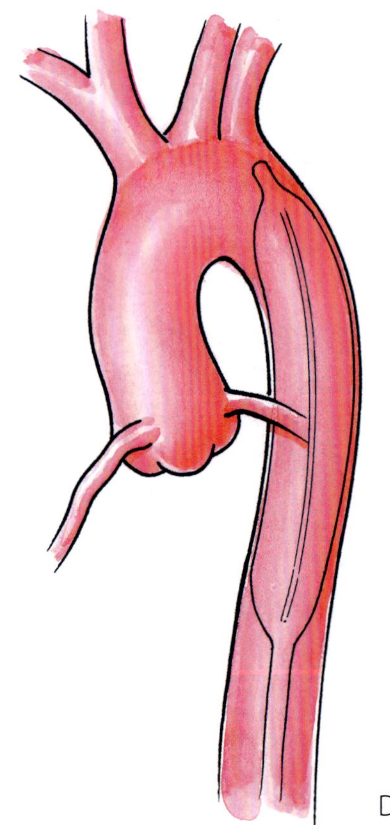

D. 将球囊导管的尖端送到降主动脉起始处，以不影响左锁骨下动脉血供为准。插入前可以将胸骨角作为标志，测量股动脉进针点到胸骨角的距离，作为球囊导管插入的长度。插入后拍 X 线胸片观察球囊导管尖端的金属标记，确定导管尖端位置。

D. The tip of the balloon catheter is sent to the origin of the descending aorta so that it does not affect the blood supply to the left subclavian artery. Before insertion, using the sternal angle as a marker, measure the distance between the sternal angle and the entry point of the femoral artery to determine the length of balloon catheter insertion. After insertion, take a chest X-ray to observe the metal mark on the tip of the balloon catheter to determine the position of the catheter tip.

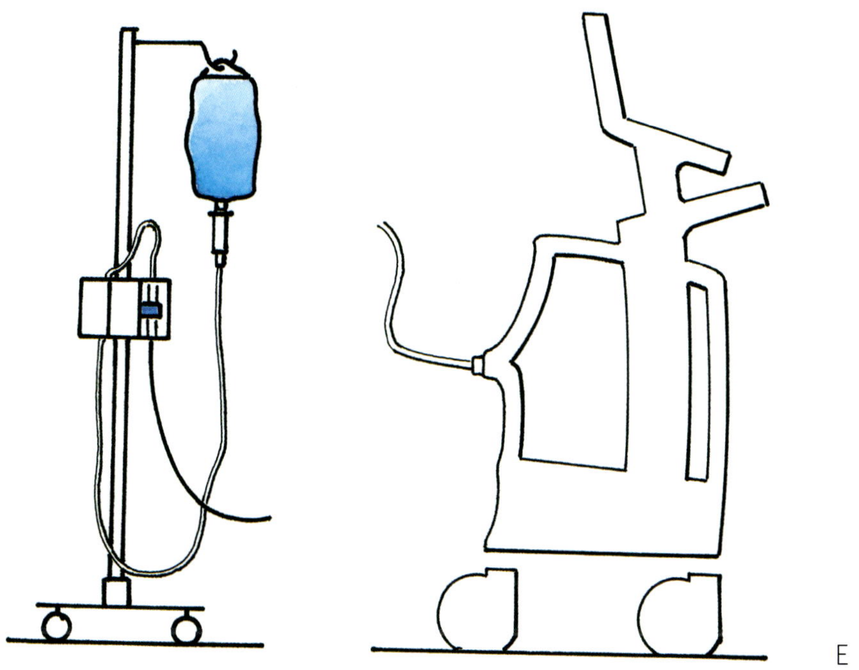

E. 将球囊导管的充放气管和测压管与反搏机相接。

E. Connect the inflation/deflation tube and pressure-measuring tube of the balloon catheter to the counterpulsation device.

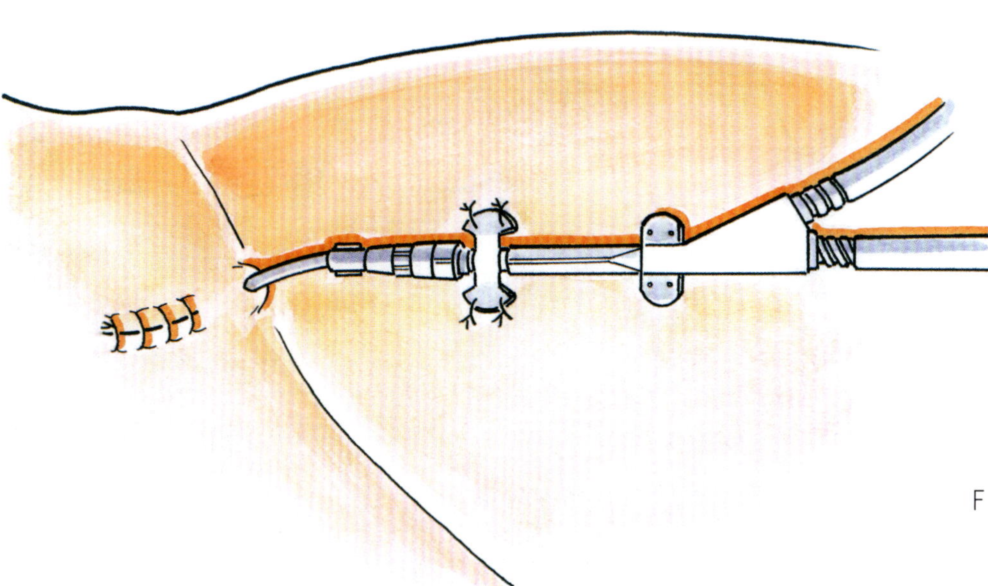

F. 缝合固定球囊导管，缝合腹股沟切口。

F. Suture to fix the balloon catheter. Suture the inguinal incision.

图 8-1-2 经锁骨下动脉插入

Figure 8-1-2 Insertion via subclavian artery

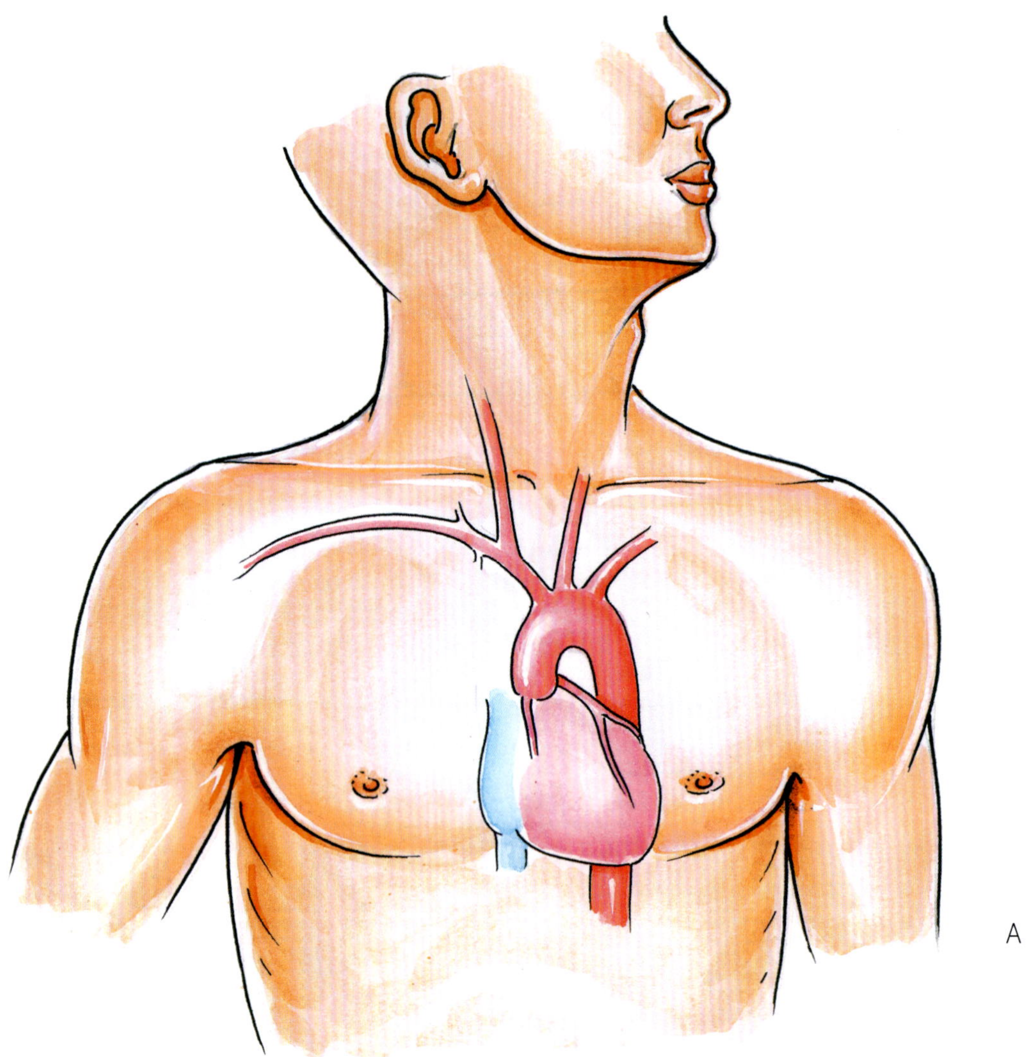

A. 仰卧位，头转向左侧。

A. The patient is positioned in the supine position with the head turning to the left.

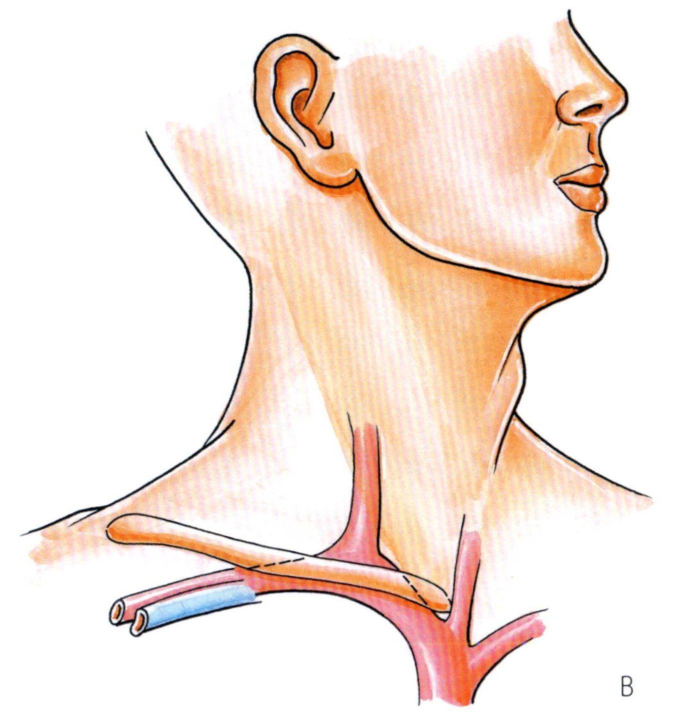

B. 右锁骨下动脉近心端作为穿刺点。

B. The right subclavian artery close to the heart serves as the puncture point.

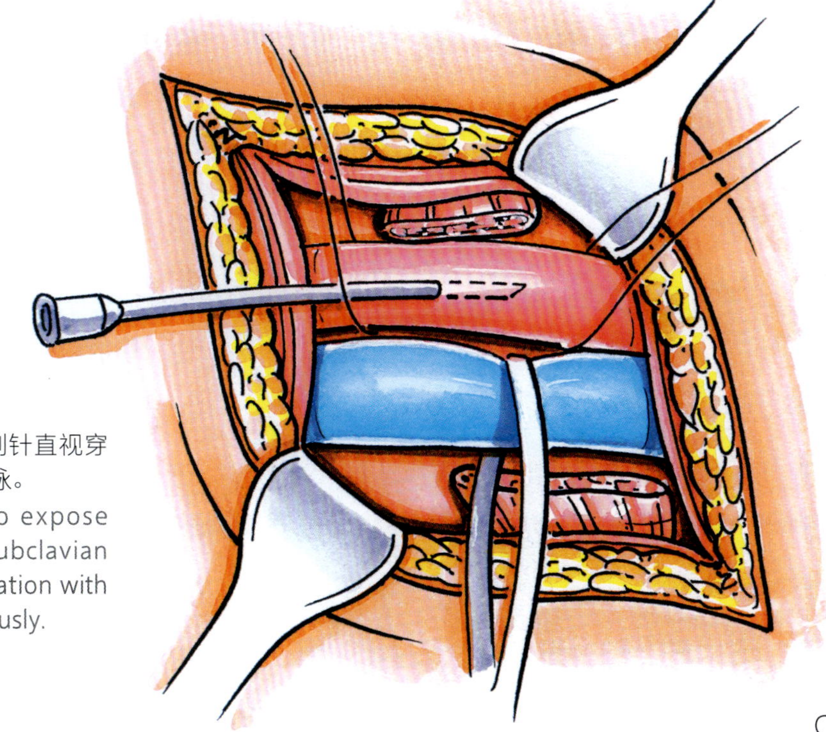

C. 锁骨下切口显露右锁骨下动脉。动脉穿刺针直视穿刺右锁骨下动脉。亦可经皮穿刺右锁骨下动脉。

C. The subclavian incision is made to expose the right subclavian artery. The right subclavian arterial is punctured under direct visualization with an arterial needle or punctured percutaneously.

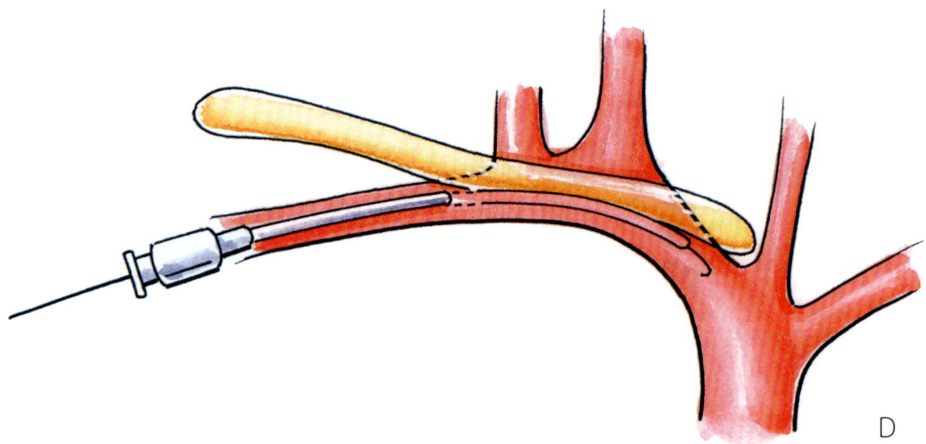

D. 经穿刺针将导引钢丝送入右锁骨下动脉，进而深入到降主动脉。

D. The guidewire is introduced by the needle into the right subclavian artery and then into the descending aorta.

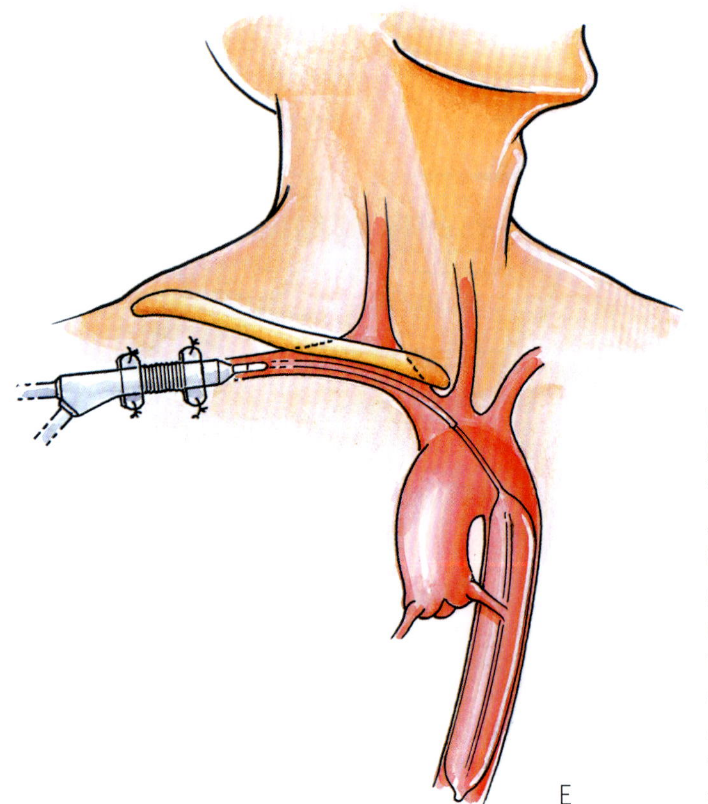

E. 退出穿刺针后，先循导引钢丝插入扩张管扩张锁骨下动脉穿刺孔，然后插入鞘管。循导引钢丝经鞘管插入球囊导管至降主动脉，球囊勿覆盖左锁骨下动脉开口以免影响其血供。

E. After withdrawing the needle, first follow the guidewire to insert the dilation tube to expand the puncture hole of the subclavian artery and then insert the sheath. Follow the guidewire to insert the balloon catheter through the sheath into the descending aorta. The balloon should not cover the opening of the left subclavian artery in order to avoid affecting the blood supply.

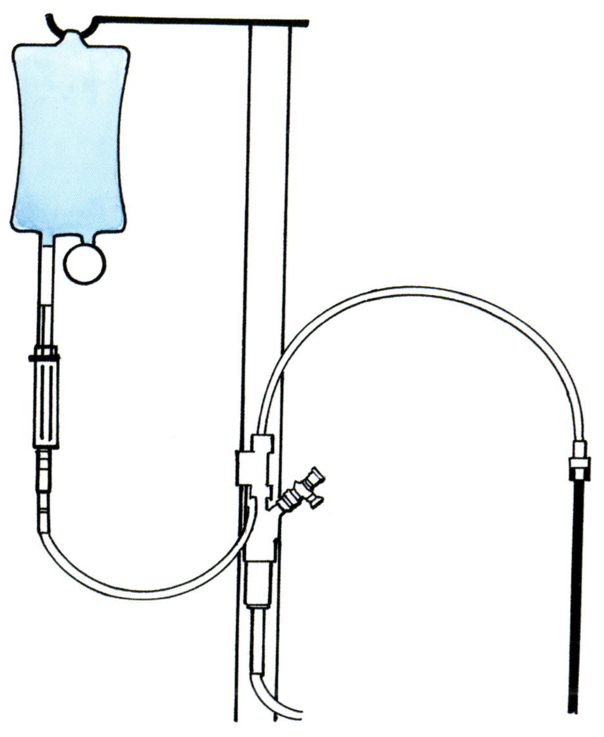

F. 连接球囊导管的测压管。

F. Connect the pressure-measuring tube of the balloon catheter.

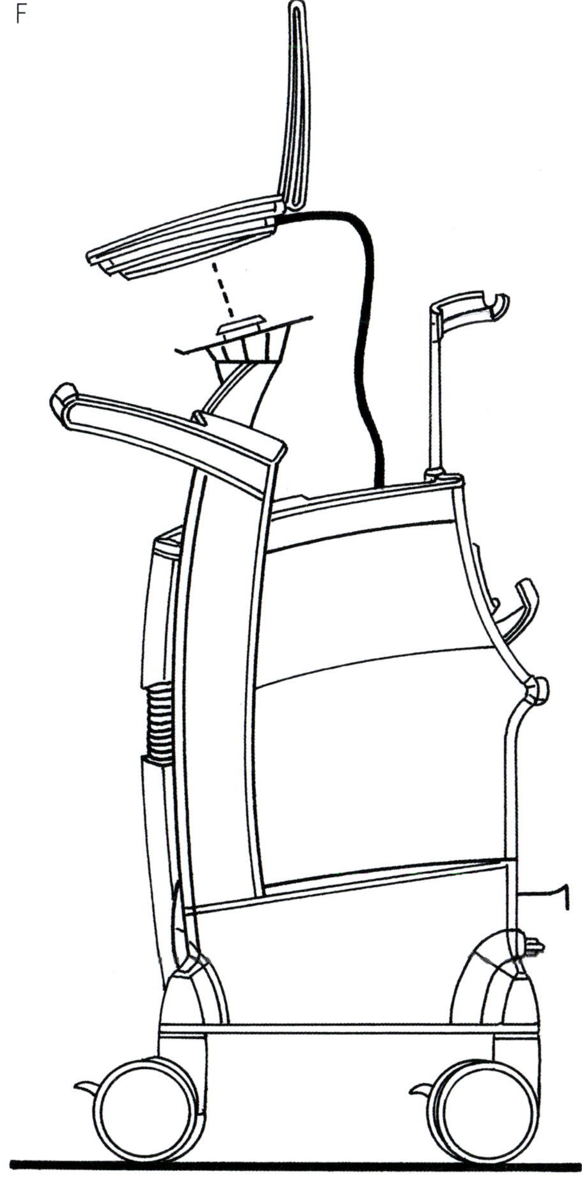

G. 将球囊导管的充放气管与反搏机相接。

G. Connect the inflation/deflation tube of the balloon catheter to the counterpulsation device.

图 8-1-3　经升主动脉插入
Figure 8-1-3　Insertion via ascending aorta

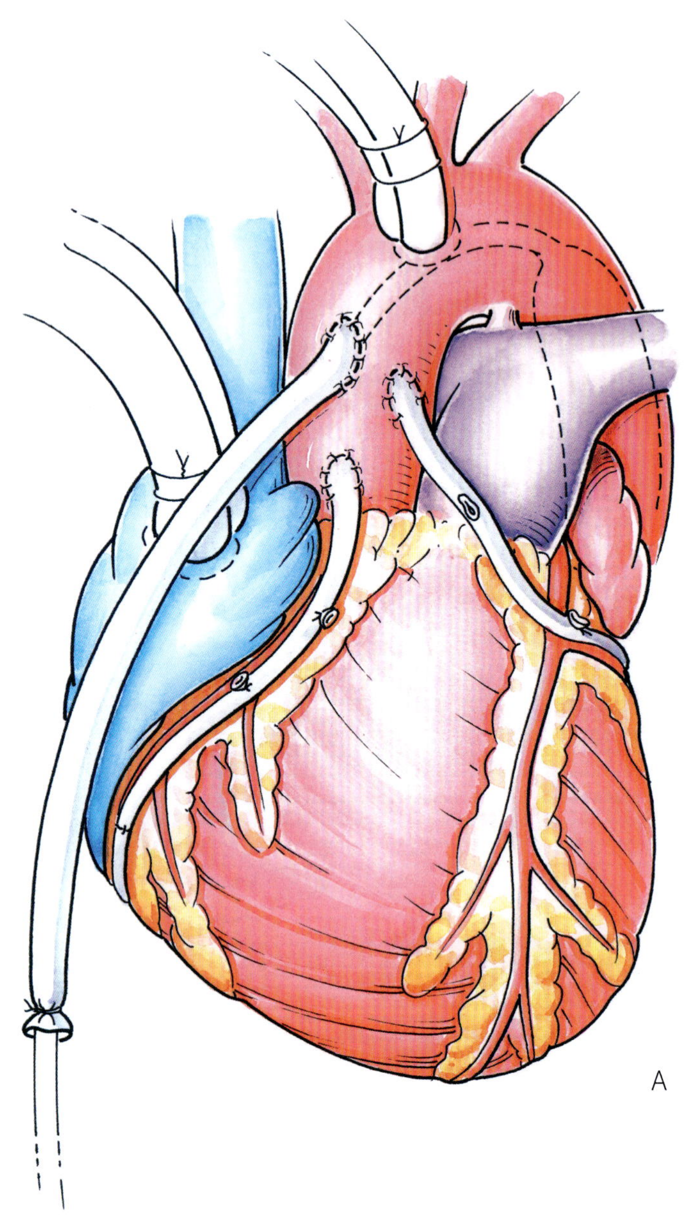

A. 体外循环心脏手术时用一段大隐静脉与升主动脉端侧吻合形成一旁路，经该旁路血管插入球囊导管至降主动脉。

A. During cardiac surgery with extracorporeal circulation support, a segment of the great saphenous vein is end-to-side anastomosed to the ascending aorta to form a bypass, through which a balloon catheter is inserted into the descending aorta.

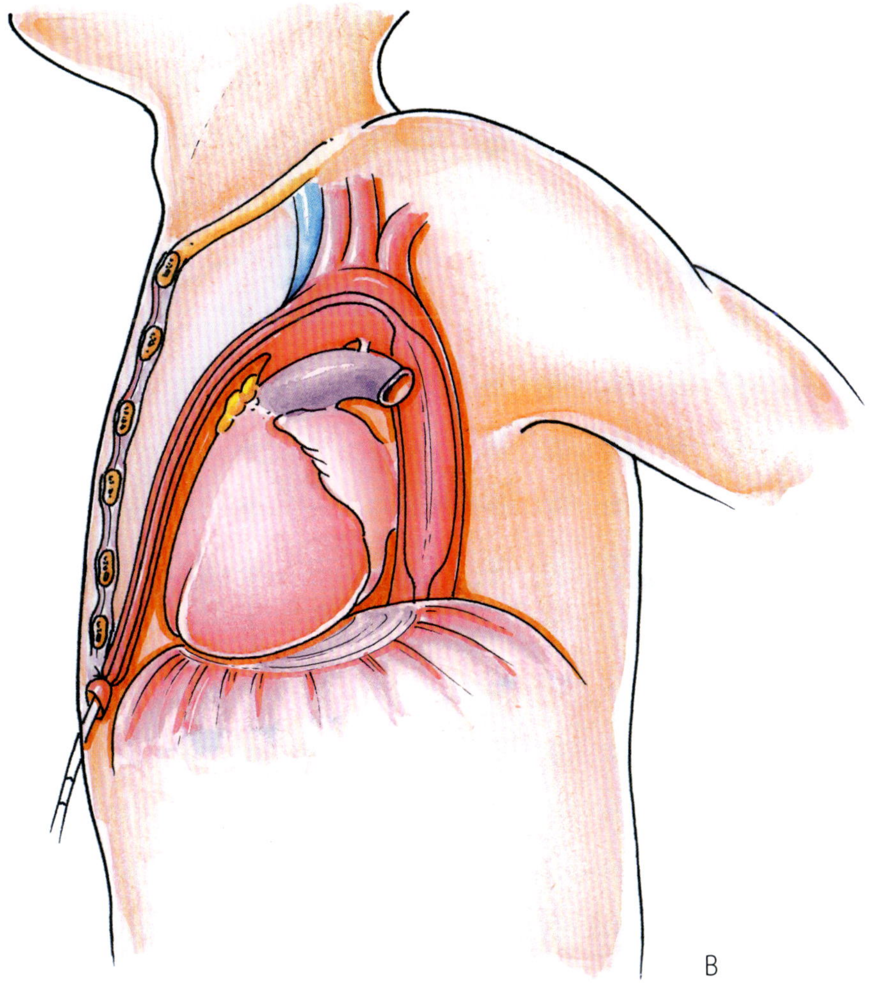

B. 球囊导管经前纵隔由剑突下戳口引出，关闭胸部切口。

B. The balloon catheter is brought out of an opening under the xiphoid process through the anterior mediastinum, and the thoracic incision is closed.

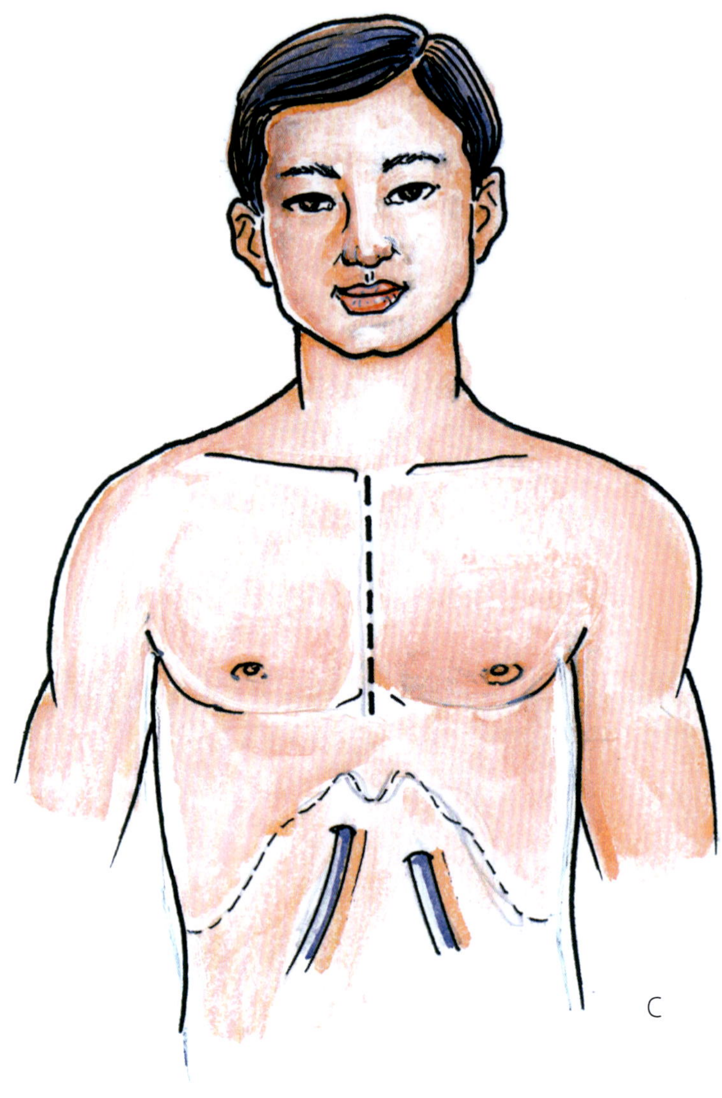

C. 右侧为球囊导管，左侧是胸腔引流管。

C. The balloon catheter is on the right side and the thoracic draining tube is on the left.

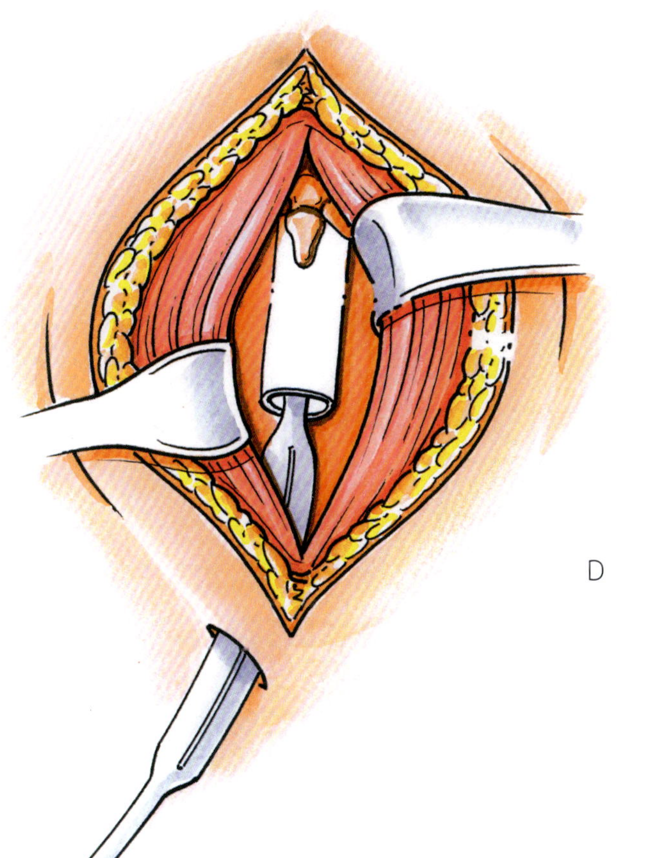

D

D. 停用主动脉内球囊反搏后再次打开原胸骨正中切口，撤出球囊导管。

D. After discontinuing the aortic balloon counterpulsation, the prior median sternal incision is opened again to withdraw the balloon catheter.

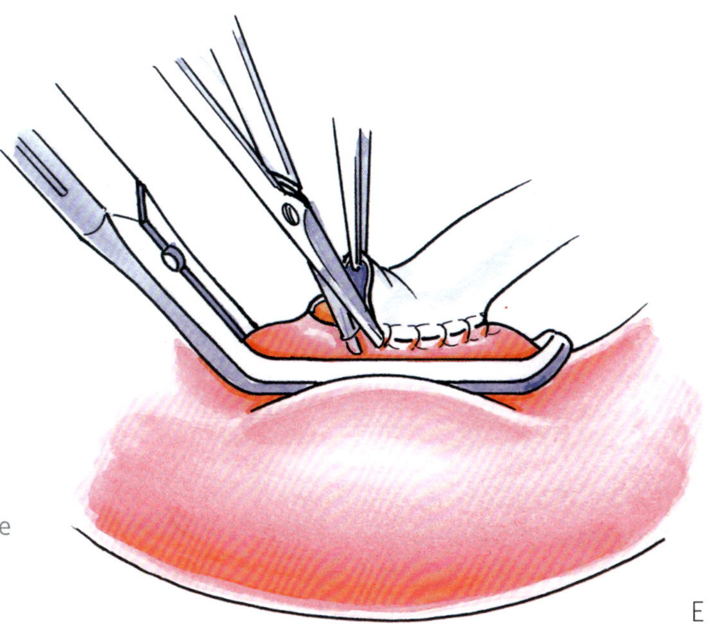

E

E. 侧壁钳钳夹升主动脉，拆除大隐静脉旁路。

E. The ascending aorta is side-clamped to remove the great saphenous vein bypass.

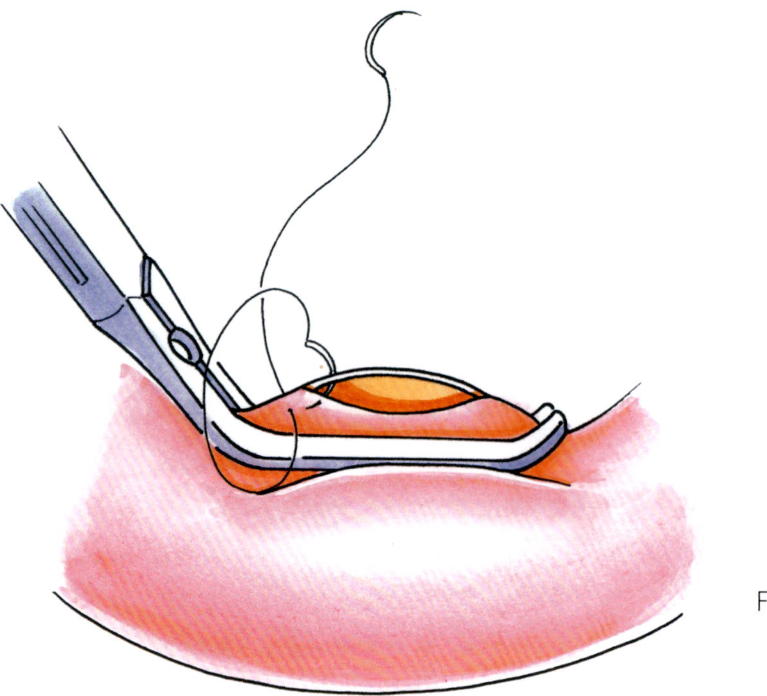

F. 缝合升主动脉遗留的孔洞。
F. Suture the holes left at the ascending aorta.

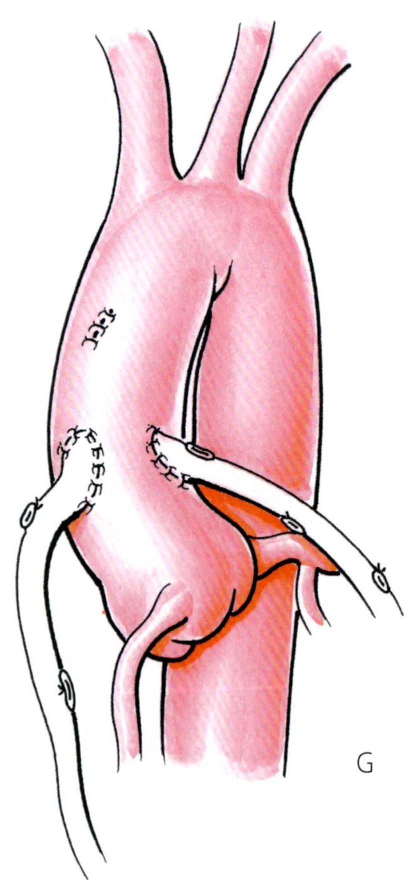

G. 升主动脉处理完毕。
G. Treatment of the ascending aorta is completed.

第 二 节　体外膜氧合
Section 2　Extracorporeal Membrane Oxygenation

图 8-2-1　**静脉-动脉体外膜氧合**
Figure 8-2-1　**Veno-arterial extracorporeal membrane oxygenation**

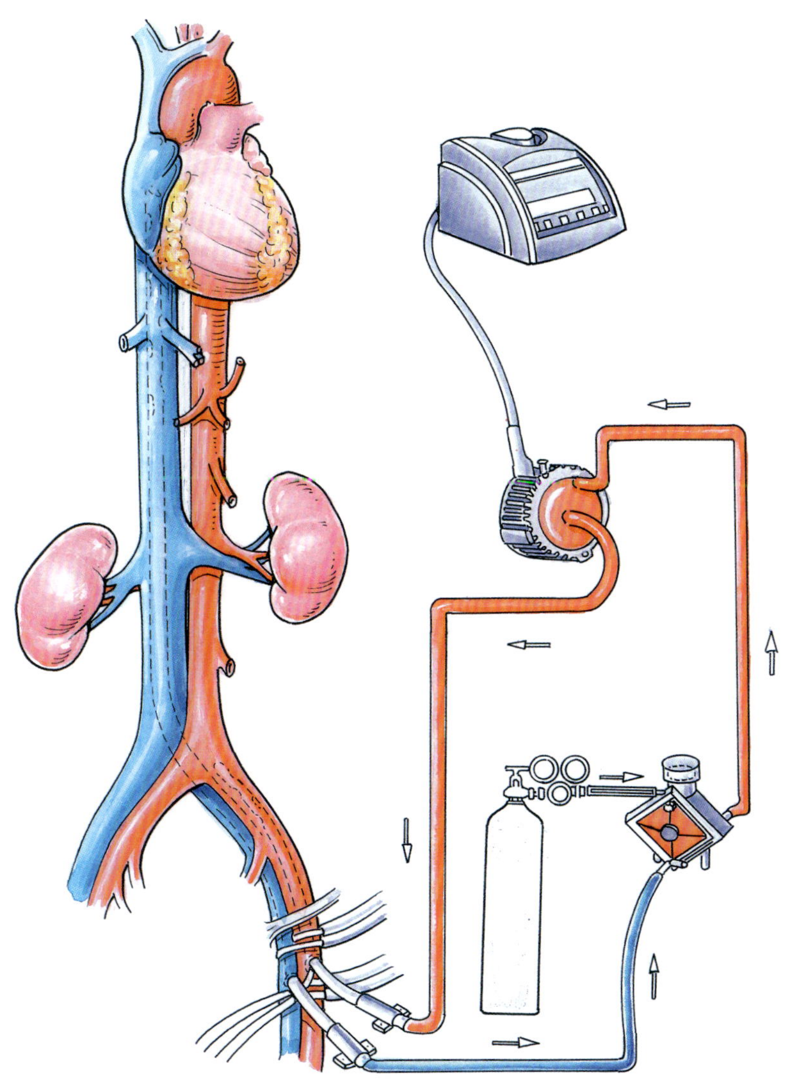

在不开胸情况下，成人经股动、静脉建立体外膜氧合（ECMO）。经股静脉将引流管插入到右心房，股动脉插供血管。静脉引流管连接至氧合器，供血管连接到血泵，建立静脉-动脉 ECMO 回路。此法股静脉回流的静脉血氧合后送入股动脉，用于循环、呼吸功能的支持。

Extracorporeal membrane oxygenation (ECMO) is established via the femoral artery and femoral vein in adults without thoracotomy. The draining cannula is inserted into the right atrium via the femoral vein and the arterial arterial cannulation is inserted into the femoral artery. The venous drainage tube is connected to the oxygenator and the arterial cannulation is connected to the blood pump to establish the veno-arterial ECMO circuit. The venous blood returning from the femoral vein is oxygenated and then sent to the femoral artery for circulatory and respiratory support.

图 8-2-2 静脉-静脉体外膜氧合
Figure 8-2-2 Veno-venous extracorporeal membrane oxygenation

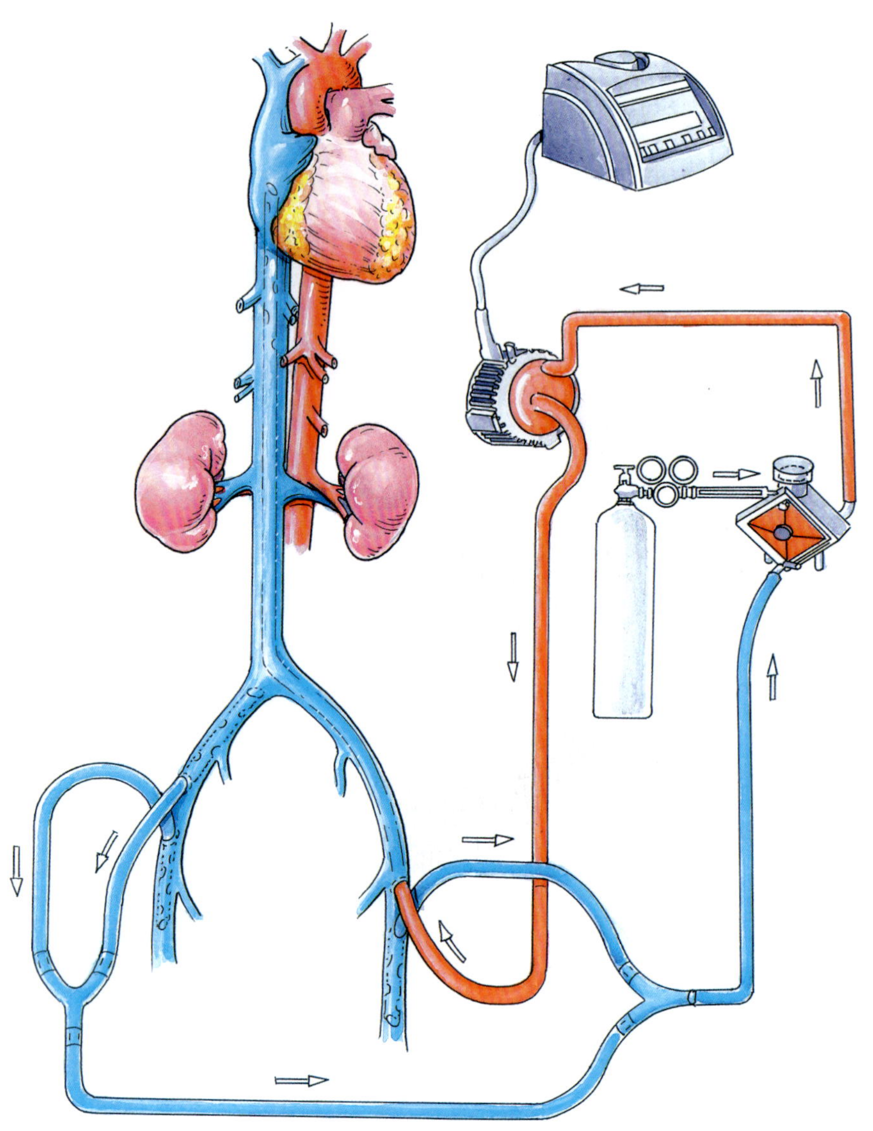

左股静脉插供血管至右心房，供血管另一端连接到血泵。左股静脉远端和右股静脉近、远端分别插入静脉引流管，再将静脉引流管用三通接头汇总后连接至氧合器，建立静脉-静脉 ECMO 回路。此法股静脉回流的静脉血氧合后送入右心房，用于呼吸功能的支持。

The arterial cannulation is inserted into the right atrium through the left femoral vein with the other end of the arterial cannulation connected to the blood pump. Insert venous draining cannulas into the distal end of the left femoral vein and the proximal and distal ends of the right femoral vein respectively. Use a three-way connector to ensure venous draining cannulas confluence, which is then connected to the oxygenator to establish a veno-venous ECMO circuit. In this approach, the venous blood returning from the femoral vein is oxygenated and returned to the right atrium for respiratory support.

图 8-2-3　ECMO 在心脏手术后的应用
Figure 8-2-3　ECMO underwent postcardiotomy

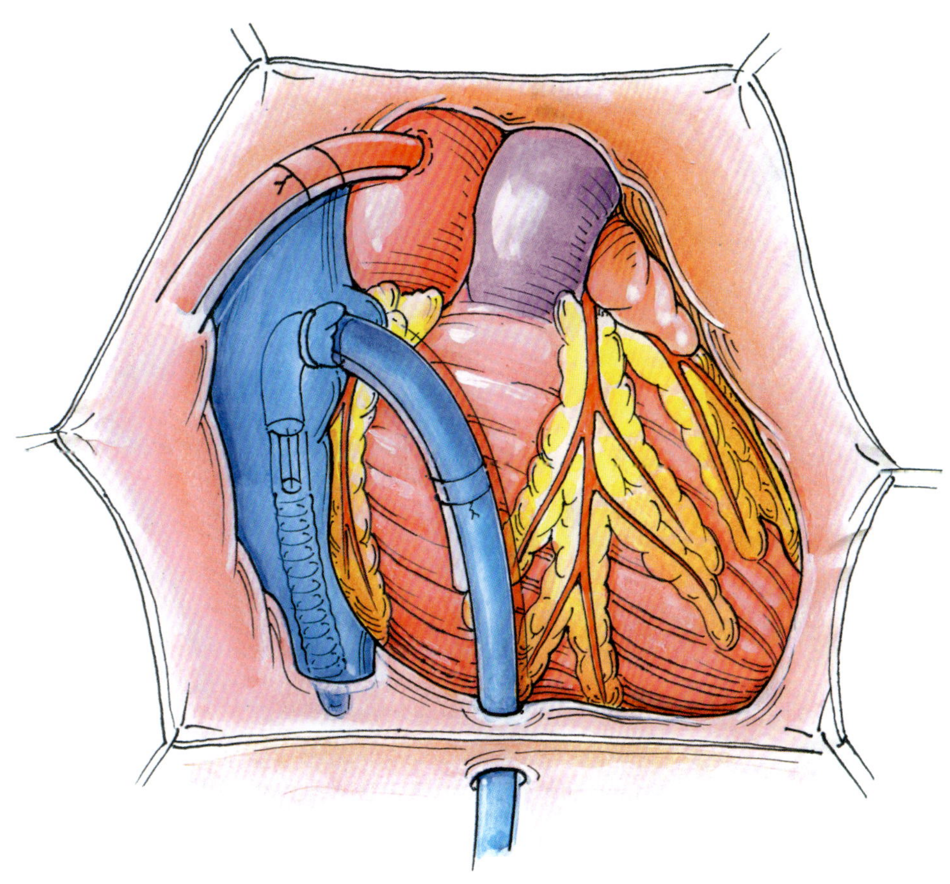

心脏手术后心脏低排脱离体外循环困难时，利用体外循环的动、静脉插管引出建立 ECMO 回路。

When it is difficult to wean the low-output heart from the extracorporeal circulation after cardiac surgery, the arterial and venous cannulas of the extracorporeal circulation are used to establish the ECMO circuit.

图 8-2-4　ECMO 与主动脉内球囊反搏同时应用
Figure 8-2-4　ECMO concomitantly intra-aortic balloon pump

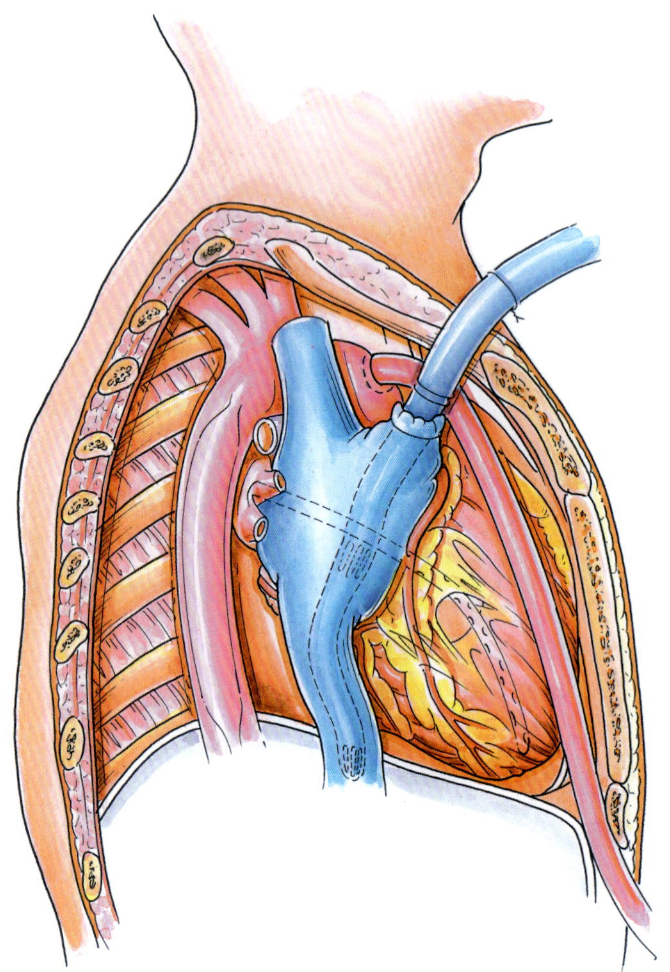

A

A. 静脉引流管经右心耳插入右心房，由胸骨上窝上方引出。升主动脉插供血管，由剑突下方引出。

A. The venous draining cannula is inserted into the right atrium through the right atrial appendage and brought out from the upper part of the sternal suprasternal fossa. The arterial arterial cannulation is inserted into the ascending aorta and brought out from below the xiphoid process.

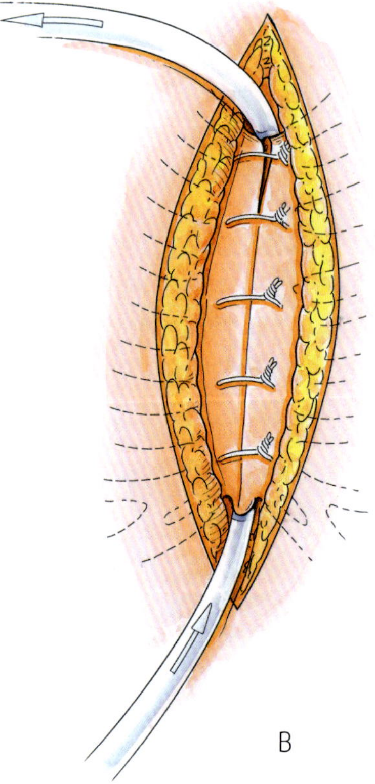

B

B. 缝合关闭胸骨正中切口。

B. Suture to close the median sternal incision.

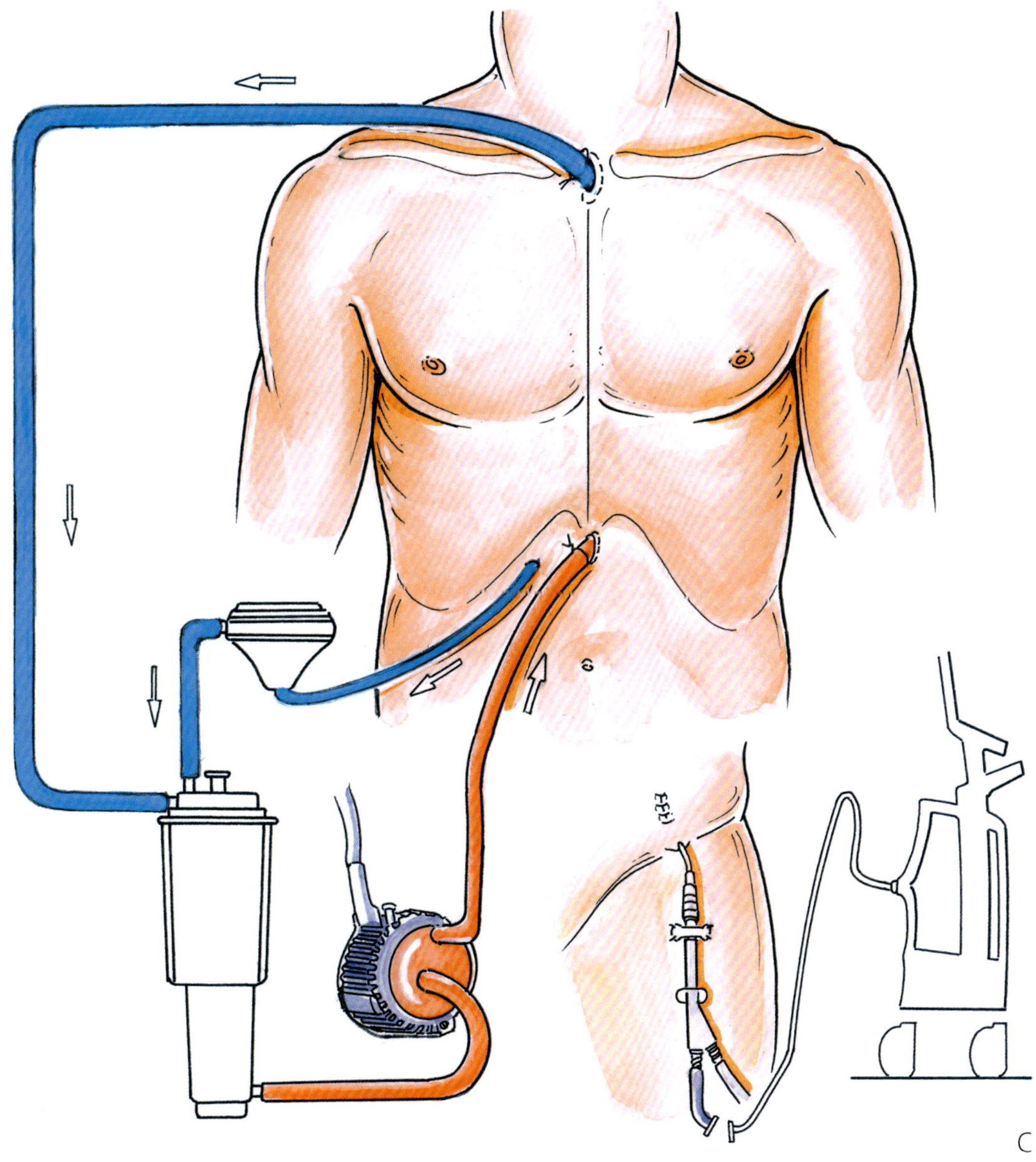

C. 静脉引流管连接至氧合器，供血管连接到血泵，建立静脉-动脉 ECMO 回路。另外一根心包引流管也通过滤器连接到氧合器，将渗出的血液氧合后回输。经股动脉插入球囊导管，建立主动脉内球囊反搏。

C. The veno-arterial ECMO circuit is established with the venous draining cannula connected to the oxygenator and the arterial cannulation connected to the blood pump. Another pericardial draining tube connected to the oxygenator through a filter returns oxygenated exudate blood. A balloon catheter is inserted through the femoral artery to establish intra-aortic balloon pump.

图 8-2-5　ECMO 在婴幼儿和儿童中的应用
Figure 8-2-5　ECMO for infants and children

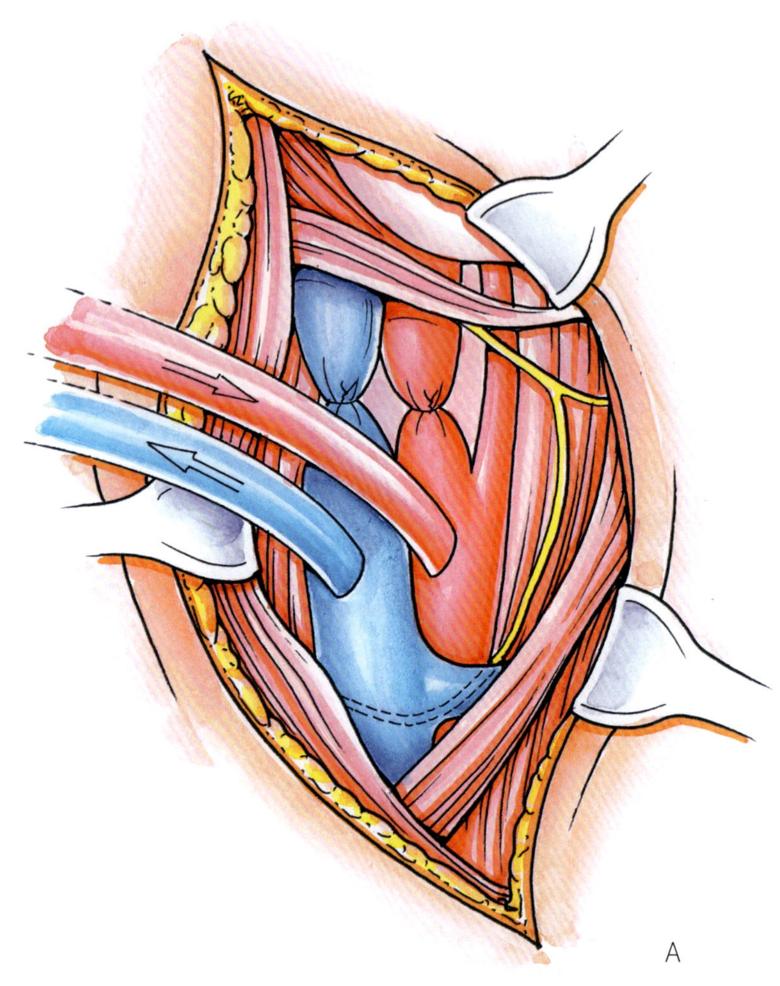

A. 在不开胸情况下，婴幼儿经外周血管建立 ECMO。婴幼儿由于股动、静脉细小，须经颈部切口显露颈总动脉和颈静脉并分别插入供血管和静脉引流管。

A. ECMO is established through peripheral vessels in infants and children without thoracotomy. Because of the small femoral arteries and veins of infants and children, the common carotid artery and jugular vein are exposed through a neck incision to be inserted with the arterial cannulation and the venous draining cannula respectively.

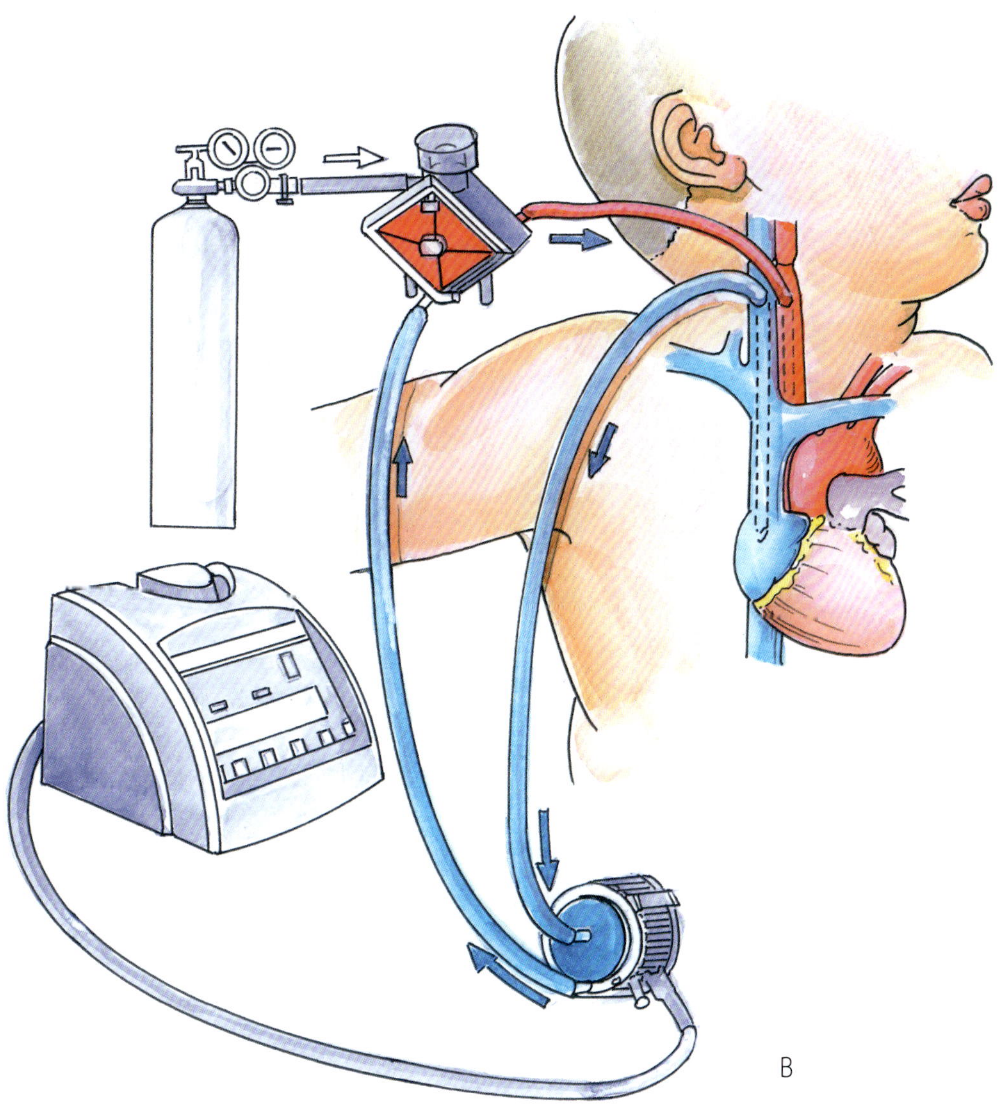

B. 供血管连接至氧合器，静脉引流管连接到血泵，实施静脉-动脉 ECMO。

B. The veno-arterial ECMO is instituted with the arterial cannulation connected to the oxygenator and the venous draining cannula connected to the blood pump.

第 三 节　心室辅助装置

Section 3　Ventricular Assist Device

Excor 心室辅助装置

Excor ventricular assist device

Excor 是柏林心脏公司设计的一个体外、气体驱动的机械式心室辅助装置（ventricular assist device，VAD），用于左心室、右心室或双心室辅助［左心室辅助装置（left ventricular assist device，LVAD）、右心室辅助装置（right ventricular assist device，RVAD）或双心室辅助装置（biventricular ventricular assist device，BVAD）］。

Excor is an extracorporeal, gas-driven, mechanical ventricular assist device (VAD) designed by Berlin Heart Corporation for left ventricular, right ventricular, or biventricular assist (left ventricular assist device [LVAD], right ventricular assist device [RVAD], or biventricular ventricular assist device [BVAD]).

整套系统包含：

The complete system consists of:

1. **血液泵**　Excor 系统最主要组件为外挂于患者体外的血液泵，其外壳由聚氨酯（PU）制成，内部以三层黑色隔膜将血液泵分隔为一个气腔和一个血腔，腔室中凡与血液接触部分都有抗凝血剂涂层。Excor 泵具有不同的容量（10ml、25ml、30ml、50ml、60ml、80ml）供选择，目的在于使其能适用于各种体型及由新生儿到老年各个年龄层的患者。

1. **Blood Pump**　The main component of the Excor system is an extracorporeal blood pump with a housing made of polyurethane (PU). The blood pump is divided into an air chamber and a blood chamber by three layers of black diaphragms with all blood-contacting surfaces of the chamber coated with anticoagulants. The Excor pumps, available in different volumes (10 ml, 25 ml, 30 ml, 50 ml, 60 ml, 80 ml), are suitable for patients of all sizes and from neonates to the elderly.

2. **插管**　分为流入插管与流出插管，由医疗级硅胶制成，具有四种不同管径尺寸及设计，以适用于各种正常及特殊情况。

2. **Cannula**　Divided into the inflow cannula and the outflow cannula, made of silicone dedicated for medical use, with four different diameters and designs to work in various normal and special settings.

3. **驱动主机**　系统配置两种不同驱动装置，分别为 Ikus 固定式驱动装置及移动式驱动装置。

3. **Drive Host**　The system is equipped with two different drive devices, namely Ikus stationary drive device and mobile drive device.

图 8-3-1　Excor 左心室辅助装置植入术
Figure 8-3-1　Implantation of Excor as a LVAD

A. 在体外循环支持下，使用侧壁钳夹住升主动脉，将升主动脉切开、打洞至适当大小，再将流出插管插入升主动脉并固定。

A. During extracorporeal circulation, with the ascending aorta side-clamped, an incision into the ascending aorta is made, and a hole of an appropriate size is made, and then the outflow cannula is inserted into the ascending aorta and fixed.

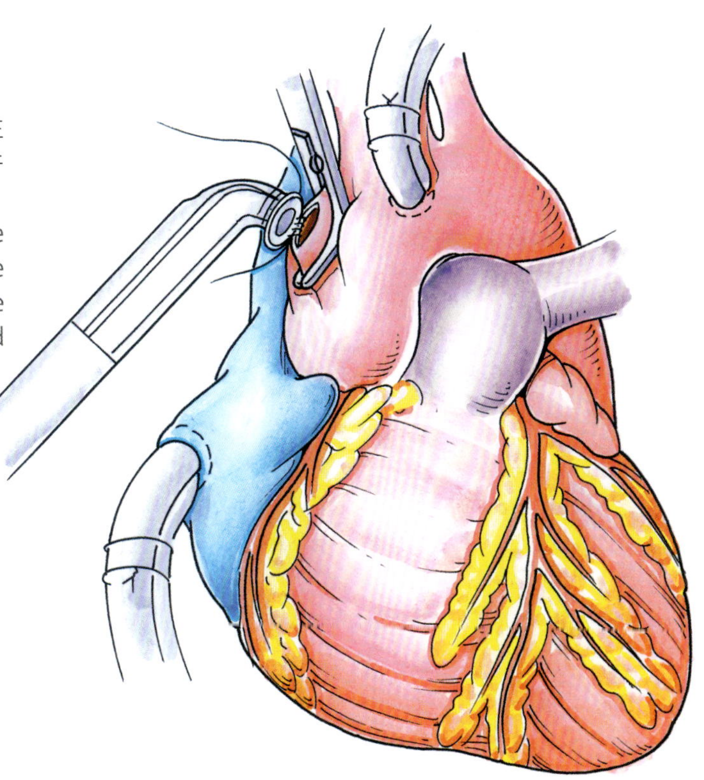

A

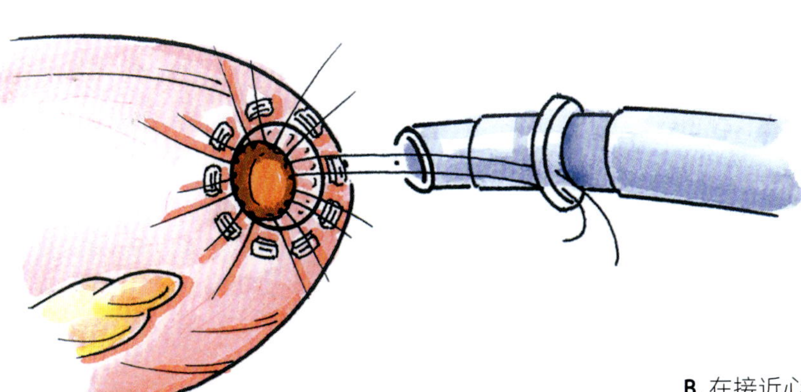

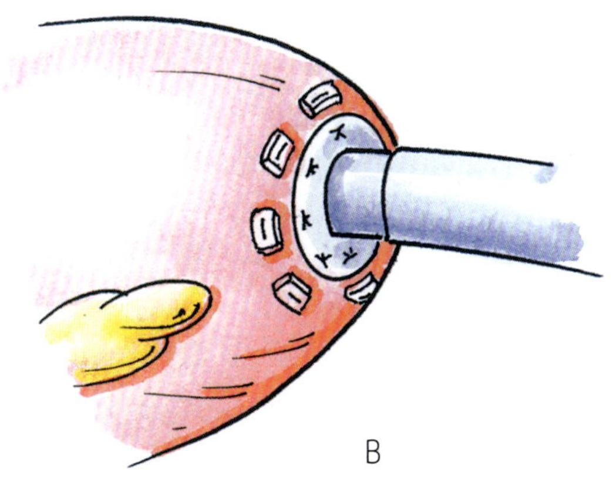

B

B. 在接近心尖的位置，以尖刀及组织剪切出略大于心室插管的圆孔，圆孔位置必须指向二尖瓣，并同时检查左心室内有无血栓。使用带垫片褥式缝线先缝入左心室心尖，大约 12 针，然后再把缝线缝入左心室插管（流入插管）的缝合环。最后将插管插入左心室并逐一打结。

B. At the position close to the heart apex, use tissue scissors and a sharp knife to cut a round hole, which is slightly larger than the ventricular cannula and must point to the mitral valve, and at the same time, check whether there is thrombus in the left ventricle. Suture the left ventricle apex, approximately 12 stitches, and then the sewing ring of the left ventricular cannula (the inflow cannula) using a pledgeted mattress suture. Knot one by one following the insertion of the cannula into the left ventricle.

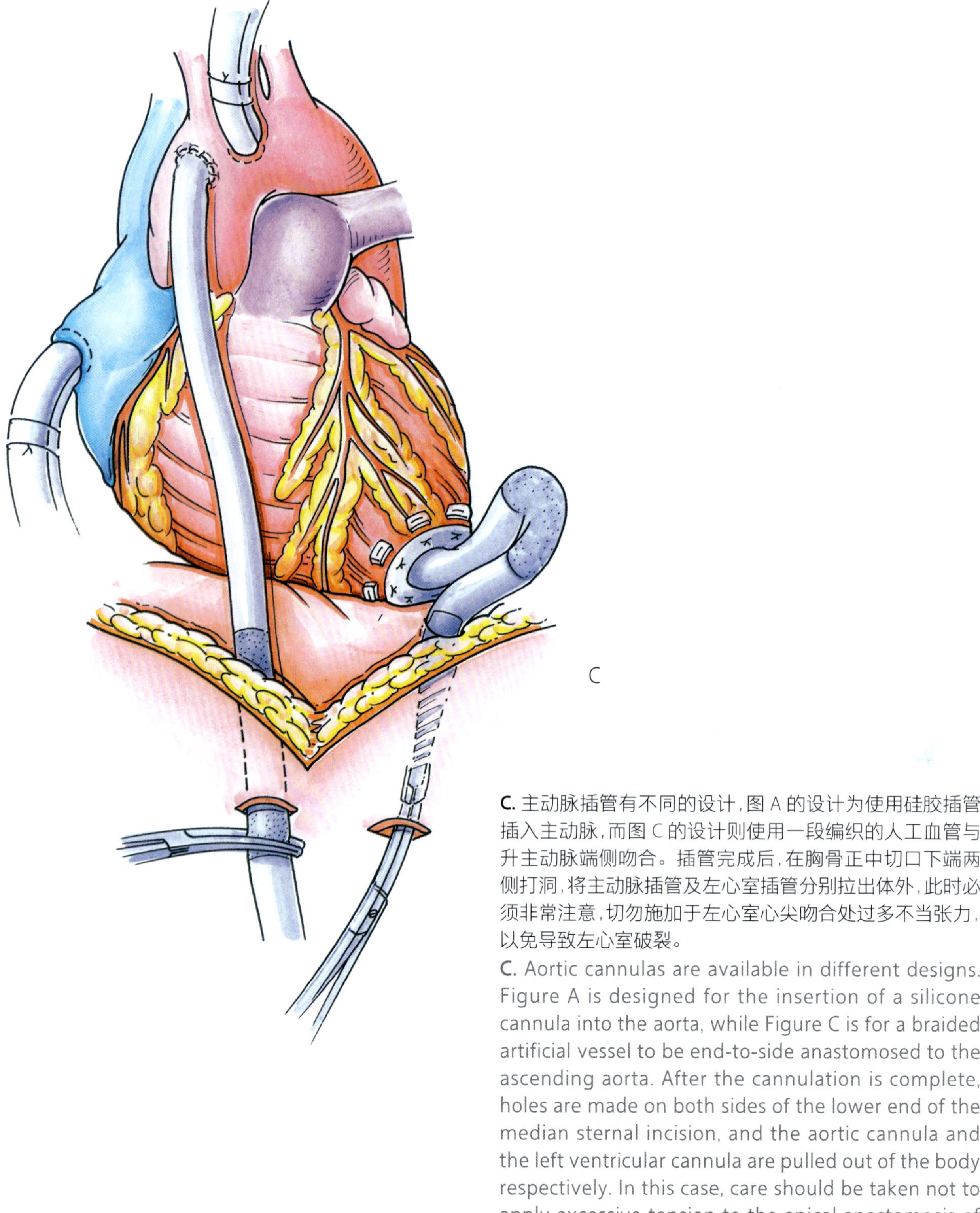

C. 主动脉插管有不同的设计，图 A 的设计为使用硅胶插管插入主动脉，而图 C 的设计则使用一段编织的人工血管与升主动脉端侧吻合。插管完成后，在胸骨正中切口下端两侧打洞，将主动脉插管及左心室插管分别拉出体外，此时必须非常注意，切勿施加于左心室心尖吻合处过多不当张力，以免导致左心室破裂。

C. Aortic cannulas are available in different designs. Figure A is designed for the insertion of a silicone cannula into the aorta, while Figure C is for a braided artificial vessel to be end-to-side anastomosed to the ascending aorta. After the cannulation is complete, holes are made on both sides of the lower end of the median sternal incision, and the aortic cannula and the left ventricular cannula are pulled out of the body respectively. In this case, care should be taken not to apply excessive tension to the apical anastomosis of the left ventricle to avoid rupture of the left ventricle.

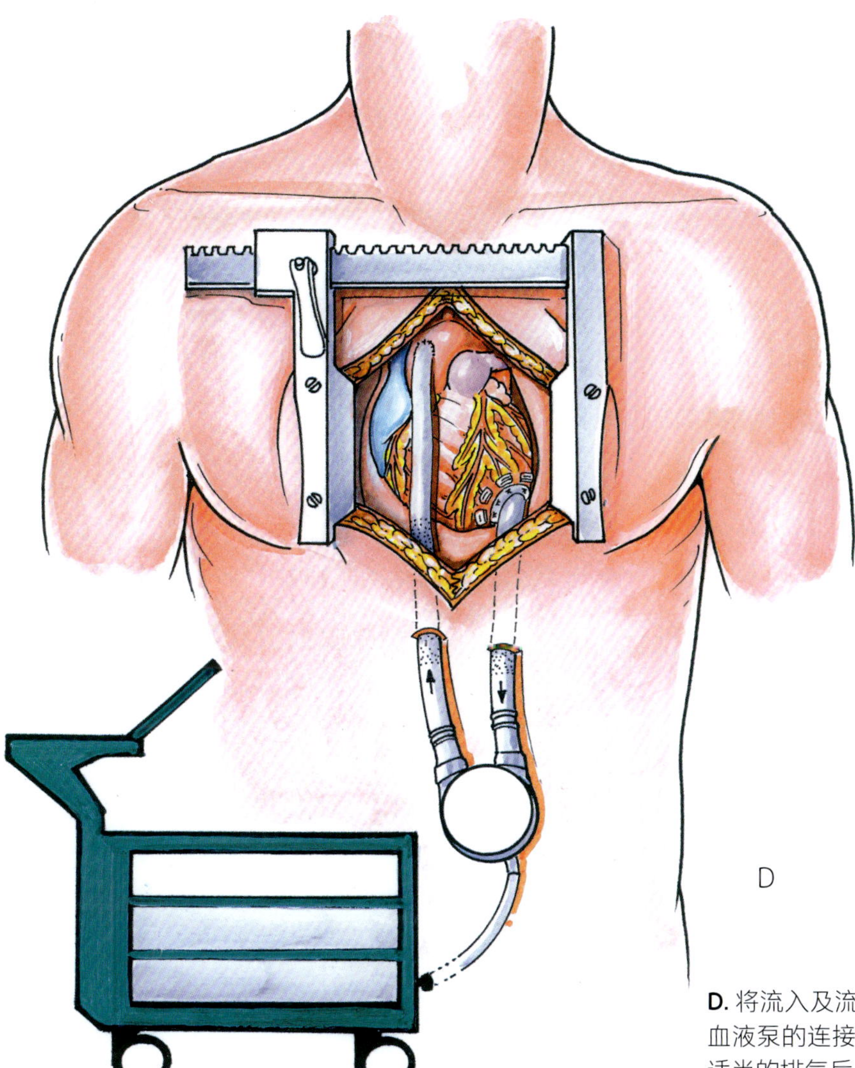

D

D. 将流入及流出插管连接至血液泵，此时必须注意管道与血液泵的连接方向必须正确。之后启动左心室辅助装置，适当的排气后，慢慢脱离体外循环，并且将体外循环插管移除，完成手术。

D. Connect the inflow and outflow cannulas to the blood pump, making sure that the tubing and the blood pump are connected in the right direction. Activate the left ventricular assist device and perform de-airing. The patient is then slowly weaned off cardiopulmonary bypass. Remove the cardiopulmonary bypass cannulas to complete the procedure.

图 8-3-2 Excor 双心室辅助装置植入术
Figure 8-3-2 Implantation of Excor as a BVAD

Excor 心室辅助装置的原始设计理念除了可以提供给不同年龄、不同体型的左心衰竭患者使用之外，它还可以辅助右心循环的插管以及驱动主机，使其可以在单独右心衰竭的患者中作为 RVAD 使用，或者是左、右心同时衰竭的患者作为 BVAD 使用。

According to the original design concept, the Excor ventricular assist device can not only be used for the left heart failure patients of different ages and body sizes, but also be used as RVAD in patients with right heart failure alone or as BVAD in patients with left and right heart failure simultaneously, because the cannula and drive frame have been designed to assist the right heart circulation.

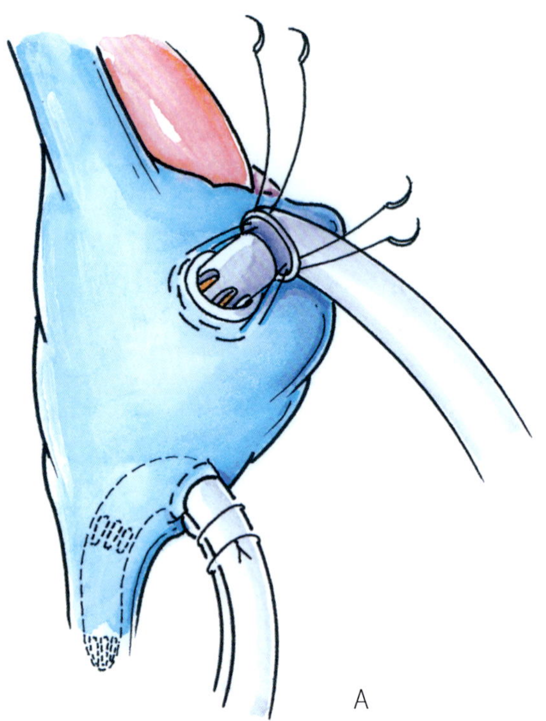

A. LVAD 部分的手术方式如图 8-3-1 所述。而在 RVAD 的部分，将右心房略靠中央位置先进行两个荷包缝合，荷包缝合的大小不能太小，以免手术后插管处出血。再将两对缝线穿过插管的缝合环并打结，打完结后使用原来的针线，以连续缝合的方法，缝合左右侧缝合环，以确保缝合处的止血及稳定。

A. The LVAD procedure is described in Figure 8-3-1. In the RVAD procedure, two purse-string sutures are first performed slightly in the center on the right atrium. The purses should not be too small to avoid postoperative bleeding at the cannulation site. Then two pairs of sutures pass through the sewing ring of the cannula and are knotted. After knotting, use the original needles and sutures to continuously suture the sewing rings at the left and right sides to ensure hemostasis and stability at the sutured site.

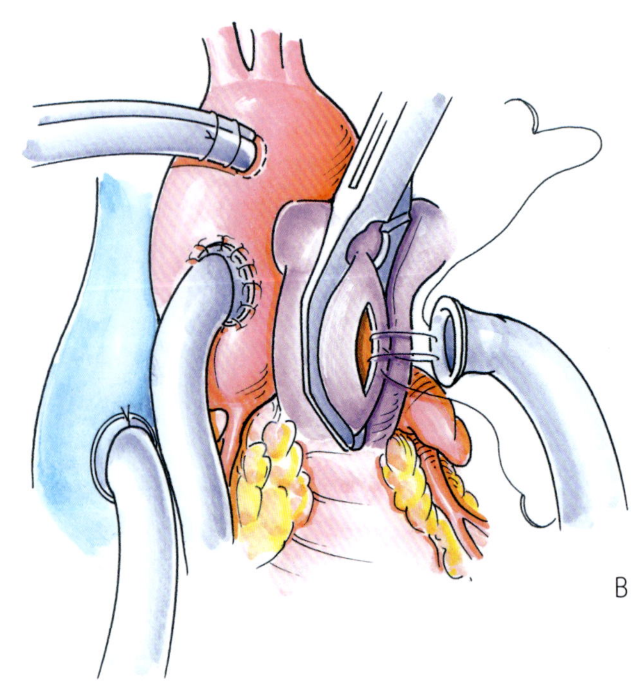

B. 肺动脉处的插管吻合做法，类似主动脉插管的方法。先以侧壁钳夹住肺动脉干，将肺动脉切开适当大小后，与流入插管进行吻合。

B. The cannulation anastomosis procedure at the pulmonary artery is similar to that for aortic cannulation. With the pulmonary trunk side-clamped, the pulmonary artery is incised to an appropriate size before anastomosis with the inflow cannula.

C. 再将 RVAD 的两根插管穿出体外。在进行 BVAD 手术的时候必须要注意，如果患者胸腔内空间比较小，升主动脉及肺动脉插管的交叉位置宜放在体外，以避免纵隔腔空间不足，造成切口缝合困难。

C. The two cannulas of RVAD are brought out of the body. When performing BVAD surgery, it must be noted that if the intrathoracic space is relatively small, the intersection of the ascending aorta and the pulmonary artery cannulas should be placed outside the body to avoid insufficient space in the mediastinal cavity resulting in difficulty in incision closing.

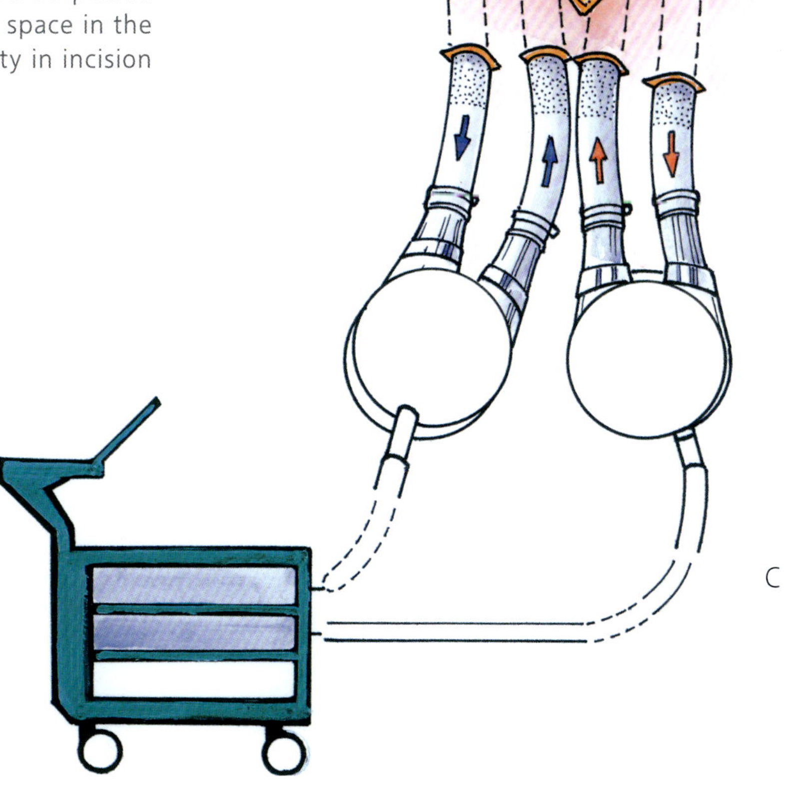

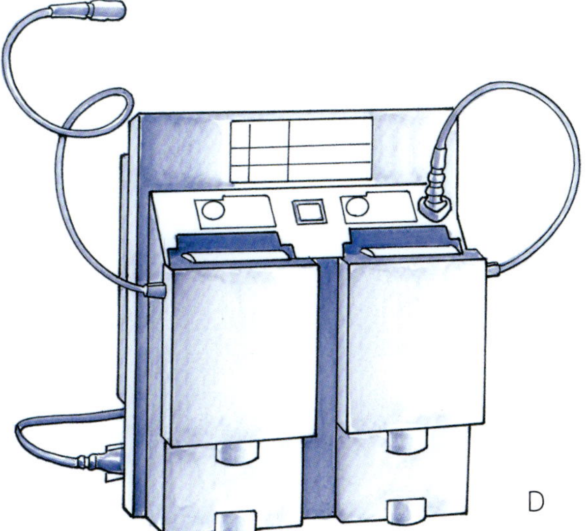

D. Excor 心室辅助的移动式驱动装置，如果配上原厂小型行李箱样推车，在行动上将会非常便利。

D. The Excor ventricular assist mobile drive device will be very convenient to move if it is accompanied by a small suitcase-like cart provided by the same manufacturer.

Impella 心室辅助装置
Impella ventricular assist device

Impella 是一个导管式微型心室辅助装置，以古希腊数学家阿基米德螺旋抽水机原理设计来支持左心室。适用于高危险性经皮冠状动脉介入治疗患者，提供小于 6 小时的暂时性心室支持。也适用于急性心肌梗死合并心源性休克的患者，提供 4~14 天的暂时性心室支持。

The Impella, a catheter-based miniaturized ventricular assist device, is designed to support the left ventricle using the spiral pump principle proposed by ancient Greek mathematician Archimedes. It is indicated in patients undergoing high-risk percutaneous coronary intervention, providing temporary ventricular support for less than 6 hours. It is also indicated in patients with acute myocardial infarction combined with cardiogenic shock, providing temporary ventricular support for 4-14 days.

Impella 启动、操作和维护简易，在临床上得到广泛地使用，但左心室血栓、主动脉瓣狭窄/钙化（相当于主动脉瓣口面积≤0.6cm^2）、使用主动脉人工机械瓣或心脏收缩装置、中度至严重的主动脉瓣关闭不全（心脏超声波评估为≥ ++）、严重的动脉疾病、心房或心室间隔缺损（包括梗死后室间隔缺损）、严重右心衰竭、左心室破裂、心脏压塞等情况，都是安装 Impella 的禁忌证。主动脉瓣膜损伤是使用 Impella 最严重的并发症，也是 Impella 在临床上只能用于暂时性心室辅助的原因。

The Impella, easy to start, operate, and maintain, is widely applied clinically, but it is contraindicated in patients with left ventricular thrombosis, aortic stenosis/calcification (i.e., aortic orifice area ≤0.6 cm^2), use of an aortic prosthetic mechanical valve or systolic device, moderate to severe aortic insufficiency (assessed by cardiac ultrasound as ≥++), severe arterial disease, atrial or ventricular septal defects (including post-infarction ventricular septal defects), severe right heart failure, left ventricle rupture, cardiac tamponade, etc. Aortic valve injury is the most severe complication in Impella use and the reason why the Impella can only be used clinically for temporary ventricular assistance.

整套系统包含：

The complete system consists of:

1. Impella 导管 是一个血管内微轴血液泵，导管远端的“猪尾巴”将导管稳定在左心室的正确位置。血液入口区域位于插管的远端，可将血液由左心室吸入。不透射线的标记物，可以通过 X 线检查看到，当其出现在主动脉瓣环水平时，表明导管放置位置正确。血液出口区域是插管的近端，血液由此注入主动脉。

1. Impella Catheter An intravascular micro axial blood pump with a “pigtail” at the distal end of the catheter, which stabilizes the catheter in the correct position in the left ventricle. The blood inlet, located at the distal end of the cannula, draws blood from the left ventricle. A radiopaque marker, which can be seen on X-ray, when present at the level of the aortic annulus, indicates the correct catheter placement. The blood outlet is located at the proximal end of the cannula from which blood is injected into the aorta.

2. 自动控制器 是 Impella 导管主要的控制界面。它控制 Impella 导管的性能，监控导管是否发出警报，并提供有关导管在主动脉瓣上位置的即时信息。面板显示器会呈现使用的压力及血液泵每分钟的实际转数。充满电后，控制器可以使用交流电源供电或使用内部电池电源运行至少 60 分钟。

美国阿比奥梅德公司设计出 Impella 2.5、Impella 5.0、Impella LD、Impella CP（Shock）、Impella CP（HRPCI）等机型。Impella 2.5、Impella 5.0 和 Impella CP 导管可由股动脉或腋动脉置入，Impella LD 则由升主动脉插入。其置入流程如下。

2. Automatic Controller As the main control interface for the Impella catheter, it controls the Impella catheter performance, monitors whether the catheter gives the alarm, and provides instant information about the position of the catheter on the aortic valve. The panel displays the pressure used and the actual revolutions per minute for the blood pump. When fully charged, the controller can operate with alternating current (AC) power or internal battery power for at least 60 minutes.

American ABIOMED designed Impella 2.5, Impella 5.0, Impella LD, Impella CP (Shock), Impella CP (HRPCI), and other models. Catheters in Impella 2.5, Impella 5.0, and Impella CP could be inserted through the femoral artery or the axillary artery, while Impella LD may be inserted through the ascending aorta. The insertion process is as follows.

图 8-3-3　Impella 左心室辅助装置植入术

Figure 8-3-3　Implantation of Impella as a LVAD

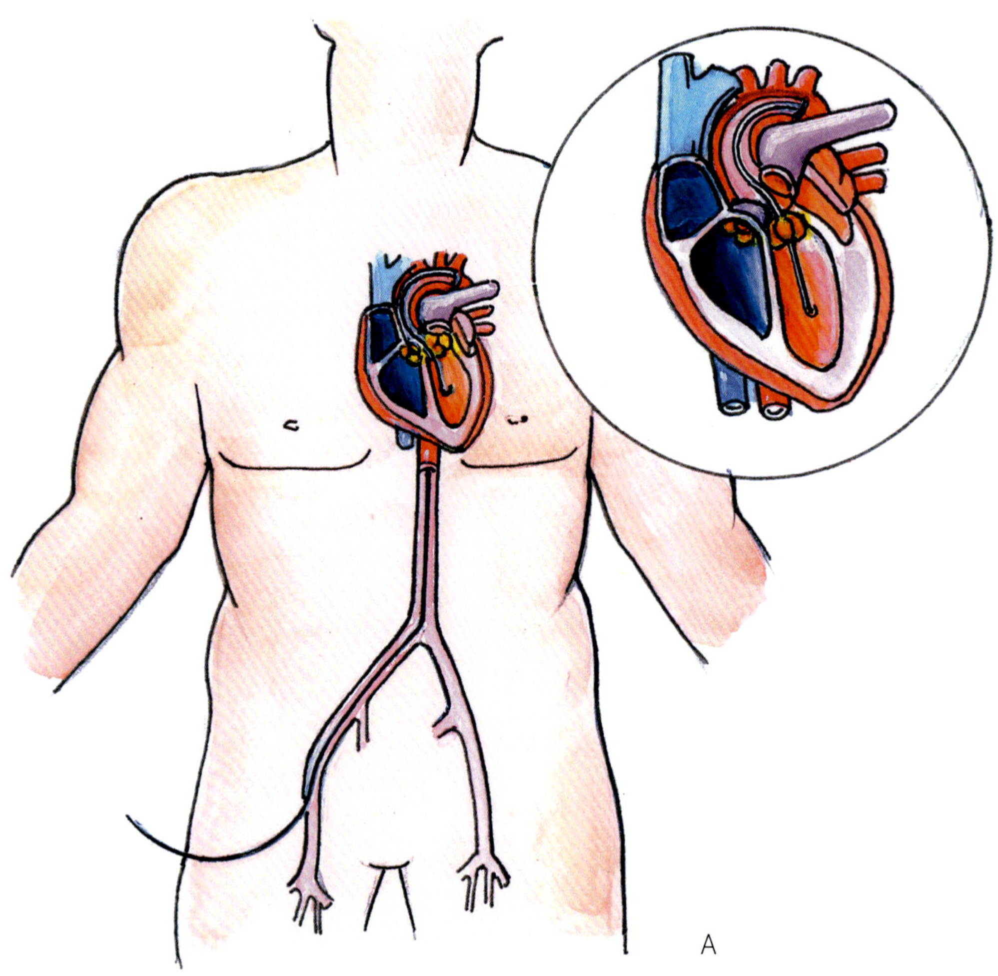

A. 由股动脉插入导管，在 X 线透视或心脏超声心动图的导引下，通过主动脉瓣到达左心室。Impella LD 直接由升主动脉插入后，置放在左心室。

A. An Impella catheter is inserted through the femoral artery and reaches the left ventricle through the aortic valve under fluoroscopy or echocardiography guidance. The Impella LD, inserted directly from the ascending aorta, is placed in the left ventricle.

B. 当导管上的"猪尾巴"到达左心室，自动控制器确认位置正确后，血液泵开始运转。由导管远端血液入口区，连续性地将左心室的血液抽吸进入导管通道，再通过近端的出口区把血液排入升主动脉。

B. When the "pigtail" on the catheter reaches the left ventricle and is confirmed by the automatic controller to be in the correct position, the blood pump starts running. The blood from the left ventricle is continuously drawn into the catheter through the inlet at the distal end of the catheter and discharged into the ascending aorta through the outlet at the proximal end of the catheter.

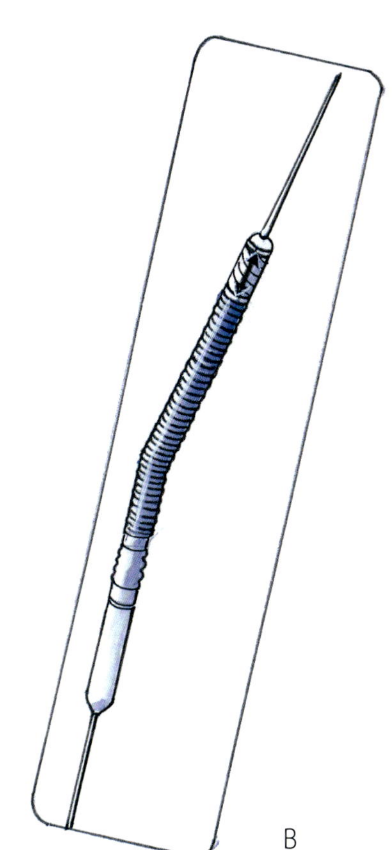

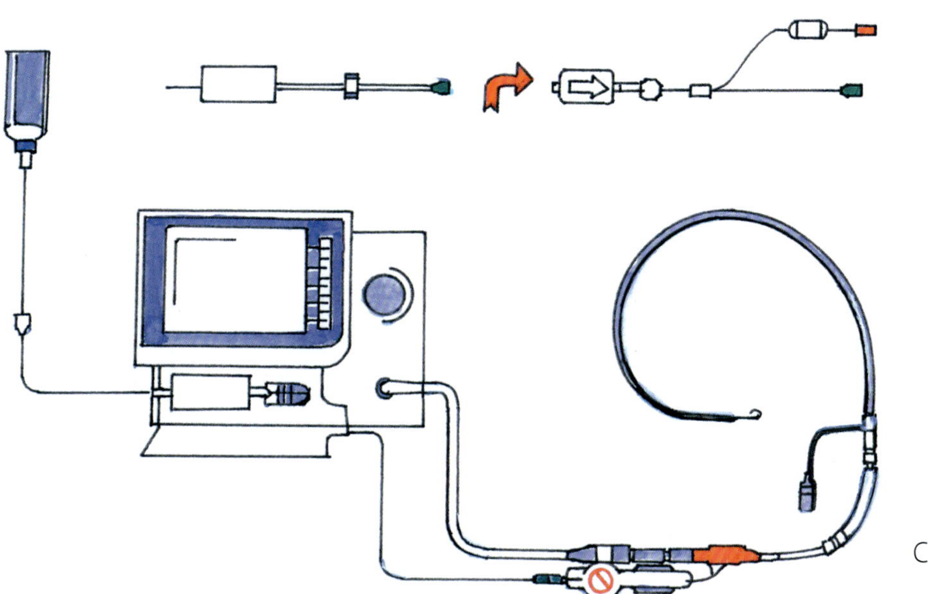

C. 从左心室向主动脉输送的血流量约 2.5~5L/min，以供应全身的血液循环。不同型号的装置输出不同的流量：2.5L/min（Impella 2.5）、3.7L/min（Impella CP）、5.0L/min（Impella 5.0 和 Impella LD）。

C. The blood volume delivered from the left ventricle to the aorta is approximately 2.5-5 L/min to supply systemic blood circulation. Different models have different outputs: 2.5 L/min (Impella 2.5), 3.7 L/min (Impella CP), 5.0 L/min (Impella 5.0 and Impella LD).

图 8-3-4 Impella 右心室辅助装置植入术
Figure 8-3-4 Implantation of Impella as a RVAD

在少数的情况之下，Impella 也可以作为单一的右心室辅助装置，其适应证包括先天性心脏病、右心室心肌梗死、肺栓塞合并右心衰竭或者是严重肺炎合并右心衰竭且并用静脉-静脉 ECMO 的患者。

The Impella, used as the only right ventricular assist device in rare cases, is indicated in patients with congenital heart disease, right ventricular myocardial infarction, pulmonary embolism combined with right heart failure, or severe pneumonia combined with right heart failure on veno-venous extracorporeal membrane oxygenation.

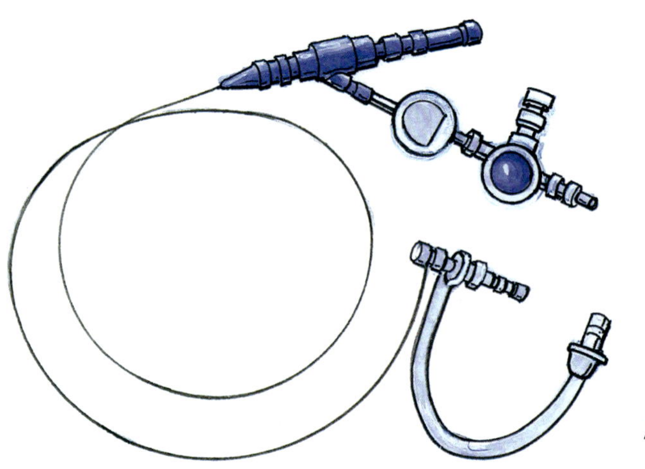

A. 心脏手术后使用的 Impella 右心辅助导管，多应用于小儿患者。

A. Impella catheter used after cardiac surgery as an RVAD is mostly applied in the pediatric population.

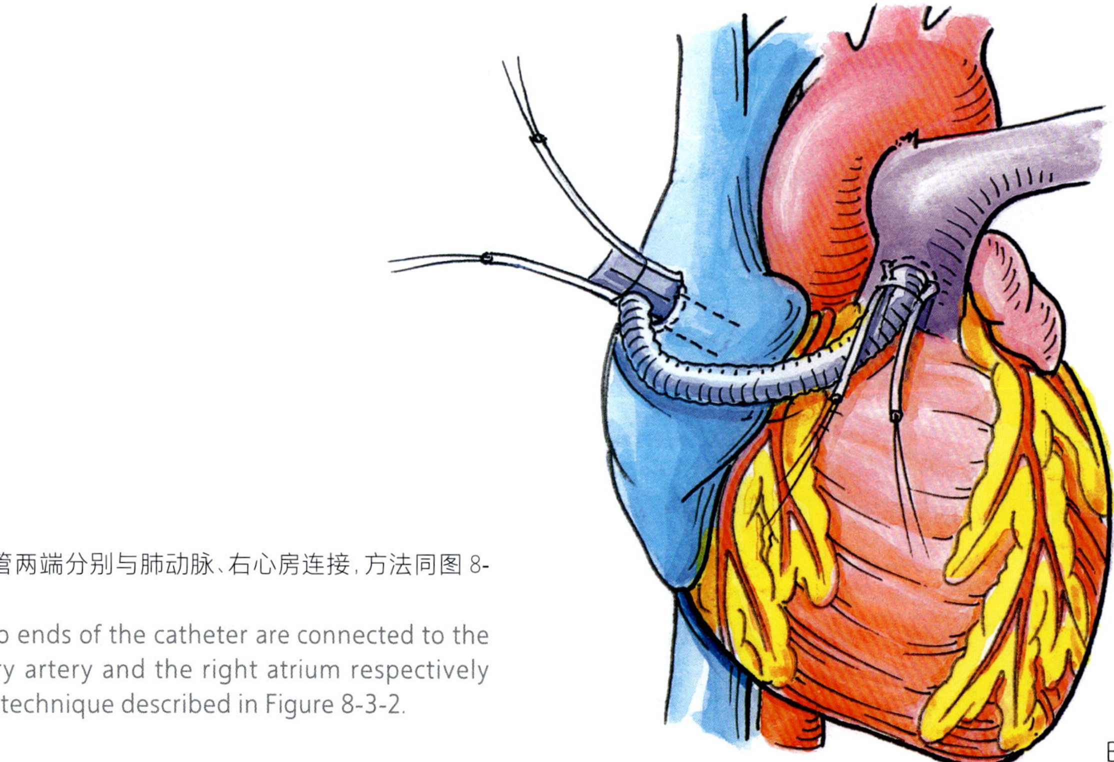

B. 将该导管两端分别与肺动脉、右心房连接，方法同图 8-3-2 所述。

B. The two ends of the catheter are connected to the pulmonary artery and the right atrium respectively using the technique described in Figure 8-3-2.

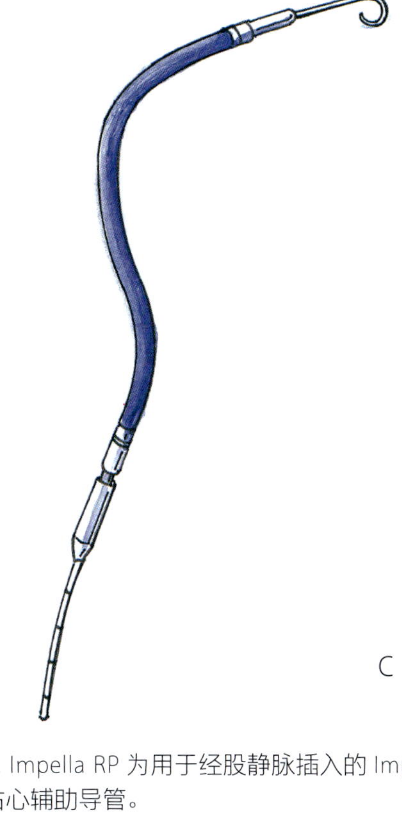

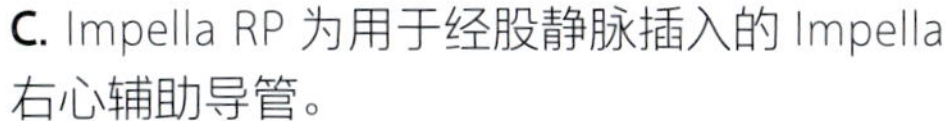

C. Impella RP 为用于经股静脉插入的 Impella 右心辅助导管。

C. Impella RP is an Impella catheter for insertion via the femoral vein.

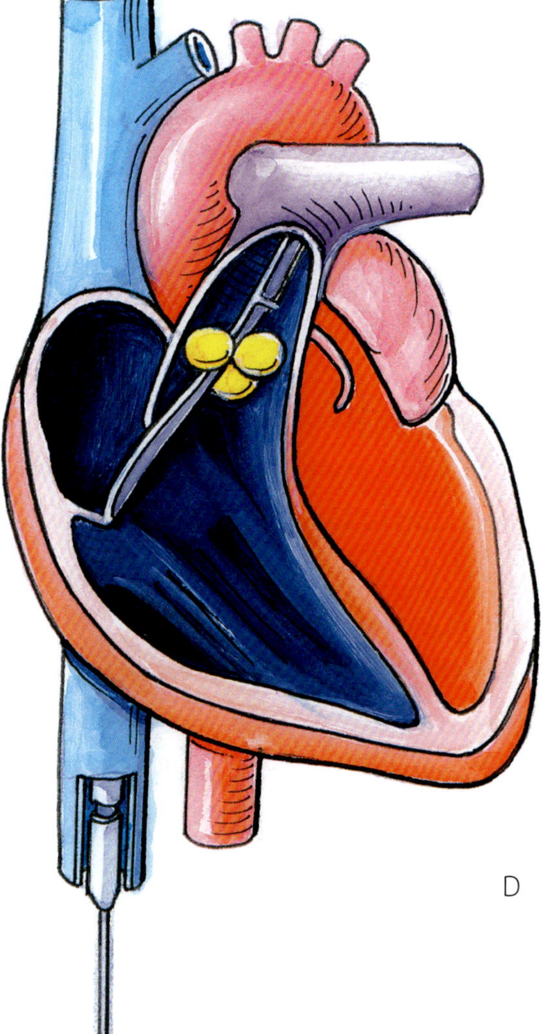

D. 由腹股沟经皮穿刺股静脉插入 Impella RP 导管，经右心房进入右心室，再由右心室通过肺动脉瓣置放在肺动脉干。该装置亦属于短效期的右心室辅助装置，对于严重右心衰竭的患者，建议置放时间不超过 2 周。

D. An Impella RP catheter is inserted into the femoral vein via the inguinal percutaneous puncture, entering the right ventricle through the right atrium, and then placed on the pulmonary trunk through the pulmonary valve from the right ventricle. This right heart assist device is short-acting. In patients with severe right heart failure, it is recommended that the placement time should not exceed two weeks.

HeartMate 心室辅助装置

HeartMate ventricular assist device

HeartMate Ⅰ 心室辅助装置

HeartMate I ventricular assist device

HeartMate Ⅰ 是一种左心室辅助装置，有气动式[HeartMate IP(implantable pneumatic)]，可携带气动式[HeartMate VE(vented electric)]及电动式[HeartMate XVE(extended vented electric)]三种机型。

HeartMate Ⅰ, a left ventricular assist device, has three models: pneumatic (HeartMate IP [implantable pneumatic]), portable pneumatic (HeartMate VE [vented electric]), and electric (HeartMate XVE [extended vented electric]).

大约从 20 世纪 70 年代中期，美国得克萨斯州休斯敦的德州心脏中心开始研发 HeartMate 左心室辅助装置。而在 1985 年 8 月 HeartMate 正式获得美国食品药品监督管理局(Food and Drug Administration，FDA)的通过，准许可作为等待心脏移植的过渡手段应用于临床上严重心力衰竭的患者，并于 1986 年有了全世界首例的使用。

From about the mid-1970s, the Texas Heart Institute in Houston, Texas, began to develop the HeartMate left ventricular assist device. In August 1985, the US FDA officially approved the HeartMate (Thermo Cardiosystem, Inc, Woburn, MA), allowing the HeartMate to be used in patients with clinically severe heart failure as a bridge to heart transplantation. It was first used worldwide in 1986.

研发 HeartMate 的目的就是建立一个长期的左心室辅助系统，希望患者能够在等待心脏移植的漫漫长路之中，有一个安全稳定的依靠。由于等待心脏移植的患者日益增加，而供心并没有成比例增加，可以预期的是每一位等待心脏移植的患者，等待供心的时间将会愈来愈长。因此，此种长期性的左心室辅助装置在临床上所扮演的角色将会愈来愈重要。

The purpose of developing the HeartMate is to establish a long-term left ventricular assist system to provide safe and stable support for patients during their long road of awaiting heart transplantation. As the number of patients waiting for heart transplantation is increasing and the donor’s heart does not increase proportionally, it can be expected that each patient awaiting heart transplantation will wait longer and longer for a heart donor. Therefore, such long-term left ventricular assist device clinically plays an increasingly important role.

其装置包含：

The device comprises:

1. **全植入式的血液泵** 血液泵的外壳为钛合金，其内部含有一片以聚氨酯（PU）所制成的隔膜，此隔膜将此血液泵区隔成空气室及血液室两部分。经由隔膜的压缩，可达到将血液泵内之血液抽入或排出的目的，进而推动血液循环，代替左心室功能。在血液泵的出入口，各有一个猪瓣膜以维持血液的单向流动。

1. **Totally Implantable Blood Pump** The housing of the blood pump is made of titanium alloy, and the blood pump contains a diaphragm made of polyurethane (PU), which divides the blood pump into two parts, the air chamber and the blood chamber. Through the compression of the diaphragm, the purpose of drawing or discharging the blood in the blood pump can be achieved, thereby promoting blood circulation and replacing the function of the left ventricle. At the inlet and outlet of the blood pump, there is a porcine valve to maintain the unidirectional flow of blood.

2. **经皮肤通到体外的驱动管路。**

2. **Extracorporeal drive tubing through the skin.**

3. **体外控制装置。**

3. **Extracorporeal control device.**

图 8-3-5 HeartMate Ⅰ 植入术
Figure 8-3-5 Implantation of HeartMate Ⅰ

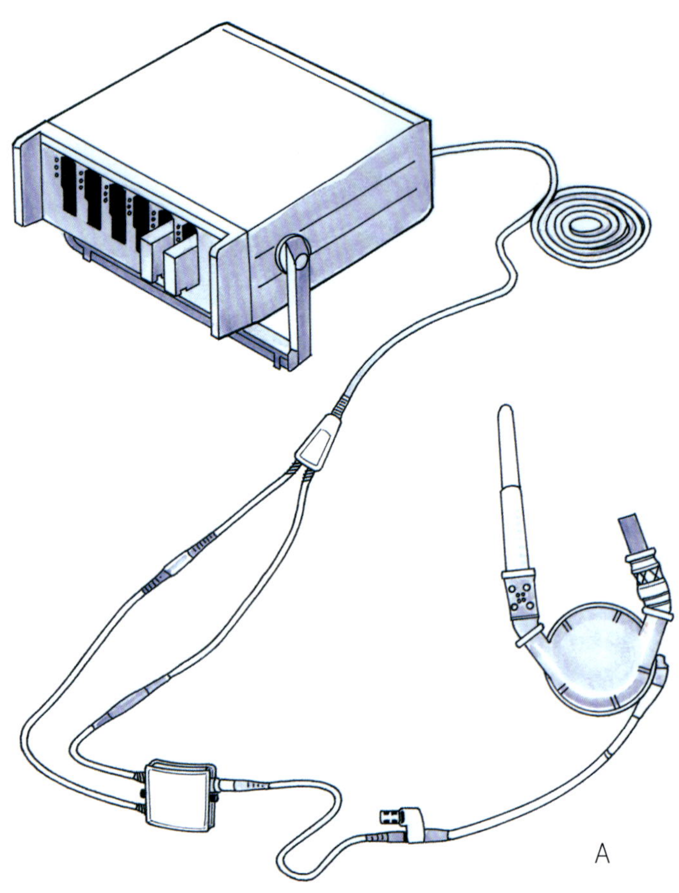

A. 整套 HeartMate XVE 装置连接充电系统的示意图。

A. The figure illustrates how to connect the complete HeartMate XVE device to the charging system.

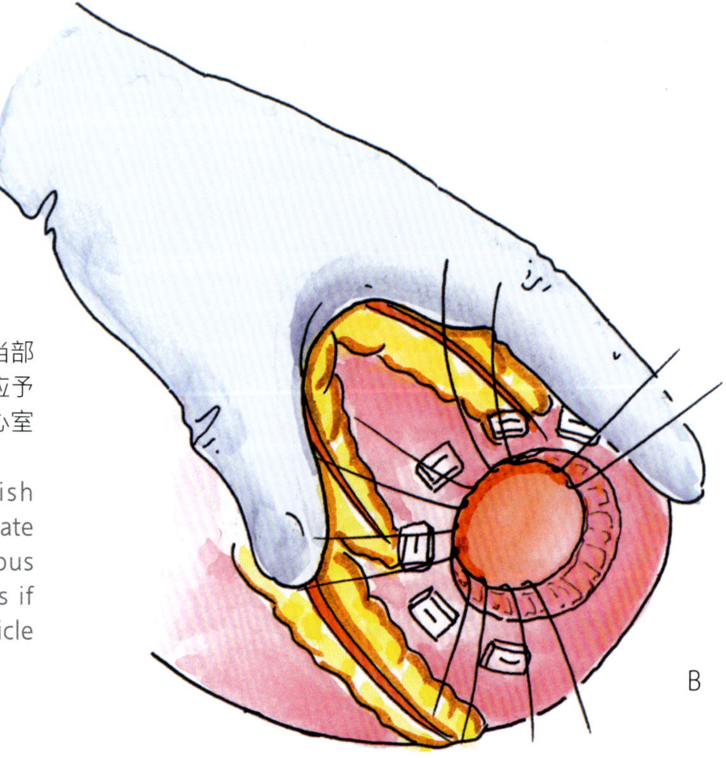

B. 胸骨正中切口开胸建立体外循环。将左心室心尖适当部位挖出一个洞，先检查左心室内部有无血栓，如有血栓应予以清除干净，然后再用带垫片的褥式缝线均匀缝在左心室开口。

B. Perform a median sternotomy to establish extracorporeal circulation. Dig a hole in the appropriate part of the left ventricle apex to check for thrombus inside the left ventricle, remove the thrombus if there is any, and then evenly suture the left ventricle ostium with pledgeted mattress sutures.

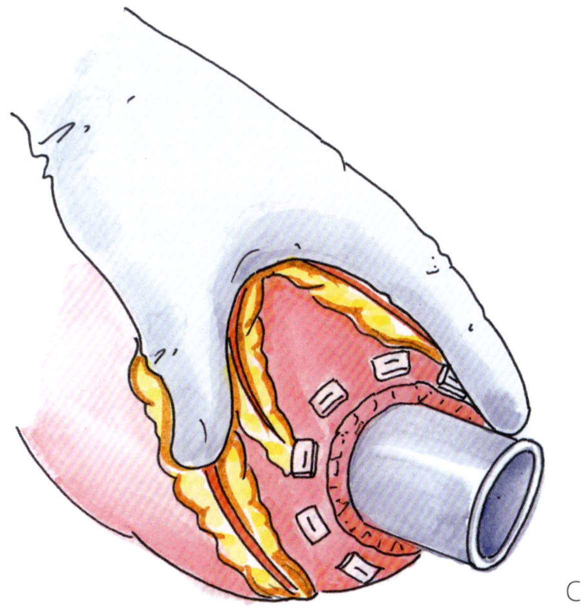

C. 将硅胶流入管接头缝合环吻合固定在心尖开口上。
C. The sewing ring of the silicone inflow connector is anastomosed and secured to the apical opening.

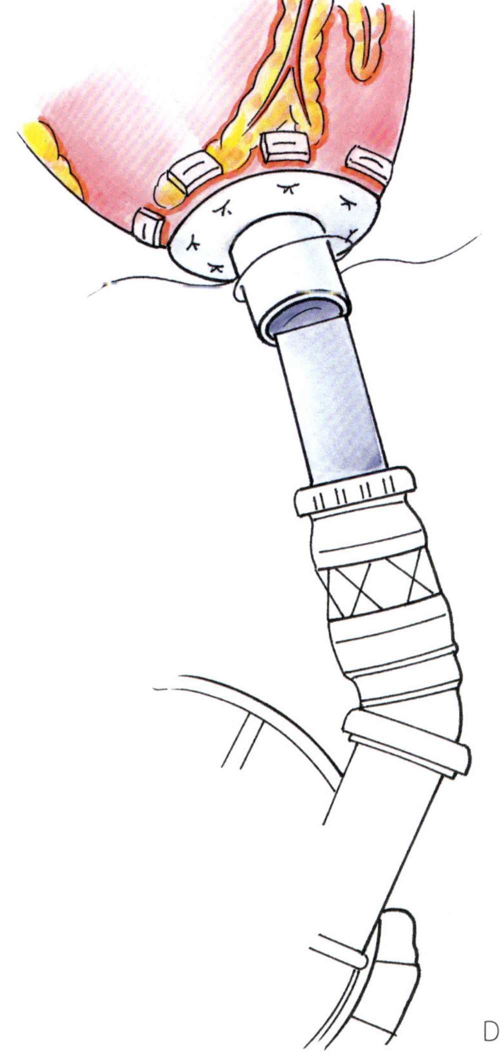

D. 血液泵流入口之金属接头与硅胶流入管接头相连接并以束带固定。
D. The metal connector at the blood pump inlet is connected to the silicone inflow connector and fixed by banding.

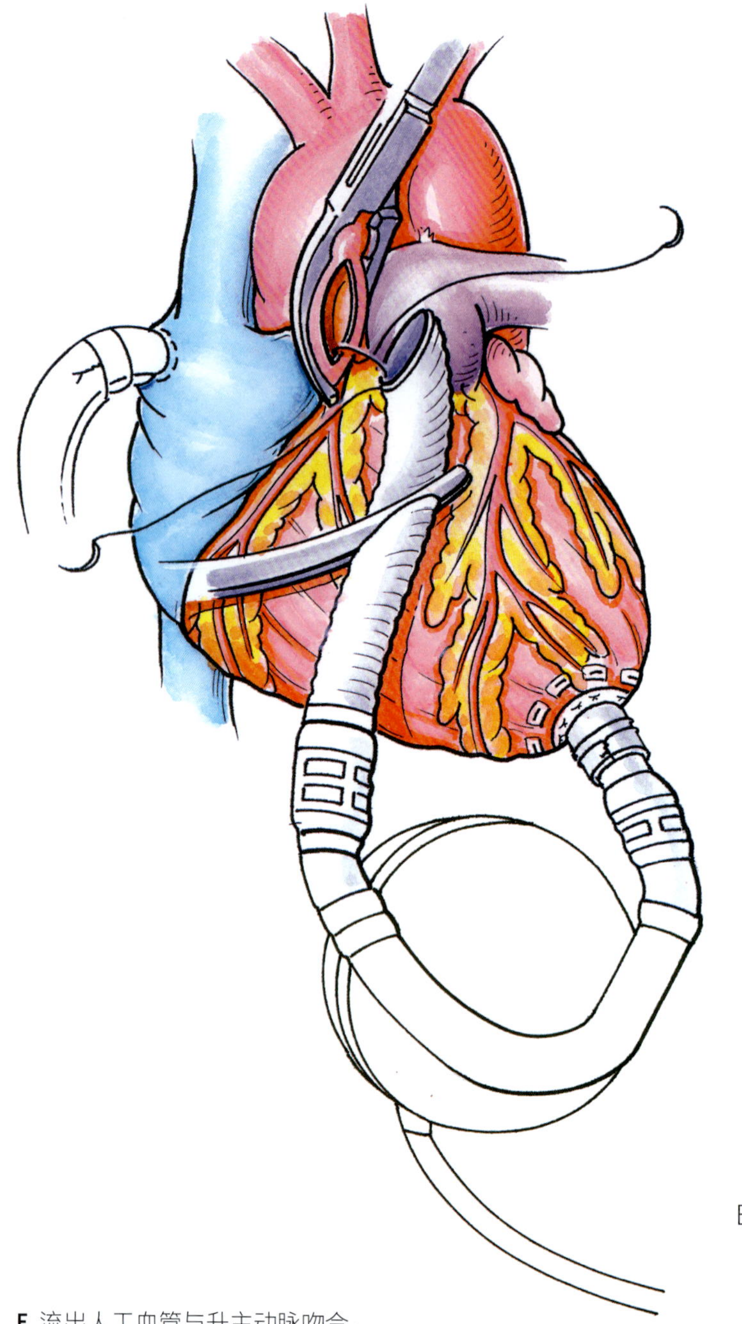

E. 流出人工血管与升主动脉吻合。

E. The artificial outflow conduit is anastomosed to the ascending aorta.

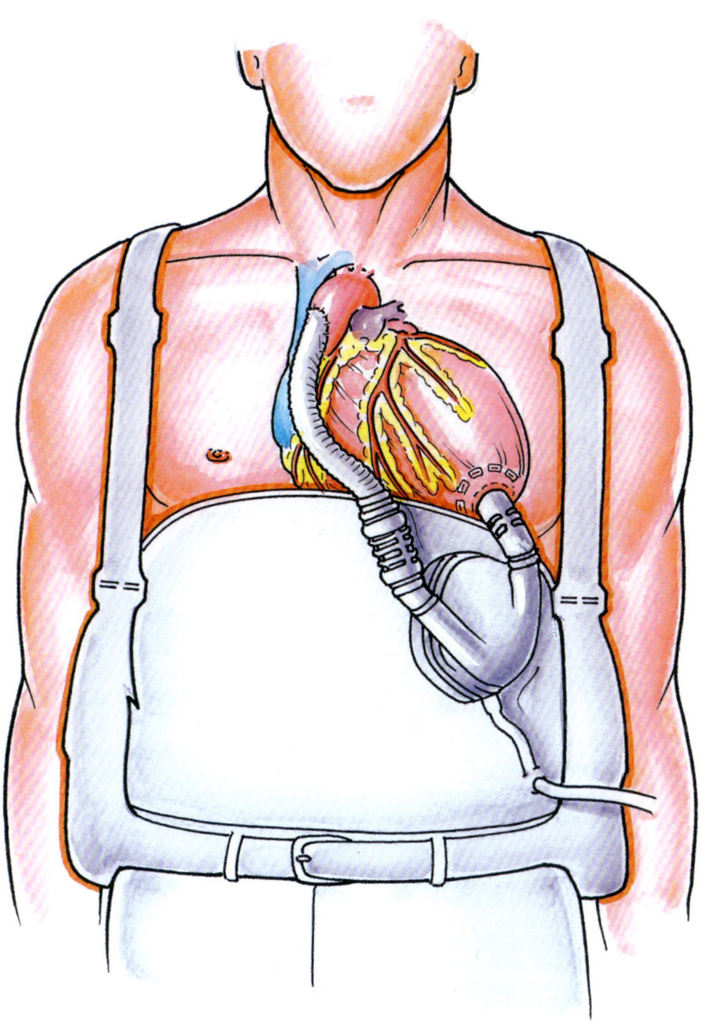

F

F. 将电力驱动电线与体外电池及控制器相连，植入完成。血液经由左心室心尖的流入人工管道流入血液泵的血液室中，经血液泵挤压推动之后，再经由流出人工管道，将血液送至升主动脉，以供应身体所需。

F. Connect the electric wires to the extracorporeal battery and the controller to complete the implantation. Blood flows into the blood chamber of the blood pump through the artificial inflow conduit at the left ventricle apex. After being squeezed and pushed by the blood pump, the blood is delivered to the ascending aorta through the artificial outflow conduit to supply the body.

G

G. 整套 HeartMate XVE 装置连接电池之示意图。

G. The figure illustrates how to connect the complete HeartMate XVE device to the batteries.

HeartMate Ⅱ 心室辅助装置

HeartMate Ⅱ ventricular assist device

HeartMate Ⅱ 左心室辅助装置适用于等待心脏移植的患者，以避免不可逆左心室衰竭造成死亡；也可适用于纽约心脏协会心功能分级ⅢB 级或Ⅳ级左心室衰竭、在最近 60 天内已接受至少 45 天适当药物治疗的患者；还可以用于救护车、飞机或直升机转运的患者。

The HeartMate Ⅱ left ventricular assist device is indicated in patients awaiting heart transplantation to avoid death from irreversible left ventricular failure. It is also indicated in patients with New York Heart Association class Ⅲ B or class Ⅳ left ventricular failure who have received appropriate medical treatment for at least forty-five days in the last sixty days. It may also be used in ambulances, planes, or helicopters to transport patients.

整套系统包括：

The complete system consists of:

1. **血液泵** HeartMate Ⅱ 左心室辅助装置是轴流旋转式泵，重 176g，直径 40mm，可产生高达 10L/min 的流量。泵内部的表面包括转子、薄壁导管、输入端启动子与输出端启动子，均由钛制成。两端分别衔接流入及流出人工血管。内部转子组合包含一个磁铁，并以电力驱动转子旋转提供动力，把血液由左心室推进到 HeartMate Ⅱ 左心室辅助装置，再回到自体的循环中。泵经由穿皮式导线连接外部系统控制器与电源进行控制与供电。

1. **Blood Pump** The HeartMate Ⅱ left ventricular assist device, an axial flow rotary pump with 176 g in weight and 40 mm in diameter, produces up to 10 L/min flow. The internal surfaces of the pump, consisting of the rotor, thin-walled conduit, input and output actuators, are made of titanium. The two ends are respectively connected to the artificial inflow conduit and artificial outflow conduit. The internal rotor assembly contains a magnet and is powered by electrically driven rotor rotation, delivering blood from the left ventricle to the HeartMate Ⅱ left ventricular assist device and back to the patient's native circulation. The pump is controlled by an external system controller via a percutaneous wire. The power is supplied through a percutaneous wire.

2. **系统控制器** 是一组电脑微处理器模组，可控制其运转与管理。系统控制器传送动力与操作信号到泵，并收集及解读回传的数据。在启动泵运作前，要预先设定调控，以维持所选择的心脏支持功能。其电力由电源模组或可重复充电的电池供应。

2. **System Controller** A set of computer microprocessor modules that can control the operation and management. The system controller transmits power and operation signals to the pump and collects and interprets the data sent back. Before starting the pump, preset controls to maintain the selected cardiac support function. Its power is supplied by power modules or rechargeable batteries.

3. 电源模组 连接于血液泵上，正常操作时提供电源给系统监视器或显示模组。

3. Power Modules It is connected to the blood pump and provides power to the system monitor or the display module during normal operation.

4. 系统监视器 监控系统参数、改变速度设定、储存数据及检视已储存的数据。系统监视器连接系统控制器，经由泵电源模组提供泵与系统状态的显示。

4. System Monitor Monitor system parameters, change speed settings, store data, and view stored data. The system monitor, connecting to the system controller,displays the status of the pump and the system via the pump power modules.

5. 电池与电池匣 不使用电源模组装置时，其电源则来自泵上的两个置于电池匣的 14V 直流电池。

5. Batteries and Battery Case When the power module unit is not in use, power comes from two 14-volt direct current (DC) batteries in the battery case on the pump.

图 8-3-6 HeartMate Ⅱ植入术

Figure 8-3-6 Implantation of HeartMate Ⅱ

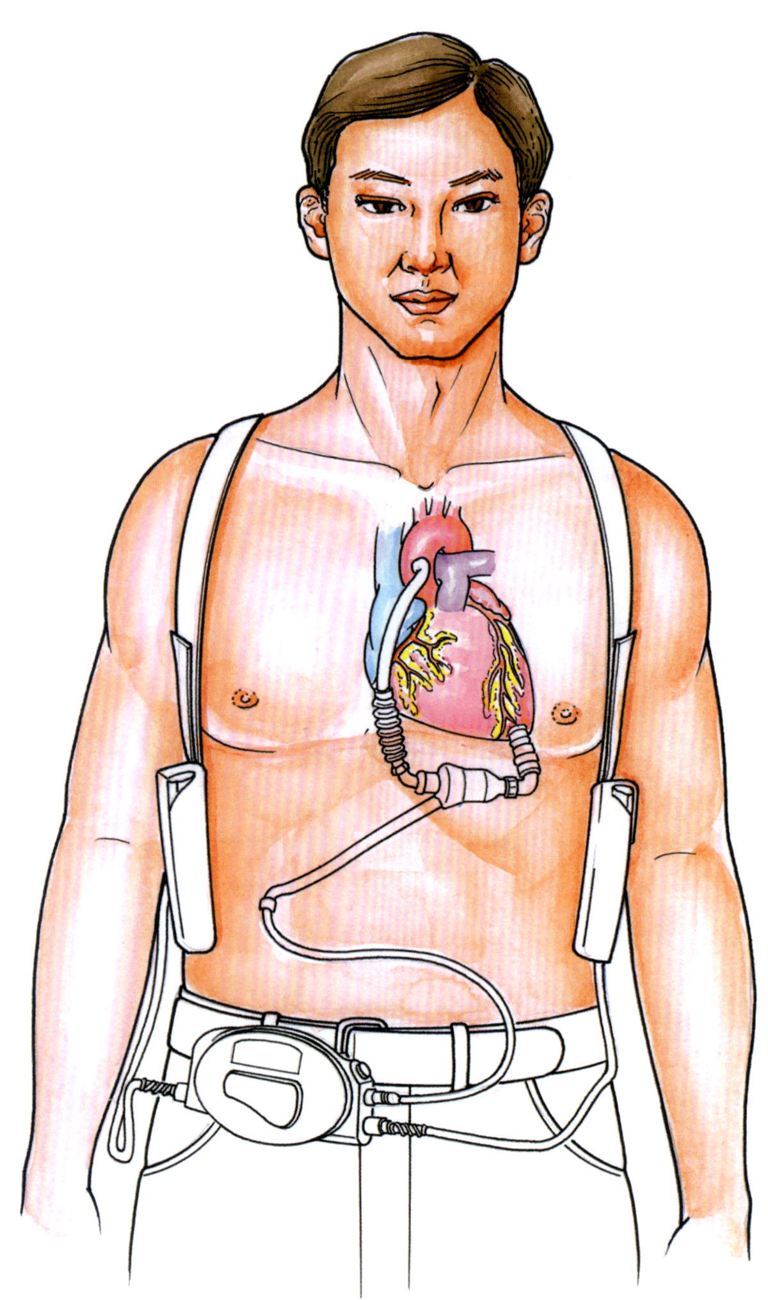

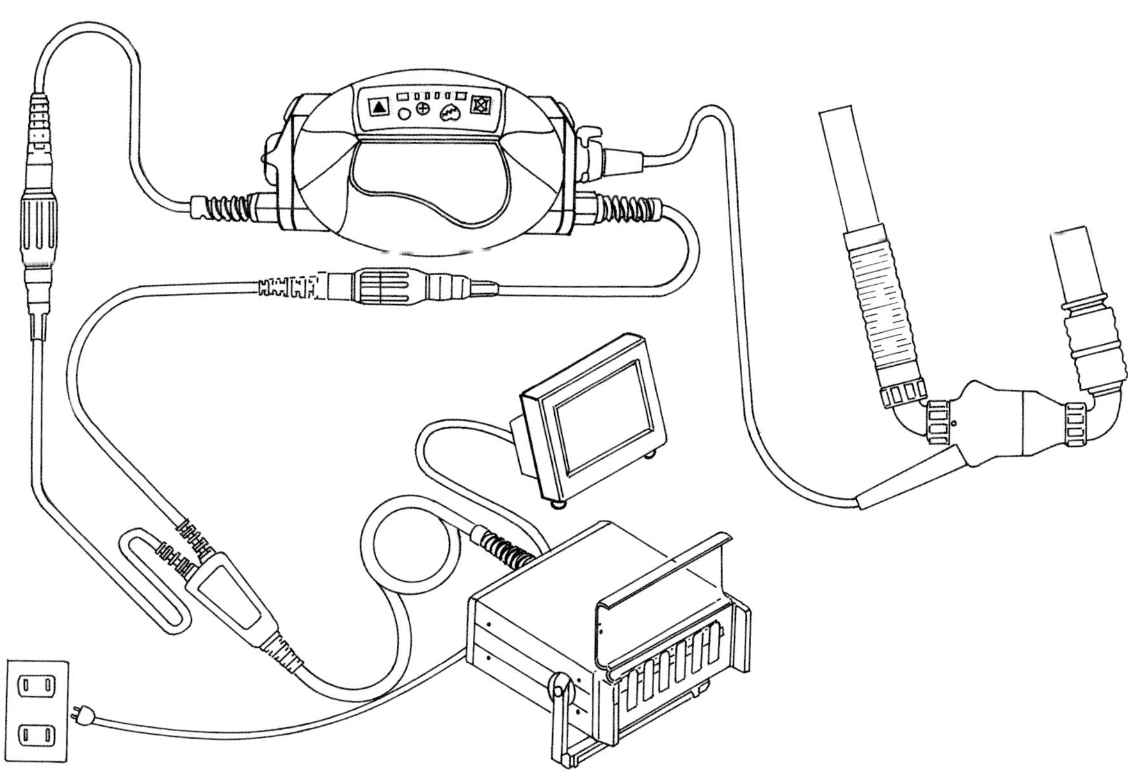

全身麻醉、体外循环下取胸骨正中切口。先在左心室心尖上做一切口，缝入缝合环加强。缝合流入插管于缝合环上，连接 HeartMate Ⅱ 泵流入端。泵另一端接上流出插管与升主动脉端侧吻合。将泵缆线由腹壁穿洞引出，接上系统控制器。泵正常启动后，脱离体外循环。缝合切口，手术完成。

A median sternotomy is performed under general anesthesia and *extracorporeal circulation*. First, an incision is made on the left ventricle apex, and a sewing ring is sutured for reinforcement. The inflow cannula, sutured to the sewing ring, is connected to the inflow end of the HeartMate Ⅱ pump. The other end of the pump, connected to an outflow cannula, is end-to-side anastomosed to the ascending aorta. Bring the pump cable out through the hole in the abdominal wall and connect it to the system controller. After the pump starts normally, the cardiopulmonary bypass is weaned off. The incision is sutured and the procedure is concluded.

HeartMate Ⅲ 心室辅助装置

HeartMate Ⅲ ventricular assist device

HeartMate Ⅲ 左心室辅助系统的设计，是为了治疗严重心力衰竭的患者，左心室辅助系统承担左心室部分或全部工作，提供患者全身的血液灌注量。目前而言，HeartMate Ⅲ 为全世界最新型、手术长期效果最好、合并症最少。从目前临床实践来看，有非常多的患者在植入 HeartMate Ⅲ 后，因其提供的优异生活品质，决定不再接受心脏移植手术，而愿意戴着 HeartMate Ⅲ 终其一生。在多个国家 HeartMate Ⅲ 除了可作为心脏移植前之桥梁以外，也被许可作为不适合接受心脏移植（例如年龄大于 65 岁）的心力衰竭患者永久治疗之用。

The HeartMate Ⅲ left ventricular assist system, designed to treat patients with severe heart failure, undertakes part or all of the work of the left ventricle to provide systemic blood perfusion. At present, as the latest left ventricular assist system in the world, the HeartMate Ⅲ has the best long-term surgical outcomes, the fewest complications, and the highest market share. The current clinical practice shows that many patients, after implanting the HeartMate Ⅲ, decide not to undergo heart transplantation because of the excellent quality of life it provides, but are willing to carry the HeartMate Ⅲ for the rest of their lives. In addition to being used as a bridge to heart transplantation, the HeartMate Ⅲ is also licensed as a permanent treatment for heart failure patients who are not suitable for heart transplantation (e.g., older than 65 years) in several countries.

整套系统包含：

1. LAVD　适用于长期植入胸腔的磁悬浮离心式血液泵，包含流入插管、马达、血泵室、转子、流出人工血管和电缆线。心室血液沿着中心轴线被吸入流入插管内，并在围绕中心轴线旋转的转子叶轮叶片之间以直角排出。血流切线向进入流出人工血管中。转子由磁悬浮支持，两个驱动和悬架都是由一个包含铁极片、背铁、铜线圈和位置传感器的定子所完成的。通过测量转子中永磁体的位置，适当地控制驱动和悬浮线圈中的电流，转子的径向位置和转速被主动地控制。控制马达驱动及悬浮所需的电力和软件，被整合到定子泵中，所有组件和转子一起组成马达。

流入插管是一个圆柱形导管，其外形尺寸和 HeartMate Ⅱ 左心室辅助装置类似，固定在泵盖上。在植入过程中，流入插管经由左心室心尖接入左心室。流出人工血管组件由密封的编织聚酯人工血管和连接到泵盖所需的接头所组成。这样的连接方式，让临床医师在置入过程执行系统的排气，并且可以在置入进行的任何时间点，将流出人工血管附接到泵上。流出人工血管的末端是可修剪或切割的设计，以便裁取适合的长度缝合到升主动脉。弯曲离隙是围绕在流出人工血管的套管，用来预防管路的扭折和磨损，更换血泵时，可以将流出人工血管与泵分离，无须重新吻合。

The complete system consists of:

1. LAVD　It is a magnetic suspension centrifugal blood pump indicated for long-term thoracic implantation, consisting of an inflow cannula, a motor, a blood pump chamber, a rotor, an artificial outflow conduit, and a cable. Ventricular blood is drawn into the inflow cannula along the central axis and discharged at right angles between the rotor impeller and blades rotating around the central axis. The blood flow tangentially enters the artificial outflow conduit. The rotor is supported by magnetic levitation, and both drives and suspensions are completed by a stator consisting of iron pole pieces, back iron, copper coils, and position sensors. By measuring the position of the permanent magnets in the rotor and appropriately controlling the currents in the drive and suspension coils, the radial position and speed of the rotor are actively controlled. The power and software required to control the motor drive and the levitation are integrated into the stator pump, and all components, together with the rotor, form the motor.

The inflow cannula, a cylindrical catheter with a similar shape and size to the HeartMate Ⅱ left ventricular assist device, is secured to the pump cover. During implantation, the inflow cannula accesses the left ventricle via the left ventricle apex. The artificial outflow conduit consists of a sealed braided polyester arterial blood vessel and fittings required to connect to the pump cover. This connection allows the clinician to vent the system and to attach the artificial outflow conduit to the pump at any time during the placement process. The end of the artificial outflow conduit is designed to be trimmable or incisable so that the appropriate length can be cut and sutured to the ascending aorta. The curved relief is reserved for the cannula around the artificial outflow conduit, which is used to prevent the kink and wear of the pipeline. When the blood pump is replaced, the artificial outflow conduit can be separated from the pump without re-anastomosing.

电缆线通过密封的通道固定在泵头，并与封闭的马达建立电器接合。电缆线穿过腹部皮下组织，通过皮肤与体外的模组电缆线进行扩展，并连接到系统控制器。电缆线和模组电缆线组成驱动系统，包含三个导体电源、地线和通信。

The cable is secured to the pump head through a sealed channel and establishes electrical engagement with the sealed motor. The cable passes through the abdominal subcutaneous tissue, extends through the skin to the extracorporal modular cable, and connects to the system controller. The cable and the modular cable make up the drive system, consisting of three conductors for power, ground wire, and communications.

2. **系统控制器** 是一台控制和监控系统操作的小型电子计算机，驱动系统将植入的血泵连接到系统控制器，使用时控制器上会有灯号、声音和信息显示。

2. System Controller The system controller is a small electronic computer that controls and monitors the operation of the system. The drive system connects the implanted blood pump to the system controller, which displays lights, sounds, and information when in use.

3. **系统监视器** 临床医生通过系统监视器，监测系统设定的参数，评估和追踪警报状态，并可查看和保存执行的数据。

3. System Monitor Clinicians use the system monitor to monitor the set parameters, assess and track alarm status, and view and save execution data.

4. **电源系统** 包括 14V 锂离子电池和电池匣、行动电源单位和充电器。

4. Power Supply System The power supply system consists of 14-volt lithium-ion battery and battery case, mobile power supply unit, and charger.

图 8-3-7　HeartMate Ⅲ植入术
Figure 8-3-7　Implantation of HeartMate Ⅲ

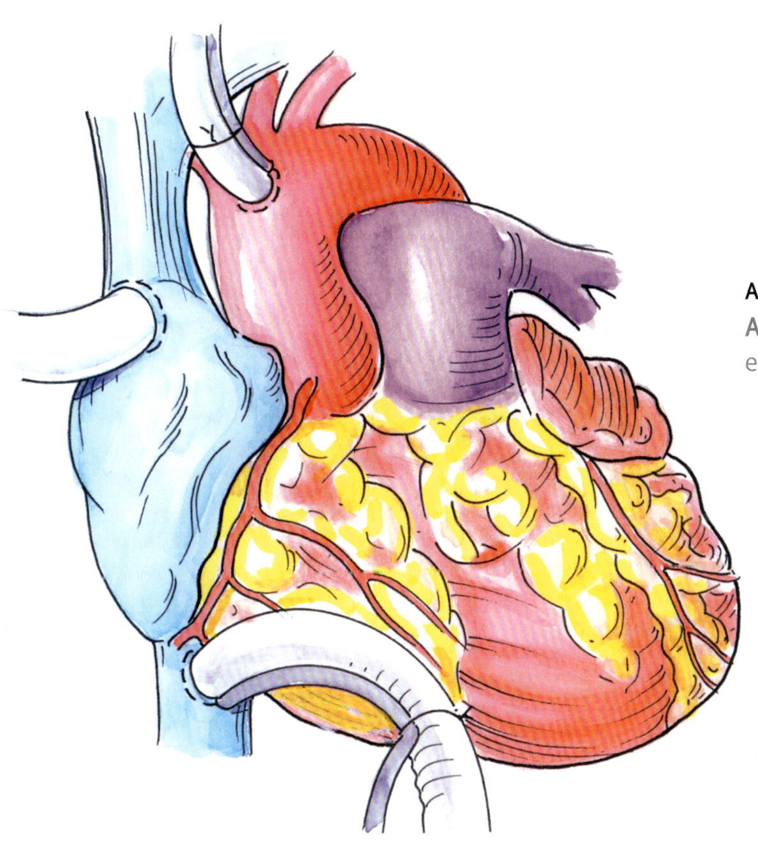

A

A. 胸骨正中切口，建立体外循环。

A. A median sternotomy is performed to establish extracorporeal circulation.

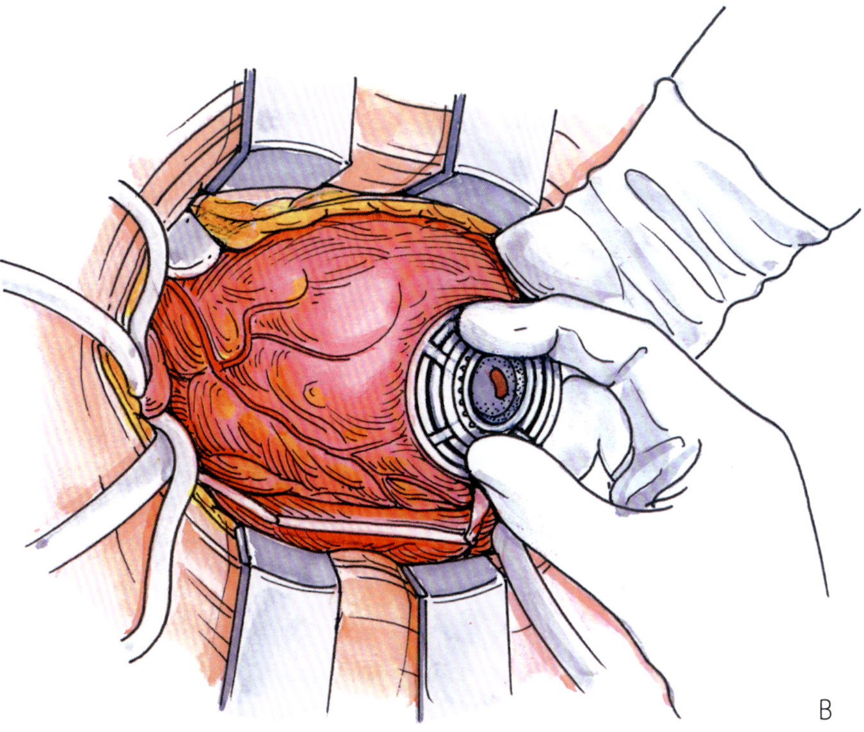

B

B. 心脏抬起后检视心脏，心尖打孔位置做出标记。HeartMate Ⅲ有特殊设计的缝合环，在与心尖缝合后能够很容易地与血泵相连接。

B. Lift the heart for inspection and make a mark where the apex is punched. With a specially designed sewing ring, the HeartMate Ⅲ can be easily connected to the blood pump after being sutured to the cardiac apex.

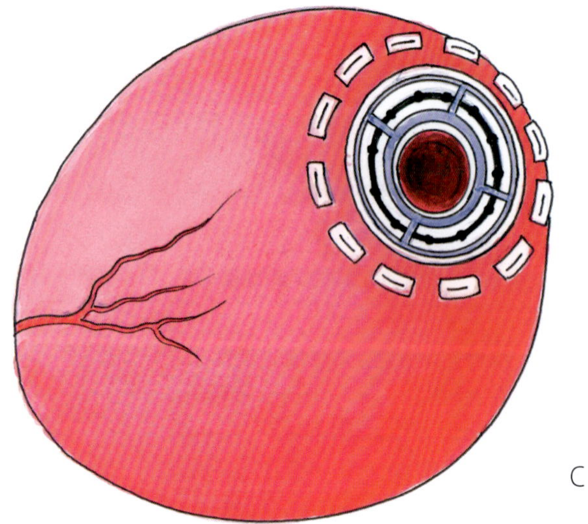

C. 常规缝合方式，用带垫片褥式缝合将缝合环固定于心尖。
C. Secure the sewing ring to the cardiac apex with pledgeted mattress sutures using a routine suturing way.

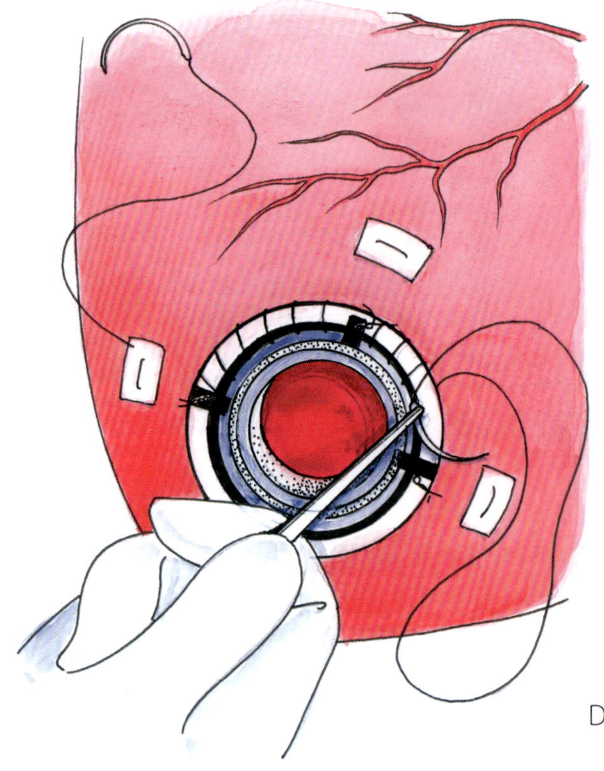

D. 另外一种新型缝合法，先做 4 针带垫片褥式缝合，将缝合环缝在心尖上面，并打结固定。再用 3-0 Prolene 缝线以连续缝合的方式，加强缝合环的固定。
D. In another new type of suturing method, four stitches are first made with pledgeted mattress sutures to suture the sewing ring on the cardiac apex, and then tie the knot for fixation. The 3-0 Prolene suture is then continuously sutured to reinforce the fixation of the sewing ring.

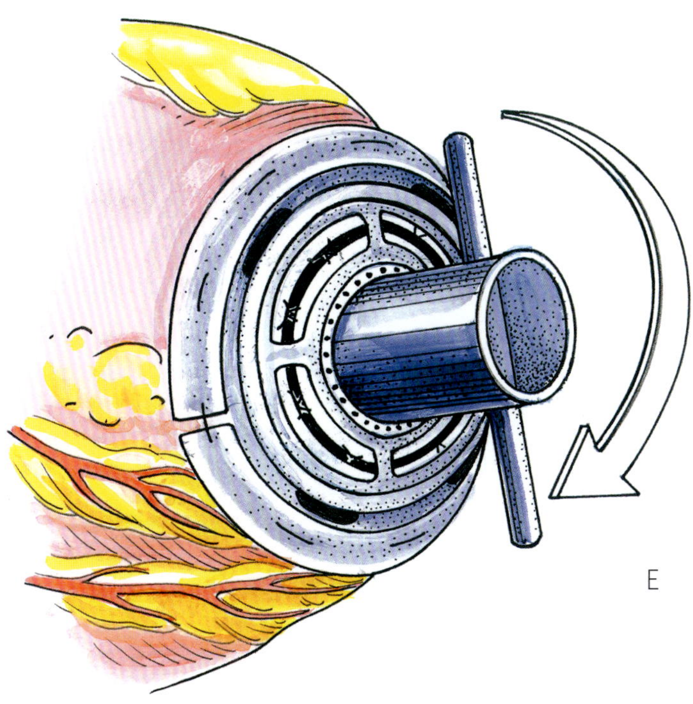

E. 也可使用环状长条形垫片，做心尖与缝合环的间断褥式缝合。缝合环缝合完成后以特制的心尖锥形刀在心尖打洞。

E. Interrupted mattress sutures between the cardiac apex and the sewing ring can also be performed using an annular strip pledget. After the sewing ring is sutured, a hole is made in the cardiac apex with a specially designed apical conical knife.

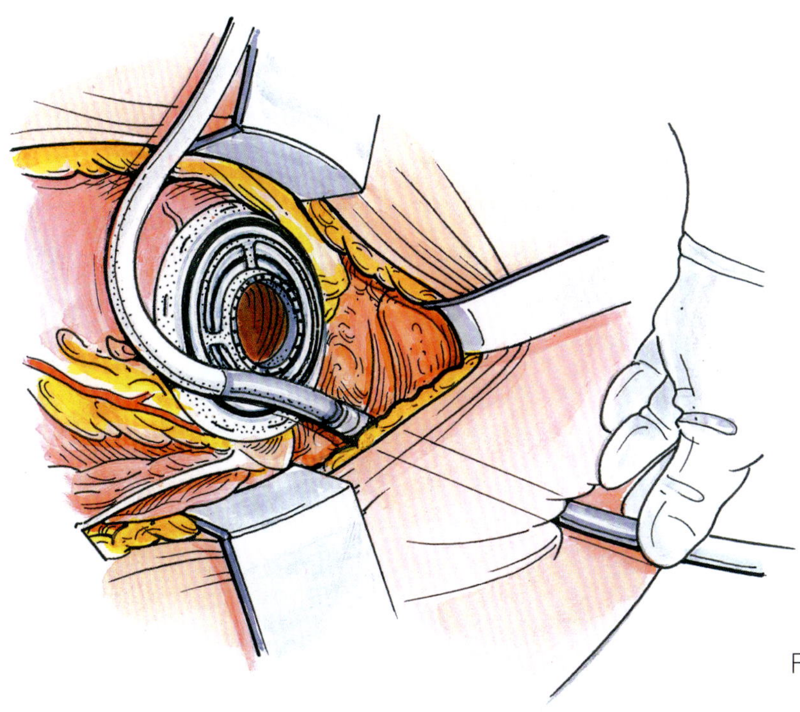

F. 以特制的穿孔器将电缆线从纵隔腔穿出至身体一侧（左侧或右侧均可），大致在脐的高度穿出皮肤。

F. The cable is pulled out through the mediastinal cavity to one side of the body (either left or right) with a specially designed perforator, exiting the skin at approximately the height of the umbilicus.

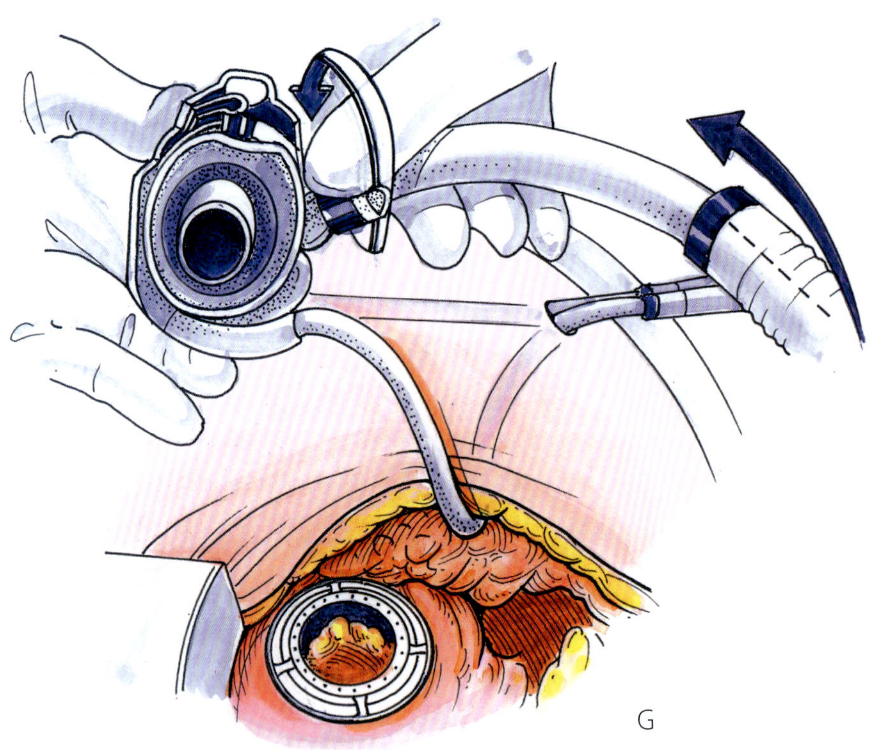

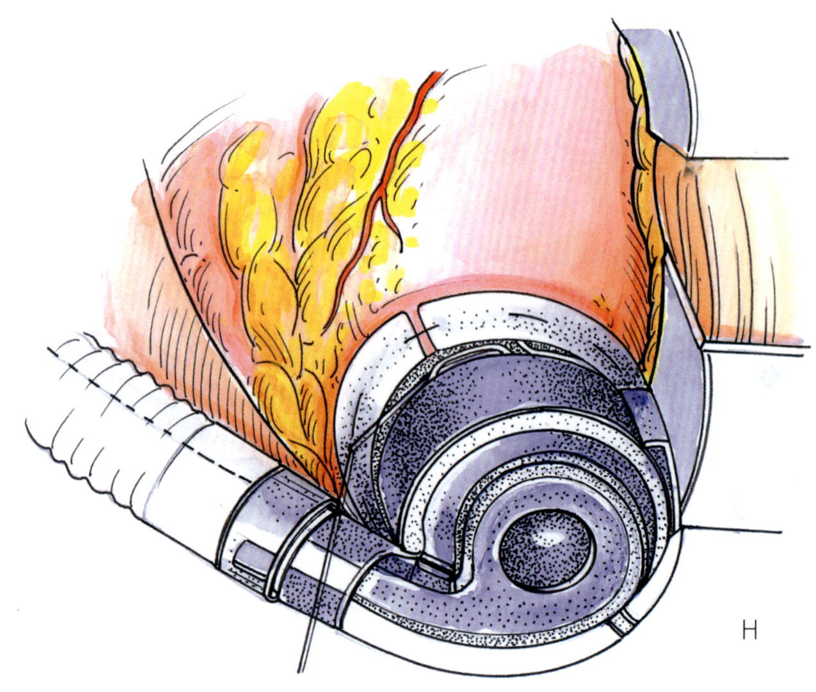

G、H. 此时将 HeartMate Ⅲ泵与缝合环扣合，并将心脏放入心包膜腔内。

G, H. At this time, the HeartMate Ⅲ pump is snapped into the sewing ring and the heart is placed into the pericardial cavity.

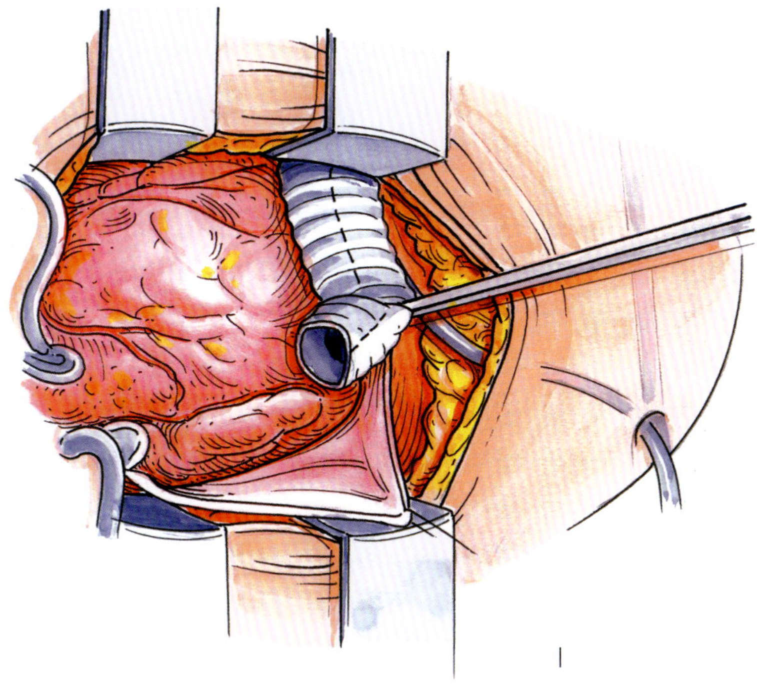

I. 再将流出血管与升主动脉吻合。

I. The outflow graft conduit is then anastomosed to the ascending aorta.

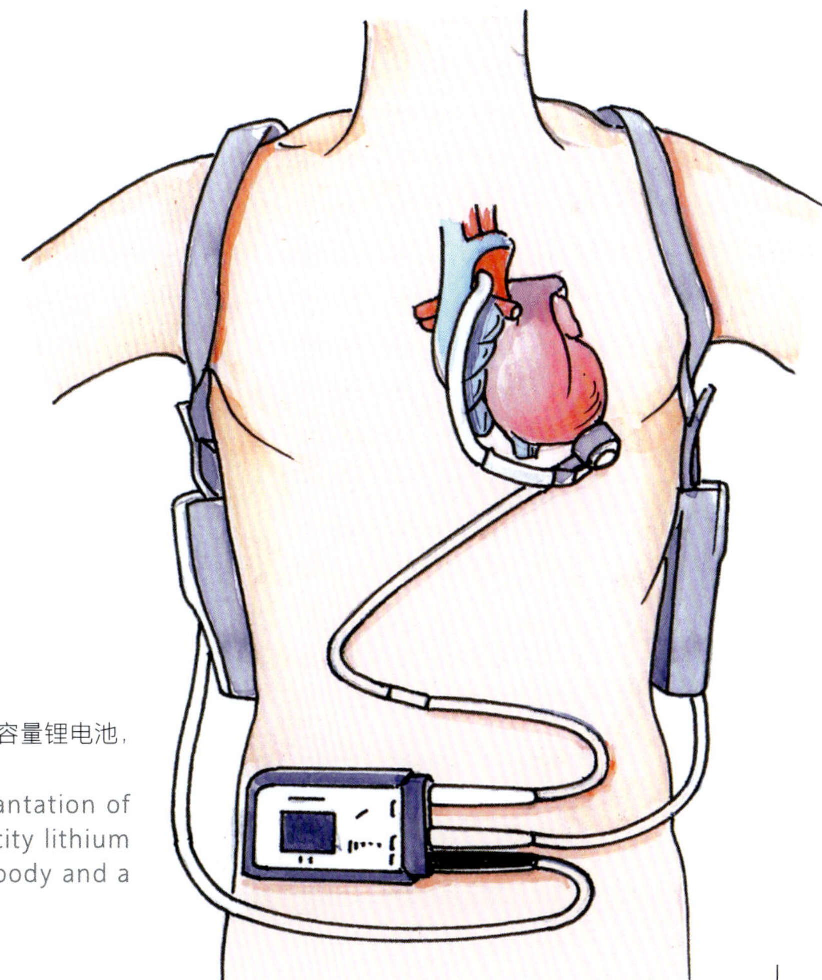

J. HeartMate Ⅲ植入后示意图，身体两侧为高容量锂电池，前方为微电脑控制器。

J. The figure illustrates the post-implantation of the HeartMate Ⅲ. There are high-capacity lithium batteries on both sides of the human body and a microcomputer controller in the front.

Novacor 心室辅助装置

Novacor ventricular assist device

Novacor 左心室辅助系统（left ventricular assist system，LVAS）是第一代的左心室辅助装置，也是第一个成功用作心脏移植前桥梁的心室辅助装置。Novacor 本身只有一种电子式的系统，而没有气动式的系统。

The Novacor left ventricular assist system (LVAS), a first-generation left ventricular assist device, was the first ventricular assist device to be successfully used as a bridge to transplantation. Novacor itself is just an electronic system, not a pneumatic one.

整套装置包含：

The complete device consists of:

1. **植入部件** 与经皮植入的控制线与电源线连接的血液泵/驱动装置、生物人工瓣膜导管、流入人工血管、流出人工血管。其血液泵内的压缩隔膜为两片式，可以产生 9L/min 的脉动血流。在流入和流出人工血管中使用生物人工瓣膜以实现血液单向流动，并且需要使用抗凝药物预防血栓发生。

1. **Implanted Components** Blood pump/drive device, biological artificial valve conduit, artificial inflow conduit and artificial outflow conduit, which are connected to the percutaneously implanted control and power lines. The compressed diaphragm within its blood pump is a two-piece type that produces 9 L/min pulsatile blood flow. Bioprosthetic valves are used in both inflow and outflow graft conduits to achieve unidirectional blood flow and anticoagulants are required to prevent thrombosis.

2. **控制盒** 放置于体外，可用肩带或腰带随身携带，独立操作与监测血液泵/驱动装置。控制盒计算及显示血液泵流量与灌注速率，基于这些数据调整血液泵的运转，从而与自体心脏的活动匹配。调节电流到驱动装置，控制血液泵的启动。监测左心室辅助系统的运作，对超出限制或不正常操作，发出警告。

2. **Control Box** It is placed outside the body with a shoulder strap or belt, which is convenient to carry around. The control box is independently operated to monitor the blood pump/drive device. The control box calculates and displays the blood pump flow and perfusion rate, which are the basis for coordinating the operation of the blood pump with the activity of the patient's heart. Adjust the current to the drive device to control the activation of the blood pump. Monitor the operation of the left ventricular assist system and issues alarms if limits are exceeded or the left ventricular assist system does not operate properly.

3. **可携带电力套组** 供应电力给控制盒，连接充电监控电路系统、充电状态指示灯及声音和视觉低电量警报。让 Novacor 的使用者能够自由活动。由单独的电源充电器充电，最多可同时为三个电源充电器充电。

3. Portable Power Kit This power kit supplies power to the control box and is connected to the charging monitoring circuit system, charging status indicator lights, and audible and visual low-battery alarms. Allow users of the Novacor to move freely. Charged by a separate mains charger, up to three mains chargers can be charged simultaneously.

4. **左心室辅助系统监视器** 由监视器或控制器电缆线连接控制盒，能评估左心室辅助系统的功能，设定及调整控制参数和警示限制。在屏幕上显示血液泵容量和流量波形、速度、心搏出量和输出量，当连接心电图装置时，屏幕上也会出现 Novacor 使用者的心电图波形和心率。连接时提供电力给控制盒，可由直流电线充电或由内部可再充电电池充电。

4. Left Ventricular Assist System Monitor The left ventricular assist system monitor, connected to the control box through the monitor cable or the controller cable, can evaluate the function of the left ventricular assist system, set and adjust control parameters and alarm limits. The blood pump volume and flow waveforms, speed, stroke volume, and output are displayed on the screen, and when the electrocardiogram (ECG) device is connected, the ECG waveform and heart rate of the Novacor user are also displayed on the screen. When connected, the left ventricular assist system monitor supplies power to the control box, which can be charged by the DC cable or by the internal rechargeable batteries.

5. **个人监视器** 小机型设计，可放置在桌上或床头柜上，用于手术后期，当 Novacor 使用者已经稳定、不需要再调整参数或诊断时，支持系统操作。提供血液泵运作和系统警示状态的信息，由监测器/控制器电缆线连接控制盒。

5. Personal Monitor The personal monitor is small in size and can be placed on the table or bedside table. It is used in the post-operative period. When the Novocor user's condition has been stabilized and no further parameter adjustment or diagnosis is required, it supports the system operation. The personal monitor, connected to the control box through the monitor/controller cable, provides information on blood pump operation and system alarm status.

图 8-3-8　Novacor 植入术
Figure 8-3-8　Implantation of Novacor

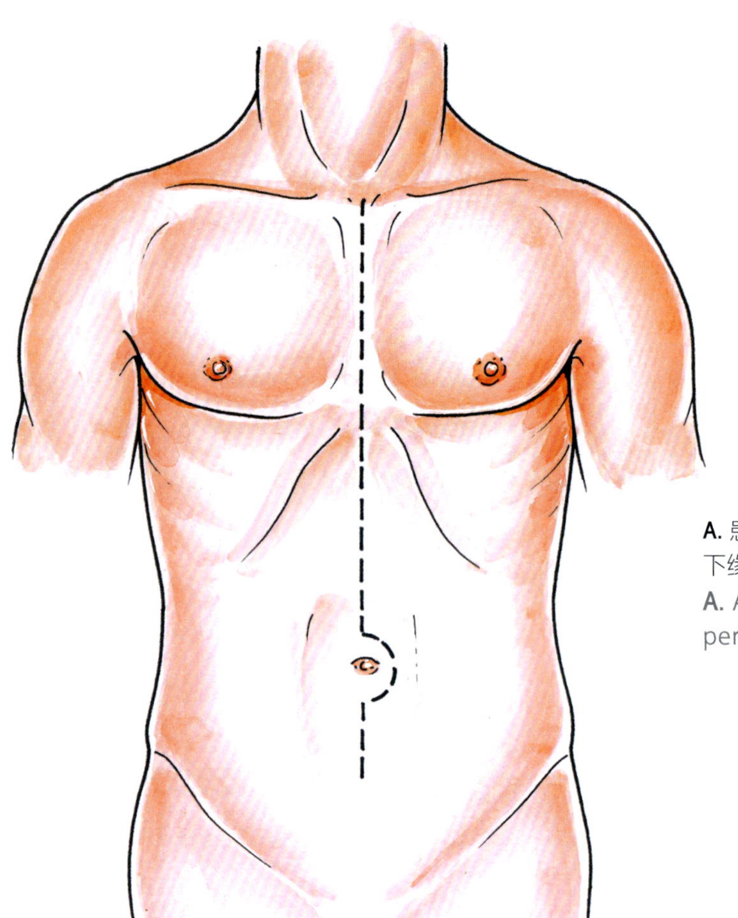

A

A. 患者在全身麻醉之后，胸部正中切口切开，一路延伸至脐下缘。

A. After general anesthesia, a median thoracotomy is performed, extending to the lower umbilical border.

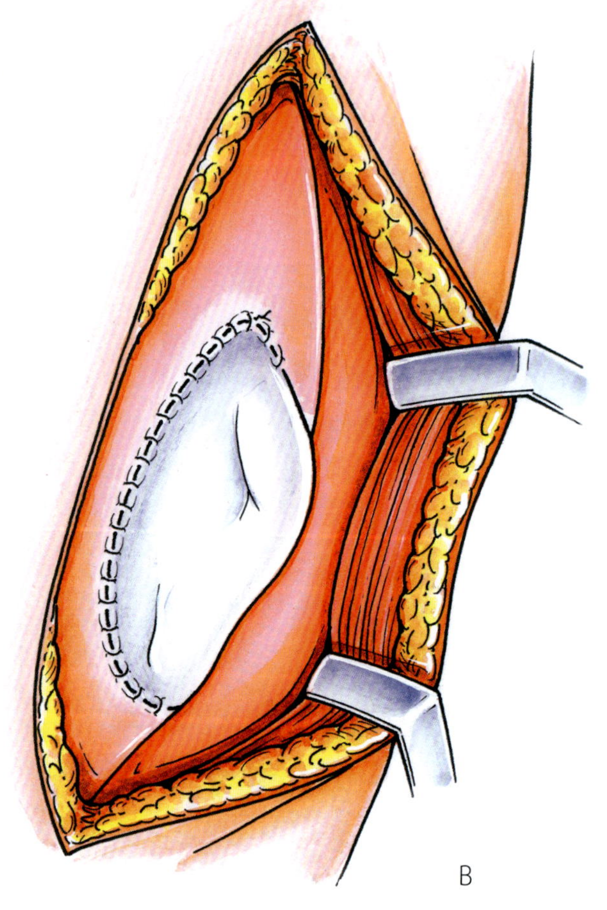

B

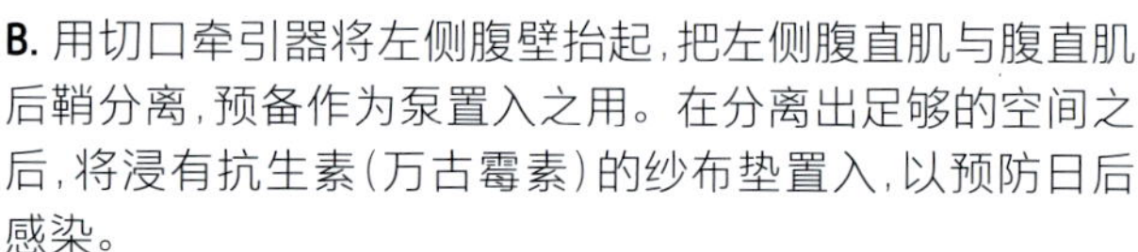

B. 用切口牵引器将左侧腹壁抬起，把左侧腹直肌与腹直肌后鞘分离，预备作为泵置入之用。在分离出足够的空间之后，将浸有抗生素（万古霉素）的纱布垫置入，以预防日后感染。

B. Lift the left abdominal wall with an incision retractor, separate the left rectus abdominis from the posterior sheath of the rectus abdominis, and prepare it for pump placement. After enough space has been isolated, a gauze pad soaked with antibiotics (vancomycin) is placed to prevent future infection.

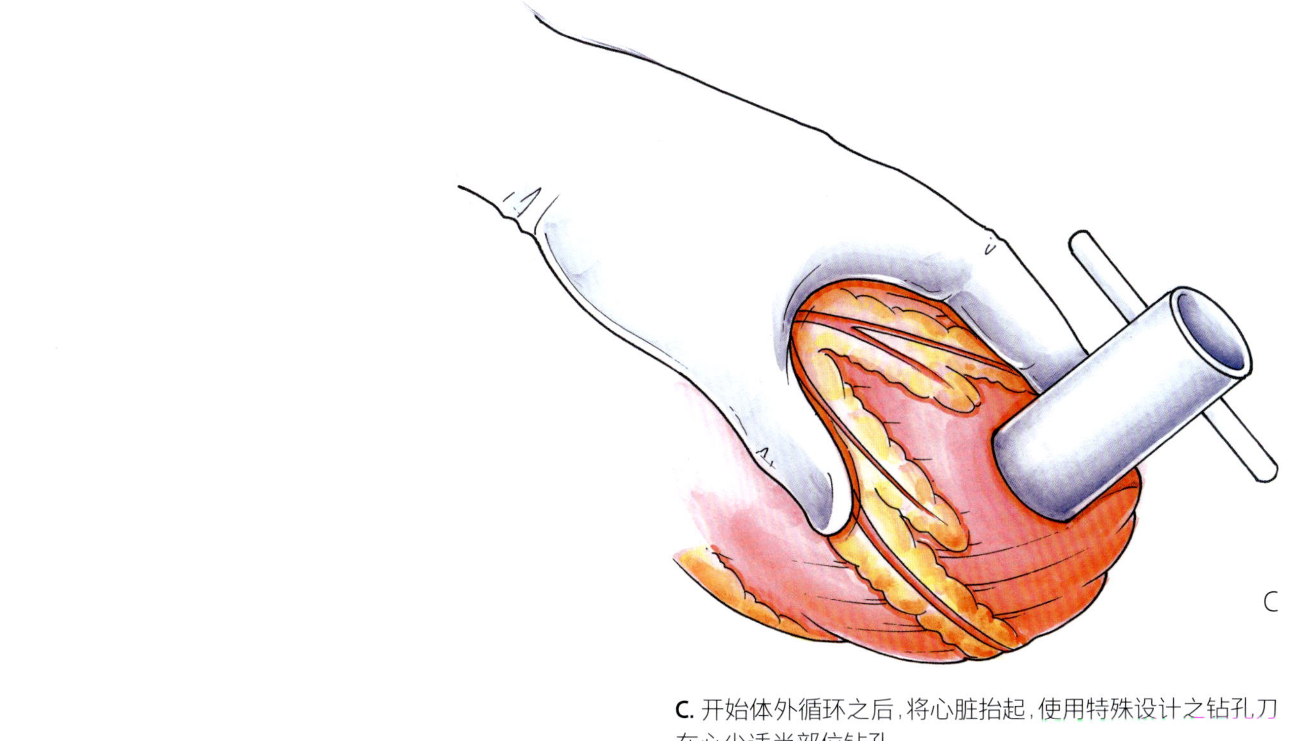

C. 开始体外循环之后，将心脏抬起，使用特殊设计之钻孔刀在心尖适当部位钻孔。

C. After the cardiopulmonary bypass is initiated, the heart is lifted and a specially designed drill knife is used to drill a hole in the appropriate part of the cardiac apex.

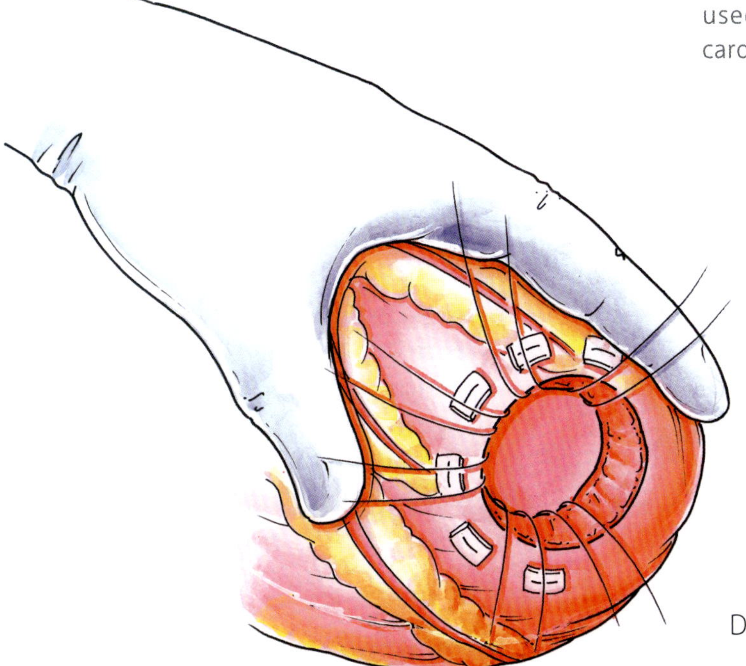

D. 先检查左心室内部有无血栓，如有血栓应予以清除干净，然后用带垫片褥式缝线均匀缝在左心室流出口。

D. First, check whether there is a thrombus inside the left ventricle. If there is any, it should be removed, and then the left ventricular outflow port is evenly sewn with pledgeted mattress sutures.

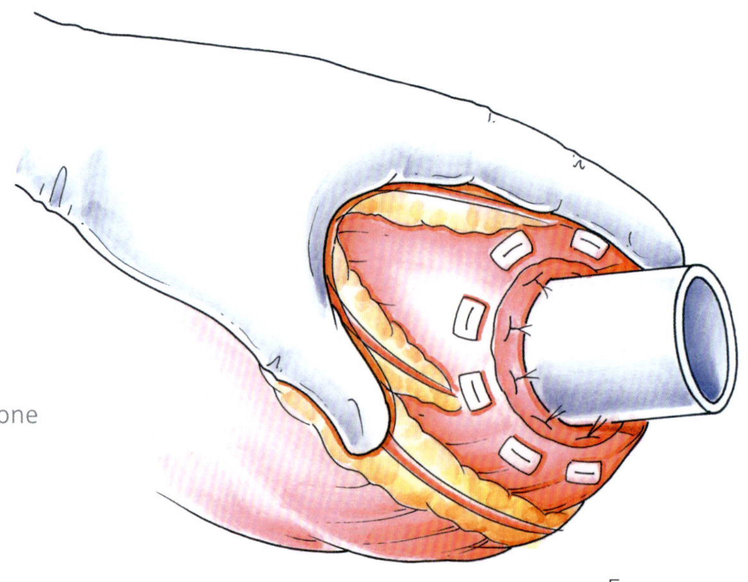

E. 将流入口缝合环及硅胶管接头缝合在心尖之上。

E. Suture the inflow port sewing ring and the silicone tube adapter on the cardiac apex.

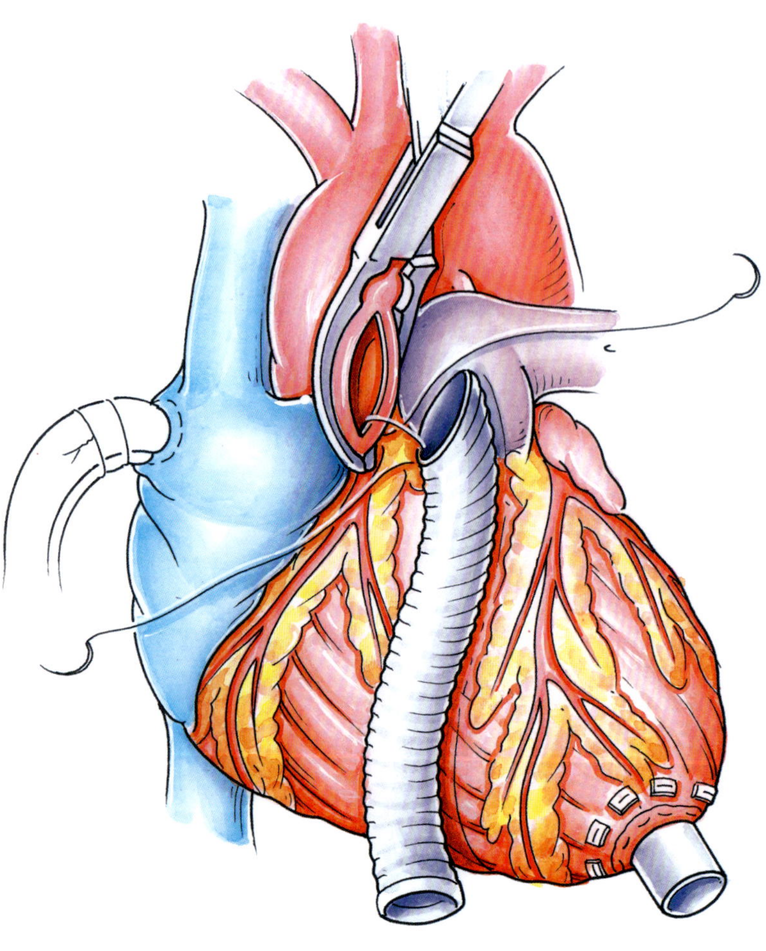

F. 侧壁钳钳夹升主动脉，将一段人工血管与升主动脉进行端侧吻合。

F. With the ascending aorta side-clamped, a segment of the artificial blood vessel is end-to-side anastomosed to the ascending aorta.

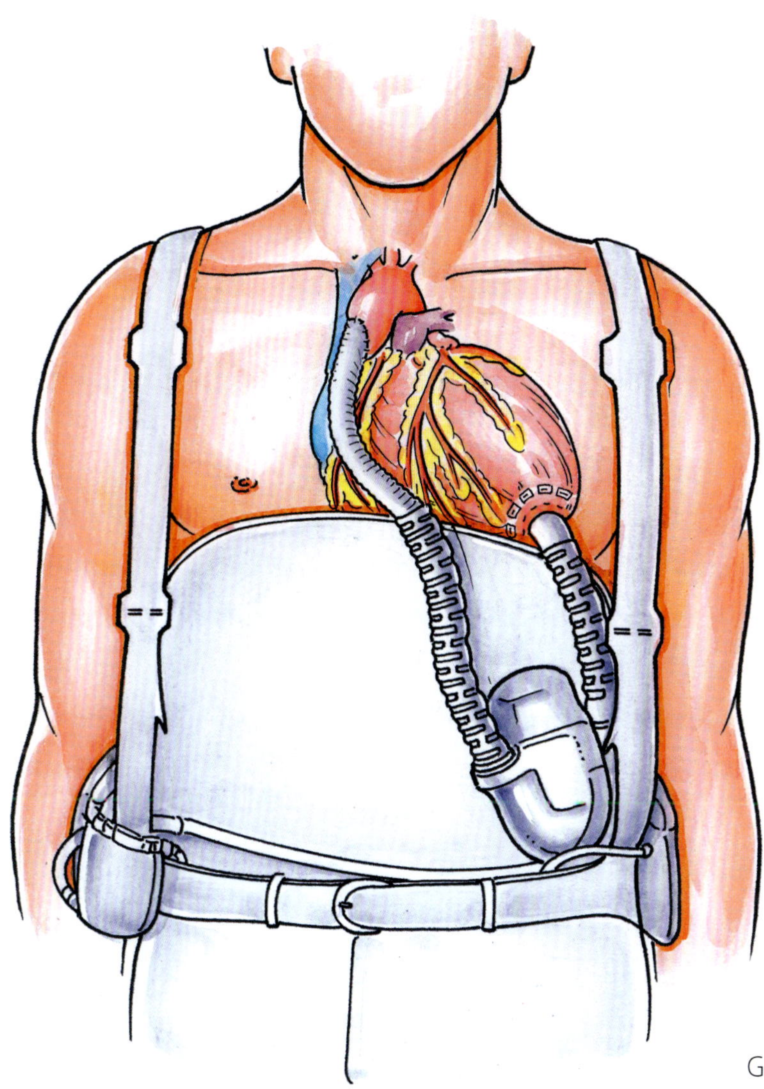

G. Novacor 泵与左心室流入口之接管接合，以及与流出口接管、人工血管相连接，完成手术。

G. The Novacor pump is connected with the connection tube of the left ventricular inflow port and with both the outflow tube and the artificial blood vessel to complete the operation.

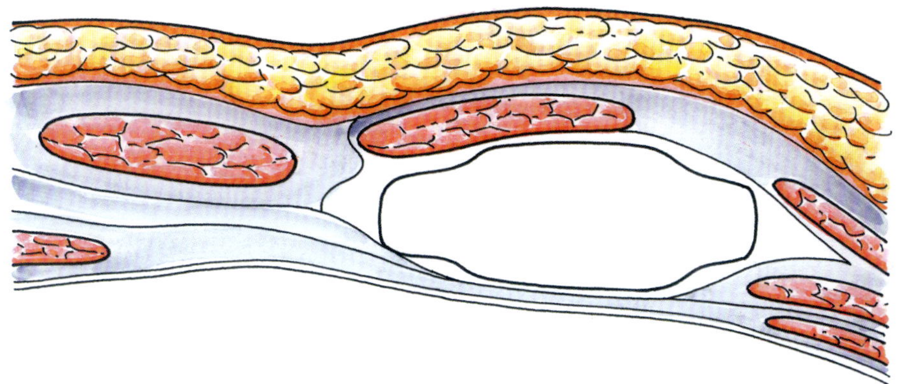

H. Novacor 泵放在腹直肌后方与腹直肌鞘之间，白色空白部分为 Novacor 泵。

H. The Novacor pump is placed between the posterior rectus abdominis and the rectus abdominis sheath, with the white blank part indicating a Novacor pump.

LionHeart 心室辅助装置

LionHeart ventricular assist device

LionHeart 是全世界第一个完全植入人体的永久治疗性左心室辅助装置，身体表面完全看不到任何的导管或连接器。

整套系统包含：

1. **血液泵** 外壳由钛制成，有流入和流出的导管组件。由滚柱螺杆和连接推板的电机驱动，螺杆的线性运动让血囊通过连接推板往复压缩在壳体上。霍尔效应感应器安装在装配箱内，并允许系统控制器持续监控推板位置。血囊和推板之间没有粘接，可确保在心脏舒张期顺利地填满血液泵。通过两个 Delrin 圆盘单支撑阀（入口 27mm，出口 25mm）保持单向血流。血液通过流入导管进入泵，流出导管由 Hemashield 人工血管所组成，吻合固定在升主动脉上。最大泵流量约为 8L/min，动态心排血量为 64ml。

2. **电力控制器** 外壳由钛制成，控制系统依舒张末期容积的连续监测确定泵的灌注量。随后调整泵，以确保完全填充泵。控制器有一组充电电池，可提供应急电源，在断电的情况下，可继续运转约 30 分钟。

The LionHeart is the world's first permanent therapeutic left ventricular assist system that is fully implanted in the human body, with no catheters or connectors visible on the surface of the body.

The complete system consists of:

1. **Blood Pump** The blood pump housing, made of titanium, has inflow and outflow conduit assemblies. Driven by a roller screw and a motor connected to the push plate, the linear movement of the screw allows the blood sac, which connects to the push plate, to be compressed reciprocally on the housing. The Hall effect sensor, installed in the assembly box, allows the system controller to continuously monitor the push plate position. There is no adhesion between the blood sac and the push plate, which ensures smooth filling of the blood pump during the diastolic phase. Unidirectional flow is maintained through two Delrin disc single support valves (inlet 27 mm, outlet 25 mm). The blood enters the pump through the inflow conduit. The outflow conduit, consisting of a Hemashield artificial vessel, is anastomosed to the ascending aorta. The maximum pump flow is approximately 8 L/min, and the dynamic cardiac output is 64 ml.

2. **Power Controller** The power controller housing is made of titanium, and the control system determines pump perfusion based on continuous monitoring of end-diastolic volume. The pump is then adjusted to ensure the complete filling. The controller has a set of rechargeable batteries, which can provide emergency power, and can continue to operate for about 30 minutes when the power is cut off.

3. 经皮能量传输系统 外部直流电被转换成交流电，通过感应连接，交流电可将能量经皮传输至植入的次级线圈。随后将该能源整流为直流电，该直流电又驱动电动机及其相关的电子硬件。

3. Transcutaneous Energy Transfer System External direct current is converted to alternating current, which, through an inductive connection, can percutaneously transfer energy to the implanted secondary coil. The energy is then rectified to direct current, which in turn drives the motor and the associated electronic hardware.

4. 缓冲室 充气式的缓冲室由圆形的聚合物囊和连接皮下通口的输注系统组成，经由输液通口对系统压力进行间歇性监控，也可经由相同的通口排出空气。

4. Buffer Chamber The inflatable buffer chamber consists of an infusion system with a circular polymer capsule connected to the subcutaneous port, and the system pressure is intermittently monitored through the infusion port, through which the air can be vented.

5. 其他外在组件 动力组、电力传输器、充电电池组、遥测棒、系统监视器和多种电力供应选择。这些组件都是为了确保使用的安全、泵的操作具有足够的灵活性，让患者出院后能够恢复正常的生活方式。

5. Other External Components Power pack, power transmitter, rechargeable battery pack, telemetry stick, system monitor, and multiple power supply options. These components are designed to ensure safe use and sufficient flexibility in pump operation to allow patients to return to their normal lives after discharge.

图 8-3-9　LionHeart 植入术
Figure 8-3-9　Implantation of LionHeart

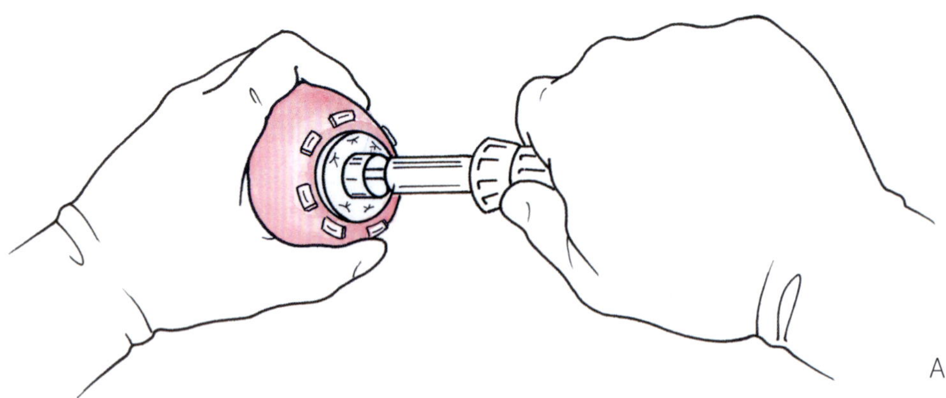

A. 体外循环开始后，先在膈肌上开一个 3cm 的开口，以便流入导管通过。将缝合环及接管缝合在左心室心尖上，再用圆刀钻孔。

A. After initiating extracorporeal circulation, cut a 3 cm opening in the diaphragm to allow the inflow conduit to pass. Suture the sewing ring and the connecting tube to the left ventricular apex and drill a hole with a circular knife.

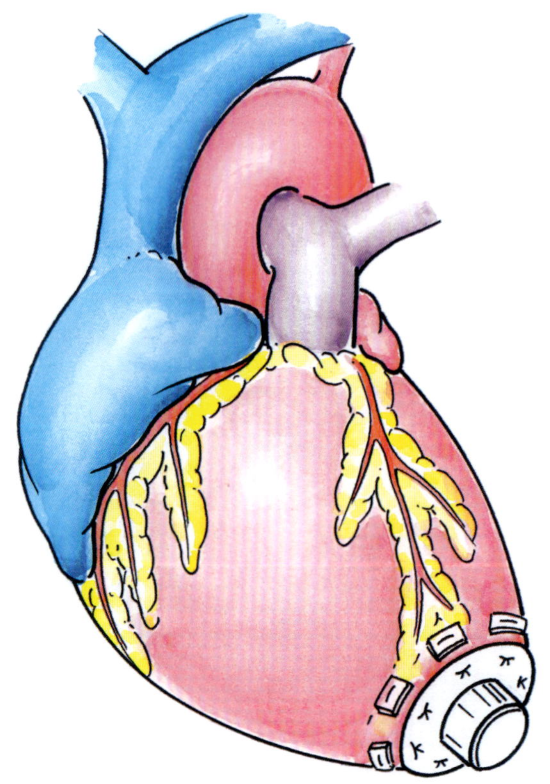

B. 心尖部位缝合完成。

B. Suturing at the apex is completed.

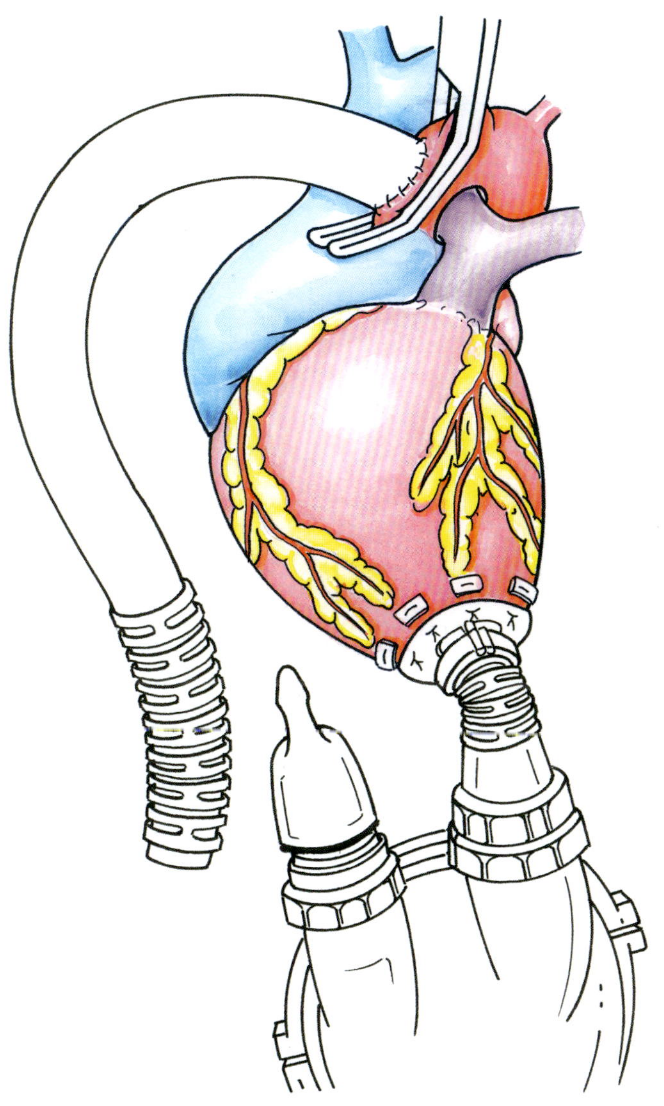

C. 将泵放置在腹直肌与后鞘之间分离出来的间隙里，再把泵的流入导管向上穿过膈肌的开口并放置在心尖开口中。在将流入导管中的小弯头调整到最好的位置后，使用定制夹具将其固定到先前放置的缝合环上。流出人工血管与升主动脉端侧吻合，其近端连接到已灌注并排空的泵上，控制器也放入腹直肌与后鞘之间分离出来的间隙里。

C. The pump is placed in the separated space between the rectus abdominis and the posterior sheath, and the inflow conduit is pulled upward through the diaphragm opening to be placed in the cardiac apex opening. After adjusting the small elbow in the inflow conduit to its best position, secure it to the previously placed sewing ring using a customized clamp. The artificial outflow conduit is end-to-side anastomosed to the ascending aorta with the proximal end connected to the perfused and emptied pump, and the controller is also placed in the separated space between the rectus abdominis and the posterior sheath.

C

D. 以束带固定缝合环接头及流入导管。

D. Secure the sewing ring connector and the inflow conduit with a strap.

D

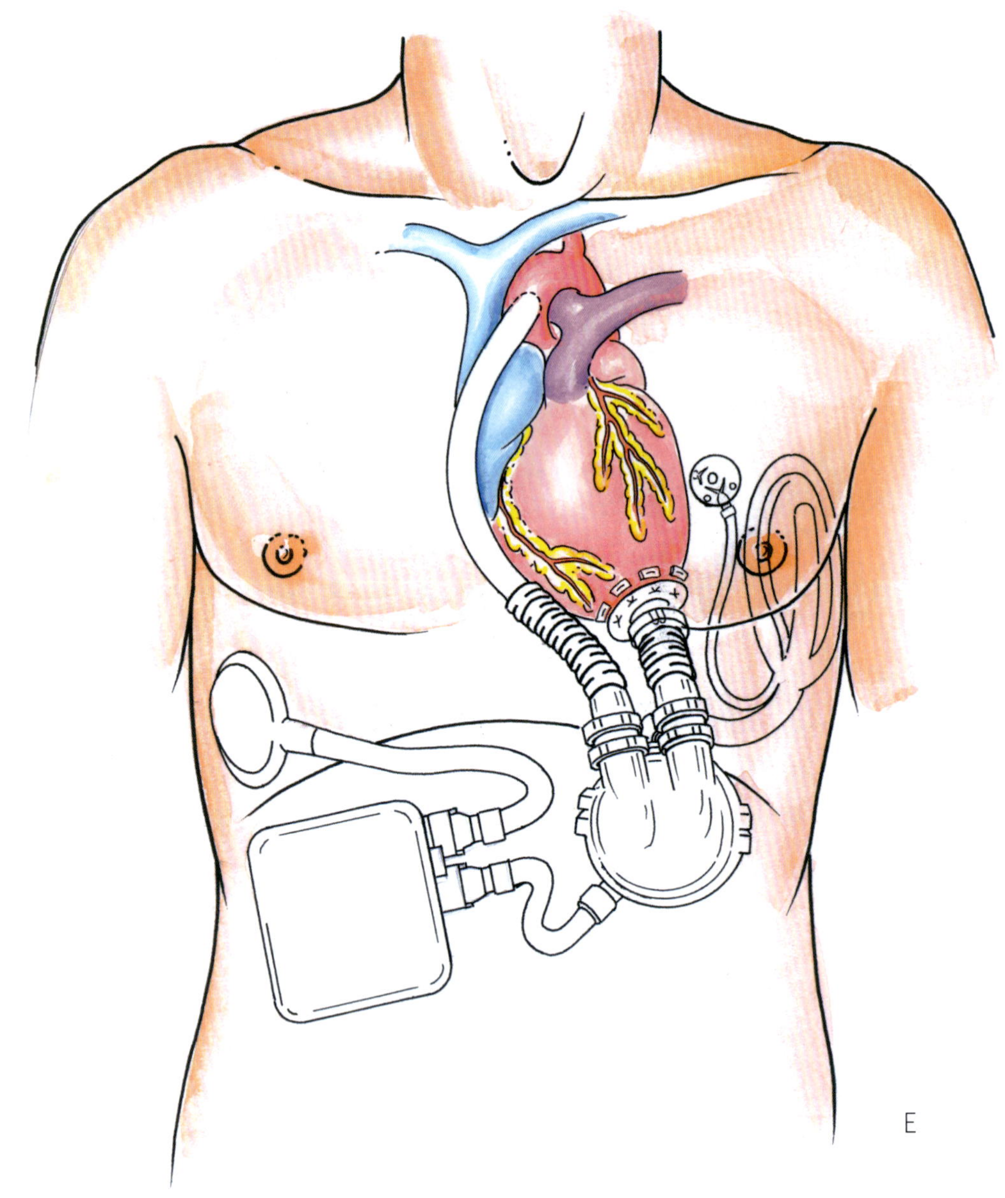

E. LionHeart 植入手术完成图，含充电线圈、马达控制器、电池等设备。

E. The figure illustrates a completed LionHeart implantation procedure, including charging coils, the motor controller, batteries, etc.

DeBakey 心室辅助装置

DeBakey ventricular assist device

DeBakey 左心室辅助装置是一个重约 93g，长 86mm，宽 25mm 的微型轴流式心室辅助装置。相较于脉动式心室辅助装置，DeBakey 左心室辅助装置的优点是没有血袋、表面小、体积小、没有阀门。只有一个运动组件、低电力消耗、无噪声，可以使用在体格较小的成人及儿童。

The DeBakey left ventricular assist device, about 93 g in weight, 86 mm in length and 25 mm in width, is a miniaturized axial flow ventricular assist device. Compared with the pulsatile ventricular assist device, the DeBakey left ventricular assist device has the advantages of no blood bag, small surface, small volume, and no valve. With only one motion component, low power consumption, and no noise, it can be applied to smaller-sized adults and children.

整套系统包括：

The complete system consists of:

1. **血液泵** 泵内部包括叶轮、叶轮前轴的整流器、叶轮后轴的扩散器，都是由钛制成。扩散器通过轴向改变来缓和快速的血流速，此一动作导致流体压力差的形成。叶轮上的叶片在泵内转动，因为是轴向流动，不需要有阀门控制。叶轮的转速可以设定为 7 500~12 000r/min。10 000r/min 时相当于 100mmHg 压力，会产生 5~6L/min 的血流量。在临床上，只需要在术后早期做转速的调整，转速设定在 9 500~10 000r/min，心脏指数可达到 2.8~3.5L/(min·m^2)。

1. **Blood Pump** Inside the blood pump are the impeller, the rectifier of the impeller front shaft, and the diffuser of the impeller rear shaft, all of which are made of titanium. That the diffuser moderates the rapid blood flow through axial change, resulting in a fluid pressure differential. The vanes on the impeller turn inside the pump, and since this is axial flow, there is no need for valve control. The impeller speed can be set in the range of 7 500-12 000 r/min. When the impeller rotates at 10 000 r/min, a pressure of 100 mmHg is generated, resulting in a blood flow of 5-6 L/min. The rotational speed, clinically, only needs to be adjusted in the early postoperative period. With the rotational speed is set between 9 500-10 000 r/min, the cardiac index can reach 2.8-3.5 L/(min·m^2).

2. **导管** 导管衔接在泵的两端。流入导管本身是钛制成，与左心室上的心尖套环连接。流出导管则是由聚酯纤维制成的人工血管所组成，衔接在升主动脉上。

2. **Conduits** The conduits are connected to both ends of the pump. The inflow conduit, made of titanium, is attached to the apical collar on the left ventricle. The outflow conduit is an artificial blood vessel made of polyester fiber, which is connected to the ascending aorta.

3. 流量探测器 固定在流出导管周围，用来探测泵的血流量，提供即时心排血量。马达电缆线和流量探测器的导线通过皮肤引出并连接到外部控制器。流量探头的导线由控制器模块、电池组和电池充电器组成。为了方便移动和返家照顾，可以用两个 12V 的直流电电池供电，运作 4~6 小时。

3. Flow Probe A flow probe, fixed around the outflow conduit, is used to detect the blood flow of the pump, providing immediate cardiac output. The motor cable and the flow probe wires are percutaneously brought out and connected to the external controller. The wire of the flow probe consists of the controller module, the battery pack, and the battery charger. A flow probe can run for 4-6 hours on two 12-volt DC batteries, achieving easy mobility and home care.

4. 监视器 流量曲线、速度、电流和功率显示在床头监控器单元（或临床数据采集系统）中，可以用来调节泵速率。

4. Monitor The flow curve, speed, current, and power are displayed in the bedside monitor unit (or clinical data acquisition system). The monitor can be used to adjust the pump rate.

图 8-3-10 DeBakey 左心室辅助装置植入术

Figure 8-3-10 Implantation of DeBakey as a LVAD

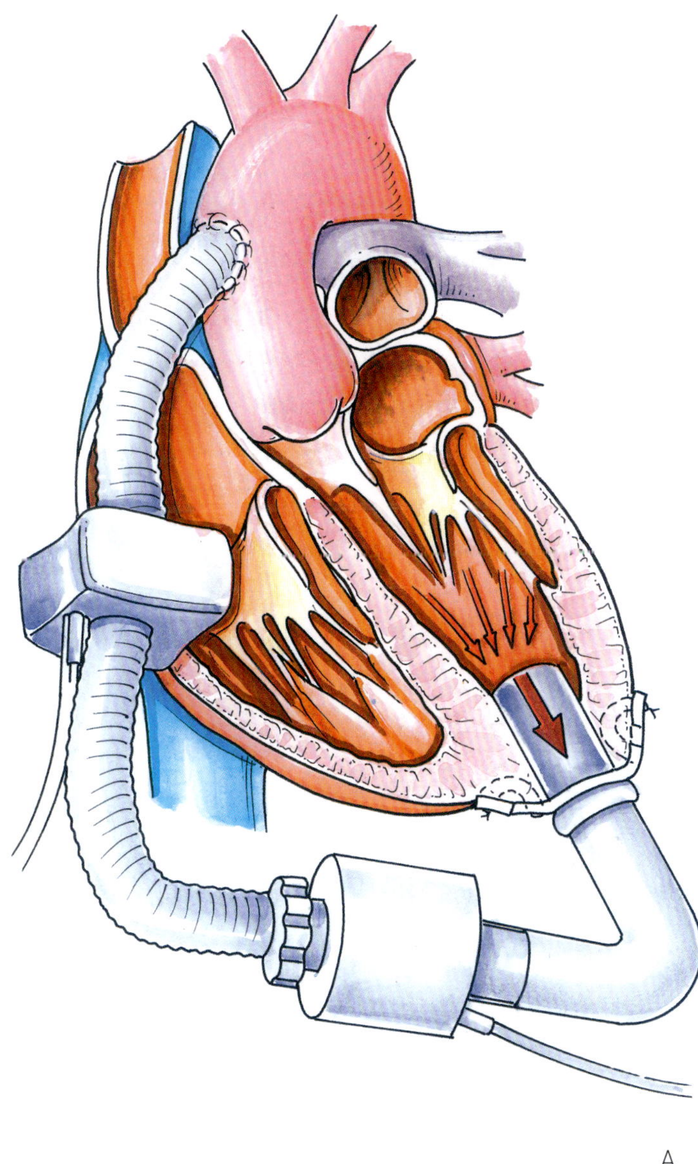

A

A. 通过标准的胸骨正中切口暴露心脏，插管建立体外循环。在大多数情况下，植入过程不用停止心脏跳动。通常常规使用经食管超声心动图（transesophageal echocardiography，TEE）来排除主动脉瓣关闭不全、心内血栓和/或房间隔缺损（或卵圆孔未闭）。此外，TEE 可以导引心脏内排气，并提供流入插管放置、右心室功能和左心室减压的影像。无须延长正中胸骨切开术切口，就能在左肋弓下缘创建一个小的腹膜前袋来容纳泵。左心室的心尖上缝入缝合环。流入人工血管插入左心室腔并固定至心尖缝合环。泵放在左肋下缘的腹膜前，在其左下方做一个小切口，传动管线由此经皮穿出并连接到控制器。接下来，流出人工血管吻合到升主动脉。对于需要重复开胸的复杂患者，流出人工血管可以通过左侧开胸吻合到降主动脉。流出人工血管排气，启动装置之后，脱离体外循环。手术完成。

A. The heart is exposed through a standard median sternotomy and cannulated to establish extracorporeal circulation. In most cases, the implantation procedure does not require the heart to stop beating. Transesophageal echocardiography (TEE) is routinely used to examine for the presence of aortic insufficiency, intracardiac thrombus, and/or atrial septal defect (or patent foramen ovale). In addition, the TEE can guide intracardiac venting and provide images of inflow cannula placement, right ventricular function, and left ventricular decompression. A small anterior peritoneal pocket can be created at the inferior border of the left costal arch to accommodate the pump without lengthening the median sternotomy incision. The sewing ring is sutured into the left ventricle apex. The artificial inflow conduit is inserted into the left ventricular chamber and secured to the apical sewing ring. The pump is placed in front of the peritoneum on the left subcostal border, and a small incision is made in the lower left of the peritoneum, through which the transmission line is percutaneously pulled out and connected to the controller. The artificial outflow conduit is then anastomosed to the ascending aorta. In complex cases requiring repeated thoracotomy, the artificial outflow conduit can be anastomosed to the descending aorta via a left thoracotomy. After the artificial outflow conduit is vented and the device is activated, the cardiopulmonary bypass is weaned off. The procedure is complete.

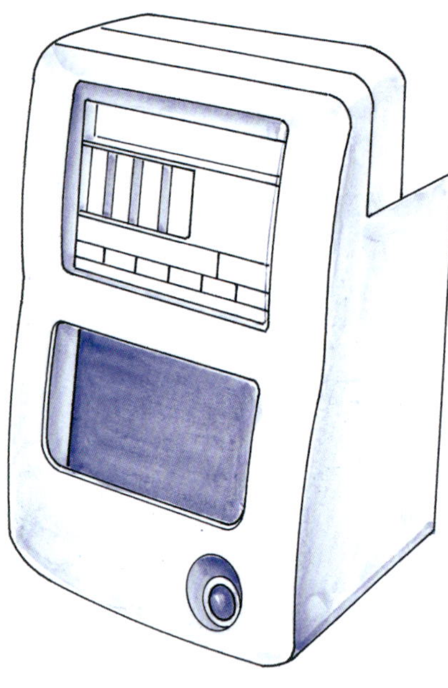

B

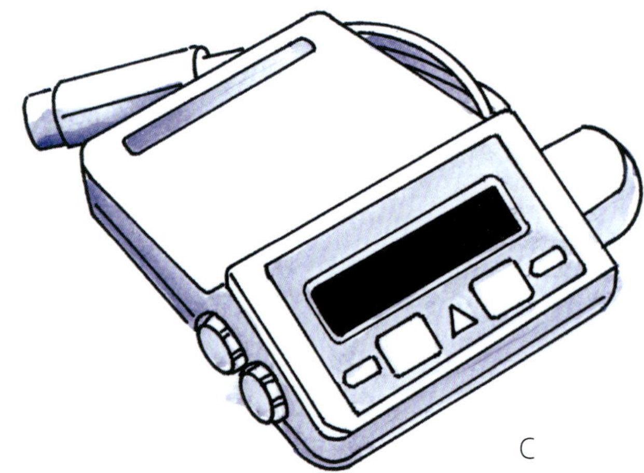

C

B、C. 控制器及充电系统。

B, C. The controller and the charging system.

Incor 心室辅助装置

Incor ventricular assist device

Incor 是第三代长期植入电磁力驱动的轴流连续泵，重 200g，直径 3cm。所有组件经过流体动力学计算设计，优化流速和降低血液损伤，耗电量低。它能够产生高达 6L/min 的流量，叶轮的转速约 7 500r/min。

Incor is the third-generation long-term implanted electromagnetic force-driven axial flow continuous pump, with 200 g in weight and 3 cm in diameter. All components are specially designed based on hydrodynamic calculations to optimize flow rate and reduce blood damage and power consumption. It is capable of producing up to 6 L/min flow with an impeller rotating at about 7 500 r/min.

整套系统包括：

The complete system consists of:

1. **导管** 流出导管和流入导管是由医疗等级的硅胶制成。

1. **Conduits** Outflow and inflow conduits are made of silicone dedicated to the medical field.

2. **轴流泵** 由钛制成，泵与血液接触表面有 Carmeda 生物活性涂层。

2. **Axial Flow Pump** Made of titanium with a bioactive coating of Carmeda on the surface where the pump contacts the blood.

3. **电力供应系统** 由主要及备用电池所组成，连接控制器，Incor 系统也可以通过交流电源进行操作。

3. **Power Supply System** It consists of main and backup batteries and is connected to the controller. The Incor system can also be operated through an AC power supply.

4. **控制器。**

4. **The controller.**

5. **泵连接线。**

5. **The pump connection line.**

6. **驱动管线。**

6. **The drivelines.**

图 8-3-11 Incor 植入术
Figure 8-3-11 Implantation of Incor

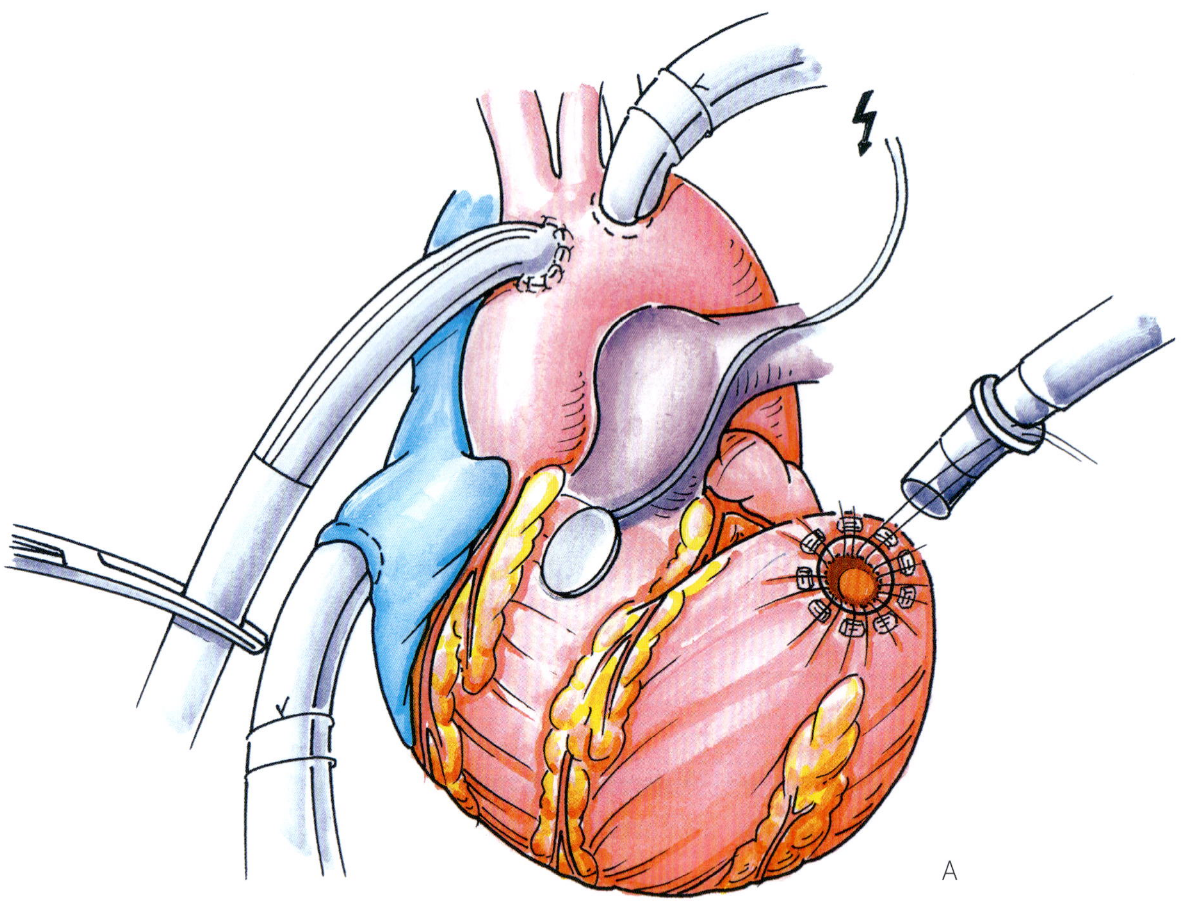

A. 在体外循环支持之下开胸，将流出导管吻合在升主动脉上。而后抬起心脏在左心室心尖处钻孔，进行左心室心尖与流入插管的吻合。

A. Perform a thoracotomy and anastomose the outflow conduit to the ascending aorta during extracorporeal circulation support. Then lift the heart to drill the left ventricle apex, and perform an anastomosis between the left ventricle apex and the inflow cannula.

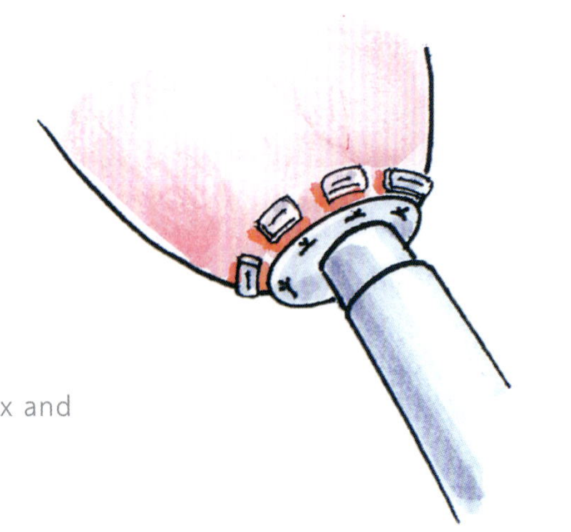

B. 心尖与流入插管吻合完成。

B. The anastomosis between the cardiac apex and the inflow cannula is completed.

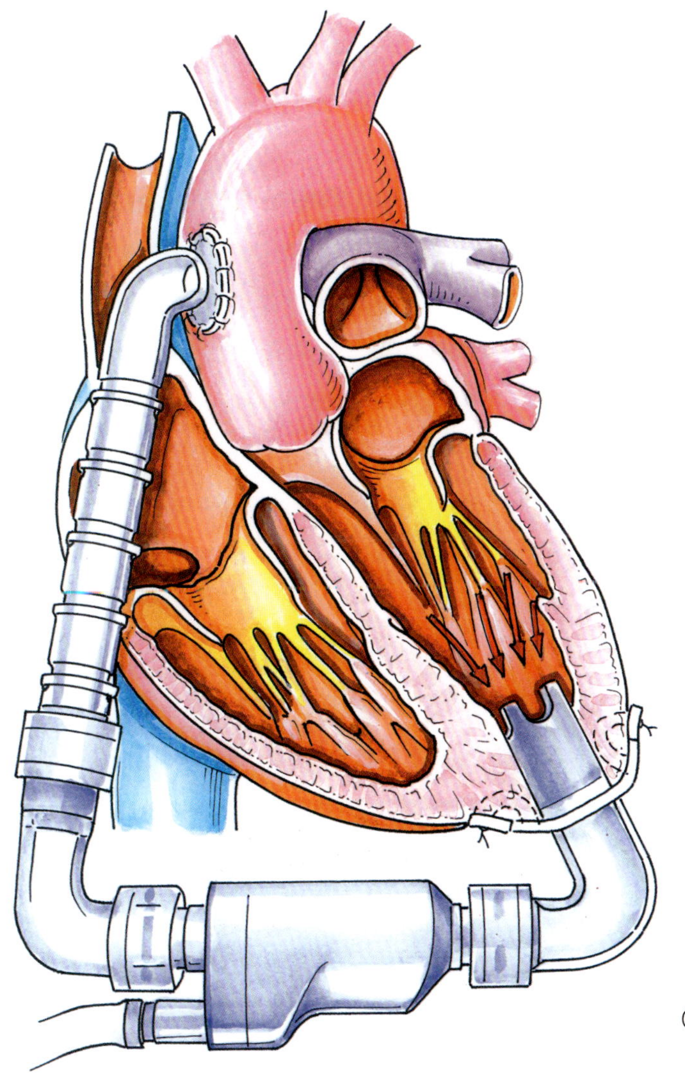

C. Incor 左心辅助手术完成，流入导管由左心室把血液输送到泵，再经由流出直角插管衔接流出导管，与升主动脉吻合。流出导管也可与降主动脉直接吻合不需要使用流出直角插管。经皮置入驱动管路连接泵到控制器。

C. The Incor left heart assist surgery is completed. Blood is delivered through the inflow conduit from the left ventricle to the pump. The outflow conduit is connected to the pump through an outflow right-angle cannula and anastomosed to the ascending aorta or the descending aorta. When performing an anastomosis to the descending aorta, the outflow right-angle cannula is not required. The pump is connected to the controller through a percutaneously inserted driveline.

DuraHeart 心室辅助装置

DuraHeart ventricular assist device

DuraHeart 左心室辅助装置，是全世界第一个通过市场认证的第三代植入式左心室辅助装置，由三个主要的可植入组件组成。

The DuraHeart left ventricular assist system, the first market-approved third-generation implantable left ventricular assist device in the world, consists of three main implantable components.

1. 血液泵 系钛和不锈钢制成的植入式离心泵，由磁性轴承、叶轮、壳体和直流电动机四个部分组成。利用磁悬浮将旋转的叶轮悬挂在血腔内，叶轮通过叶轮和电机之间的磁联结而旋转，并被三个电磁体磁悬浮。每个电磁体的电流通过三个位置传感器进行控制，使叶轮在泵壳体的中心自由浮动。该泵既不需要旋转轴，也不需要轴封。钛制外壳将电气组件密封，以防止与血液或组织接触。DuraHeart 泵的直径为 72mm，厚度为 45mm，重约 540g。排出量为 196ml，比第一代脉冲式泵少 30%~50%。包括泵在内，流入和流出导管的水平长度比轴向流左心室辅助装置的长度短 50%~60%。泵能够在 120mmHg 的压力差下提供 8L/min 的血流量，并且能够产生从 1 200r/min 的 50mmHg 到 2 400r/min 的 180mmHg 的宽压力范围脉动泵的能力。由电磁轴承控制的泵稳定叶轮位置，还具有维持血液路径内的连续冲洗从而减少了血栓形成可能性的优势。

1. Blood Pump An implantable centrifugal pump made of titanium and stainless steel, consisting of four parts: magnetic bearing, impeller, housing, and DC motor. The rotating impeller is suspended in the blood chamber by magnetic levitation. The impeller rotates by the magnetic connection between the impeller and the motor and is magnetically suspended by three electromagnets. The current to each electromagnet is controlled using three position sensors, allowing the impeller to float freely in the center of the pump housing. The pump requires neither a rotating shaft nor a shaft seal. The titanium-made housing seals the electrical components to prevent contact with blood or tissue. The DuraHeart pump has a diameter of 72 mm, a thickness of 45 mm, and a weight of approximately 540 g. The discharge volume is 196 ml, which is 30%-50% smaller than that of the first-generation pulsatile pump. The horizontal length of the inflow and outflow conduits (including pumps) is approximately 50%-60% shorter than the length of the axial flow left ventricular assist device. The pump can deliver a blood flow of 8 L/min at a differential pressure of 120 mmHg and of produce a wide pressure range of pulsation from 50 mmHg at 1 200 r/min to 180 mmHg at 2 400 r/min. The pump, controlled by an electromagnetic bearing, stabilizes the impeller position and also has the advantage of maintaining continuous irrigation within the blood path, thereby reducing the potential for thrombosis.

2. 控制器 用于建立、维护和监视泵的正常运行。控制器控制电动机和悬浮电路的电源输入，监视相关参数及输出信号中的错误情况，并有 30 天的数据储存容量，以进行故障检测和数据记录。由可穿戴电池、医院控制台或电池充电器供电。

2. Controller The controller is used to establish, maintain and monitor the normal operation of the pump. The controller controls the power input of the motor and the levitated circuit, monitors the relevant parameters and errors in the output signal, and has a 30-day data storage capacity to facilitate fault detection and data recording. The controller is powered by wearable batteries, hospital console, or battery charger.

3. 电池组 穿戴式电池由可充电锂离子电池组成，两个备用电池，在正常情况下可以提供控制器和泵 7 个小时使用。

3. Battery Pack The wearable battery consists of a rechargeable lithium-ion battery and has two backup batteries, providing the controller and pump for seven hours of continuous use under normal conditions.

图 8-3-12 DuraHeart 植入术

Figure 8-3-12 Implantation of DuraHeart

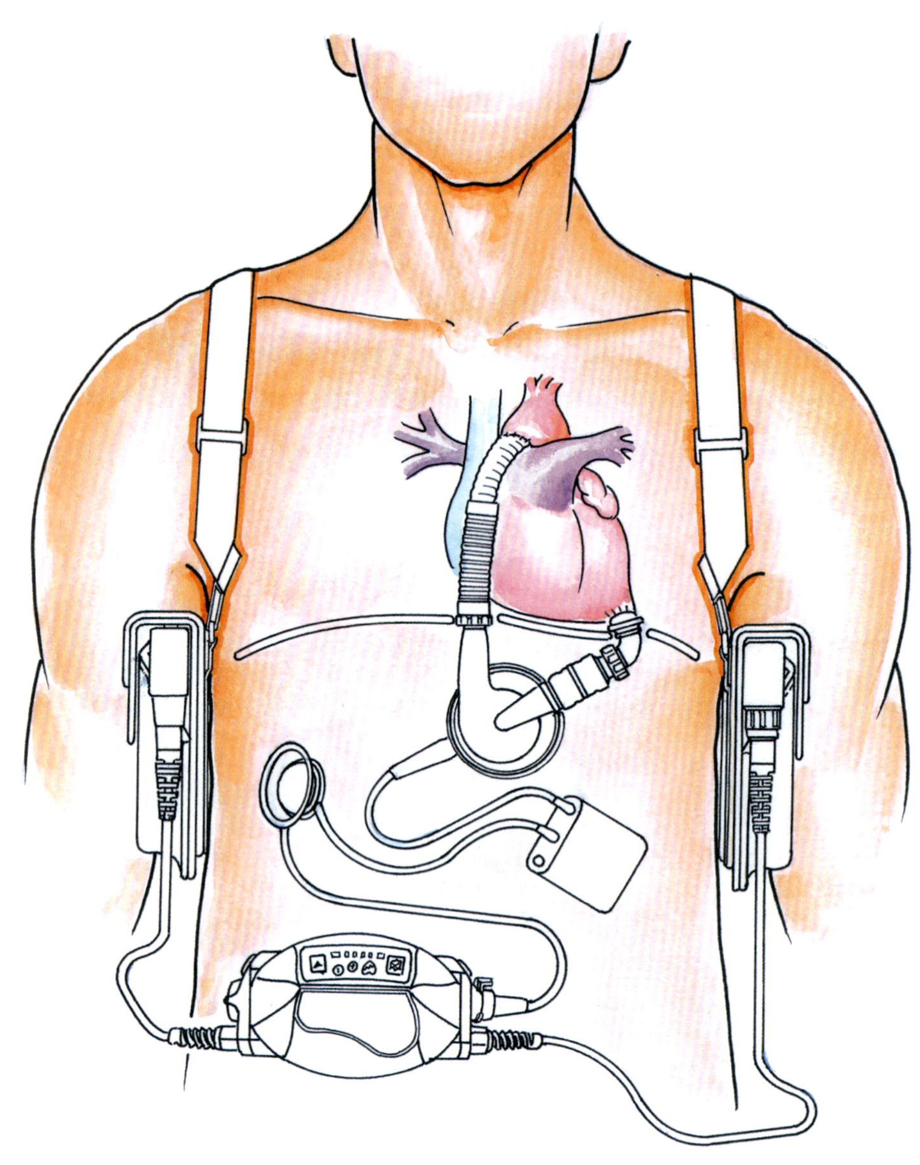

VentraAssist 心室辅助装置
VentraAssist ventricular assist device

VentraAssist 是第三代离心式的左心室辅助装置，泵的设计使血液在所有与血液接触的表面上的流动最大化，从而避免淤滞和血栓形成的可能性。

The VentraAssist, the third-generation centrifugal left ventricular assist device, whose pump is designed to maximize blood flow on all blood-contacting surfaces, thereby avoiding the potential for stasis and thrombosis.

主要的组成组件包括：

The main components are as follows:

1. **血液泵** 泵重约 300g，直径为 2.5 英寸（1 英寸=2.54 厘米），在正常设置下以 1 800~3 000r/min 的速度运行。流体动力悬挂叶轮是其唯一的运动部件。叶轮包括四个嵌入永磁体的小叶片，当电流在泵的三对线圈之间顺序切换时，叶轮叶片旋转。叶轮由薄薄的血液垫悬挂在八个液压轴承的间隙中，四个轴承的每个面上各有一个。八个水动轴承力、流体力和重力之间的动态相互作用，可防止旋转的叶轮接触泵壳体的任何部分。使用流体动力轴承消除了血液泵与壳体之间的摩擦磨损，并且使血液畅通无阻地流经血液泵系统，降低设备磨损和血栓形成的风险。

1. **Blood Pump** The blood pump, approximately 300 g in weight, 2.5 inches (1 inch = 2.54 cm) in diameter, runs at 1 800-3 000 r/min under normal settings. The hydrodynamic suspension impeller is its only moving part. The impeller consists of four small blades embedded in permanent magnets, which rotate when current is switched sequentially between the three pairs of coils of the pump. The impeller is suspended by a thin blood pad in the clearance of eight hydraulic bearings, one on each face of the four bearings. The dynamic interaction among eight hydrodynamic bearing forces, fluid forces, and gravity prevents the rotating impeller from contacting any part of the pump housing. The use of hydrodynamic bearings eliminates friction and wear between the blood pump and the housing, and reduces the risk of equipment wear and the risk of thrombosis by allowing unobstructed blood flow through the blood pump system.

2. **血液导管** 所有植入物件均由完全生物相容性材料组成，包括钛合金。这些材料重量轻，强度高，无毒且对体内降解具有高度抵抗力。

2. **Blood Conduits** All implants consist of fully biocompatible materials, including titanium alloy. These materials are light in weight, high in strength, non-toxic, and highly resistant to in vivo degradation.

3. **系统控制器** 控制器记录和显示系统参数，例如泵速率、功率和估计流量。控制器由穿戴在外部皮带或背包上的可充电镍氢电池供电。控制器管理电池，具有声响和可见的用户警报。

3. **System Controller** The controller records and displays system parameters such as pump rate, power, and estimated flow. The controller is powered by a rechargeable nickel-metal hydride (Ni-MH) battery worn on an external belt or backpack. The controller manages the battery with audible and visible user alarms.

图 8-3-13　VentraAssist 植入术
Figure 8-3-13　Implantation of VentraAssist

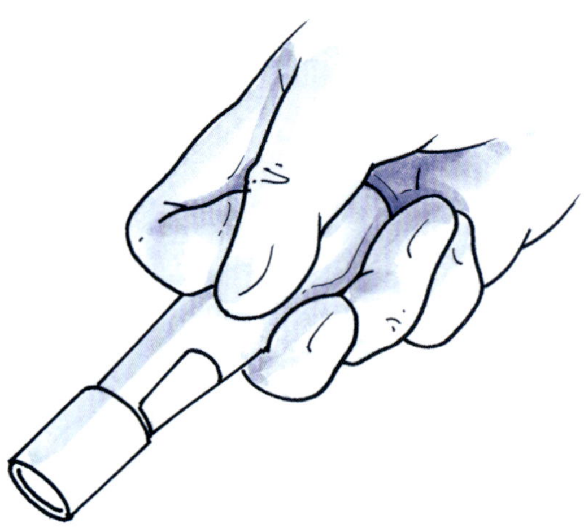

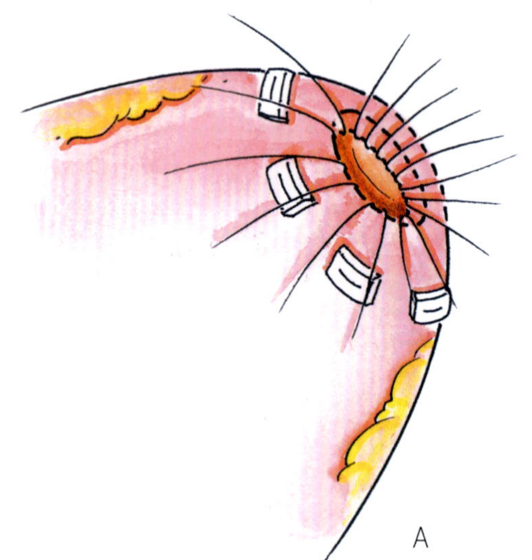

A

A. 在体外循环的支持下，将左心室心尖钻孔，置入带垫片褥式缝线。

A. With extracorporeal circulation support, the left ventricular apex is drilled and pledgeted mattress sutures are placed.

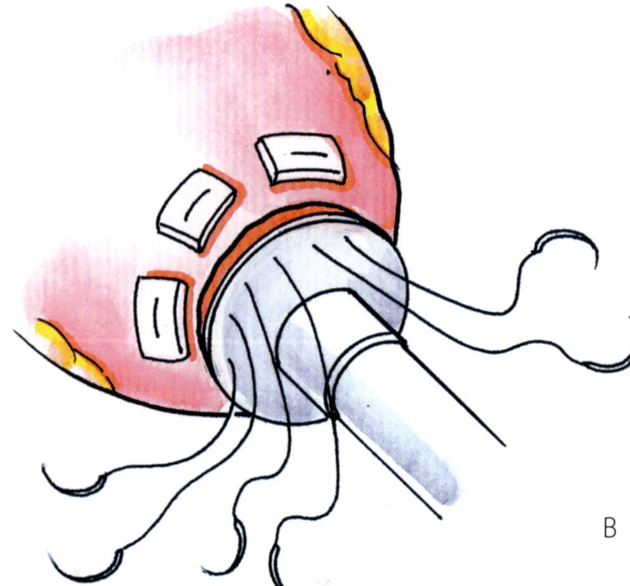

B

B. 用上述褥式缝线将缝合环缝到心尖上。

B. Suture the sewing ring to the apex with the mattress sutures mentioned above.

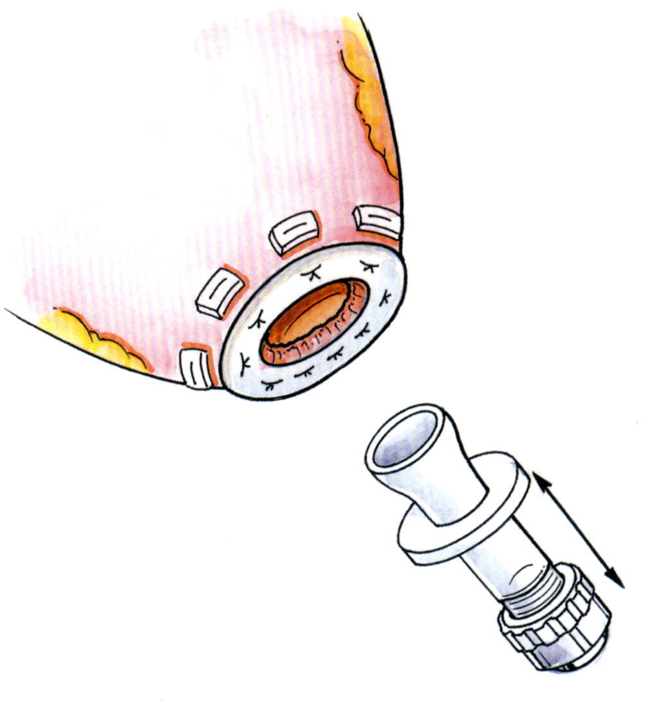

C. 将流入口接管与缝合环进行吻合。

C. The inflow connector is anastomosed with the sewing ring.

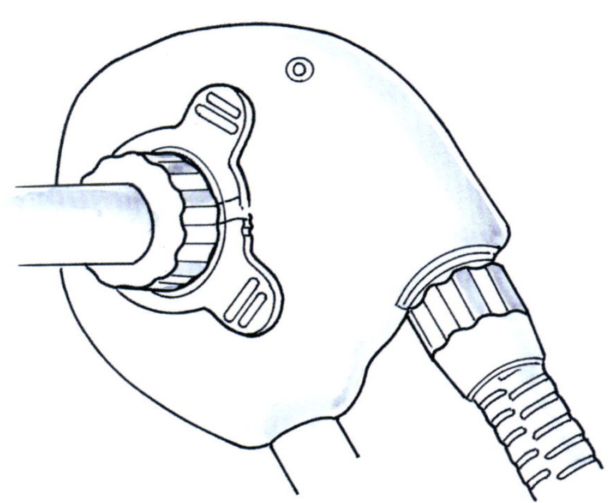

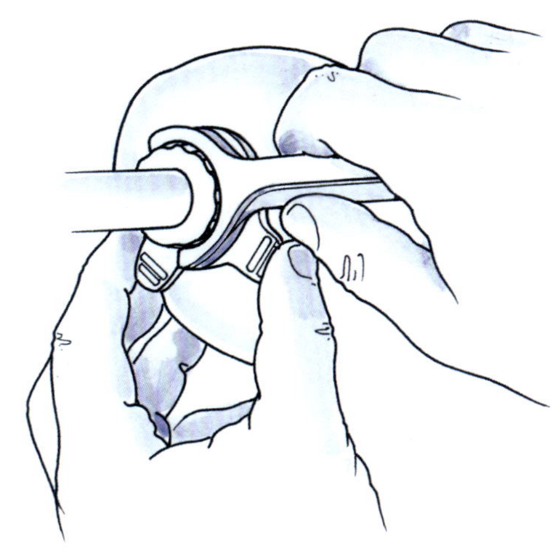

D~F. 装入 VentraAssist 泵，血液泵被植入一个小袋中，小袋位于人体左侧，膈肌下方，腹直肌鞘后面。流入导管与泵连接。

D-F. The VentraAssist pump is implanted, with the blood pump implanted in a pocket located on the left side of the body, below the diaphragm, and behind the rectus abdominis sheath. The inflow conduit is connected to the pump.

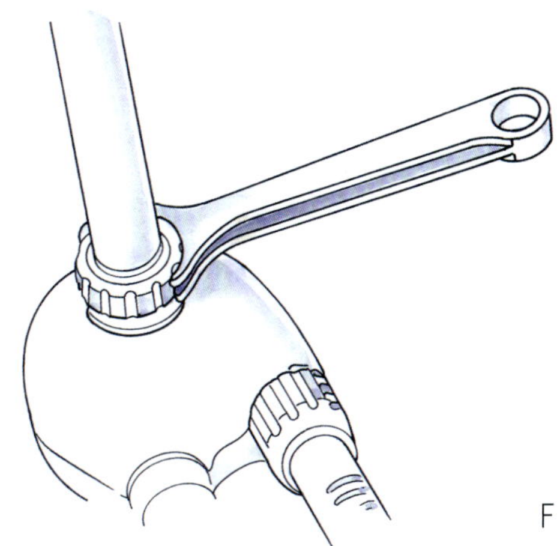

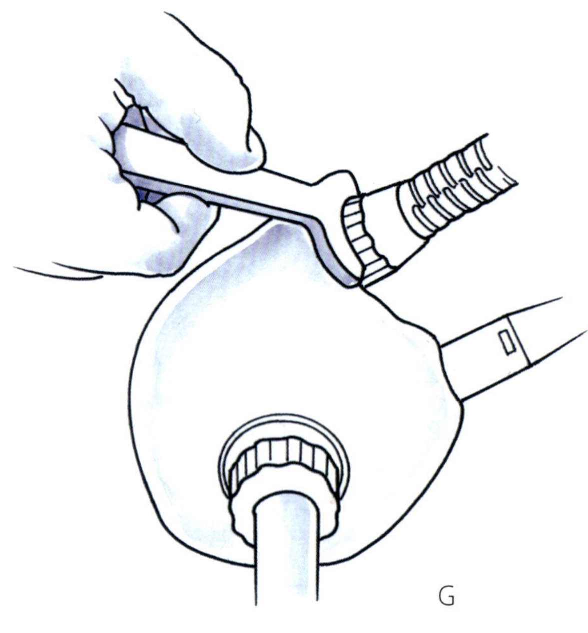

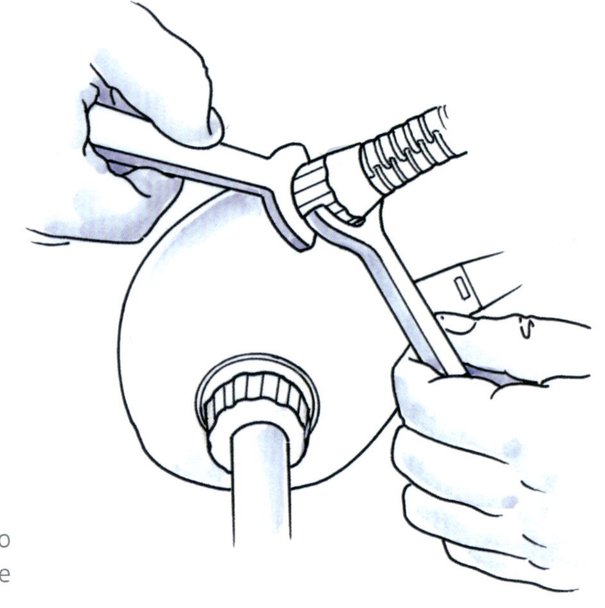

G、H. 流出导管与升主动脉端侧吻合，另一端与泵连接。

G, H. The outflow conduit is end-to-side anastomosed to the ascending aorta with the other end connected to the pump.

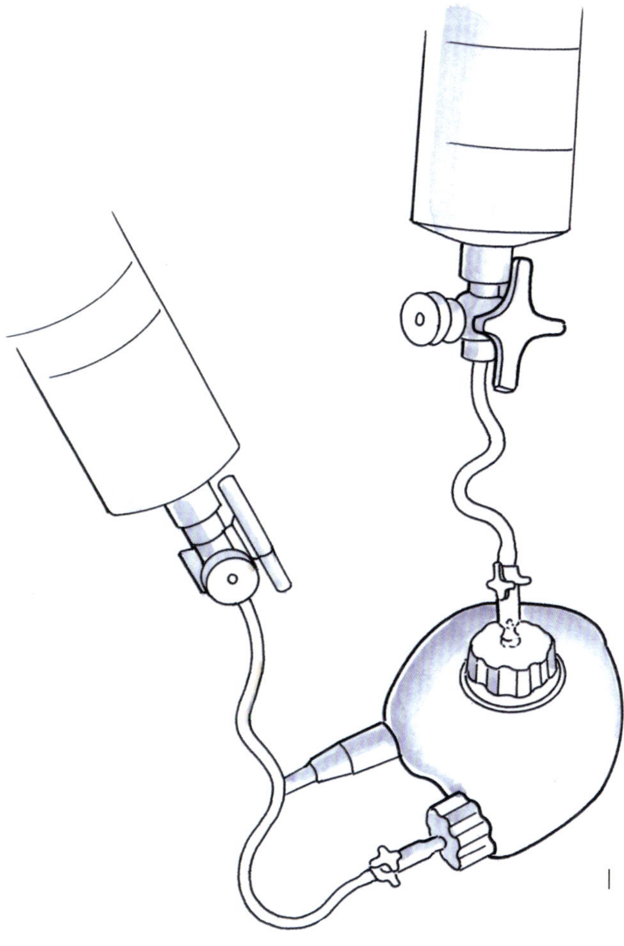

I. VentraAssist 泵排气。

I. VentraAssist pump deairing.

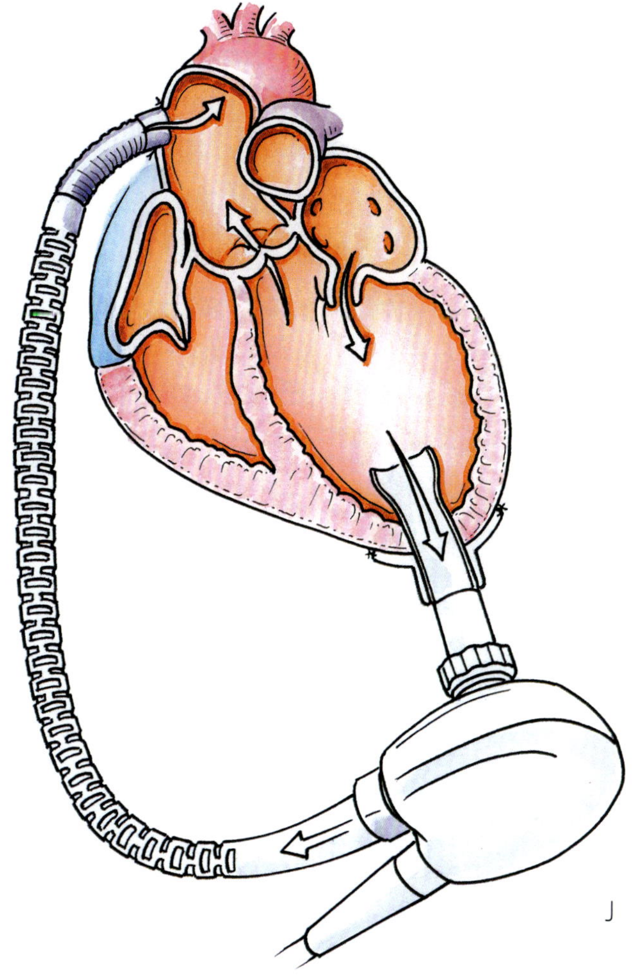

J. 来自泵的一根细的经皮导线从身体的右上象限引出，连接到系统控制器。启动系统，血液从衰竭的左心室经由流入导管输送到泵，再经流出导管送到升主动脉。

J. A thin percutaneous wire from the pump is brought out from the upper right quadrant of the body and connected to the system controller. The system is activated and blood is delivered from the failing left ventricle through the inflow conduit to the pump and then through the outflow conduit to the ascending aorta.

Jarvik 2000 心室辅助装置
Jarvik 2000 ventricular assist device

Jarvik 2000 是一种可植入式微型轴流式心室辅助装置，通过单个旋转的叶片式叶轮产生血流。依照驱动电缆线置入的位置，分成耳后型和腹部型两种。

The Jarvik 2000, an implantable miniaturized axial flow ventricular assist device, produces blood flow through a single rotating vane impeller. According to the position where the drive cable is placed, it is divided into two types: postauricular type and abdominal type.

其装置包含：

The device comprises:

1. **血液泵** 泵非常小，大约相当于 2 号电池的大小（高度 49.5mm，直径 25.3mm）。泵内所有与血液接触的表面均由光滑的钛所制成。叶轮由钕铁硼磁体和流体动力钛叶片组成，通过两个陶瓷轴承固定。流体动力叶片位于叶轮的外表面，流出的定子叶片位于叶轮的下游。

1. **Blood Pump** The pump is very small, approximately the size of an AA battery (49.5 mm in height, 25.3 mm in diameter). All surfaces in the pump that contact the blood are made of smooth titanium. The impeller consists of a neodymium-iron-boron magnet and hydrodynamic titanium blades fixed by two ceramic bearings. The hydrodynamic blades are located on the outer surface of the impeller and the outflow stator blades are located downstream of the impeller.

2. **泵速度控制器** 电动机产生的电磁力，使叶轮以 8 000~12 000r/min 的转速旋转，在 4~6W 的功率下，相对于生理压力，平均流量为 3~6L/min。

2. **Pump Speed Controller** The electromagnetic force generated by the motor drives the impeller to rotate at a speed of 8 000-12 000 r/min, with an average flow of 3-6 L/min relative to the physiological pressure at a power of 4-6 watts.

3. **流出导管是一个直径 16mm 的人工血管。**

3. **The outflow conduit is an artificial blood vessel with a diameter of 16 mm.**

4. **电力电缆线** 由节律型电线构成，这些电线用聚氨酯绝缘，部分包裹有尼龙纤维。

4. **Power Cable** Power cable consists of rhythmic wires that are insulated with polyurethane and partially wrapped with nylon fibers.

5. **直流电源** 通过可充电铅酸或锂离子电池为控制器和泵提供持续电力。

5. **DC Power Supply** The controller and the pump are continuously powered by rechargeable lead-acid or lithium-ion batteries.

图 8-3-14　Jarvik 2000 植入术

Figure 8-3-14　Implantation of Jarvik 2000

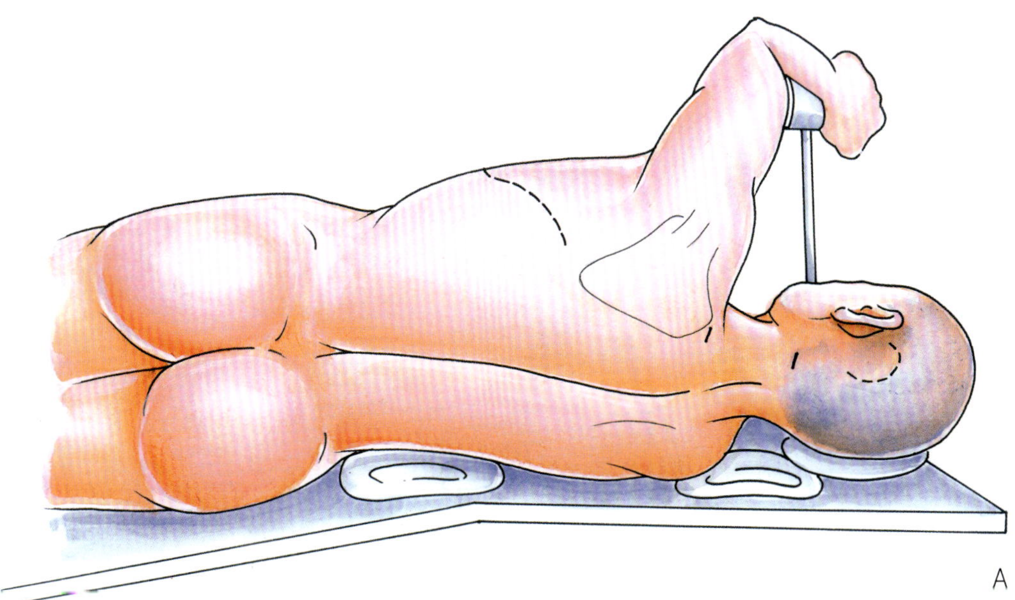

A. 全身麻醉后取右侧卧位进行手术。从左侧胸壁切口进胸，切开心包腔。也可采用胸骨正中切口入路。

A. The operation is performed with the patient in the right lateral decubitus position under general anesthesia. Open the pericardial cavity via a left lateral thoracotomy approach. Median sternotomy access may be used.

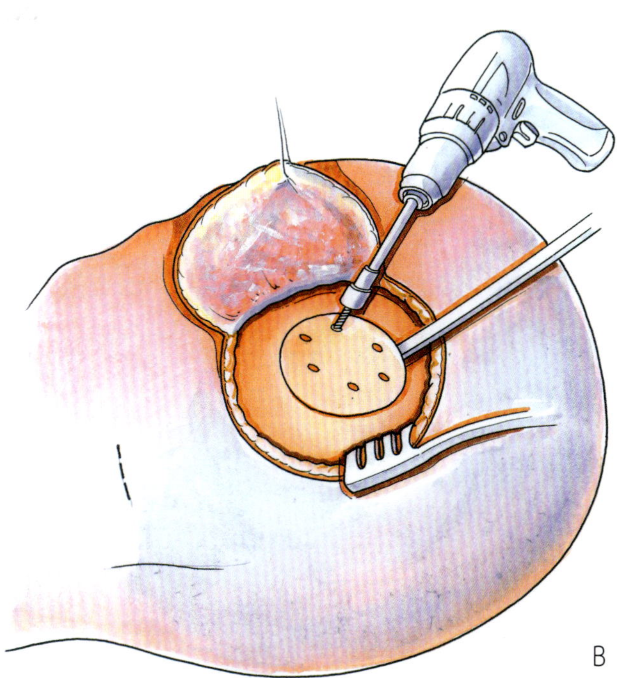

B. 耳后部位做一个半圆形的切口。

B. A semicircular incision is made in the retroauricular area.

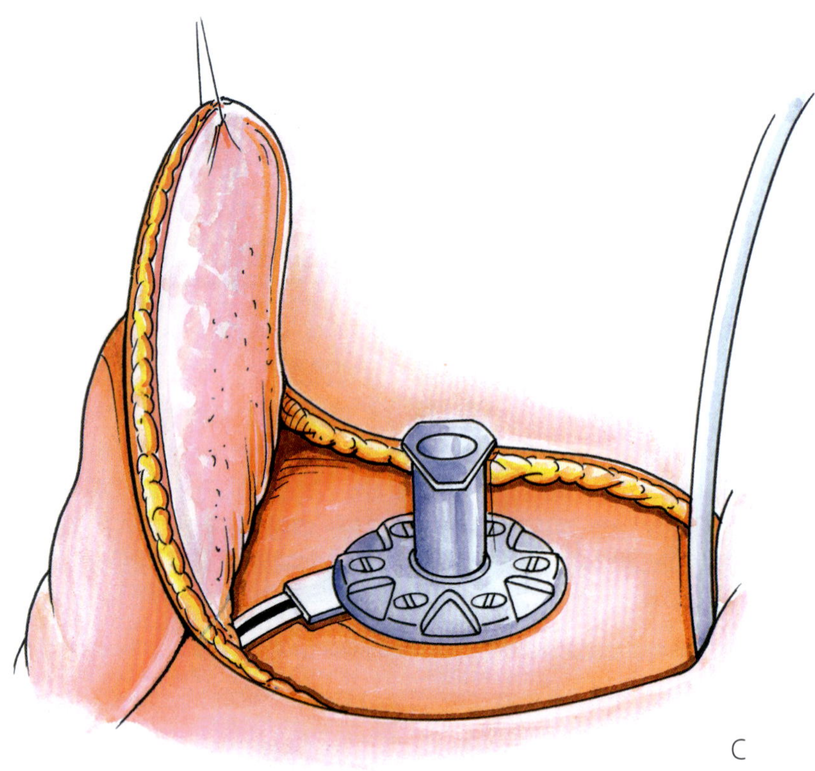

C. 将连接体外驱动电缆线的底座固定于颅骨上。

C. Secure the pedestal connecting the extracorporeal driveline on the skull.

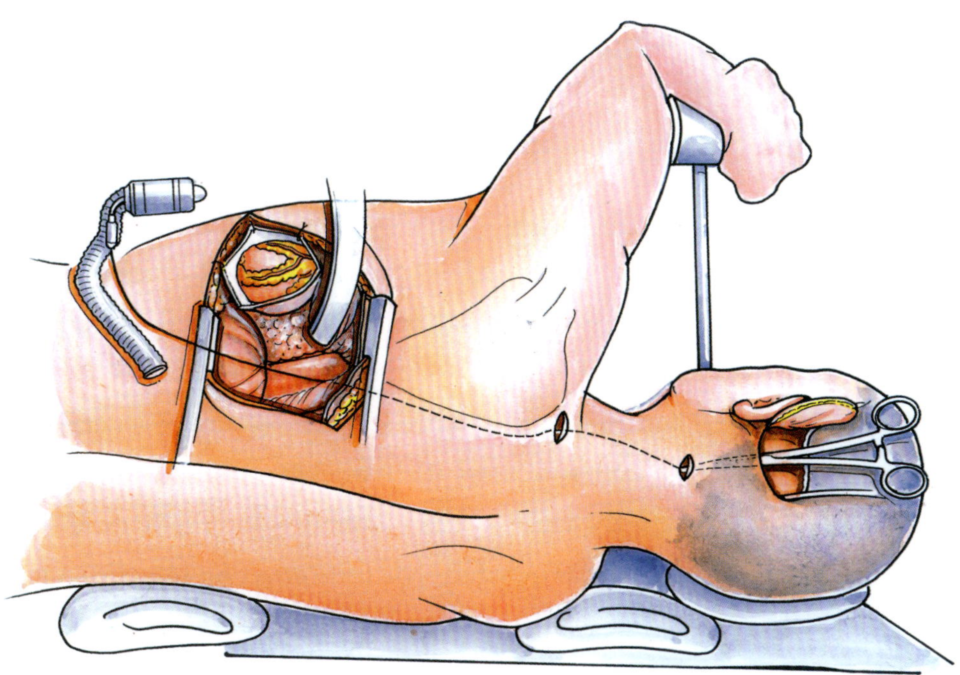

D

D. 在部分体外循环下于左心室心尖顶点装一个硅橡胶套环，通过该套环将泵置入并固定在左心室内。电缆线从泵拉到左胸顶，然后穿入颈部，经皮下隧道到左耳后的底座，再将驱动电缆线接头固定在底座之上。电缆线也可以通过腹部的右侧外延。流出人工血管吻合于胸部降主动脉，经胸骨正中切口进入时流出人工血管则吻合到升主动脉。

D. A silicone rubber cuff is placed at the left ventricle apex under partial cardiopulmonary bypass, through which the pump is placed and fixed in the left ventricle. The cable is pulled from the pump to the left thoracic top, then runs into the neck, subcutaneously tunneled towards the left retroauricular pedestal, and fixed on the pedestal via the driveline connector. The cable can also extend through the abdominal right side. The artificial outflow conduit is anastomosed to the descending thoracic aorta. Instead, the artificial outflow conduit is anastomosed to the ascending aorta when median sternotomy access is used.

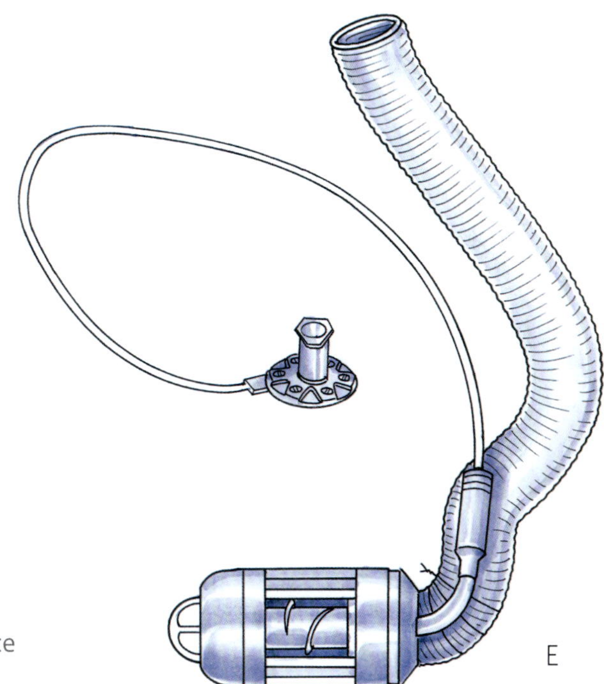

E

E. Jarvik 2000 VAD 主要装置图。

E. The figure illustrates Jarvik 2000 VAD main device

图 8-3-15 Jarvik 2000 非体外循环下植入术
Figure 8-3-15 Implantation of Jarvik 2000 with off-pump technique

Jarvik 2000 由于其特殊的设计，接头的部分就是泵的部分，让它一旦置入左心室后，马上就可以很方便地开始运转。在以左侧胸切开的植入方法中，心脏不需要被抬高，患者在全身麻醉的情况之下，血流动力学及血压影响较小。同时流出人工血管也可以使用侧壁钳直接吻合在胸部降主动脉上面，对血液循环及血压影响也不大。因此可以使用非体外循环的方式进行手术。

The Jarvik 2000 connector is part of the pump. Due to this special design, it can be easily activated once placed in the left ventricle. In the implantation via a left thoracotomy, the heart does not need to be elevated, and the patient's hemodynamics and blood pressure are less affected under general anesthesia. At the same time, the artificial outflow conduit can also be directly anastomosed on the descending thoracic aorta using a side clamp, which has little effect on blood circulation and blood pressure. Therefore, the surgery can be performed without cardiopulmonary bypass support.

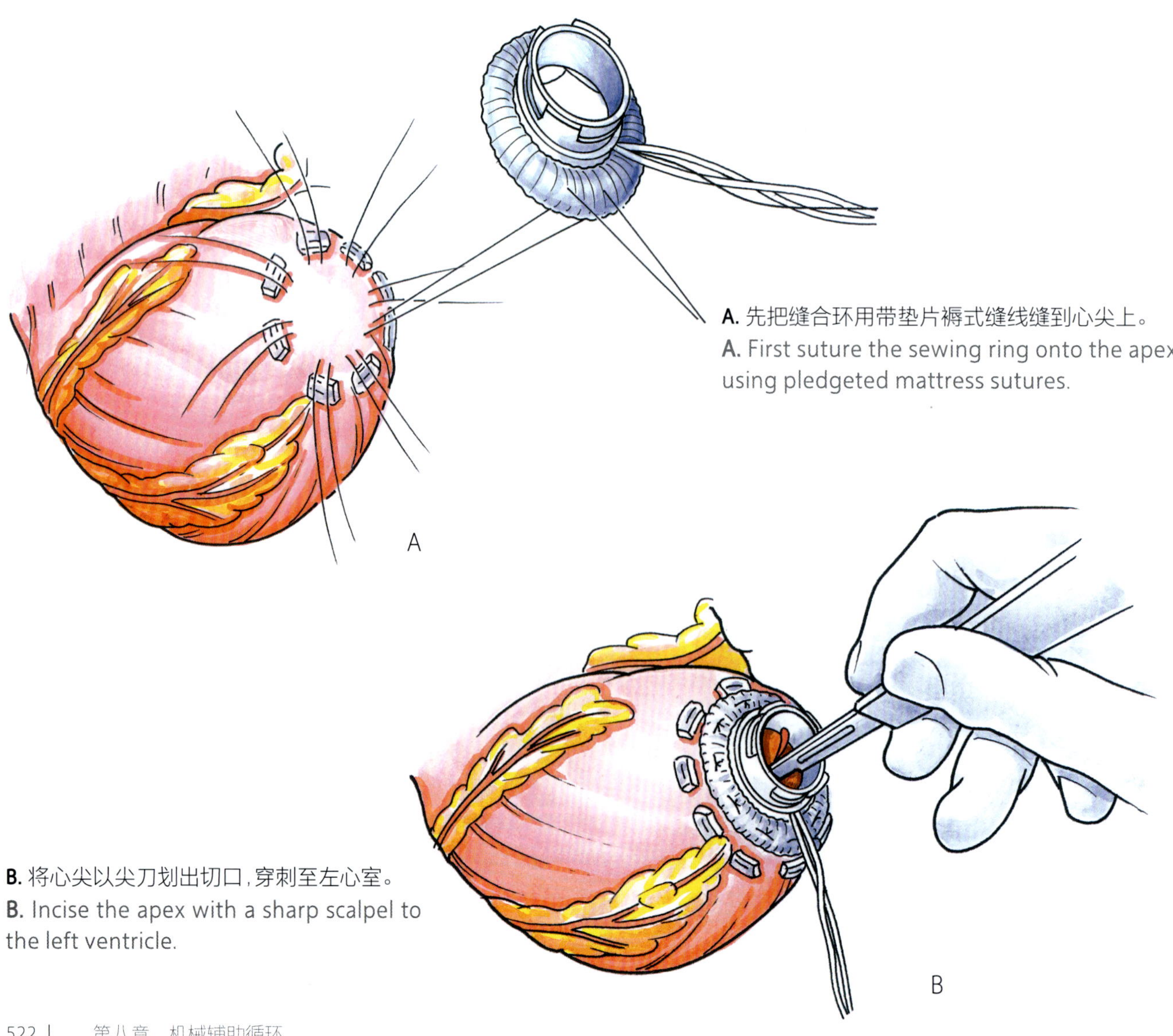

A. 先把缝合环用带垫片褥式缝线缝到心尖上。
A. First suture the sewing ring onto the apex using pledgeted mattress sutures.

B. 将心尖以尖刀划出切口，穿刺至左心室。
B. Incise the apex with a sharp scalpel to the left ventricle.

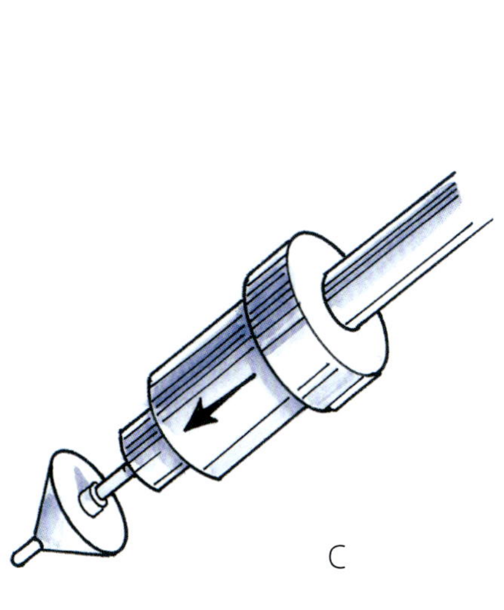

C. 专用的心肌打孔器。
C. Dedicated myocardial perforator.

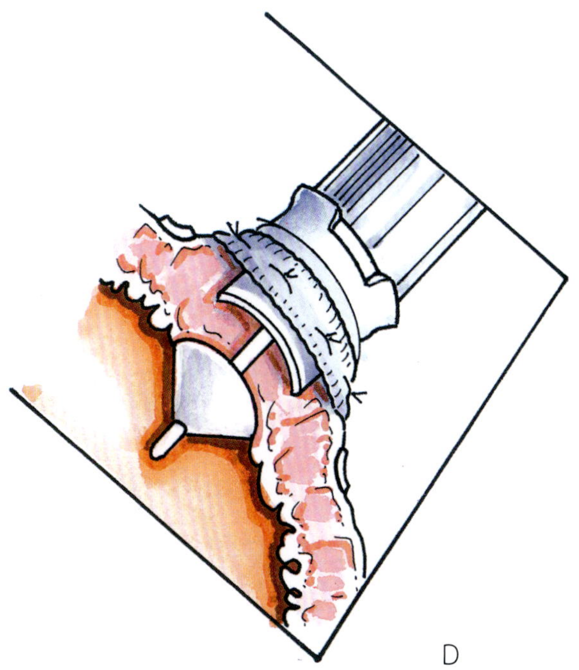

D. 心肌打孔器经心尖穿刺口插入左心室，将心尖部分肌肉切除后取出。
D. The myocardial perforator is inserted into the left ventricle through the apical puncture site, and part of the apical muscle is excised and removed.

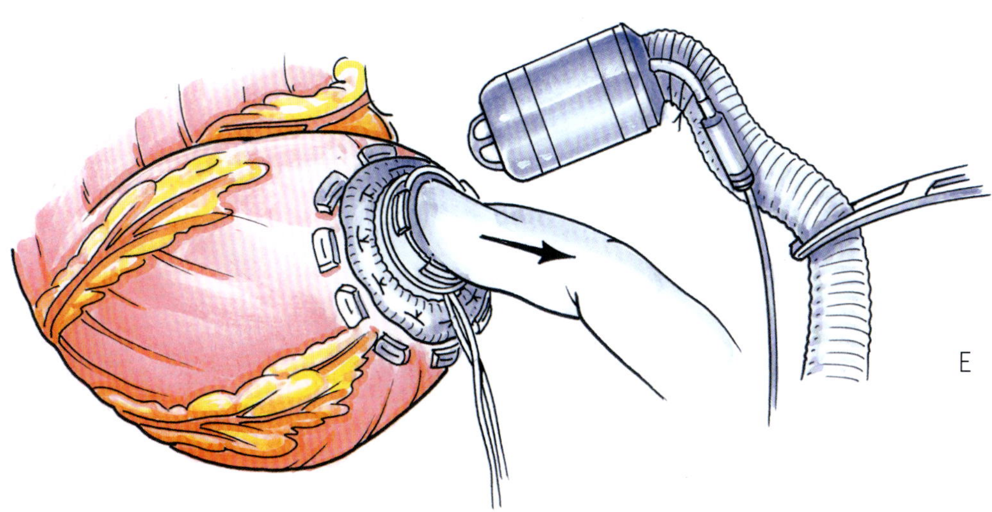

E. 将泵立即塞入缝合环中，并且直接将连接头固定。箭头代表泵头由心尖塞入左心室后血液在流出人工血管中的流动方向。
E. Insert the pump into the sewing ring immediately and secure the connector directly. The arrows indicate the direction of blood flowing through the artificial outflow conduit after the pump head is inserted into the left ventricle from the cardiac apex.

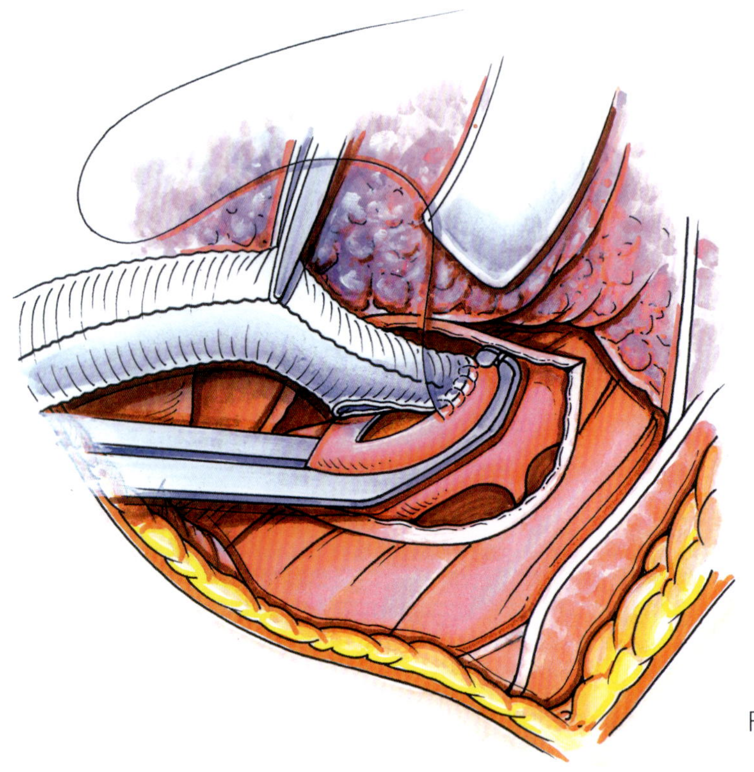

F. 用牵引器挡开肺叶，暴露出降主动脉，流出人工血管与降主动脉端侧吻合。

F. The lung lobe is blocked with a retractor to expose the descending aorta, and the artificial outflow conduit is end-to-side anastomosed to the descending aorta.

图 8-3-16　Jarvik 2000 左心室辅助装置植入术和双心室辅助装置植入术
Figure 8-3-16　Implantation of Jarvik 2000 as a LVAD and a BVAD

Jarvik 2000 由于泵头本身非常的小，因此在手术操作上可以采用不同的方式。除了可以用传统的方法从胸骨正中切开植入之外，也可以从左侧胸腔切开植入。可以用来当作右心室辅助装置，或者同时植入两个泵作为 BVAD。

Different surgical approaches can be used for the Jarvik 2000 implantation due to the small size of the pump head itself. In addition to the conventional median sternotomy, the implantation can also be performed via a left thoracotomy. It can be used as a right ventricular assist system, or two pumps can be simultaneously implanted as a BVAD.

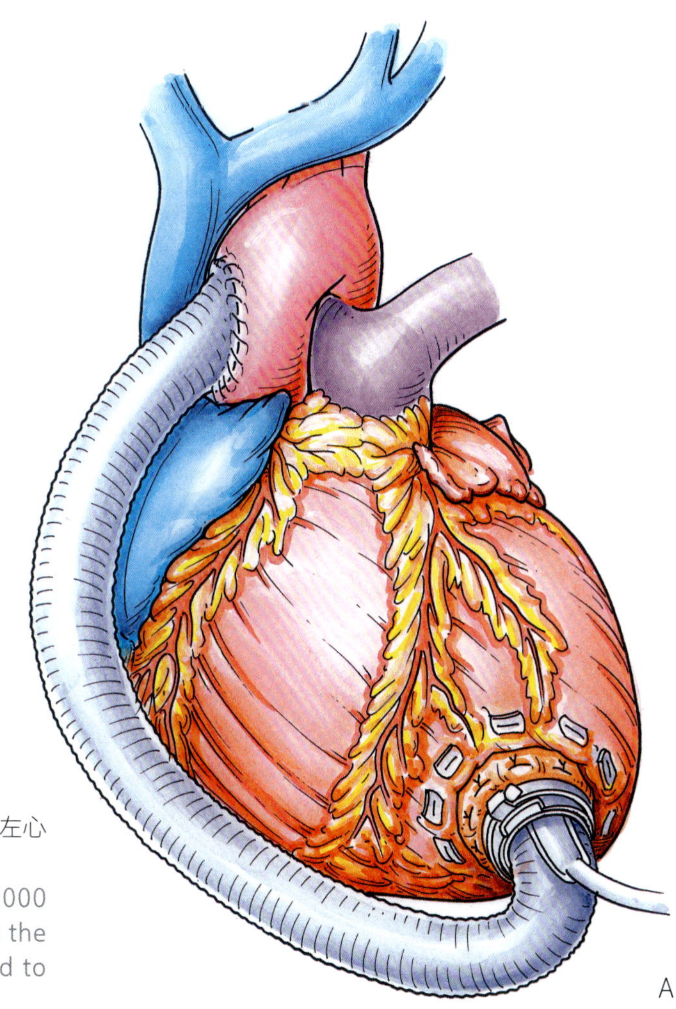

A. 传统方法的 LVAD 植入术，Jarvik 2000 的泵头经心尖插入左心室，流出人工血管与升主动脉吻合。

A. In conventional LVAD implantation, the Jarvik 2000 pump head is inserted into the left ventricle through the apex with the artificial outflow conduit anastomosed to the ascending aorta.

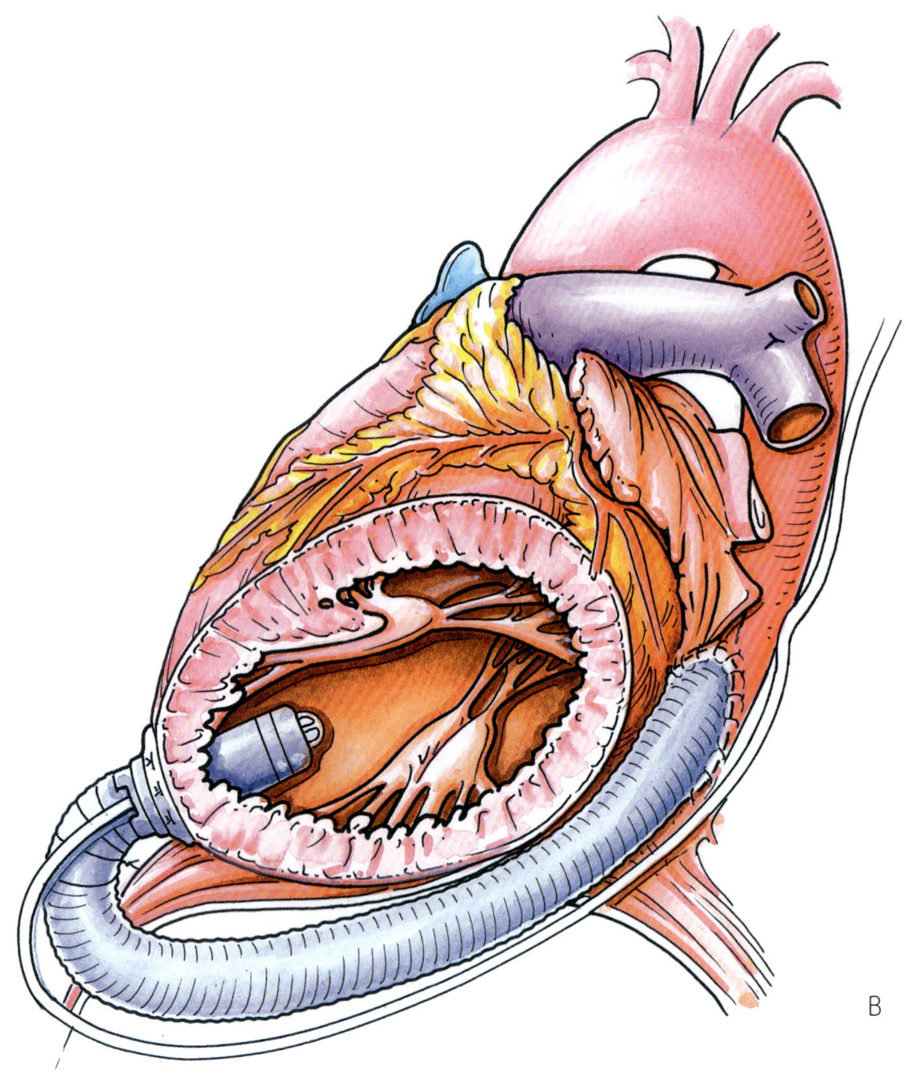

B. 从左侧胸壁切开的 LVAD 植入术，泵头经心尖插入左心室，流出人工血管与降主动脉吻合。
B. In LVAD implantation via a left thoracotomy, the pump head is inserted into the left ventricle through the apex with the artificial outflow conduit anastomosed to the descending aorta.

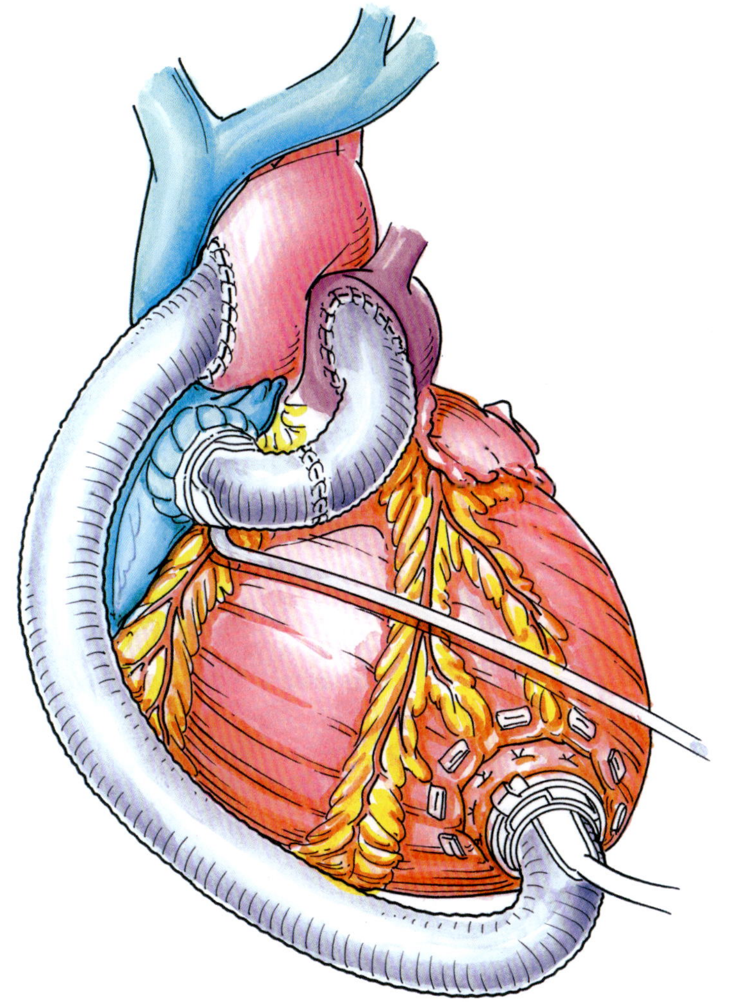

C. Jarvik 2000 作为双心室辅助装置植入。右心辅助装置植入时，将泵头吻合在右心房内，右心流出人工血管则吻合在肺动脉干上。左心辅助装置植入仍按传统方法施行。

C. The Jarvik 2000 is implanted as a biventricular assist device. The pump head is anastomosed in the right atrium, and the right heart artificial outflow conduit is anastomosed on the pulmonary trunk during right ventricular assist device implantation while it is implanted conventionally during left ventricular assist device implantation.

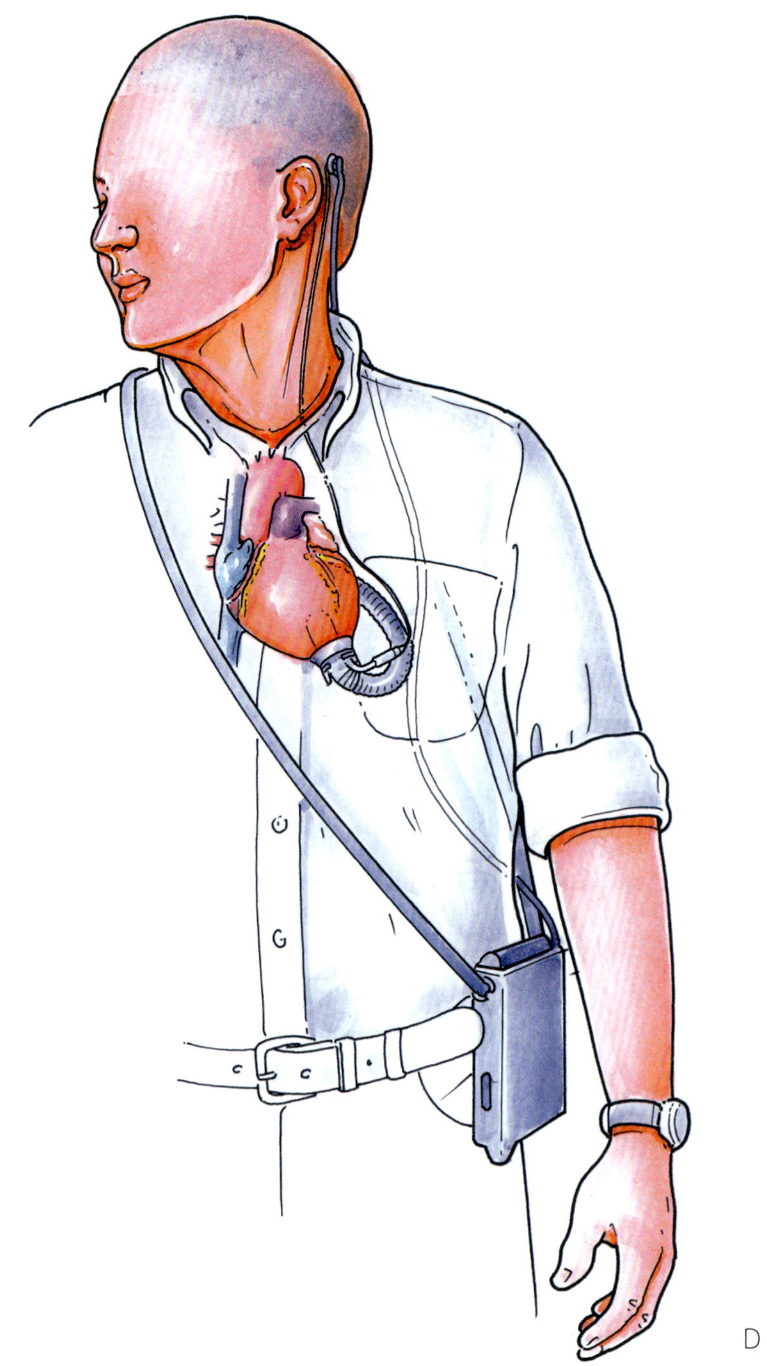

D. Jarvik 2000 传统植入方式最特殊的地方在于电缆线固定在耳后颅骨上，由于固定的地方不会晃动，再加上头皮的血液循环很丰富，因此电缆线皮肤引出处感染率几乎为零。

D. In Jarvik 2000 conventional implantation, the most notable feature is that the cable is fixed on the retroauricular skull. Due to the stable fixation and the rich blood circulation of the scalp, the infection rate of the site where the cable is percutaneously brought out is almost zero.

HeartWare 心室辅助装置

HeartWare ventricular assist device

HeartWare 心室辅助系统是最小的第三代可植入式的心室辅助系统，适用于等待心脏移植的患者，以避免不可逆左心室衰竭造成死亡。

The HeartWare ventricular assist system, the smallest third-generation implantable ventricular assist system, is indicated for patients awaiting heart transplantation to avoid death from irreversible left ventricular failure.

整套系统包括：

The complete system consists of:

1. **HeartWare 心室辅助系统** 包含一个直径 10cm、重 160g 的流体动力离心血液泵，一支流出人工血管及一条经皮传导电缆线。流出人工血管外套有抗压力套管，用以预防人工血管褶皱。传导缆线包覆聚酯纤维织物，可促进皮肤出口位置的组织往内生长。泵内的叶轮可转动血液并产生最大可达 10L/min 的流量。泵内置两个马达，其中一个为备用马达。连接到心肌的缝合环由钛制成，便于手术过程中调整泵方向。

1. **HeartWare Ventricular Assist System** The HeartWare ventricular assist system consists of a hydrodynamic centrifugal blood pump (10 cm in diameter, 160 g in weight), an artificial outflow conduit, and a percutaneous conductive cable. There is an anti-pressure sleeve outside the artificial outflow conduit to prevent wrinkling. The conductive cables are covered with polyester fabric that promotes tissue ingrowth at the exit site of the skin. The impeller inside the pump turns the blood and produces a flow of up to 10 L/min. The pump has two built-in motors, one of which is a backup motor. The sewing ring attached to the heart muscle is made of titanium, which facilitates the easy adjustment of the pump direction during surgery.

2. **外部控制器** 是一组微处理组件，控制并管理 HeartWare 心室辅助系统的运作，可将电力与操作信息送至血液泵，并搜集泵的数据。经皮传导缆线从体内引出后连接控制器，并随时连接两种电源——交流转接器或直流转接器及/或可重复充电的电池。控制器内装有无法更换但可重复充电的电池，可在两种电源均中断时，供应“无电源”警铃所需的电力。控制器与荧幕显示器通过资料连接埠连接。

2. **External Controller** The external controller is a set of microprocessor components that controls and manages the operation of the HeartWare ventricular assist system, sends power and operational information to the blood pump, and collects pump data. The percutaneous conductive cable, when pulled out of the body, is connected to the controller and is ready to be connected to two sources of power at any time-AC adapter or DC adapter and/or rechargeable batteries. The controller contains a non-replaceable but rechargeable battery that supplies the power required for the “no power” alarm when both power sources are off. The controller and the screen display are connected through the data connection port.

3. 荧幕显示器 是含有触控画面的台式电脑，采用专属软件，可显示系统性能信息并可调整选定的控制器参数。荧幕连接控制器时，会接收控制器持续提供的血液泵信息，并显示即时和旧有数据。荧幕显示器也会显示警铃状态。

3. Display Screen A desktop computer with a touch screen and proprietary software to display system performance information and adjust the selected controller parameters. When connected to the controller, the screen will continuously receive the blood pump information from the controller and display both real-time and prior data. The display screen also shows the alarm status.

4. 控制器电源 控制器需要有两种电源才能确保安全运作，可以是两颗电池或一颗电池搭配一个交流转接器或直流转接器。处于活动状态时，患者通常会使用两颗电池。休息或睡觉时，应使用电源插头（交流转接器）提供的电源，如此在使用上没有时间限制。电池的电力低于25% 时即应更换。手边应随时有备用、电量充足的电池。

4. Controller Power Supply The controller requires two power sources for safe operation, which can be two batteries or one battery with an AC adapter or a DC adapter. When active, patients typically use two batteries. When resting or sleeping, patients should use the power provided by the power plug (AC adapter), so there is no time limit on the use. The battery should be replaced when the power falls below 25%. A spare, fully charged battery should be available at all times.

图 8-3-17 HeartWare 植入术
Figure 8-3-17 Implantation of HeartWare

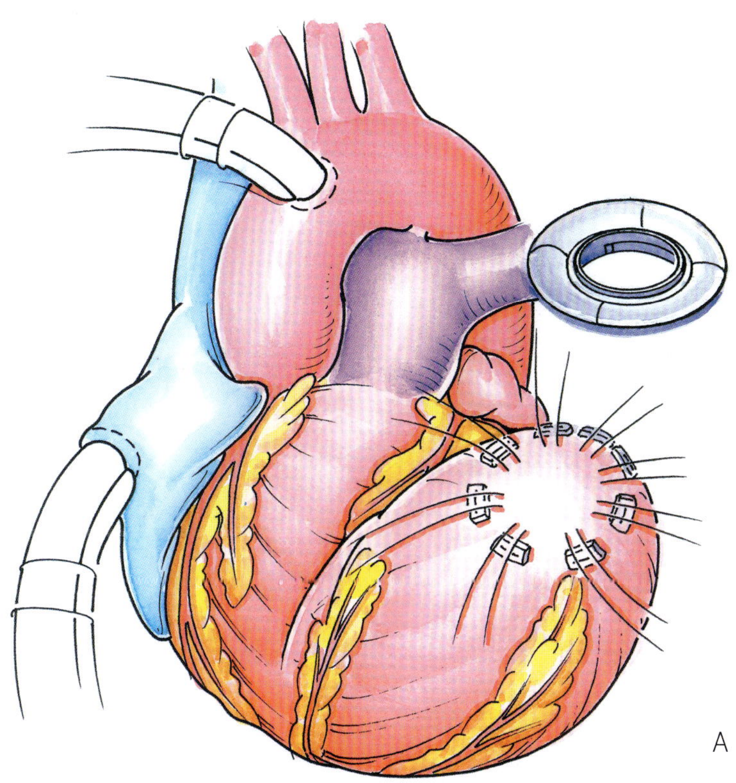

A. 在体外循环下，将缝合环固定在心尖之上。

A. Fix the sewing ring on the apex under extracorporeal circulation.

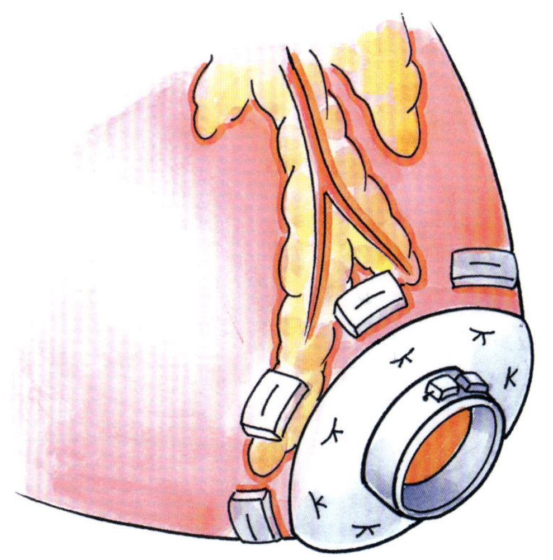

B. 缝合环固定完毕。钛制成的缝合环连接到心肌以便于手术过程中调整泵方向。

B. The sewing ring is fixed. The sewing ring made of titanium is attached to the heart muscle to facilitate adjustment of the pump direction during surgery.

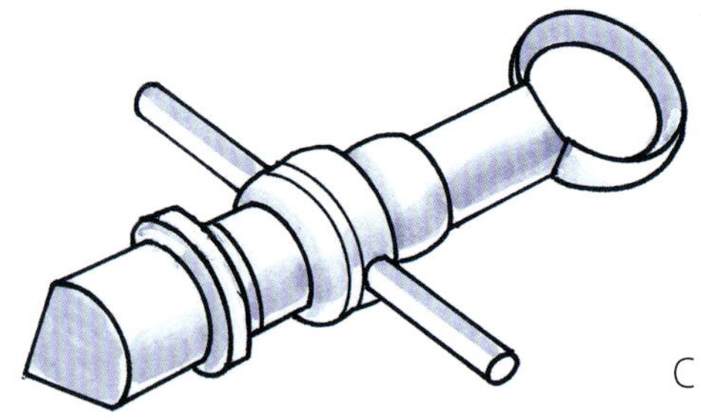

C. 特殊设计之钻孔器。
C. Specially designed drill.

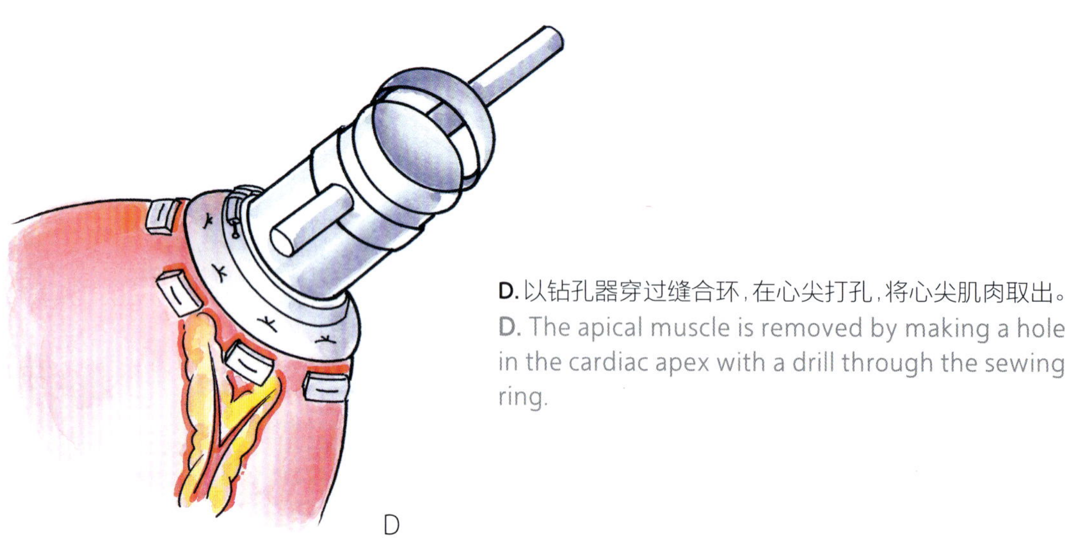

D. 以钻孔器穿过缝合环，在心尖打孔，将心尖肌肉取出。
D. The apical muscle is removed by making a hole in the cardiac apex with a drill through the sewing ring.

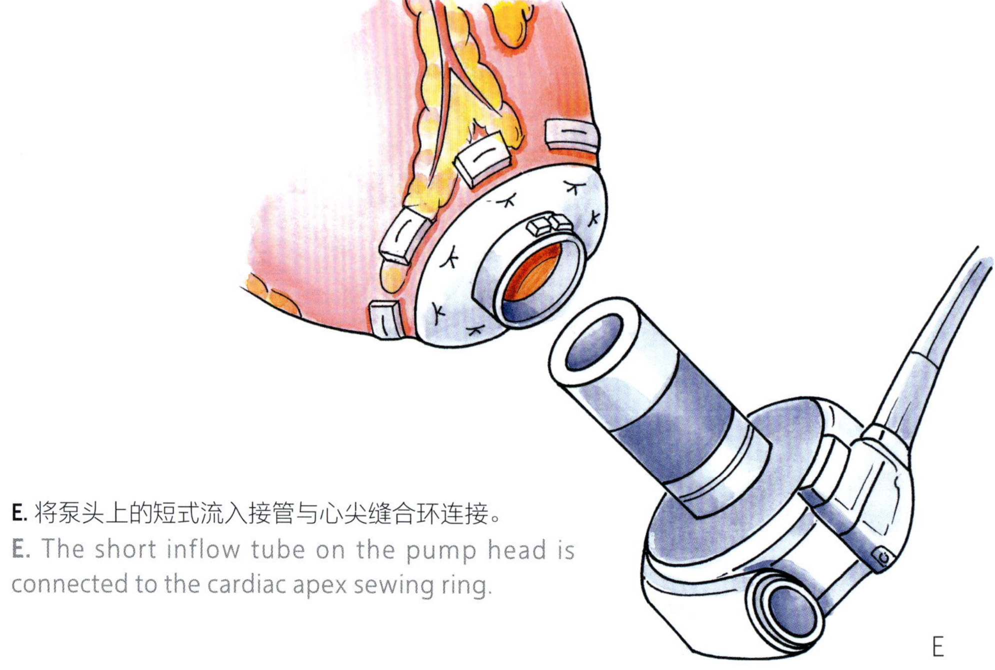

E. 将泵头上的短式流入接管与心尖缝合环连接。
E. The short inflow tube on the pump head is connected to the cardiac apex sewing ring.

F. 再将流出人工血管与升主动脉端侧吻合。

F. The artificial outflow conduit is then end-to-side anastomosed to the ascending aorta.

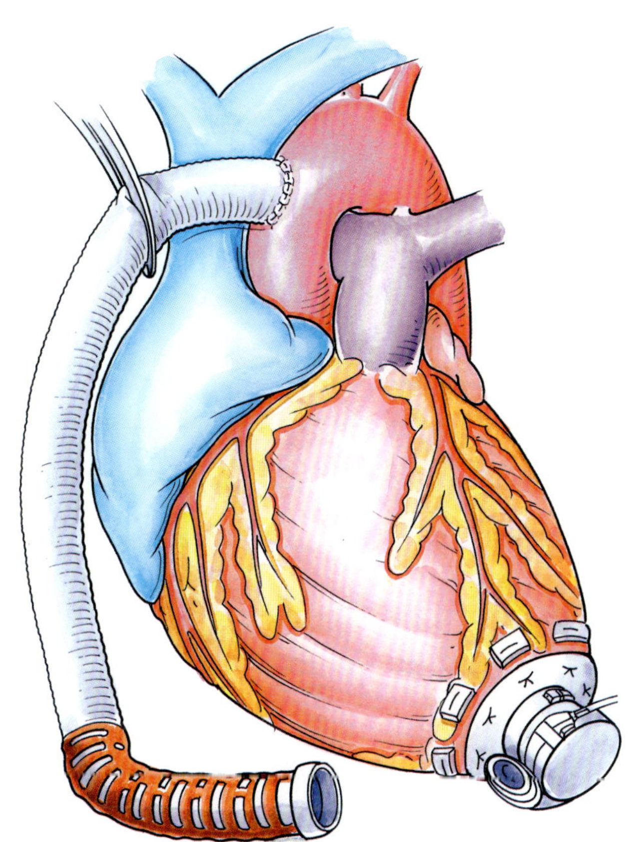

F

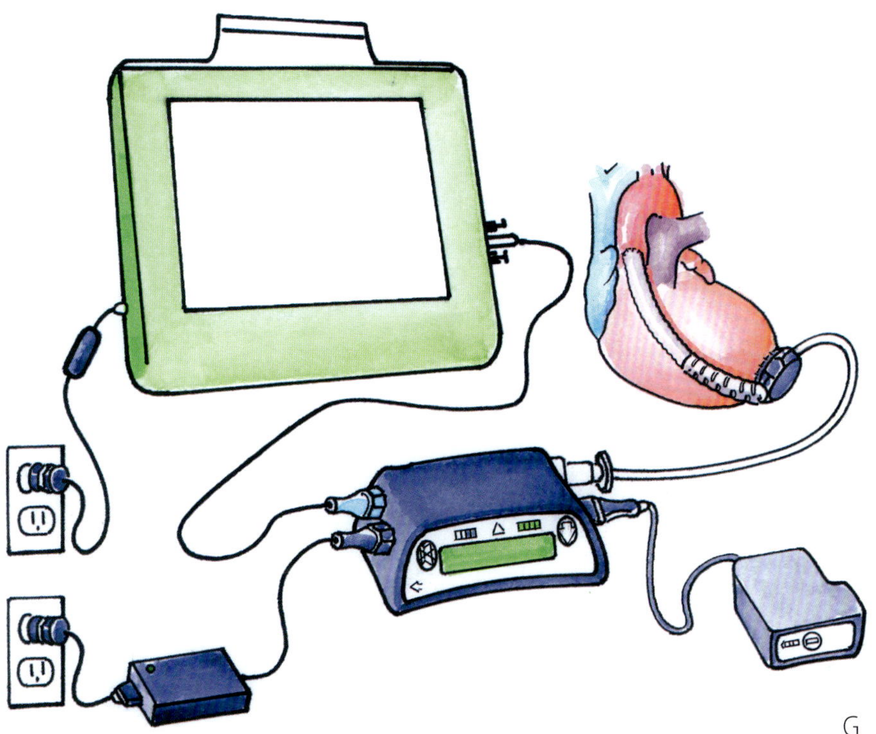

G

G. 整套 HeartWare 心室辅助装置包含微电脑控制器、电池、监控荧幕等。

G. The whole set of the HeartWare ventricular assist device includes a microcomputer controller, batteries, a monitoring screen, etc.

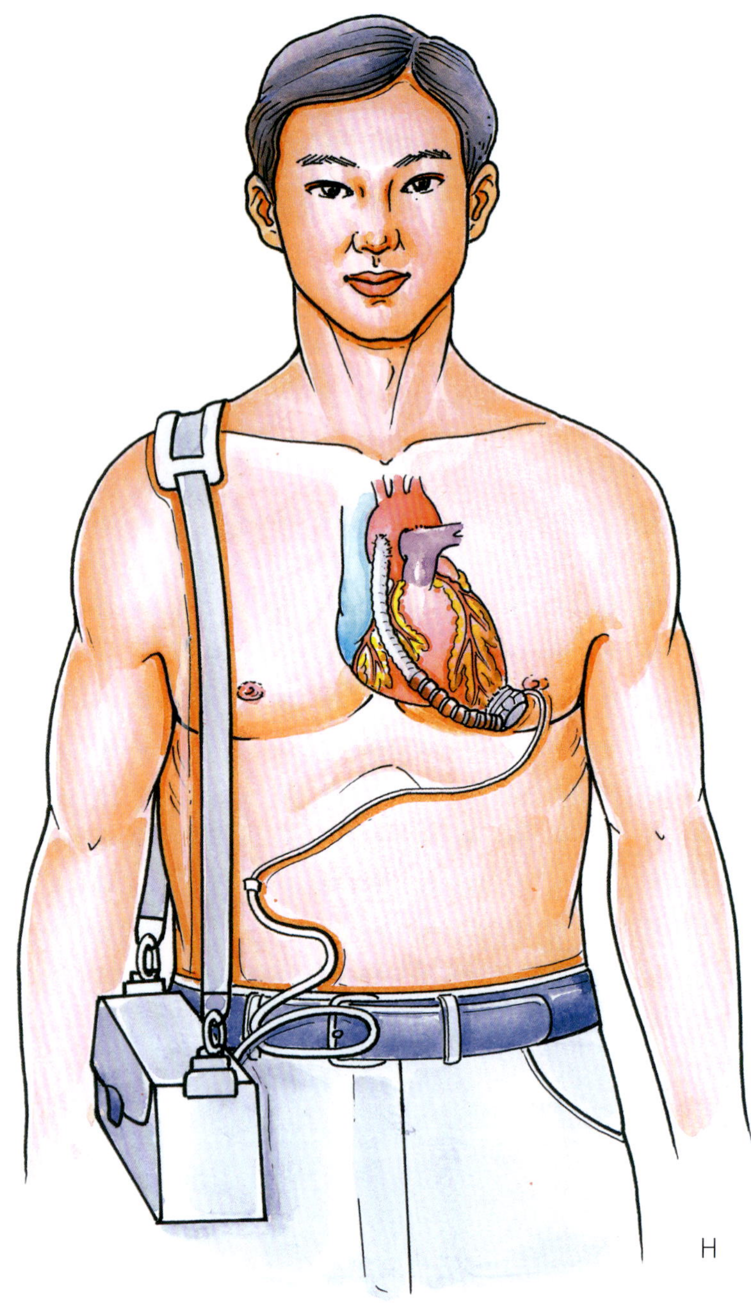

H. HeartWare泵及其短式流入管路，可放置在心脏周围，而不需另行腹部切口和分离出装置囊袋。电缆线从右侧肋下腹壁穿出连接至控制器及电池。

H. The HeartWare pump, together with its short inflow conduit, can be placed around the heart without the need for an additional abdominal incision and the separation of the device pocket. The cable running from the right subcostal abdominal wall is connected to the controller and batteries.

图 8-3-18　HeartWare 微创植入术
Figure 8-3-18　Minimally invasive implantation of HeartWare

由于心室辅助系统的发展已经超过 30 年，因此患者选择、手术技术、术前术后处理以及长期的照顾都有长足的进步。心室辅助装置的微创植入术就是进步之一。此种手术之好处除了减少胸骨发炎的机会外，最大的优点是在未来要进行心脏移植时，可以大幅度减少粘连的问题。

As ventricular assist systems have been developed for more than 30 years, great progress has been made in patient selection, surgical techniques, preoperative and postoperative management, and long-term care. Minimally invasive implantation of ventricular assist device is one of such advancement. In addition to reducing the risk of sternum inflammation, the biggest advantage of this type of surgery is that it can greatly reduce adhesions when heart transplantation is to be performed in the future.

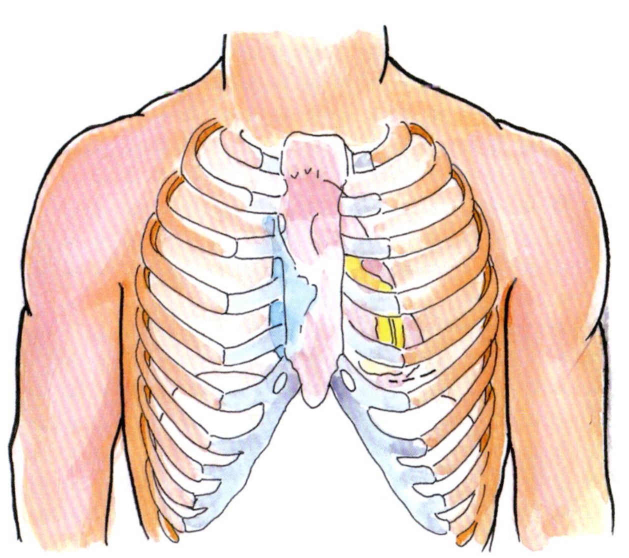

A. 心尖部位的手术是从左胸前外侧切口第 5 肋间进入左胸。

A. The apical surgery is performed through the fifth intercostal space via the left anterolateral thoracotomy.

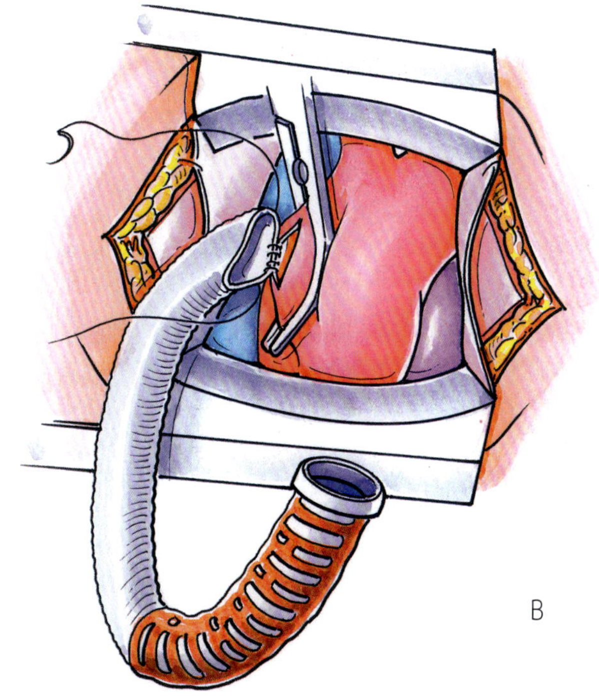

B. 升主动脉的吻合则从胸骨右侧第 2 肋间切开，同样打开心包膜之后，以侧壁钳夹住升主动脉，流出人工血管与升主动脉端侧吻合。

B. A thoracotomy is performed through the second intercostal space on the right side of the sternum for the ascending aorta anastomosis. With the pericardium opened and the ascending aorta side-clamped, the artificial outflow conduit is end-to-side anastomosed to the ascending aorta.

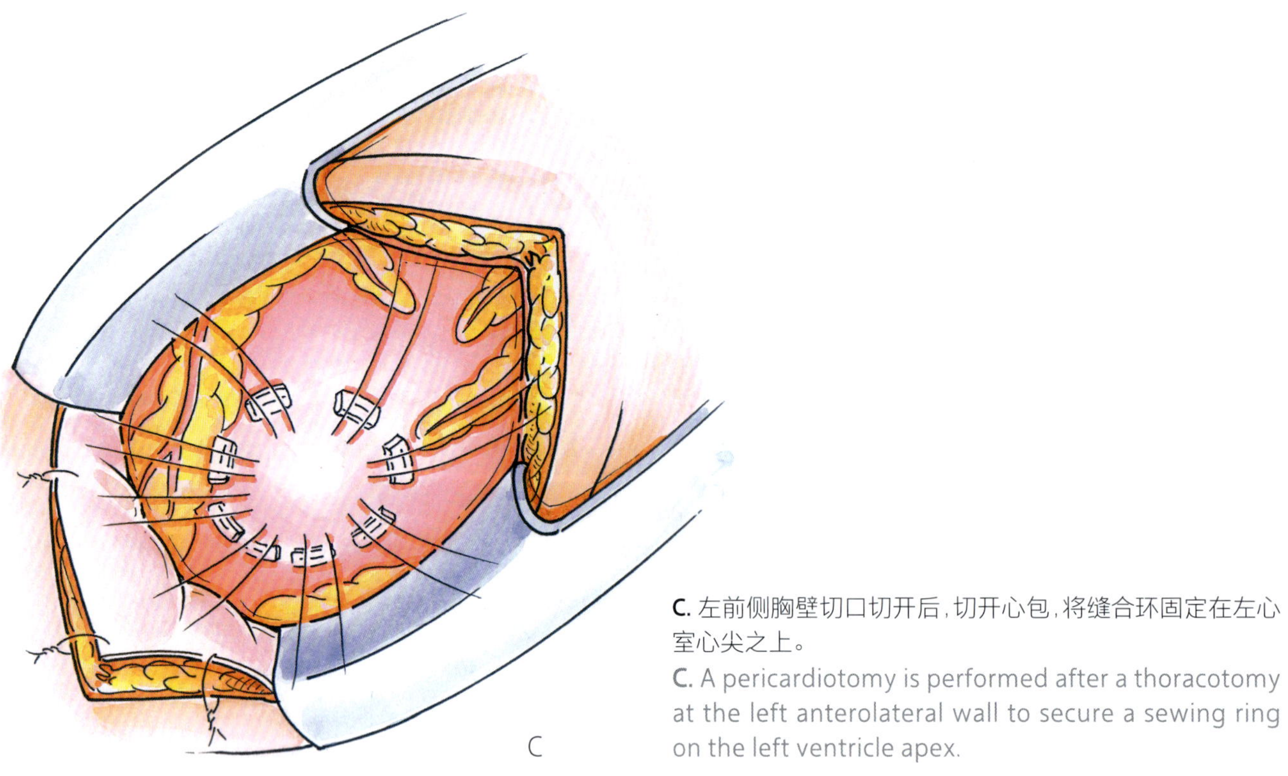

C. 左前侧胸壁切口切开后，切开心包，将缝合环固定在左心室心尖之上。

C. A pericardiotomy is performed after a thoracotomy at the left anterolateral wall to secure a sewing ring on the left ventricle apex.

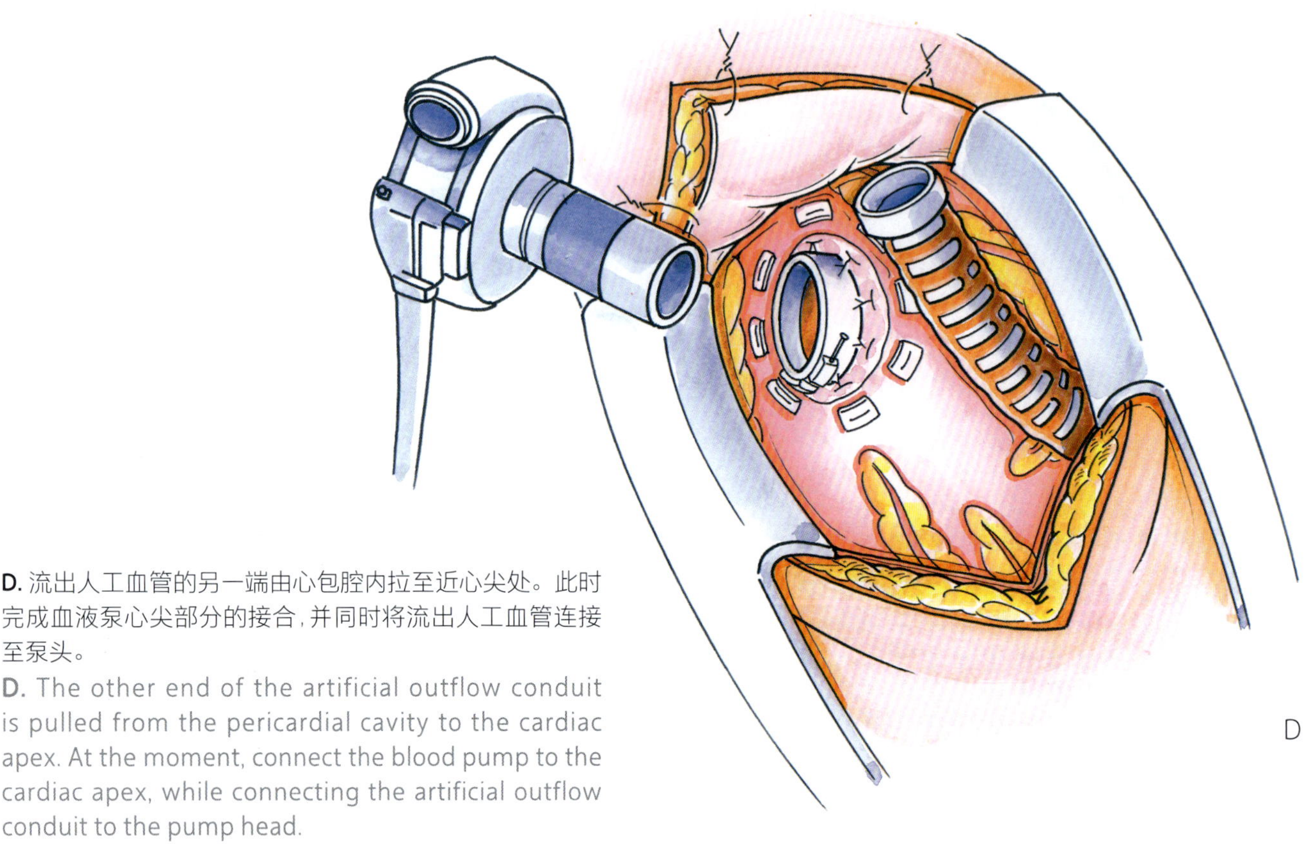

D. 流出人工血管的另一端由心包腔内拉至近心尖处。此时完成血液泵心尖部分的接合，并同时将流出人工血管连接至泵头。

D. The other end of the artificial outflow conduit is pulled from the pericardial cavity to the cardiac apex. At the moment, connect the blood pump to the cardiac apex, while connecting the artificial outflow conduit to the pump head.

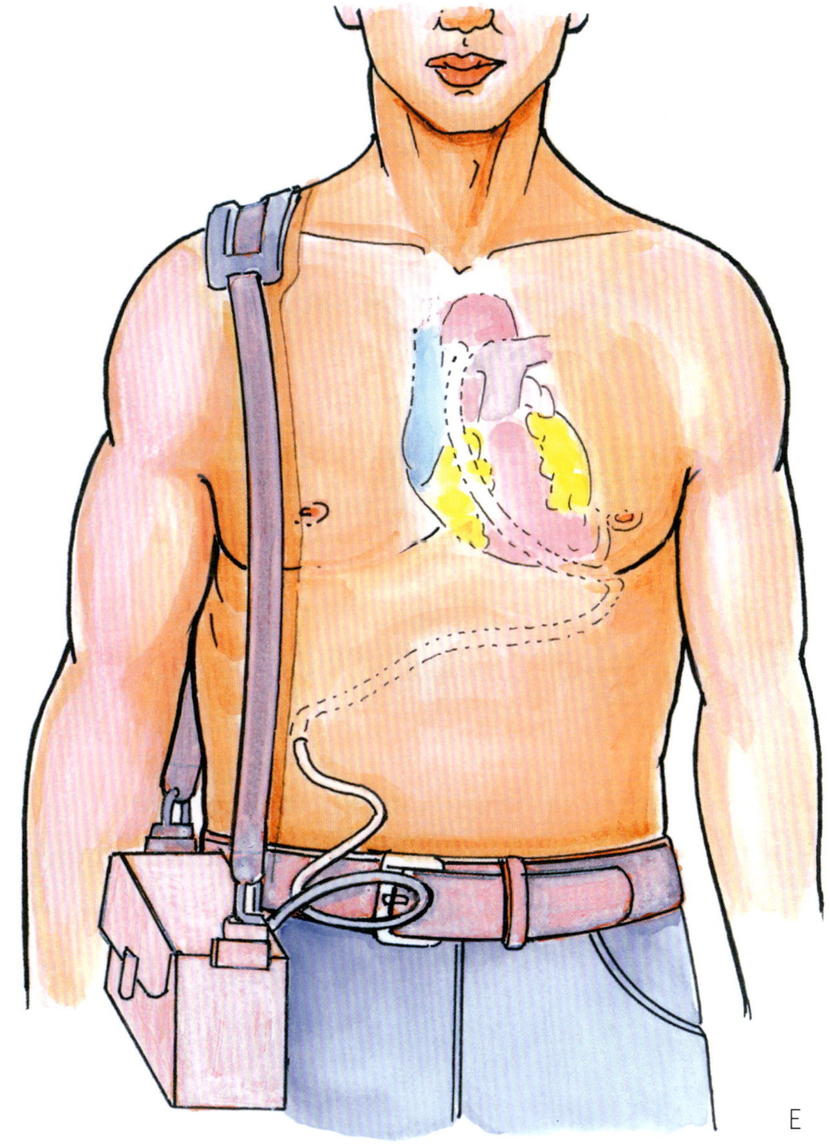

E. 缝合切口。电缆线从右侧肋下穿出连接至控制器及电池。

E. Suture the incision. The cable brought out from underneath the right rib is connected to the controller and battery.

Levitronix 心室辅助装置
Levitronix ventricular assist device

Levitronix 心室辅助装置用于30天之内的临时机械辅助循环支持，可用在单心室或双心室辅助系统，以及 ECMO 系统。

The Levitronix ventricular assist device is used for temporary mechanical circulatory support for up to 30 days and can be used in single or biventricular assist systems, as well as in ECMO systems.

整套系统包含：

The complete system consists of:

1. **血液泵** 采用无轴承电动机技术的电子驱动式离心泵，使用聚碳酸酯材质。叶轮在定子的磁场内悬浮并旋转，通过旋转叶轮所产生的离心力输送血液。用磁性使叶轮悬浮以及消除密封和平轴来减少血细胞的损伤。Levitronix 泵的最大流量可以达到 10L/min，最大压力为 600mmHg。

1. **Blood Pump** The blood pump, made of polycarbonate, is an electronically driven centrifugal pump using bearingless motor technology. The impeller suspends and rotates in the magnetic field of the stator, delivering blood by the centrifugal force generated by the rotating impeller. Reduce blood cells damage with impeller magnetic suspension and elimination of seals and flat shafts. The maximum flow of the Levitronix pump can reach 10 L/min and the maximum pressure is 600 mmHg.

2. **血流探头** 是一种可以重复使用、不接触患者的超声波流量计。第二代机有两款血流探头，分别可提供流量测定范围是 0~10L/min、0~3L/min。

2. **Blood Flow Probe** It is a reusable ultrasonic flowmeter that does not touch the patient. The second-generation machine has two blood flow probes, which can provide flow measurement ranges of 0-10 L/min and 0-3 L/min respectively.

3. **操控台** 主操控台是一种微处理器为基础的控制装置，使用单相交流电。微处理器产生马达控制信号，监视系统感应器，输出监视显示屏信号，并且提供警报功能。

3. **Console** The main console is a microprocessor-based control device that uses a single-phase alternating current. The microprocessor generates motor control signals, monitors system sensors, outputs signals on the display screen, and provides alarms.

4. **马达** 承载可抛弃式的血液泵并驱动血液泵中的转子。

4. **Motor** The motor carries the disposable blood pump and drives the rotor in the blood pump.

5. 监视器 显示操控台的数据，并且提供控制操控台另一方式。通过在显示器的软触控按键，显示器的荧幕可用来显示操作的数据系统选项和选单。操作者设定的警报和参数，两台主操控台的数据可以同时显示在同一台显示器上。备用操控台的主要功能是当主操控台故障时，提供基本的维持生命功能，直到另一部主操控台更换为止。

5. Monitor The monitor displays the console data and provides another way to control the console. The monitor screen can display the operating data system options and menus through soft-touch buttons on the monitor. The alarms and parameters set by the operator, the data of the two main consoles can be displayed on the same screen at the same time. The primary function of the backup console is to provide basic life-sustaining support when the primary console fails until the failed primary console is replaced.

图 8-3-19 Levitronix 左心室辅助装置植入术
Figure 8-3-19 Implantation of Levitronix as a LVAD

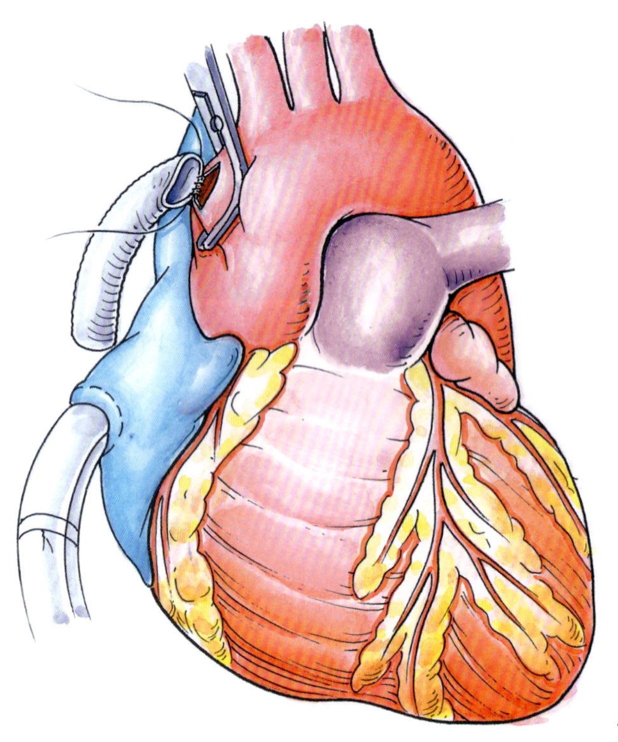

A. 在体外循环下，侧壁钳钳夹升主动脉，将一段人工血管吻合至升主动脉。

A. Under extracorporeal circulation, the ascending aorta, clamped by the side clamp, is anastomosed with a segment of the artificial blood vessel.

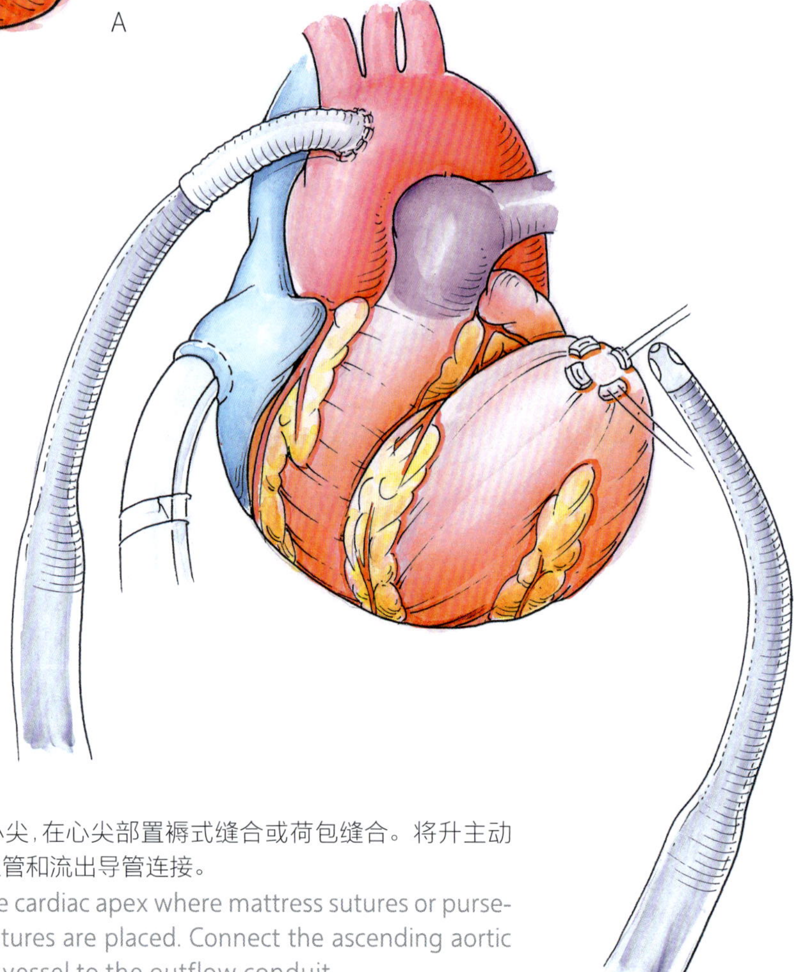

B. 托出心尖，在心尖部置褥式缝合或荷包缝合。将升主动脉人工血管和流出导管连接。

B. Lift the cardiac apex where mattress sutures or purse-string sutures are placed. Connect the ascending aortic artificial vessel to the outflow conduit.

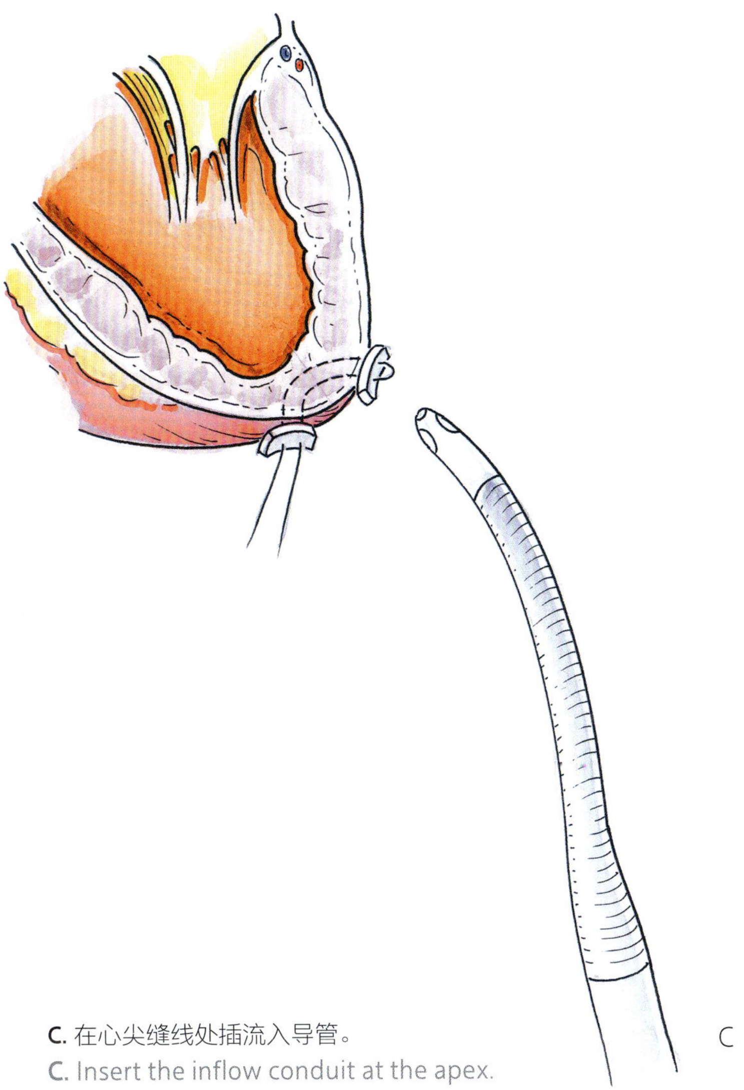

C. 在心尖缝线处插流入导管。

C. Insert the inflow conduit at the apex.

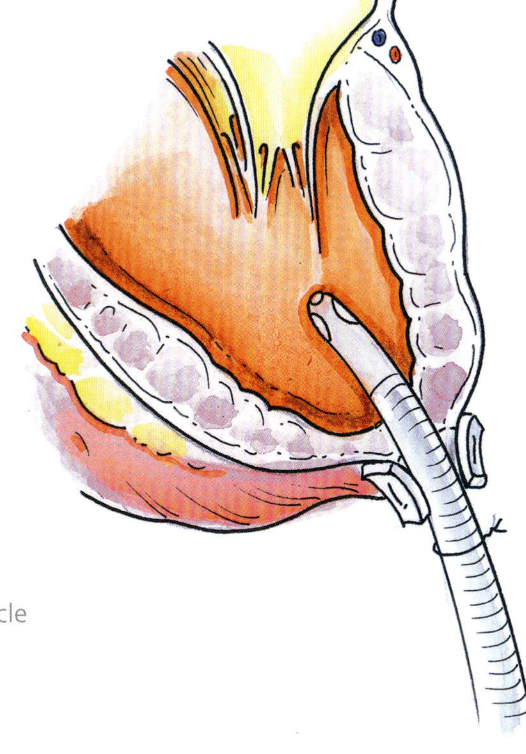

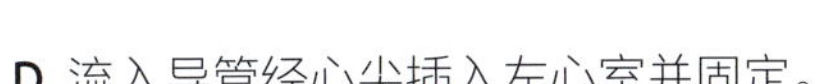

D. 流入导管经心尖插入左心室并固定。

D. The inflow conduit is inserted into the left ventricle through the apex and fixed.

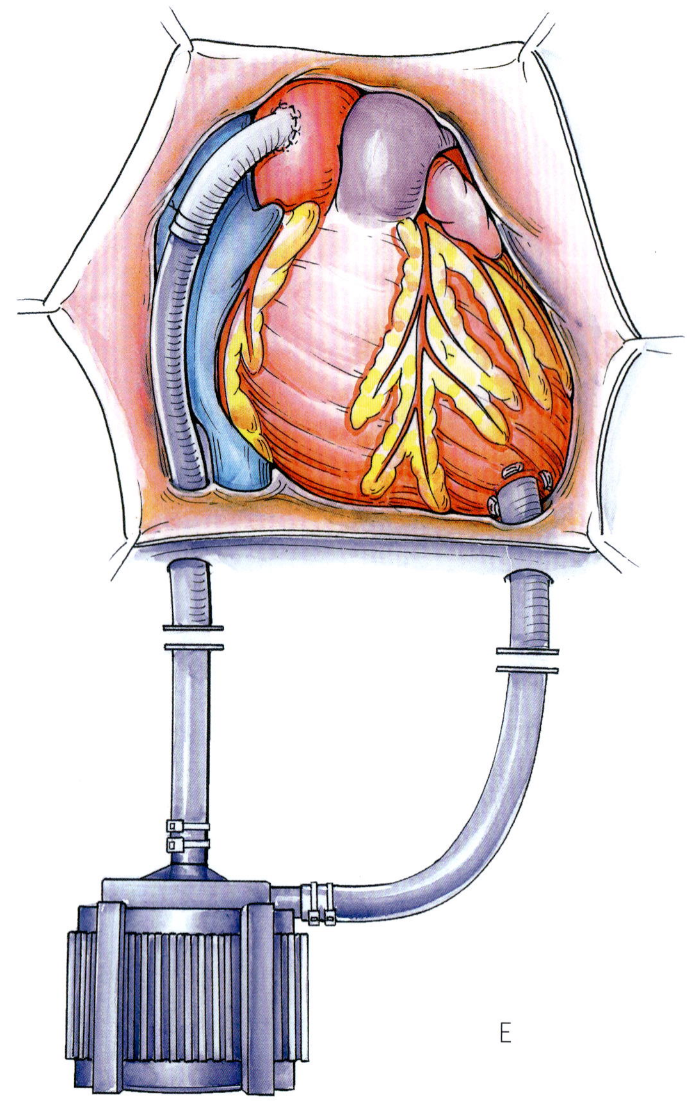

E. 流入导管、流出导管分别连接到 Levitronix 泵，手术完成。

E. The inflow and outflow conduits are connected to the Levitronix pump, respectively, and the procedure is completed.

图 8-3-20　Levitronix 右心室辅助装置和双心室辅助装置植入术
Figure 8-3-20　Implantation of Levitronix as a RVAD and a BVAD

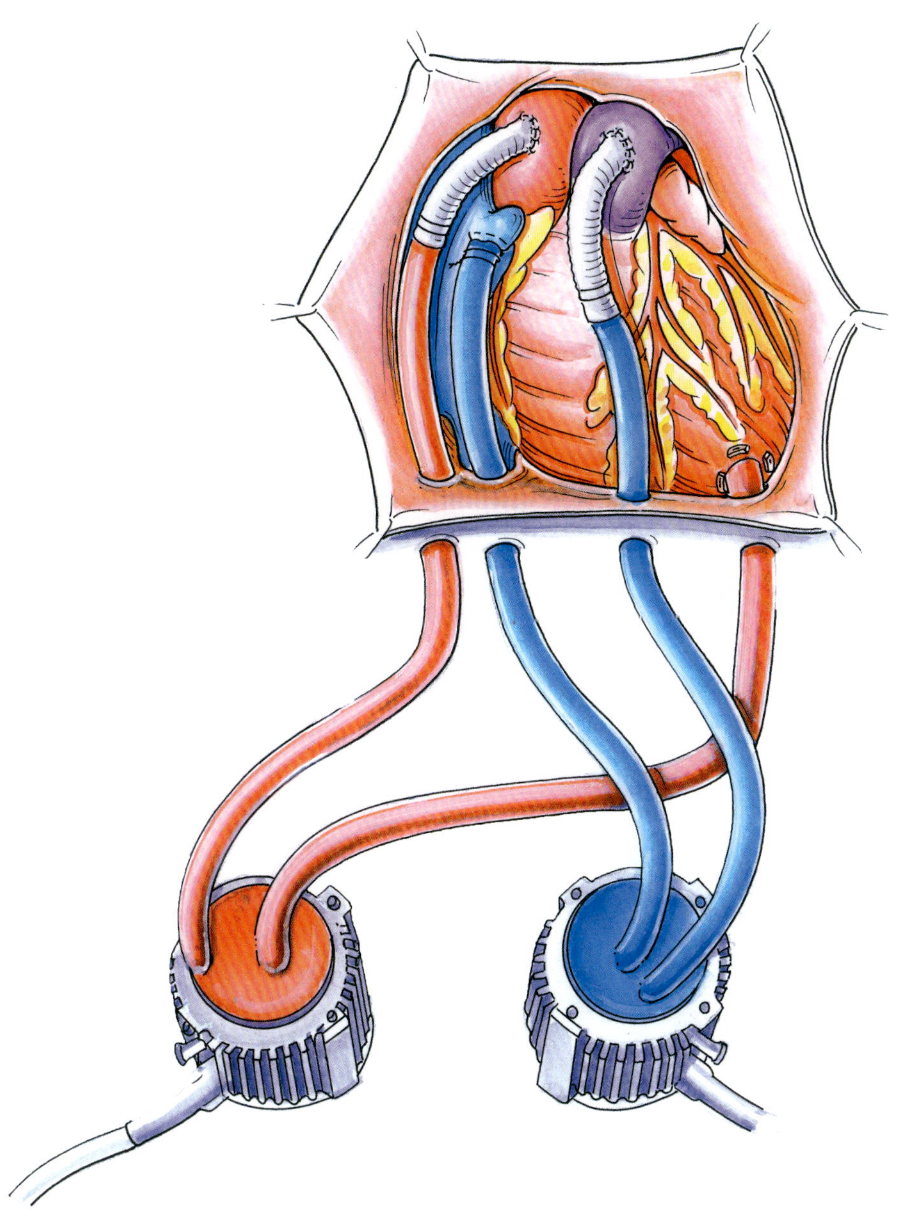

Levitronix 心室辅助装置植入方法与常规建立体外循环的方式非常类似。如果患者只有严重右心衰竭，可以单独将装置装于右心，流入导管从右心房插入，流出导管插入肺动脉，成为 RVAD。全心衰竭时 Levitronix 心室辅助装置也可以支持双心室变成双心室辅助装置。

The implantation of the Levitronix ventricular assist system is very similar to the way cardiopulmonary bypass is routinely established. For patients with severe right heart failure alone, the device, used as a RVAD, can be installed in the right heart alone with an inflow conduit inserted from the right atrium and an outflow conduit inserted into the pulmonary artery. The Levitronix ventricular assist system can also be used as a biventricular assist device to support both ventricles in the case of total heart failure.

第四节 儿童心室辅助装置
Section 4 Ventricular Assist Device for Children

图 8-4-1 新生儿和儿童 Excor 植入术
Figure 8-4-1 Implantation of Excor for neonates and children

新生儿或者是儿童心力衰竭而需要心室辅助装置的时候，Excor 心室辅助系统是目前全世界唯一得到美国 FDA 及欧盟 CE 认证的医疗装备。成人的装置方法见上一章，而新生儿及儿童的装置方法则与成人略有不同。

When neonates or children with heart failure need a ventricular assist device, the Excor ventricular assist system is the only medical device in the world that has been certified by the US FDA and EU CE. The Excor implantation method for adults is described in the previous chapter, while the Excor implantation method for neonates and children is slightly different from that for adults.

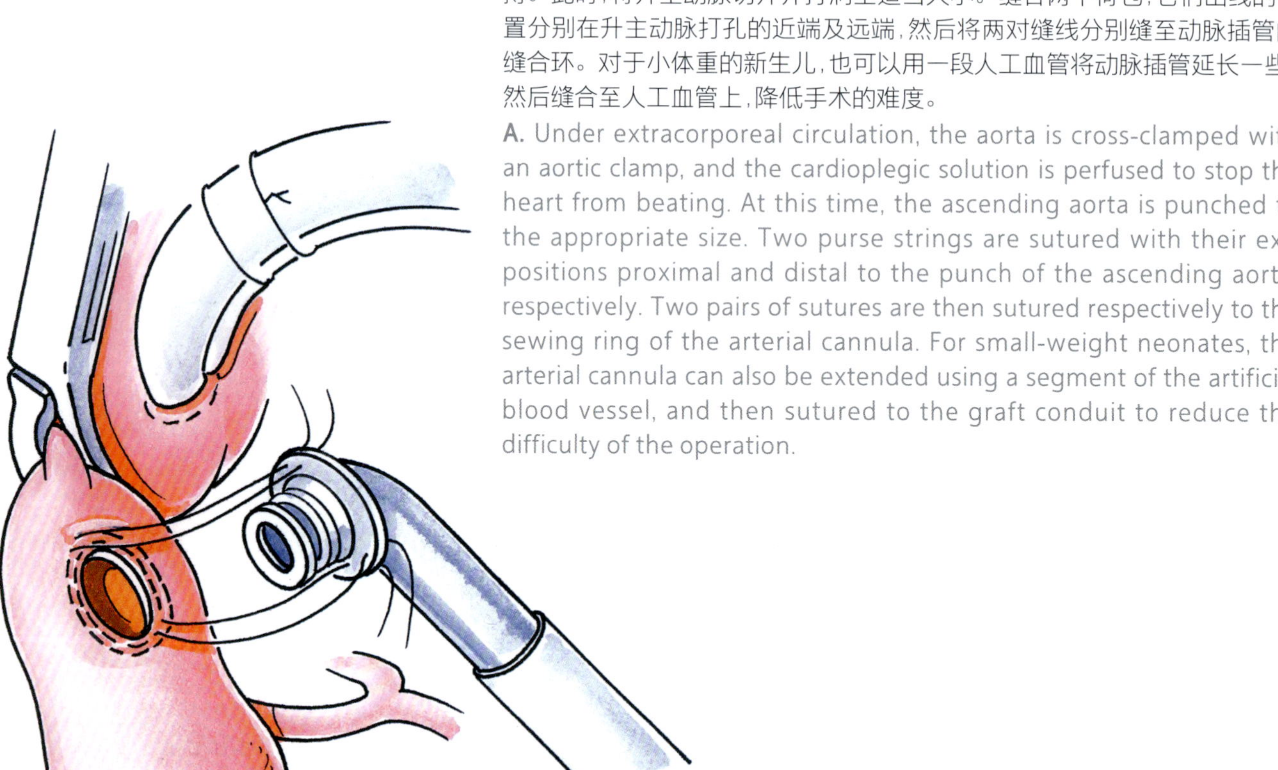

A. 在体外循环下，先用主动脉阻断钳将主动脉阻断，灌入心肌保护液心脏停搏。此时，将升主动脉切开并打洞至适当大小。缝合两个荷包，它们出线的位置分别在升主动脉打孔的近端及远端，然后将两对缝线分别缝至动脉插管的缝合环。对于小体重的新生儿，也可以用一段人工血管将动脉插管延长一些，然后缝合至人工血管上，降低手术的难度。

A. Under extracorporeal circulation, the aorta is cross-clamped with an aortic clamp, and the cardioplegic solution is perfused to stop the heart from beating. At this time, the ascending aorta is punched to the appropriate size. Two purse strings are sutured with their exit positions proximal and distal to the punch of the ascending aorta, respectively. Two pairs of sutures are then sutured respectively to the sewing ring of the arterial cannula. For small-weight neonates, the arterial cannula can also be extended using a segment of the artificial blood vessel, and then sutured to the graft conduit to reduce the difficulty of the operation.

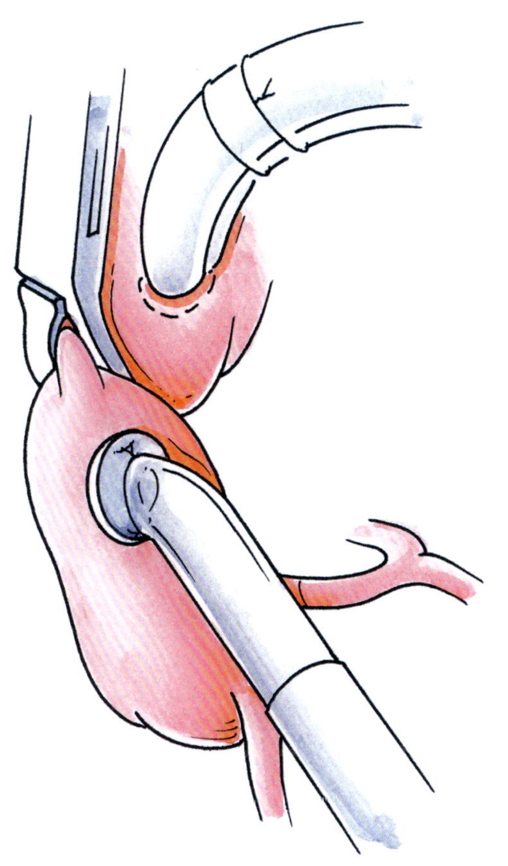

B. 将动脉插管插入升主动脉，缝线打结，并继续完成左右两侧的缝合。

B. Insert the arterial cannula into the ascending aorta, knot the sutures, and continue to complete the sutures on the left and right sides.

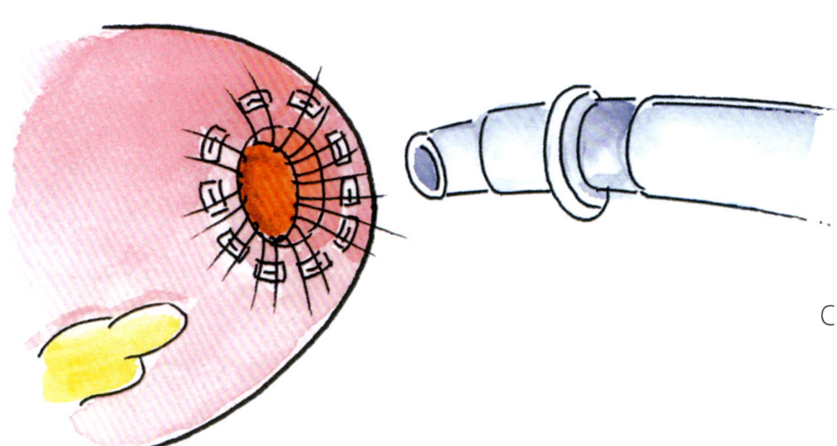

C. 在接近心尖的位置，以尖刀及组织剪切出略大于心室插管的圆孔，圆孔位置必须指向二尖瓣，并同时检查左心室内有无血栓。再用带垫褥式缝线缝合心尖左心室侧，大约 8 针，褥式缝线再缝入左心室插管的缝合环。

C. At the position close to the heart apex, use a sharp knife and tissue scissors to cut a round hole, which is slightly larger than the ventricular cannula and must point to the mitral valve, and at the same time, check whether there is thrombus in the left ventricle. Use pledgeted mattress sutures to suture the left ventricle apex, approximately eight stitches, and then the sewing ring of the left ventricular cannula.

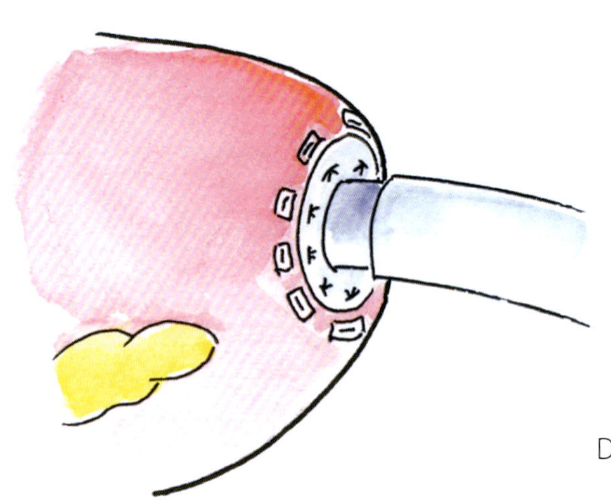

D. 全部缝线均与缝合环缝合后，再将插管插入左心室，并逐一打结完成缝合。

D. After the sewing ring is sutured with all sutures, the cannula is inserted into the left ventricle. Knot one by one to complete the suture.

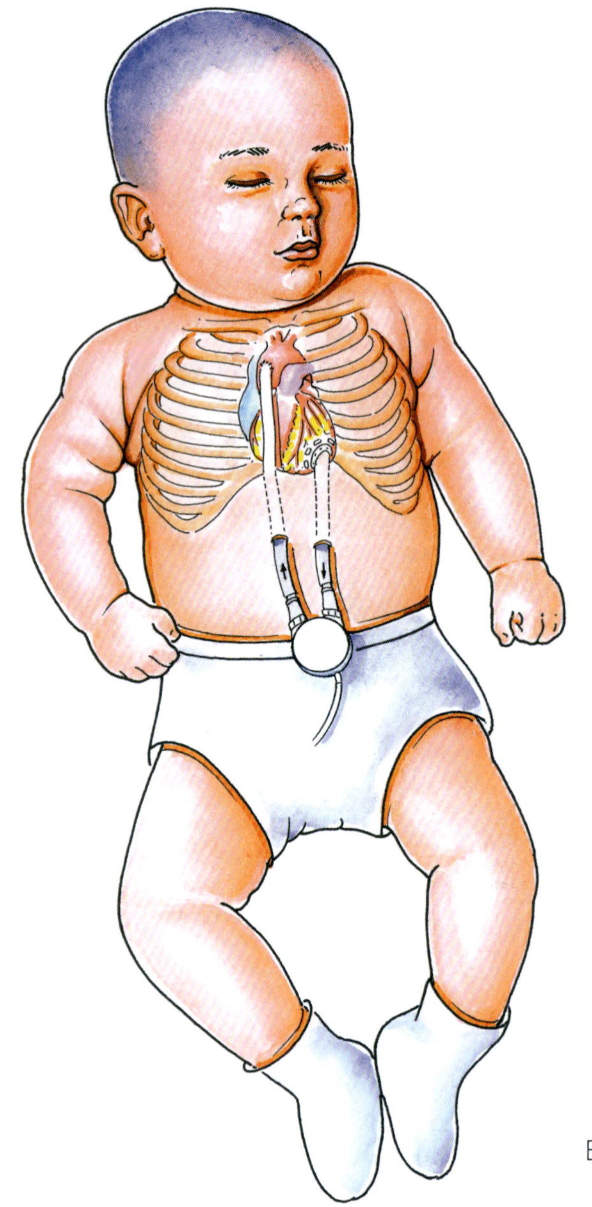

E. 将左心室插管及主动脉插管引出体外，与血液泵相连接，排完气后，脱离体外循环，完成手术。

E. The left ventricular cannula and aortic cannula are brought out of the body and connected to the blood pump. After the exhaust, the cardiopulmonary bypass is weaned off. The surgery is complete.

第五节 全人工心脏
Section 5 Total Artificial Heart

CardioWest 全人工心脏
CardioWest total artificial heart

CardioWest 适用于全心衰竭、心源性休克、多器官功能衰竭或有左心室辅助装置植入风险的患者，植入后取代人体的心室和瓣膜。植入 CardioWest 后，患者不再需要使用正性肌力药或抗心律失常药，并且避免了肺动脉高压、右心衰竭以及与心肌和瓣膜有关的问题。

The CardioWest is indicated in patients with total heart failure, cardiogenic shock, multiple organ failure, or patients who are risky to implant a left ventricular assist device, which replaces the human ventricle and valve. Implantation of CardioWest eliminates the need for inotropic drugs or antiarrhythmics and avoids pulmonary hypertension, right heart failure, and problems related to myocardium and valves.

主要的组成组件包括：

The main components are:

1. CardioWest 重 160g，被植入者体表面积的下限认为是 1.7m^2，适用于大多数成年人和一些较大的青少年。CardioWest 由两个独立的气动涤纶聚酯纤维心室组成，具有单向流入和流出阀，总容积为 750ml，属气动式脉动血泵。聚氨酯隔膜将血液与由外部驱动器控制的气压脉冲分开。驱动器通过驱动线将气动脉冲传递到心室的气室中，使隔膜张开并喷射血液。从机体引出来的 2m 气动驱动线由涤纶聚酯丝绒覆盖，以使组织向内生长，并避免沿线传播感染。

1. The CardioWest weighs 160 g, and since the lower limit of the body surface area for the recipient is considered to be 1.7 m^2, it is mostly applied to adults and some larger-size adolescents. The CardioWest consists of two independent pneumatic polyester fiber ventricles with one-way inflow and outflow valves. It is a pneumatic pulsatile blood pump with a full ejection volume of 750 ml. The polyurethane diaphragm separates the blood from the air pressure pulses controlled by an external driver. The driver delivers a pneumatic pulse through a drive wire into the air chambers in the ventricle, causing the diaphragm to open and eject blood. The 2 m pneumatic drive wire leading from the organism is covered with polyester velour to allow tissue ingrowth and avoid spreading infection along the wire.

2. 驱动器控制台包含两个压缩空气罐和一个备用电源（电池），以方便移动。电源中断的任何情况下，电池都会自动激活。控制台上的便携式计算机会计算并提供非侵入式监视信息。计算机屏幕显示设备速率、心搏出量、心排血量、驱动压力和流量波形、心排血量趋势以及与患者相关的警报。

2. The driving console contains two compressed air tanks and a backup power source (batteries) for easy movement. The battery is automatically activated whenever the power supply is off. A laptop computer at the console computes and provides non-intrusive monitoring information. Device rate, stroke volume, cardiac output, driving pressure and flow waveforms, cardiac output trends, and patient-related alarms are displayed on the computer screen.

3. 具有最短的血液流动路径，从而降低了血栓栓塞的风险。它还具有最大的流入导管面积，可实现高心排血量，流量可高达 9.5L/min。较大的流入直径和较短的血液流经设备的距离，会降低中心静脉压，而高的心排血量会增加全身压力，改善器官灌注和功能。该设备每分钟的搏动范围为 100~130 次，心室容积为 70ml。通常将其设置为部分填充，并以固定的收缩率和每分钟 120~130 次搏动的固定搏动速率运行，搏出量为 50~60ml。节拍率保持在预设值，直到在设备上将其重置后才波动。70ml 的静脉回流血液尚未完全把心室充满，在运动或增加负荷时，心排血量会像正常心脏一样自动增加。

3. The blood flow route is the shortest, thus reducing the risk of thromboembolism. It also has the largest inflow conduit area to achieve high cardiac output, and the flow rate can be as high as 9.5 L/min. Larger inflow diameters and shorter distances for blood flowing through the device reduce central venous pressure, while high cardiac output increases systemic pressure and improves organ perfusion and function. The device beats in a range of 100-130 beats per minute with a ventricular volnme of 70 ml. It is typically set to partially fill and runs at a fixed systole rate and a fixed beat rate of 120-130 beats per minute, with a stroke volume of 50-60 ml. The beat rate remains at the preset value and does not fluctuate until it is reset on the device. The venous return blood of 70 ml has not completely filled the ventricle, and the cardiac output will automatically increase like a normal heart during exercise or when the load increases.

图 8-5-1 CardioWest 全人工心脏植入术

Figure 8-5-1 Implantation of CardioWest total artificial heart

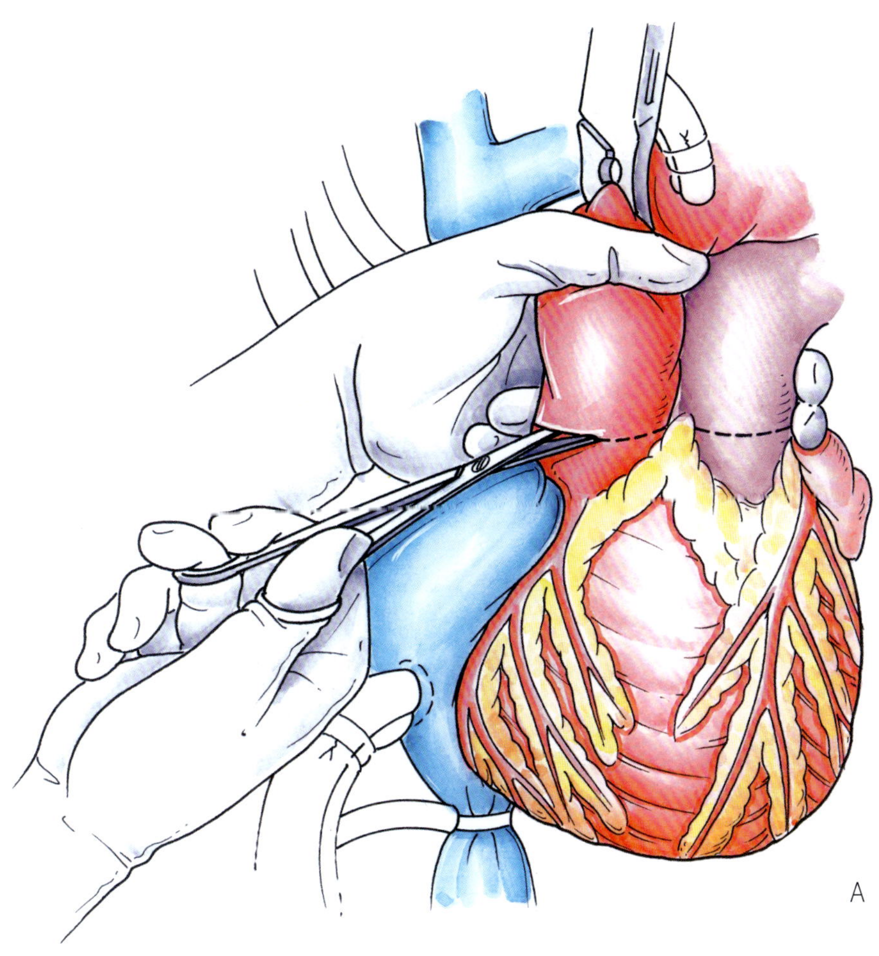

A. 胸骨正中切口，建立体外循环，静脉插管按照心脏移植方式由上、下腔静脉分别插入。比照心脏移植方式将升主动脉、肺动脉干、左心房及右心房切除。

A. A median sternotomy is made to establish extracorporeal circulation, and venous cannulas are inserted through the superior and inferior vena cava, respectively, in a similar way in heart transplantation. Ascending aorta, the pulmonary trunk, the left atrium and the right atrium are resected similarly in heart transplantation.

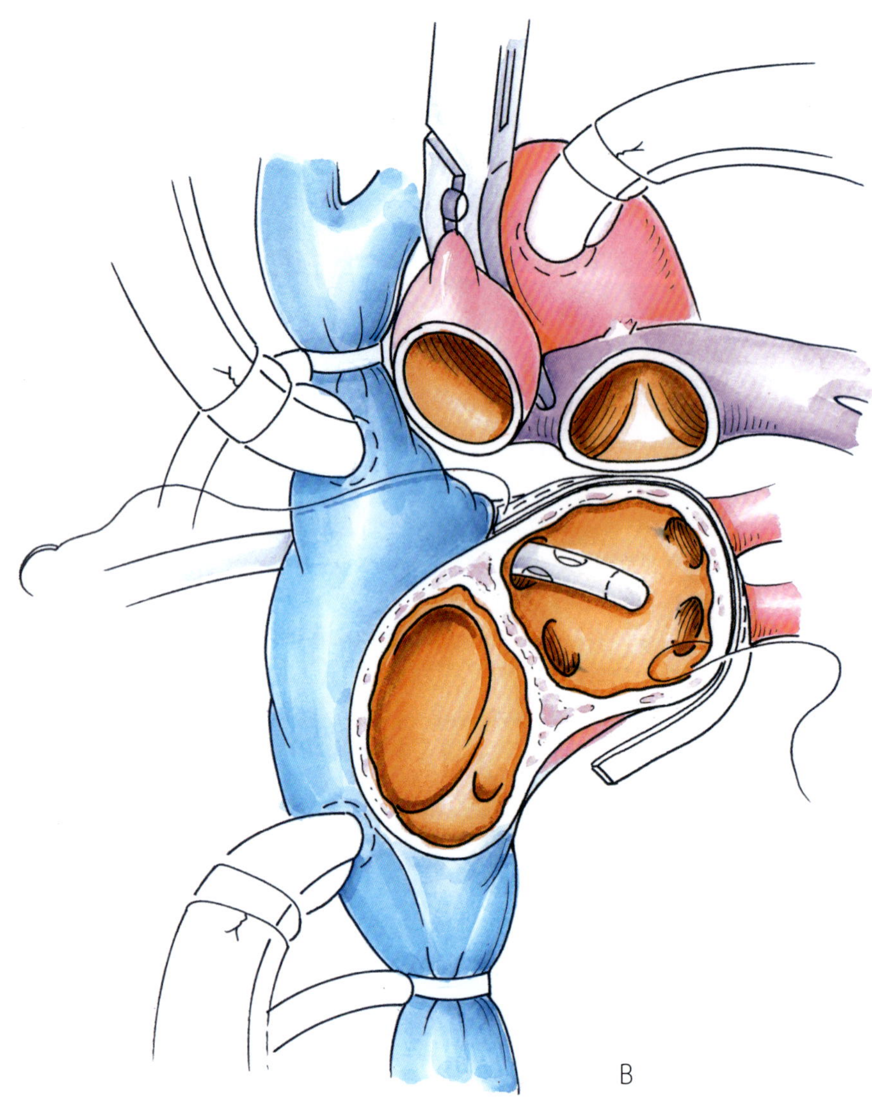

B. 患者心脏切除后，在左右心房切端外侧以聚四氟乙烯（Teflon）毡片条加强，同时避免出血。

B. After excision of the patient heart, reinforcement is achieved with polytetrafluoroethylene (Teflon) felt strips on the lateral sides of the left and right atrial incisal ends while avoiding bleeding.

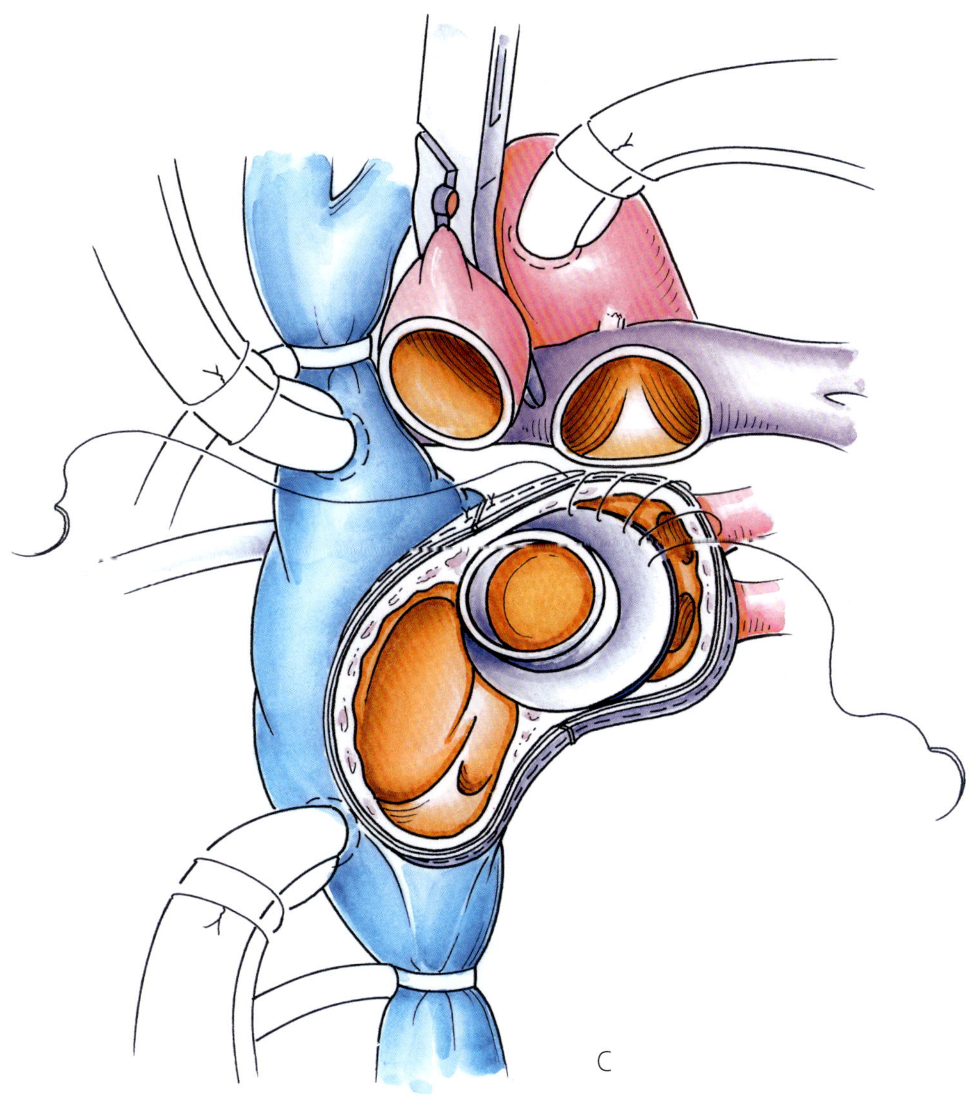

C. 将心房接合器与左心房吻合。

C. The atrial connector is anastomosed to the left atrium.

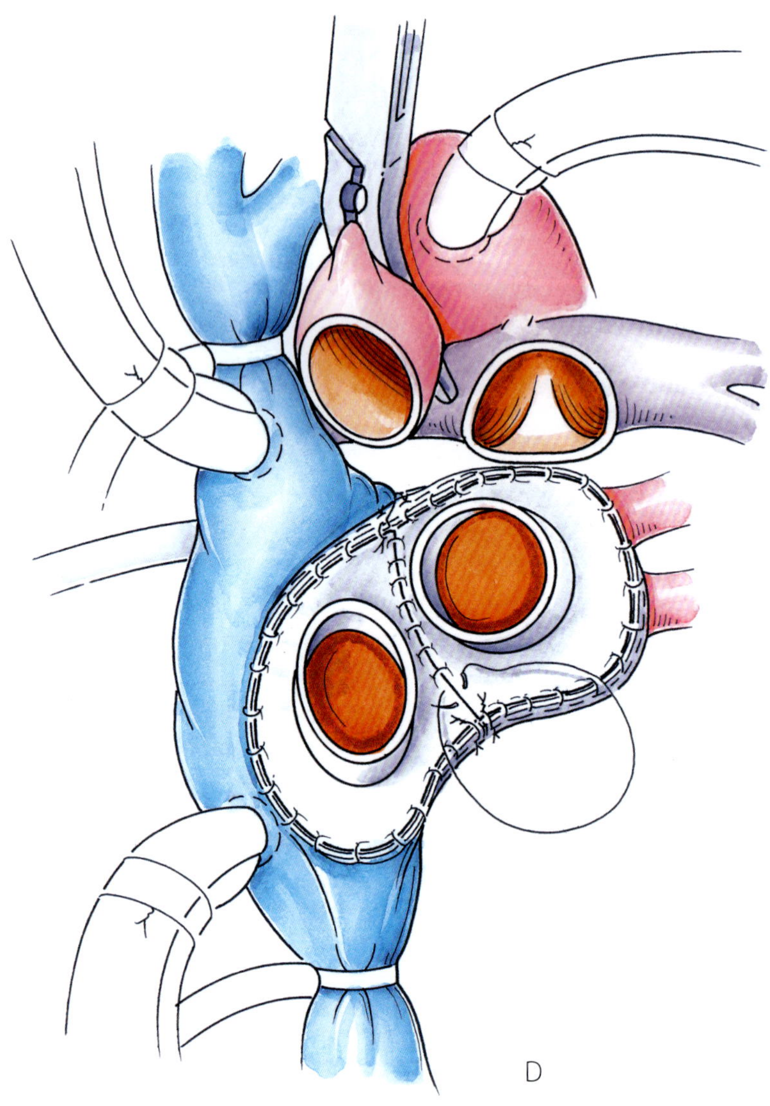

D. 心房接合器与右心房吻合。

D. The atrial connector is anastomosed to the right atrium.

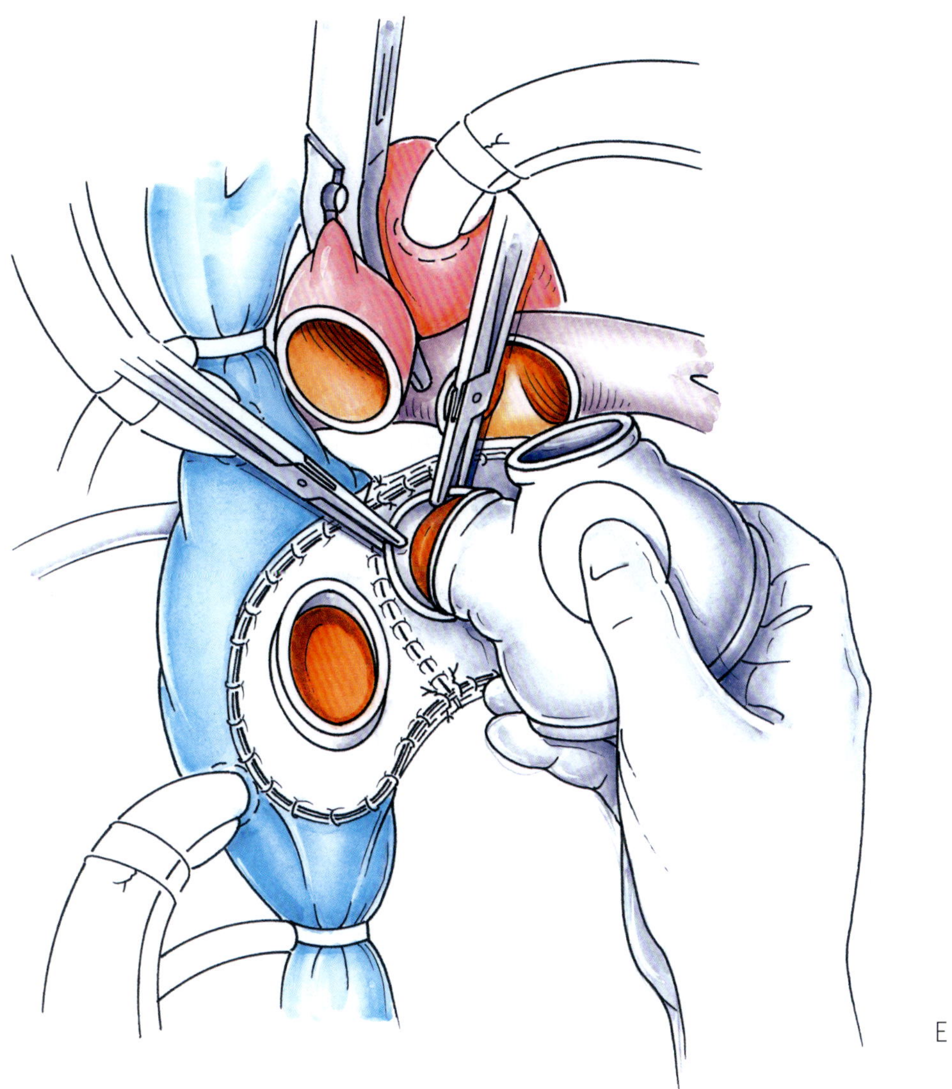

E. 将 CardioWest 全人工心脏左心室与左心房连接器接合。

E. Engage the CardioWest total artificial heart left ventricle with the left atrium connector.

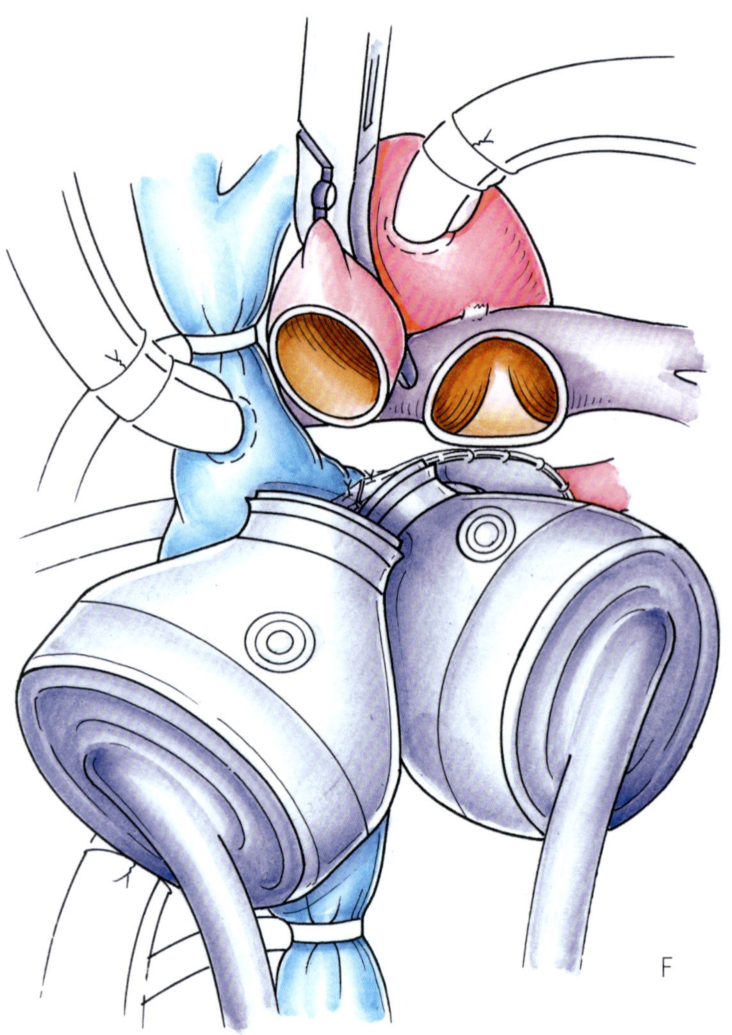

F. 将 CardioWest 全人工心脏右心室与右心房连接器接合。

F. Engage the CardioWest total artificial heart right ventricle with the right atrium connector.

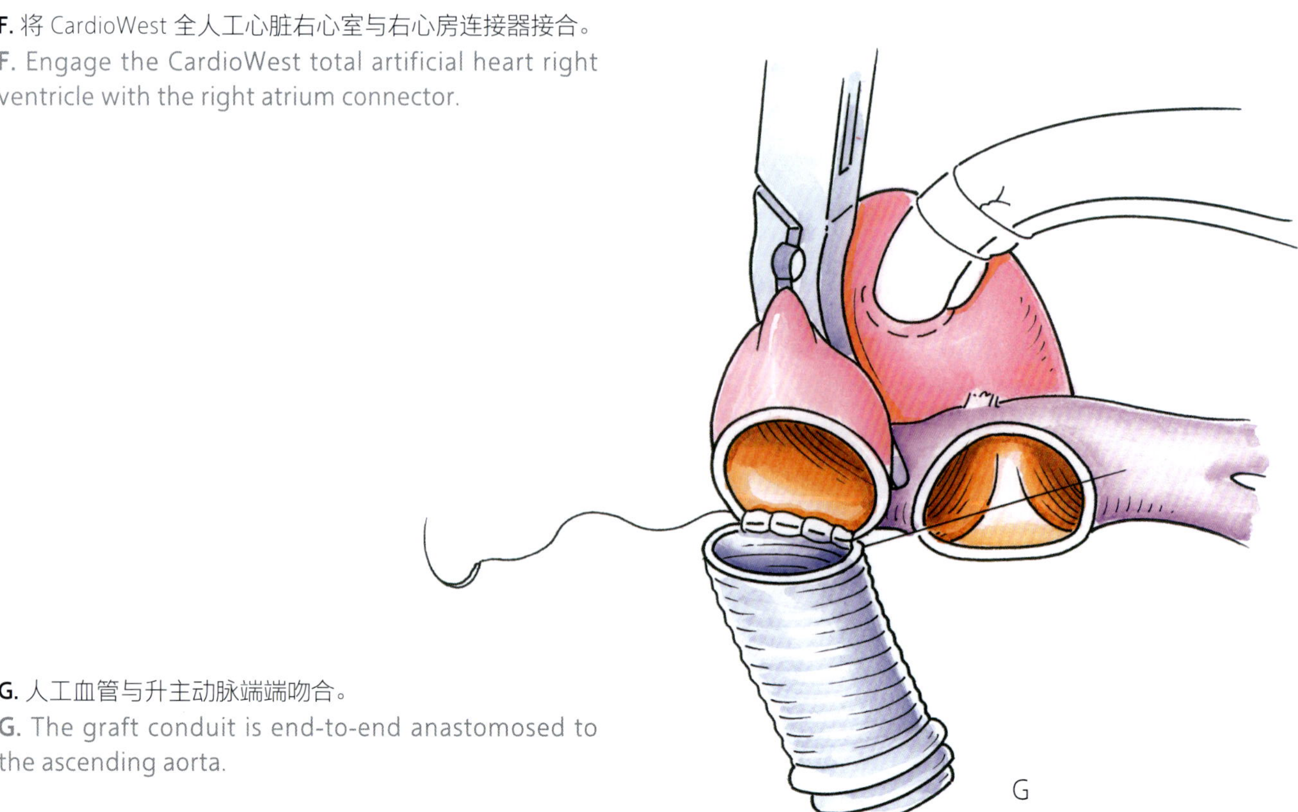

G. 人工血管与升主动脉端端吻合。

G. The graft conduit is end-to-end anastomosed to the ascending aorta.

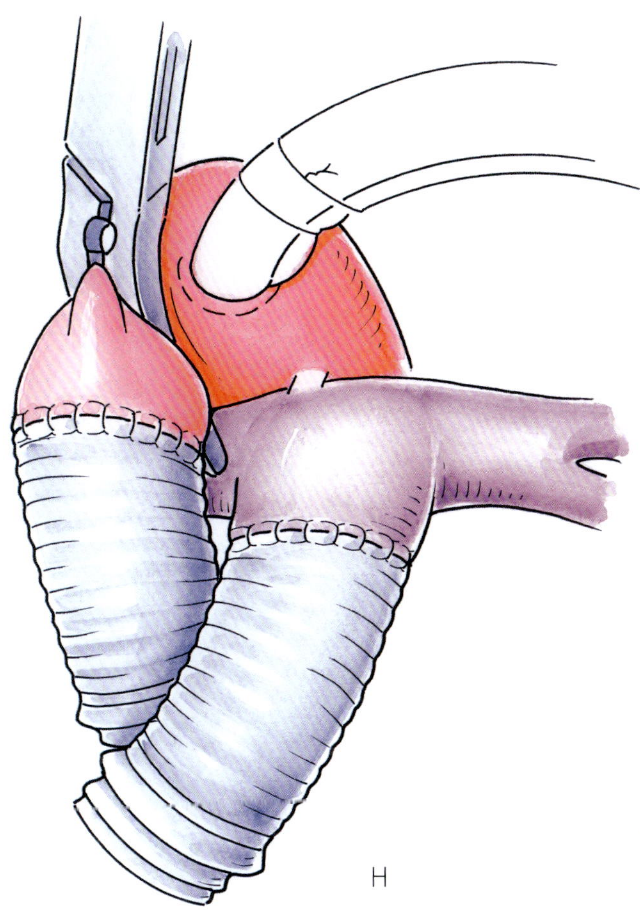

H. 人工血管与肺动脉干端端吻合。

H. The graft conduit is end-to-end anastomosed to the pulmonary trunk.

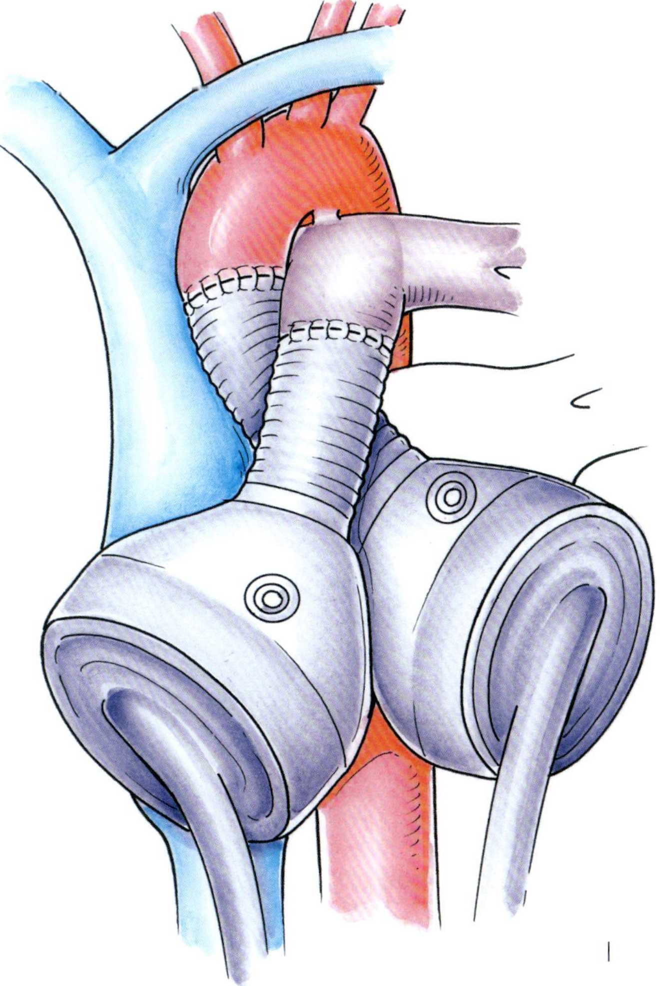

I. 人工血管分别与 CardioWest 左心室及右心室相连接，并完成手术。

I. Connect the graft conduit to the CardioWest left ventricle and right ventricle, respectively, and complete the operation.